Tendinopathy

Kentaro Onishi
Michael Fredericson • Jason L. Dragoo
Editors

Tendinopathy

From Basic Science to Clinical Management

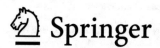 Springer

Editors
Kentaro Onishi
Department of Physical Medicine and
Rehabilitation
Department of Orthopedic
Surgery, University of Pittsburgh
Pittsburgh, PA
USA

Michael Fredericson
Department of Orthopedic Surgery
Division of PM&R
Stanford University
Redwood City, CA
USA

Jason L. Dragoo
Department of Orthopedic Surgery
University of Colorado Denver
Denver, CO
USA

ISBN 978-3-030-65337-8   ISBN 978-3-030-65335-4   (eBook)
https://doi.org/10.1007/978-3-030-65335-4

Preface

The only source of knowledge is experience.

– Albert Einstein

Tendinopathy is a pervasive and debilitating condition that affects all walks of life, from a young athlete to an older adult. Because these injuries affect one's ability to execute basic daily movements and the propensity for incomplete healing and recurrence are common, this condition's societal burden is enormous. Successful treatment requires in-depth knowledge about tendon biology, pathophysiology, region-specific anatomy/biomechanics, as well as current evidence surrounding various treatment options. Ultimately, the care for a person affected by tendinopathy should be personalized based on severity, location, and individual goals.

Over the last 30+ years of our combined practice, treatment of tendinopathy has been challenging and very rewarding. Healing painful tendinopathy after months to years of unsuccessful therapy is immensely satisfying when we see the patient can run and play the sport he/she enjoys better, their pain resolves, and their overall function improves. We wrote this book to reference the basic understanding of tendon biology, tendon pathophysiology, clinical evaluation and diagnosis, and management based on currently available evidence. Chapters are divided by anatomical areas for ease of use in clinical practice. The book also features chapters that discuss evolving basic science and select topics of interest in evolving treatment options for tendinopathy.

The contributors range from basic scientists to both surgical and non-surgical clinical experts. They were selected based on their expertise. The peer-reviewed literature along with the author's experience has become the knowledge provided in this book. We hope that it gives the reader a better understanding of this difficult condition.

Pittsburgh, PA, USA
Redwood City, CA, USA
Denver, CO, USA

Kentaro Onishi
Michael Fredericson
Jason L. Dragoo

Contents

Contributors

Svetlana Abrams, DO Department of Rehabilitation and Human Performance, Icahn School of Medicine at Mount Sinai, New York, NY, USA

Zachary Bailowitz, MD Department of Orthopedics, Podiatry, & Sports Medicine, Kaiser Permanente Medical Center, Oakland, CA, USA

Joanne Borg-Stein, MD Department of Physical Medicine and Rehabilitation, Harvard Medical School, Spaulding Rehabilitation Hospital, Charlestown, MA, USA

Mary E. Caldwell, DO Department of Physical Medicine and Rehabilitation, Virginia Commonwealth University, Richmond, VA, USA

Eliana Cardozo, DO Department of Rehabilitation and Human Performance, Icahn School of Medicine at Mount Sinai, New York, NY, USA

Jesse Charnoff, MD Department of Physiatry, Hospital for Special Surgery, New York, NY, USA

David J. Cormier, DO, DPT Department of Physical Medicine and Rehabilitation, Harvard Medical School, Spaulding Rehabilitation Hospital, Charlestown, MA, USA

Daniel Dean, MD Department of Orthopedic Surgery, MedStar Health, Washington, DC, USA

Arthur Jason De Luigi, DO Department of Physical Medicine and Rehabilitation, Mayo Clinic, Scottsdale, AZ, USA

Jeanne M. Doperak, DO Department of Orthopedic Surgery, University of Pittsburgh, Pittsburgh, PA, USA

Lauren Elson, MD Department of Physical Medicine and Rehabilitation, Harvard Medical School, Spaulding Rehabilitation Hospital, Charlestown, MA, USA

David R. Espinoza, MD The San Antonio Orthopedic Group (TSAOG), San Antonio, TX, USA

Gregory V. Gasbarro, MD Department of Orthopedic Surgery, Mercy Medical Center, Baltimore, MD, USA

Stephanie A. Giammittorio, DO Riverside Medical Group Orthopedics and Sports Medicine, Williamsburg, VA, USA

Marc Gruner, DO Department of Rehabilitation Medicine, Georgetown University, Washington, DC, USA

Lawrence V. Gulotta, MD Shoulder and Elbow Division, Sports Medicine Institute, Hospital for Special Surgery, New York, NY, USA

Mark A. Harrast, MD Department of Rehabilitation Medicine, University of Washington, Seattle, WA, USA

Todd R. Hayano, DO Department of Physical Medicine and Rehabilitation, Harvard Medical School, Spaulding Rehabilitation Hospital, Charlestown, MA, USA

Eric R. Helm, MD Department of Physical Medicine and Rehabilitation, University of Pittsburgh, Pittsburgh, PA, USA

Joseph E. Herrera, DO Department of Rehabilitation and Human Performance, Icahn School of Medicine at Mount Sinai, New York, NY, USA

Ma Calus V. Hogan, MD Department of Orthopedic Surgery, University of Pittsburgh, Pittsburgh, PA, USA

Melody Hrubes, MD Rothman Orthopedics, New York, NY, USA

Jerry Huang, MD Department of Orthpaedics and Sports Medicine, University of Washington, Seattle, WA, USA

Joseph Ihm, MD Shirley Ryan Ability Lab, Northwestern University, Chicago, IL, USA

David Impastato, MD UW Medicine Sports Medicine Center at Husky Stadium, University of Washington, Seattle, WA, USA

Abdullah Kandil, MD Department of Physical Medicine and Rehabilitation, University of California Irvine, Orange, CA, USA

Abdurrahman Kandil, MD Department of Orthopedic Surgery, Stanford University, Redwood City, CA, USA

Jonathan S. Kirschner, MD Department of Physiatry, Hospital for Special Surgery, New York, NY, USA

Bryson P. Lesniak, MD Department of Orthopedic Surgery, University of Pittsburgh, Pittsburgh, PA, USA

Brian C. Liem, MD UW Medicine Sports Medicine Center at Husky Stadium, University of Washington, Seattle, WA, USA

Albert Lin, MD Department of Orthopedic Surgery, University of Pittsburgh, Pittsburgh, PA, USA

Nicola Maffulli, MD, PhD Department of Musculoskeletal Disorders, School of Medicine and Surgery, University of Salerno, Salerno, Italy

Mary University of London, Barts and the London School of Medicine and Dentistry, Centre for Sports and Exercise Medicine, Mile End Hospital, London, UK

Gerard A. Malanga, MD New Jersey Regenerative Institute, Cedar Knolls, NJ, USA

Kenneth Mautner, MD Department of Orthopedic Surgery, Emory University, Atlanta, GA, USA

Ashley McCann, MD Department of Family Medicine, Morehouse School of Medicine, Atlanta, GA, USA

Christopher McCrum, MD Department of Orthopedic Surgery, University of Texas Southwestern, Dallas, TX, USA

Francis Xavier McGuigan, MD Department of Orthopedic Surgery, MedStar Health, Washington, DC, USA

Alex Miner, DO Department of Physical Medicine and Rehabilitation, University of California Irvine, Orange, CA, USA

Gerardo Miranda-Comas, MD Department of Rehabilitation and Human Performance, Icahn School of Medicine at Mount Sinai, New York, NY, USA

Katherine Nanos, MD Strive Physiotherapy and Sports Medicine, Toronto, ON, Canada

Usker Naqvi, MD Las Vegas, Nevada, USA

Rohit Navlani, DO Department of Anesthesiology and Perioperative Medicine, University of Pittsburgh, Pittsburgh, PA, USA

Alyssa Neph, MD Department of Physical Medicine and Rehabilitation, University of Pittsburgh, Pittsburgh, PA, USA

Michael O'Connell, DO Department of Physical Medicine and Rehabilitation, University of Pittsburgh, Pittsburgh, PA, USA

Francesco Oliva, MD, PhD Department of Musculoskeletal Disorders, School of Medicine and Surgery, University of Salerno, Salerno, Italy

Kentaro Onishi, DO Department of Physical Medicine and Rehabilitation, Department of Orthopedic Surgery, University of Pittsburgh, Pittsburgh, PA, USA

Department of Orthopedic Surgery, University of Pittsburgh, Pittsburgh, PA, USA

Kevin Pelletier, MD Department of Physical Medicine and Rehabilitation, University of California Irvine, Orange, CA, USA

Miguel Pelton, MD Tidewater Orthopedics, Suffolk, VA, USA

Joseph M. Powers, MD Northside Hospital Orthopedic Institute, Atlanta, GA, USA

Lindsay Ramey Argo, MD Department of Physical Medicine and Rehabilitation, University of Texas Southwestern, Dallas, TX, USA

Joshua B. Rothenberg, DO Orthopedic Group, Baptist Health North Medical Group, Boca Raton Regional Hospital, Boca Raton, FL, USA

Mark J. Sakr, DO Northside Hospital Orthopedic Institute, Atlanta, GA, USA

Stephen Schaaf, MD Department of Physical Medicine and Rehabilitation, University of Pittsburgh, Pittsburgh, PA, USA

Caroline Schepker, DO Department of Physical Medicine and Rehabilitation, Weill Cornell Medical College, New York, NY, USA

Allison Schroeder, MD Department of Physical Medicine and Rehabilitation, University of Pittsburgh, Pittsburgh, PA, USA

Ryan S. Selley, MD Department of Orthopedic Surgery, Northwestern University, Chicago, IL, USA

Jason J. Shin, MD Department of Orthopedic Surgery, University of Pittsburgh, Pittsburgh, PA, USA

Vince Si, MD Department of Sports Medicine, Redwood City Medical Center, Redwood City, CA, USA

Scott Joshua Szabo, MD Department of Orthopedic Surgery, University of Pittsburgh, Pittsburgh, PA, USA

Ronald Takemoto, MD Department of Physical Medicine and Rehabilitation, University of California Irvine, Orange, CA, USA

Adam S. Tenforde, MD Department of Physical Medicine and Rehabilitation, Harvard Medical School, Cambridge, MA, USA

Bhavani P. Thampatty, PhD MechanoBiology Laboratory, Department of Orthopaedic Surgery, University of Pittsburgh, Pittsburgh, PA, USA

Terrence Thomas, MD Department of Physiatry, Hospital for Special Surgery, New York, NY, USA

Vehniah K. Tjong, MD Department of Orthopedic Surgery, Northwestern University, Chicago, IL, USA

Christopher Urbanek, DO Department of Family Medicine, East Carolina University, Greenville, NC, USA

Alessio Giai Via, MD Department of Musculoskeletal Surgery, San Camillo-Forlanini Hospital, Rome, Italy

Christopher Visco, MD Department of Rehabilitation and Regenerative Medicine, Columbia University, New York, NY, USA

James H-C. Wang, PhD MechanoBiology Laboratory, Department of Orthopaedic Surgery, University of Pittsburgh, Pittsburgh, PA, USA

Departments of Physical Medicine and Rehabilitation, and Bioengineering, University of Pittsburgh, Pittsburgh, PA, USA

Xiaoning Yuan, MD Department of Physical Medicine and Rehabilitation, Uniformed Services University of the Health Sciences, Bethesda, MD, USA

Biological and Biomechanical Adaptation of Young and Aging Tendons to Exercise

James H-C. Wang and Bhavani P. Thampatty

Abbreviations

AGEs	Advanced glycation end products
bFGF	Basic fibroblast growth factor
CSA	Cross-sectional area
CTGF	Connective tissue growth factor
ECM	Extracellular matrix
ERK	Extracellular signal-regulated kinases
GAG	Glycosaminoglycans
GFP	Green fluorescent protein
GH	Growth hormone
IGF-1	Insulin growth factor-1
IL-6	Interleukin-6
ITR	Intensive treadmill running
MMP-3	Matrix metalloproteinase 3
MTR	Moderate treadmill running
NS	Nucleostemin
Oct-4	Octamer binding transcription factor 4
PDGF	Platelet-derived growth factor
PPARγ	Peroxisome proliferator-activated receptor γ
SASP	Senescence-associated secretory phenotype
SSEA-1	Stage-specific embryonic antigen 1
TS	Triceps surae
TSC	Tendon stem/progenitor cell

J. H-C. Wang (✉)
MechanoBiology Laboratory, Department of Orthopaedic Surgery, University of Pittsburgh, Pittsburgh, PA, USA

Departments of Physical Medicine and Rehabilitation, and Bioengineering, University of Pittsburgh, Pittsburgh, PA, USA
e-mail: wanghc@pitt.edu

B. P. Thampatty
MechanoBiology Laboratory, Department of Orthopaedic Surgery, University of Pittsburgh, Pittsburgh, PA, USA

Introduction

The mammalian tendon is a cord of connective tissues. Highly structured type I collagen with longitudinally aligned collagen fibrils make up most (60–90%) of the dry matter of adult tendons [1, 2]. Small amounts of other types of collagen such as types III, V, and IX also constitute the structure of extra cellular matrix (ECM) [2]. A variety of proteoglycans and glycosaminoglycans (GAG) surround collagen. These highly hydrophilic molecules that can retain large amounts of water improve the elasticity of tendon against shear and compressive forces, and changes in their composition can cause dehydration and loss of function [3]. Other non-collagenous proteins of tendon ECM include fibronectin, tenascin-C, thrombospondin, and elastin. While collagen imparts structural integrity to tendon, elastin is responsible for its flexibility. The unique hierarchical structure and specific composition of ECM are critical for the proper mechanical function of tendon, namely

© Springer Nature Switzerland AG 2021
K. Onishi et al. (eds.), *Tendinopathy*, https://doi.org/10.1007/978-3-030-65335-4_1

bearing mechanical forces due to muscle contractions and transmitting the mechanical forces to the bone, thus enabling the joint movements.

Mechanically, tendons are stiff. Their stiffness depends on the tendon's Young's modulus, which largely reflects tendon's composition such as collagens, and also on tendon's geometry, including the tendon length and its cross-sectional area (CSA) [4]. Changes in collagen synthesis, fibril morphology, and levels of collagen molecular cross-linking ultimately result in tendon's structural changes [5]. Tendons are viscoelastic, a unique property that affords their ability to store, translate, and dissipate energy.

Like all tissues in body, tendons contain cells. The major cellular components of tendon are tendon fibroblasts, also called tenocytes. Inside the tendon, these cells extend numerous cytoplasmic processes into the matrix to establish intracellular contacts in the form of tight junctions and gap junctions [2]. Tenocytes synthesize and secrete the various ECM components for the maintenance of tendon homeostasis and repair of tendons when injured. In recent years, tendon stem/progenitor cells (TSCs) were identified in humans, mice, rats, and rabbits [6–8]. These cells play a vital role in normal tendon physiology by undergoing self-renewal and also differentiating into tenocytes. However, because TSCs possess multi-differentiation potential, recent studies also suggested that they may play an important role in degenerative changes in the tendon in response to excessive mechanical loading placed on the tendon [9, 10].

Since tendons are live, load-bearing tissues, mechanical loading is essential for tendon development, homeostasis, and repair [1, 11]. However, mechanical overloading of tendons, which is common in athletes, induces chronic tendon injury or tendinopathy [12, 13]. In addition, aging can predispose human tendons to develop degenerative changes [14] and make them susceptible to tendinopathy development [15]. Tendinopathy is a major socioeconomic clinical problem, and the treatment is difficult and costly. Therefore, maintaining tendon health with exercise is important not only for young and healthy but also for the increasing aging population in this country. It is known that regular exercise is beneficial to tendons in terms of promoting its anabolic response, and as a result, exercise enhances tendon structural integrity and mechanical strength [16]. However, the underlying mechanisms of tendon's mechanical adaptation are still unclear. Mechanical loading during exercise initiates a signaling cascade of cellular and molecular events, the phenomenon which is termed mechanotransduction [11, 17, 18]. Secretion of various growth factors that enhance ECM synthesis to counteract the age-related loss is proposed in this hypothesis [1, 19]. This chapter reviews the effects of exercise on animal and human tendons of both young and old and associated cellular changes. This chapter also describes the cellular and molecular mechanisms of such mechanobiological effects.

The Effects of Exercise on Young and Aging Tendons in Animals and Humans

The Effects of Aging on Tendons

Aging-related tendon structural changes limit its function and reduce the capacity to respond to stresses considerably [14, 20]. Aging-related tendon matrix changes are manifested as decreased tendon stiffness, tensile strength, and modulus of elasticity [21, 22]. Collagen turnover decreases, and the decrease in essential enzymes for collagen synthesis delays the tissue repair, and tendon matrix loses integrity [14]. Similar degenerative tendency may occur in tendon disuse and immobilization manifested by decrease in tensile strength, elastic stiffness, and total weight of tendon [20, 23, 24]. Cellular senescence which refers to cessation of cell division is a clear phenomenon in aging tendon [14]. A characteristic feature of metabolically active senescent cells is senescence-associated secretory phenotypes (SASP) that secrete inflammatory cytokines, growth factors, and proteases (IL-6, IGF-1, MMPs, etc.), and their role is implicated in many age-related diseases such as diabetes and osteoarthritis [25, 26].

At the tissue level, the cell number and vascularization in the tendon decrease with aging [27], whereas lipid deposition and accumulation of proteoglycans and calcium deposits increase with aging (Fig. 1.1) [28]. The blood supply to tendon decreases with advancing age that may lead to hypoxia and altered metabolic activity [29]. The metabolic pathway for the production of energy changes from aerobic to anaerobic [30]. Age-related decline in aerobic capacity may also

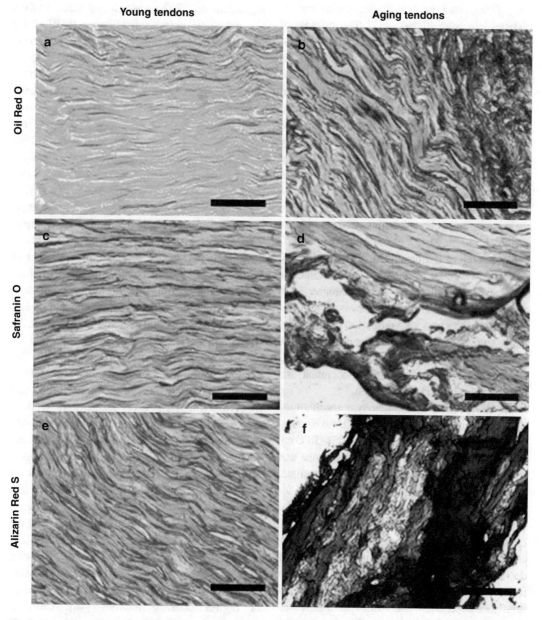

Fig. 1.1 Aging mouse (9 months) patellar tendons show increased lipid deposition, proteoglycans, and calcium deposits compared to young tendons (2.5 months). Oil Red O (**a**, **b**), Safranin O (**c**, **d**), and Alizarin Red S (**e**, **f**) detected the presence of lipids, proteoglycans, and calcium deposits, respectively. Only minimal amounts of these non-tendinous tissues were detected in young tendons; in contrast, extensive amounts of these tissues are found in aging tendons. Bar: 50 µm

impair tendon function. In addition, lipid deposition and calcium deposits may disrupt collagen fiber bundles and reduce the tendon strength.

Tendon matrix shows substantial changes due to aging that accelerate tendon injuries. The decreases in extracellular water content, collagen, GAG, and proteoglycans contribute to changes in tendon stiffness [31]. The stiffness of collagen is in part due to hydrogen bonds formed between the amino acid residues of the tropocollagen molecules and the cross-links associated with the assembly of collagen fibrils. Advanced glycation end products (AGEs) that are generated by slow collagen turnover form additional cross-links that further stiffen collagen fibrils, and they accumulate with age [32]. Thermal stability of tendons depends on the tight packing of collagen molecules that are stabilized by these cross-links. The cross-links become more stable and change their structural characteristics due to aging, thereby increasing the thermal stability and stiffening of collagen fibers [33]. The mechanical properties of collagen decrease with changes in collagen cross-links and fibril diameter with aging [34]. Collagen fibers increase in diameter and vary in thickness with reduction in the oxidative enzymes such as dehydrogenases that are essential for collagen synthesis. Increase in collagen cross-linking alters the biochemical and mechanical properties of collagen.

At the cellular level, tenocyte morphology changes – it becomes more flattened and its number decreases with increasing age [35]. To compensate for the decreasing number of cells and increasing tendon matrix, the cellular processes of tenocytes become thinner and longer. Also, the TSCs undergo distinct cellular and molecular changes in response to aging and degeneration of tendon by premature entry into cellular senescence accompanied by deficit in self-renewal, decrease in number, decreased proliferation, reduced colony formation, decreased tendon lineage gene expression, and adipocytic differentiation [36, 37]. In summary, the degenerative changes in aging tendons are evident at the tissue and cellular level, and this degeneration may predispose the aging population to eventual development of tendinopathy.

The Effects of Exercise on Young Tendons

Exercise may maintain the structural and functional integrity of young tendons in animals and humans. The development of improved measuring techniques such as ultrasound-based method and magnetic resonance imaging (MRI) have enabled reliable investigations in tendon's structural and mechanical properties, as well as its morphological properties in vivo. In some earlier studies in animals, tensile strength and stiffness, CSA, and collagen content of tendons increased with physical training in young and aging tendons [38, 39]. However, in studies using animal models, there was no consensus in terms of the effect of endurance training on tendon biomechanical properties possibly due to the differences in species, exercise type, load magnitude, intensity, frequency, and duration of the training. The overall observation suggests that tendons become larger, stronger, and more resistant to injury in response to physical training in some animals under certain conditions despite the several confounding factors such as the age of animals, rate of strain, and decreased size and tensile strength of the tendons of caged animals that are used as controls for comparison [20, 40]. For example, some studies reported increased tensile strength and/or stiffness of tendons in rabbit and rat Achilles and swine digital extensor tendons subjected to endurance training [24, 39, 41, 42]. According to the studies, increase in strength and stiffness is generally attributed to tendon hypertrophy, which may help mitigate the risk of injury. Also, inconsistencies exist in terms of tendon size changes in response to exercise in earlier studies. Some studies found no difference in the dry weights of tendon between exercised animals and control animals [43–45]. While long-term training had no effect on the dry weight of swine digital flexor tendons, it increased the dry weight of digital extensor tendons [46]. Collagen concentration did not show increase in these studies. However, the variability may be due to the differences in the nature (extensor or flexor) and age (developing/mature) of tendons, and nature of loading (endurance/intermittent). Also, conflicting results exist in terms of collagen fibril distribution and diameter. There was increase in collagen fibril diameter in Achilles tendons of rats after 10 weeks of exercise [47], and there was increase in fibril diameter, fibril distribution, and CSA in mice subjected to treadmill running for a week [48]. However, collagen fibril diameter did not show any significant changes in the digital flexor tendons of horses undergoing treadmill training program of galloping exercise [49]. Tendon regional differences and species difference may account for this variability. In response to training, CSA of digital extensor tendons of horses and swine and Achilles tendons of rats increased [42, 50, 51]. Also, proteoglycans levels increased with exercise in tendons of rats and chickens [44, 52].

Young human tendons also show definite pattern of changes in response to exercise. Measurement of the elastic properties of long distance runners showed that their tendons were approximately 20% stiffer [53]. Isometric training of healthy young adults increased the tendon stiffness and Young's modulus as well as muscle size and strength [54]. The same investigators reported that resistance and stretching training increased the stiffness and viscosity of tendons in young adults [55]. Increased Achilles tendon CSA in young trained runners compared to non-runners suggests that repetitive loading associated with running has resulted in hypertrophic tissue adaptation [56]. Increase in tensile strength and stiffness may be due to a change in the turnover of the collagen and consequently in the intermolecular cross-linking [21]. In a previous study, acute exercise increased collagen type I formation in human Achilles tendons [16]. Rapid increase in collagen synthesis was observed after strenuous non-damaging exercise (one-legged kicking exercise) in patellar tendons of healthy young men [57]. Moreover, resistance training in humans showed increases in tendon CSA [4, 58, 59]. In the Achilles tendons of young adults who underwent high strain magnitude of exercise for 14 weeks, increases in tendon stiffness, elastic modulus, and a region-specific hypertrophy [58] were found. Similar observations were true for increased rate and duration of exercise [60]. The

patellar tendons of young adults who have undergone resistance training showed similar increases in stiffness and CSA [4, 59]. High-intensity plyometric and isometric training 2–3 times for 6 weeks significantly increased medial gastrocnemius tendon stiffness [61]. Moreover, habitual loading increased human patellar tendon size and stiffness and induced tendon hypertrophy [62]. Robust changes in the tendon mechanical properties were evident in this study. When comparing the effect of habitual exercise (running) on the structural and mechanical properties of patellar tendon in men and women, the training resulted in larger patellar tendon CSA in men, not in women [63]. Also, collagen synthesis rate and mechanical strength of isolated collagen fascicles from young men surpassed that of young women after a bout of acute exercise. Moreover, patellar tendon stiffness and patellar and Achilles tendon CSA were greater in trained young men compared to trained young women [64]. Since women are more prone to connective tissue injuries than men, it is possible that hormonal influence may play a role in the differential responses [65–67]. Studies in young recreational runners showed increase in tendon aponeurosis stiffness and improved running economy in triceps surae (TS) muscle-tendon units [68, 69]. Exercised young men showed significantly increased patellar tendon stiffness and modulus after 12 weeks of exercise 3 times a week compared to non-exercised group [70]. However, human studies also suffer from several limitations such as small sample size, varied loading conditions such as intensity and duration, and different methodological approaches. A recent meta-analysis of exercise intervention studies on healthy adults provides strong statistical evidence that tendons are highly responsive to diverse loading regimens, and loading magnitude plays a key role in tendon adaptation [71]. The analysis suggests that changes in tendon stiffness can be attributed to tendon adaptation, and longer duration of exercise (>12 weeks) is beneficial to facilitate tendon adaptation. In summary, although the studies are limited and inconclusive, physical training of young animals and humans at moderate levels helps maintain the structural integrity of tendons by increasing the tendon mechanical strength and stiffness.

The Effects of Exercise on Aging Tendons

Moderate exercise may be beneficial to counteract the detrimental effects of aging tendons in animals and humans according to several studies, although there are inconsistencies. The effects of physical training on the biomechanical properties of aging rat limb muscle tendons were not affected significantly by exercise in trained animals when compared to sedentary animals [72]. However, while plantaris tendon stiffness increased with aging, stiffness decreased to levels similar to adult control values following moderate intensity exercise in aging mice [73]. Also, gene expression levels of collagen I and MMP-3 in Achilles tendon increased without changes in cell density or cell morphology. Calcification which was minimal in adult tendons increased significantly with age. However, Achilles tendon calcification was significantly reduced in old mice following exercise [73]. Although the study has limitations such as using only a single time point for evaluation and gene expression levels were not measured in the same tendons used for mechanical studies, data suggest that age-related changes in tendon can be modified with physical training.

The mechanical properties of aging human tendons show substantial improvement in response to moderate exercise. A 10% decrease in stiffness and 14% decrease in Young's modulus of patellar tendon in older population (average age of 74) could be reversed by 14 weeks of resistance training by which fascicle length and tendon stiffness increased by 10 and 64%, respectively [74]. Strength training altered the viscoelastic properties of patellar tendons in older population with significantly increased stiffness and decreased hysteresis (the amount of energy lost as heat during the recoil from the stretch) compared to non-exercised controls [75]. Their results indicate that resistance training in old age

can at least partly maintain the normal tendon properties and function. Another study supports this observation. Resistance training for 12 weeks, 3 times a week in older people has shown significant increases in patellar tendon stiffness and Young's modulus [76]. Increased tendon stiffness and CSA will decrease tendon stress and strain and may reduce the risk of tendon injuries. The differential response of young male and female tendons to exercise is also reflected in older population. Resistance training-induced tendon stiffness is higher in older males compared to older females suggesting that adaptation to exercise has hormonal influence [77]. In summary, exercise intervention at moderate-level physical loading is beneficial for greater adaptive tendon responses compared to non-exercised tendon in old animals and humans, although further standardized studies are warranted.

Cellular Changes in the Young and Aging Tendons Due to Exercise

Effects of Exercise on Young Tendon Cells

The biological response of tendon to physical loading is triggered by both tenocytes and TSCs. The transcription factor scleraxis, a marker for tenocytes that has a role in the embryonic development of limb tendons by promoting tendon cell proliferation and matrix synthesis, decreases with aging [78]. In transgenic mice (4 months old) that express green fluorescent protein (GFP) under the control of scleraxis promoter (Scx-GFP), moderate treadmill running for 6 weeks showed increase in expression of typical tenocyte-related genes, scleraxis, tenomodulin, and type I collagen compared to caged control animals [79]. Many earlier studies have shown that mechanical loading regulates stem cell proliferation and differentiation [80, 81]. In vitro experiments conducted by mechanical stretching of TSCs isolated from patellar and Achilles tendons of rabbits (4–6 month- old) under different loading conditions showed that moderate stretching promoted

TSC differentiation into tenocytes as the cells expressed higher levels of collagen I without the expression of non-tenocytes markers such as adipogenic, chondrogenic, and osteogenic [9]. However, stretching at a high magnitude induced at least some TSCs to differentiate into non-teno-cyte phenotype by expressing genes, PPARγ, collagen type II, Sox-9, and Runx-2, specific for adipocytes, chondrocytes, and osteocytes. This study suggests that moderate physical loading is beneficial in terms of maintaining the integrity of tendons at the cellular level. Additional in vivo experiments supported this observation. An in vivo mouse (2.5 month old) model that applied moderate and intensive treadmill running (MTR and ITR) to apply mechanical loads showed that while MTR upregulated tenocyte related gene expression without affecting non-tenocyte related genes in both patellar and Achilles tendon tissues, ITR induced non-tenocyte-related gene expression [10]. The results from parallel in vitro stretching experiments using tenocytes and TSCs isolated from non-treadmill running control mice confirmed the in vivo observations.

Effects of Exercise on Aging Tendon Cells

The beneficial effects of moderate mechanical loading are evident on aging animal tendons in vitro and in vivo. Compared to TSCs obtained from young mice (2.5 and 5 months old), TSCs from aging mice (9 and 24 months old) proliferated significantly slower and showed decreased expression of stem cell markers such as Oct-4, nucleostemin (NS), Sca-1, and SSEA-1 [28]. However, moderate-level stretching of aging TSCs significantly increased the expression of NS, tenocyte-related markers such as collagen I, and tenomodulin, while higher level stretching increased the expression of non-tenocyte-related genes. Interestingly, MTR not only increased the proliferation rate of aging TSCs in culture but also decreased lipid deposition, proteoglycan accumulation, and calcification and increased the expression of NS in patellar tendons (Fig. 1.2).

This study shows that moderate exercise can reverse the impaired proliferative capacity and stemness of aging tendons and help maintain the tissue integrity to decrease age-related tendon degeneration. Further studies reinforced these findings. For example, the healing of a "window"-shaped tendon defect created after 4 weeks of MTR regimen in aging rats (20 months old) was significantly accelerated by quicker defect closure [27]. MTR improved the organization of collagen fibers and decreased the senescent cells in aging rats compared to cage control. MTR also lowered vascularization, increased TSCs number and proliferation, significantly increased the expression of stem cell markers, and decreased the expression of non-tenocyte-related genes. This study brings the importance of moderate exercise in aging tendons to help alleviate age-related tendon degeneration presumably by enhancing the tendon healing via a TSC-based mechanism. In summary, moderate exercise brings many beneficial changes at the tendon cellular level in young and old animals.

Cellular and Molecular Mechanisms Responsible for the Effects of Exercises on Tendons

The precise mechanisms for tendon adaptation to exercise are still unknown. But it is beyond doubt that resident tendon cells, including tenocytes and TSCs, must play an essential role in the process of mechanical adaption to exercise. In response to exercise, these cells divide and produce more ECM components to maintain structural integrity and strengthen the tendon to meet the mechanical demands placed on the tendons. However, the roles of vascular cells and possibly other types of cells in the endotenon, epitenon, and paratenon in the mechanical adaption to exercise are currently unknown.

There are strong indications that increased synthesis of collagen that is related to the actions of various growth factors such as CTGF and TGB-β produced by tendon cells in response to mechanical loading is mainly responsible for

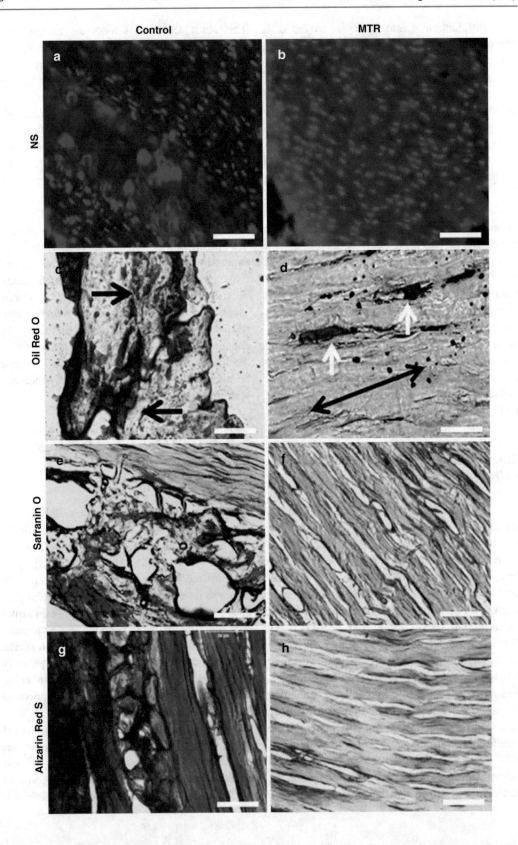

Fig. 1.2 MTR increases nucleostemin (NS), a stem cell marker, expression and decreases lipid deposition, proteogly-can accumulation, and calcification in TSCs of aging mice (9 months). NS (**a, b**) Oil Red O (**c, d**), Safranin O (**e, f**), and Alizarin Red S (**g, h**) detected the presence of nucleostemin-expressed cells, lipids, proteoglycans, and calcium deposits, respectively. Extensive lipids (**c**, arrows point to accumulated lipids), proteoglycans (**e**), and calcium deposits (**g**) are present in the control aging tendons. After MTR, less non-tendinous tissues were found in the tendon (**d**, two white arrows point to a few residual lipids and a double arrow indicates the long axis of the tendon). Bar: 50 μm

tendon adaptation [82, 83]. Mechanical loading and TGF-β increased proteoglycan synthesis in tendons [84]. Furthermore, it has been shown that mechanical loading induces increased secretion of TGF-β, PDGF, basic FGF (bFGF), and IL-6 in human tendon cells that may stimulate cell proliferation, differentiation, and matrix formation [85, 86]. The release of growth factors in response to mechanical stimulation is the result of mechanotransduction [87], which converts "mechanical stimuli" on the cell into biochemical cascade of events inside the cell. Specifically, one such mechanotransduction mechanism may involve a mechanosensory complex consisting of ECM, integrins, and cytoskeletal components. A wide range of cellular responses including the release of such growth factors by a signaling kinase cascade are presumably triggered by cell deformation in response to extrinsic mechanical load [17]. Growth factors and cytokines activate kinases such as ERK and S6, and their phosphorylation initiates gene transcription and protein synthesis. A variety of "stress-responsive" genes of ECM such as tenascin-C and collagen IX and of cytokines such as PDGF and TGF-β1 alter their gene expression by mechanical stimulation [1].

Concluding Remarks

Tendons play an essential role in transmitting muscular force to bone to enable joint movements. When young, tendons possess great mechanical strength to bear large mechanical loads; however, aging tendons gradually lose their structural integrity and become weak in its mechanical strength. As "live structures," tendons are responsive to mechanical loading such as exercise and such mechanobiological responses lead to changes in the cellular metabolism and gene/protein expression, which in turn alter the tendon's structural and mechanical properties. In young tendons, exercise increases their CSA and stiffness. However, "overuse" exercise such as in the athletic settings may actually do harm the tendons – they gradually develop tendinopathy, that is, tendon inflammation and tendon degeneration either alone or in combination. In aging tendons, the same effects take place; for example, moderate exercise "rejuvenates" aging tendons, meaning that moderate exercise makes the aging tendons "young-like" with improved structural organization and reduced presence of degenerative changes in the tendon substance such as lipid deposits, proteoglycan accumulation, and calcifications.

The mechanobiological changes in the young and aging tendons are the results of cellular mechanotransduction. This means that cells have the intricate mechanisms by which mechanical stimuli acting on them can be transduced into biochemical events inside the cells, which in turn trigger a cascade of cellular events leading to upregulation of certain genes and proteins related to ECM including collagens and proteoglycans as well as MMP and TIMP. The end results of such mechanotransduction events are modification of tendon matrix and/or repair of compromised matrix.

While much is known about the effects of exercise on the tendons, there are still much to learn. Exercise can induce production of circulating "systemic effectors" such as growth hormone (GH) and its primary downstream mediator, insulin-like growth factor I (IGF-I) [88]. These systemic effectors may alter gene and protein expression, as well as anabolic/catabolic states of local tendon cells. Together with local changes by exercise due to tendon deformation, possible micro-tears at the collagen fibrils and cellular deformation ensure remodeling of tendon matrix.

A better understanding of the interactions between systemic and local events due to mechanical loading placed on tendons is of vital importance to define appropriate exercise regimens that impart only beneficial effects on young and aging tendons. Additionally, how exercise rejuvenates aging tendons at cellular levels needs to be investigated in future research. It is likely that this involves TSCs, because they are the very cells that are responsible for replenishing lost tenocytes due to aging and at the same time producing more offspring stem cells for maintenance of the aging tendons. In particular, the effects of exercise on aging TSCs and mechanisms involving transforming "senescent tendon cells" into active cells need to be investigated in future. The findings of this research will help devise optimal exercise protocols that induce the production of more TSCs/tenocytes to effectively replenish aging tendon cells, thus reducing or preventing aging-related tendinopathy.

References

1. Kjaer M. Role of extracellular matrix in adaptation of tendon and skeletal muscle to mechanical loading. Physiol Rev. 2004;84(2):649–98.
2. Thorpe CT, Screen HR. Tendon structure and composition. Adv Exp Med Biol. 2016;920:3–10.
3. Bailey AJ. Molecular mechanisms of ageing in connective tissues. Mech Ageing Dev. 2001;122(7):735–55.
4. Kongsgaard M, Reitelseder S, Pedersen TG, Holm L, Aagaard P, Kjaer M, et al. Region specific patellar tendon hypertrophy in humans following resistance training. Acta Physiol (Oxf). 2007;191(2):111–21.
5. Heinemeier KM, Kjaer M. In vivo investigation of tendon responses to mechanical loading. J Musculoskelet Neuronal Interact. 2011;11(2):115–23.
6. Bi Y, Ehirchiou D, Kilts TM, Inkson CA, Embree MC, Sonoyama W, et al. Identification of tendon stem/progenitor cells and the role of the extracellular matrix in their niche. Nat Med. 2007;13(10):1219–27.
7. Rui YF, Lui PP, Li G, Fu SC, Lee YW, Chan KM. Isolation and characterization of multipotent rat tendon-derived stem cells. Tissue Eng Part A. 2010;16(5):1549–58.
8. Zhang J, Wang JH. Characterization of differential properties of rabbit tendon stem cells and tenocytes. BMC Musculoskelet Disord. 2010;11:10.
9. Zhang J, Wang JH. Mechanobiological response of tendon stem cells: implications of tendon homeostasis and pathogenesis of tendinopathy. J Orthop Res. 2010;28(5):639–43.
10. Zhang J, Wang JH. The effects of mechanical loading on tendons--an in vivo and in vitro model study. PLoS One. 2013;8(8):e71740.
11. Wang JH. Mechanobiology of tendon. J Biomech. 2006;39(9):1563–82.
12. Herring SA, Nilson KL. Introduction to overuse injuries. Clin Sports Med. 1987;6(2):225–39.
13. Ackermann PW, Renstrom P. Tendinopathy in sport. Sports Health. 2012;4(3):193–201.
14. Tuite DJ, Renstrom PA, O'Brien M. The aging tendon. Scand J Med Sci Sports. 1997;7(2):72–7.
15. Birch HL, Peffers MJ, Clegg PD. Influence of ageing on tendon homeostasis. Adv Exp Med Biol. 2016;920:247–60.
16. Langberg H, Rosendal L, Kjaer M. Training-induced changes in peritendinous type I collagen turnover determined by microdialysis in humans. J Physiol. 2001;534(Pt 1):297–302.
17. Banes AJ, Tsuzaki M, Yamamoto J, Fischer T, Brigman B, Brown T, et al. Mechanoreception at the cellular level: the detection, interpretation, and diversity of responses to mechanical signals. Biochem Cell Biol/Biochimie et biologie cellulaire. 1995;73(7–8):349–65.
18. Wall ME, Dyment NA, Bodle J, Volmer J, Loboa E, Cederlund A, et al. Cell signaling in tenocytes: response to load and ligands in health and disease. Adv Exp Med Biol. 2016;920:79–95.
19. Kragstrup TW, Kjaer M, Mackey AL. Structural, biochemical, cellular, and functional changes in skeletal muscle extracellular matrix with aging. Scand J Med Sci Sports. 2011;21(6):749–57.
20. Kannus P, Jozsa L, Natri A, Jarvinen M. Effects of training, immobilization and remobilization on tendons. Scand J Med Sci Sports. 1997;7(2):67–71.
21. Avery NC, Bailey AJ. Enzymic and non-enzymic cross-linking mechanisms in relation to turnover of collagen: relevance to aging and exercise. Scand J Med Sci Sports. 2005;15(4):231–40.
22. Svensson RB, Heinemeier KM, Couppe C, Kjaer M, Magnusson SP. Effect of aging and exercise on the tendon. J Appl Physiol (1985). 2016;121(6):1353–62.
23. Tipton CM, Vailas AC, Matthes RD. Experimental studies on the influences of physical activity on ligaments, tendons and joints: a brief review. Acta Med Scand Suppl. 1986;711:157–68.
24. Vilarta R, Vidal BC. Anisotropic and biomechanical properties of tendons modified by exercise and denervation: aggregation and macromolecular order in collagen bundles. Matrix. 1989;9(1):55–61.
25. Ohtani N, Hara E. Roles and mechanisms of cellular senescence in regulation of tissue homeostasis. Cancer Sci. 2013;104(5):525–30.
26. Zhu Y, Armstrong JL, Tchkonia T, Kirkland JL. Cellular senescence and the senescent secretory phenotype in age-related chronic diseases. Curr Opin Clin Nutr Metab Care. 2014;17(4):324–8.
27. Zhang J, Yuan T, Wang JH. Moderate treadmill running exercise prior to tendon injury enhances wound healing in aging rats. Oncotarget. 2016;7(8):8498–512.

28. Zhang J, Wang JH. Moderate exercise mitigates the detrimental effects of aging on tendon stem cells. PLoS One. 2015;10(6):e0130454.
29. Astrom M. Laser Doppler flowmetry in the assessment of tendon blood flow. Scand J Med Sci Sports. 2000;10(6):365–7.
30. Tipton CM, Matthes RD, Maynard JA, Carey RA. The influence of physical activity on ligaments and tendons. Med Sci Sports. 1975;7(3):165–75.
31. Wood LK, Arruda EM, Brooks SV. Regional stiffening with aging in tibialis anterior tendons of mice occurs independent of changes in collagen fibril morphology. J Appl Physiol (1985). 2011;111(4):999–1006.
32. Reddy GK. Cross-linking in collagen by nonenzymatic glycation increases the matrix stiffness in rabbit achilles tendon. Exp Diabesity Res. 2004;5(2):143–53.
33. Bailey AJ, Paul RG, Knott L. Mechanisms of maturation and ageing of collagen. Mech Ageing Dev. 1998;106(1–2):1–56.
34. Goh KL, Holmes DF, Lu HY, Richardson S, Kadler KE, Purslow PP, et al. Ageing changes in the tensile properties of tendons: influence of collagen fibril volume fraction. J Biomech Eng. 2008;130(2):021011.
35. Moore MJ, De Beaux A. A quantitative ultrastructural study of rat tendon from birth to maturity. J Anat. 1987;153:163–9.
36. Zhou Z, Akinbiyi T, Xu L, Ramcharan M, Leong DJ, Ros SJ, et al. Tendon-derived stem/progenitor cell aging: defective self-renewal and altered fate. Aging Cell. 2010;9(5):911–5.
37. Kohler J, Popov C, Klotz B, Alberton P, Prall WC, Haasters F, et al. Uncovering the cellular and molecular changes in tendon stem/progenitor cells attributed to tendon aging and degeneration. Aging Cell. 2013;12(6):988–99.
38. Kiiskinen A. Physical training and connective tissues in young mice--physical properties of Achilles tendons and long bones. Growth. 1977;41(2):123–37.
39. Simonsen EB, Klitgaard H, Bojsen-Moller F. The influence of strength training, swim training and ageing on the Achilles tendon and m. soleus of the rat. J Sports Sci. 1995;13(4):291–5.
40. Buchanan CI, Marsh RL. Effects of exercise on the biomechanical, biochemical and structural properties of tendons. Comp Biochem Physiol A Mol Integr Physiol. 2002;133(4):1101–7.
41. Viidik A. Tensile strength properties of Achilles tendon systems in trained and untrained rabbits. Acta Orthop Scand. 1969;40(2):261–72.
42. Woo SL, Ritter MA, Amiel D, Sanders TM, Gomez MA, Kuei SC, et al. The biomechanical and biochemical properties of swine tendons--long term effects of exercise on the digital extensors. Connect Tissue Res. 1980;7(3):177–83.
43. Viidik A. The effect of training on the tensile strength of isolated rabbit tendons. Scand J Plast Reconstr Surg. 1967;1(2):141–7.
44. Vailas AC, Pedrini VA, Pedrini-Mille A, Holloszy JO. Patellar tendon matrix changes associated with aging and voluntary exercise. J Appl Physiol (1985). 1985;58(5):1572–6.
45. Curwin SL, Vailas AC, Wood J. Immature tendon adaptation to strenuous exercise. J Appl Physiol (1985). 1988;65(5):2297–301.
46. Woo SL, Gomez MA, Amiel D, Ritter MA, Gelberman RH, Akeson WH. The effects of exercise on the biomechanical and biochemical properties of swine digital flexor tendons. J Biomech Eng. 1981;103(1):51–6.
47. Enwemeka CS, Maxwell LC, Fernandes G. Ultrastructural morphometry of matrical changes induced by exercise and food restriction in the rat calcaneal tendon. Tissue Cell. 1992;24(4):499–510.
48. Michna H. Morphometric analysis of loading-induced changes in collagen-fibril populations in young tendons. Cell Tissue Res. 1984;236(2):465–70.
49. Patterson-Kane JC, Firth EC, Parry DA, Wilson AM, Goodship AE. Effects of training on collagen fibril populations in the suspensory ligament and deep digital flexor tendon of young thoroughbreds. Am J Vet Res. 1998;59(1):64–8.
50. Sommer HM. The biomechanical and metabolic effects of a running regime on the Achilles tendon in the rat. Int Orthop. 1987;11(1):71–5.
51. Birch HL, McLaughlin L, Smith RK, Goodship AE. Treadmill exercise-induced tendon hypertrophy: assessment of tendons with different mechanical functions. Equine Vet J Suppl. 1999;30:222–6.
52. Yoon JH, Brooks R, Kim YH, Terada M, Halper J. Proteoglycans in chicken gastrocnemius tendons change with exercise. Arch Biochem Biophys. 2003;412(2):279–86.
53. Kubo K, Kanehisa H, Kawakami Y, Fukunaga T. Elastic properties of muscle-tendon complex in long-distance runners. Eur J Appl Physiol. 2000;81(3):181–7.
54. Kubo K, Kanehisa H, Ito M, Fukunaga T. Effects of isometric training on the elasticity of human tendon structures in vivo. J Appl Physiol (1985). 2001;91(1):26–32.
55. Kubo K, Kanehisa H, Fukunaga T. Effects of resistance and stretching training programmes on the viscoelastic properties of human tendon structures in vivo. J Physiol. 2002;538(Pt 1):219–26.
56. Rosager S, Aagaard P, Dyhre-Poulsen P, Neergaard K, Kjaer M, Magnusson SP. Load-displacement properties of the human triceps surae aponeurosis and tendon in runners and non-runners. Scand J Med Sci Sports. 2002;12(2):90–8.
57. Miller BF, Olesen JL, Hansen M, Dossing S, Crameri RM, Welling RJ, et al. Coordinated collagen and muscle protein synthesis in human patella tendon and quadriceps muscle after exercise. J Physiol. 2005;567(Pt 3):1021–33.
58. Arampatzis A, Karamanidis K, Albracht K. Adaptational responses of the human Achilles tendon by modulation of the applied cyclic strain magnitude. J Exp Biol. 2007;210(Pt 15):2743–53.
59. Seynnes OR, Erskine RM, Maganaris CN, Longo S, Simoneau EM, Grosset JF, et al. Training-induced changes in structural and mechanical properties of the patellar tendon are related to muscle hypertro-

phy but not to strength gains. J Appl Physiol (1985). 2009;107(2):523–30.

60. Bohm S, Mersmann F, Tettke M, Kraft M, Arampatzis A. Human Achilles tendon plasticity in response to cyclic strain: effect of rate and duration. J Exp Biol. 2014;217(Pt 22):4010–7.

61. Burgess KE, Connick MJ, Graham-Smith P, Pearson SJ. Plyometric vs. isometric training influences on tendon properties and muscle output. J Strength Cond Res. 2007;21(3):986–9.

62. Couppe C, Kongsgaard M, Aagaard P, Hansen P, Bojsen-Moller J, Kjaer M, et al. Habitual loading results in tendon hypertrophy and increased stiffness of the human patellar tendon. J Appl Physiol (1985). 2008;105(3):805–10.

63. Magnusson SP, Hansen M, Langberg H, Miller B, Haraldsson B, Westh EK, et al. The adaptability of tendon to loading differs in men and women. Int J Exp Pathol. 2007;88(4):237–40.

64. Westh E, Kongsgaard M, Bojsen-Moller J, Aagaard P, Hansen M, Kjaer M, et al. Effect of habitual exercise on the structural and mechanical properties of human tendon, in vivo, in men and women. Scand J Med Sci Sports. 2008;18(1):23–30.

65. Jones BH, Bovee MW, Harris JM 3rd, Cowan DN. Intrinsic risk factors for exercise-related injuries among male and female army trainees. Am J Sports Med. 1993;21(5):705–10.

66. Arendt EA. Anterior cruciate ligament injuries. Curr Womens Health Rep. 2001;1(3):211–7.

67. Yu WD, Panossian V, Hatch JD, Liu SH, Finerman GA. Combined effects of estrogen and progesterone on the anterior cruciate ligament. Clin Orthop Relat Res. 2001;383:268–81.

68. Fletcher JR, Esau SP, MacIntosh BR. Changes in tendon stiffness and running economy in highly trained distance runners. Eur J Appl Physiol. 2010;110(5):1037–46.

69. Albracht K, Arampatzis A. Exercise-induced changes in triceps surae tendon stiffness and muscle strength affect running economy in humans. Eur J Appl Physiol. 2013;113(6):1605–15.

70. Malliaras P, Kamal B, Nowell A, Farley T, Dhamu H, Simpson V, et al. Patellar tendon adaptation in relation to load-intensity and contraction type. J Biomech. 2013;46(11):1893–9.

71. Bohm S, Mersmann F, Arampatzis A. Human tendon adaptation in response to mechanical loading: a systematic review and meta-analysis of exercise intervention studies on healthy adults. Sports Med Open. 2015;1(1):7.

72. Nielsen HM, Skalicky M, Viidik A. Influence of physical exercise on aging rats. III. Life-long exercise modifies the aging changes of the mechanical properties of limb muscle tendons. Mech Ageing Dev. 1998;100(3):243–60.

73. Wood LK, Brooks SV. Ten weeks of treadmill running decreases stiffness and increases collagen turnover in tendons of old mice. J Orthop Res. 2016;34(2):346–53.

74. Reeves ND, Maganaris CN, Narici MV. Effect of strength training on human patella tendon mechanical properties of older individuals. J Physiol. 2003;548(Pt 3):971–81.

75. Reeves ND, Narici MV, Maganaris CN. Strength training alters the viscoelastic properties of tendons in elderly humans. Muscle Nerve. 2003;28(1):74–81.

76. Grosset JF, Breen L, Stewart CE, Burgess KE, Onambele GL. Influence of exercise intensity on training-induced tendon mechanical properties changes in older individuals. Age (Dordr). 2014;36(3):9657.

77. Onambele-Pearson GL, Pearson SJ. The magnitude and character of resistance-training-induced increase in tendon stiffness at old age is gender specific. Age (Dordr). 2012;34(2):427–38.

78. Murchison ND, Price BA, Conner DA, Keene DR, Olson EN, Tabin CJ, et al. Regulation of tendon differentiation by scleraxis distinguishes force-transmitting tendons from muscle-anchoring tendons. Development. 2007;134(14):2697–708.

79. Mendias CL, Gumucio JP, Bakhurin KI, Lynch EB, Brooks SV. Physiological loading of tendons induces scleraxis expression in epitenon fibroblasts. J Orthop Res. 2012;30(4):606–12.

80. Yamamoto K, Sokabe T, Watabe T, Miyazono K, Yamashita JK, Obi S, et al. Fluid shear stress induces differentiation of Flk-1-positive embryonic stem cells into vascular endothelial cells in vitro. Am J Physiol Heart Circ Physiol. 2005;288(4):H1915–24.

81. Song G, Ju Y, Soyama H, Ohashi T, Sato M. Regulation of cyclic longitudinal mechanical stretch on proliferation of human bone marrow mesenchymal stem cells. Mol Cell Biomech. 2007;4(4):201–10.

82. Schild C, Trueb B. Mechanical stress is required for high-level expression of connective tissue growth factor. Exp Cell Res. 2002;274(1):83–91.

83. Yang G, Crawford RC, Wang JH. Proliferation and collagen production of human patellar tendon fibroblasts in response to cyclic uniaxial stretching in serum-free conditions. J Biomech. 2004;37(10):1543–50.

84. Robbins JR, Evanko SP, Vogel KG. Mechanical loading and TGF-beta regulate proteoglycan synthesis in tendon. Arch Biochem Biophys. 1997;342(2):203–11.

85. Skutek M, van Griensven M, Zeichen J, Brauer N, Bosch U. Cyclic mechanical stretching modulates secretion pattern of growth factors in human tendon fibroblasts. Eur J Appl Physiol. 2001;86(1):48–52.

86. Skutek M, van Griensven M, Zeichen J, Brauer N, Bosch U. Cyclic mechanical stretching enhances secretion of Interleukin 6 in human tendon fibroblasts. Knee Surg Sports Traumatol Arthrosc. 2001;9(5):322–6.

87. Wang N, Butler JP, Ingber DE. Mechanotransduction across the cell surface and through the cytoskeleton. Science. 1993;260(5111):1124–7.

88. Nindl BC. Insulin-like growth factor-I, physical activity, and control of cellular anabolism. Med Sci Sports Exerc. 2010;42(1):35–8.

The Pathogenic Mechanisms of Tendinopathy

2

James H-C. Wang and Bhavani P. Thampatty

Abbreviations

Ach	Acetylcholine
ADAMTS	A disintegrin and metalloproteinase with a thrombospondin
CGRP	Calcitonin gene-related peptide
COX-2	Cyclooxygenase-2
ECM	Extracellular matrix
GAG	Glycosaminoglycans
HIF	Hypoxia-inducible factors
HSP	Heat shock proteins
IFNγ	Interferon γ
IGF	Insulin growth factor
IL-1β	Interlukin-1β
IL-6	Interleukin-6
MCP-1	Monocyte chemoattractant protein-1
MMP	Matrix metalloproteinase
NF-kB	Nuclear factor-kB
NMDA	N-methyl-D-aspartate
NSAID	Non-steroidal anti-inflammatory drug
PGE$_2$	Prostaglandin E$_2$
PRP	Platelet-rich plasma
SP	Substance P
STAT6	Signal transducer and activator of transcription 6
TGF-β	Transforming growth factor-β
TIMP	Tissue inhibitors of matrix metalloproteinase
TNF-α	Tumor necrosis factor-α
TSC	Tendon stem/progenitor cell
VEGF	Vascular endothelial growth factor

J. H-C. Wang (✉)
MechanoBiology Laboratory, Department of Orthopaedic Surgery, University of Pittsburgh, Pittsburgh, PA, USA

Departments of Physical Medicine and Rehabilitation, and Bioengineering, University of Pittsburgh, Pittsburgh, PA, USA
e-mail: wanghc@pitt.edu

B. P. Thampatty
MechanoBiology Laboratory, Department of Orthopaedic Surgery, University of Pittsburgh School of Medicine, Pittsburgh, PA, USA

Introduction

Tendon is a connective tissue that functions as a mechanical link to transmit forces from muscle to bone to enable body movements. As a result, tendons are constantly subjected to mechanical loads. The ability of tendon to withstand great mechanical forces is attributed to the high degree of organization of its extracellular matrix (ECM) [1]. About 95% of healthy tendon is composed of highly structured bundles of fibril-forming type I collagen intermingled with glycoproteins (fibronectin and thrombospondin) and glycosaminoglycans (GAG) such as aggrecan, decorin, biglycan, and fibromodulin [2]. The anatomical structure of a tendon is shaped in a unique hierarchical fibrillar arrangement of collagen [3]. At the very basic level, this ascending order of structural arrangement of tendons starts with the triple helical type I collagen molecules (tropocollagen)

© Springer Nature Switzerland AG 2021
K. Onishi et al. (eds.), *Tendinopathy*, https://doi.org/10.1007/978-3-030-65335-4_2

that orderly aggregate into microfibrils and form fibrils. Fibrils form a wave form or "crimp" pattern which opens out under tension that may act as mechanical safety buffer. Collagen fibrils group together to form collagen fibers, and fiber bundles then aggregate into fascicles [4, 5]. Fascicles finally form the tendon unit. Between the fascicles and fiber bundles, a thin layer of loose connective tissue that binds fascicles called endotenon facilitates the sliding movement of fascicles [6]. Endotenon carries blood vessels, lymphatics, and nerves in tendon. Fascicles have the ability to extend and recoil under tensile mechanical loads. Another sheet of connective tissue called epitenon rich in blood vessels and lymphatics surrounds the tendon as a whole. Some tendons such as Achilles and patellar have an additional connective tissue called paratenon that covers the tendon.

Tendon possesses both elastic and viscous properties that are largely controlled by the composition, such as collagens, of the tendinous tissue [6]. The cross-links of collagens of tendon tissue also increase its stiffness enabling the tendon to withstand large mechanical stress and strain [7]. Most tendons are only subjected to stresses of up to a 30 MPa, although Achilles tendon may experience stresses of up to 70 MPa [8]. Positional tendons like finger flexor tendons are generally subjected to small strains of 2–3%, while load-bearing tendons such as human Achilles tendon can withstand strain of up to 8% without micro-damage [9].

Tendons contain fibroblast-like cells termed tenocytes, which are the dominant resident tendon cells exhibiting elongated morphology with spindle-shaped nuclei. Tenocytes are responsible not only for ECM synthesis but also for its maintenance and degradation through MMPs and TIMPs [10]. There is no single cell marker that defines tenocytes; however, the transcription factors scleraxis and tenomodulin are considered the two relatively specific markers of tenocytes [11].

There are gap junctions between the tenocytes and also between rows of these cells, and these gap junctions allow rapid exchange of ions and signaling molecules. Tendon stem/progenitor cells (TSCs) were identified in recent years, and these cells, which constitute less than 5% of the total tendon cells, possess clonogenicity, self-renewal, and multi-differentiation potential [12]. The TSCs play a vital role in maintaining the homeostasis of normal tendons and repair in injured tendons [13].

Despite its ability to withstand large mechanical forces, tendons are prone to injuries due to intrinsic and extrinsic factors [14]. Some of the major intrinsic factors include age, sex, body weight, diabetes, and rheumatologic diseases, and extrinsic factors mainly include sports- and occupation-related activities [15]. Chronic tendon injuries due to repetitive mechanical loading placed on the tendons present a highly prevalent medical problem in orthopedics and sports medicine.

Tendon conditions including inflammation, degeneration, and injury are often described using various yet confusing terms such as tendonitis, tendinosis, and tendinopathy. Once used to describe any tendon pain, tendinitis (or tendon inflammation) is used to describe inflammation of the tendon as the suffix "itis" indicates inflammation. It generally refers to a clinical symptom, not to a specific histopathological entity. Patients with tendinitis may experience localized pain, swelling, and warmth. Tendinosis (or tendon degeneration) refers to non-inflammatory degeneration of the tendon without histological signs of inflammation [16, 17]. Tendon rupture may occur without symptoms especially in Achilles tendon that often results from repetitive microtrauma. Tendinopathy (etiologically less specific) is an umbrella term used to describe tendon inflammation, various degrees of tears, and/or degeneration and is now used to describe a chronic painful tendon condition that fails to heal [18]. Although earlier histopathological examinations failed to detect the presence of inflammation, more recent studies show the presence of inflammatory mediators in the chronic tendinopathic tendons [19, 20].

Clinical treatments of tendinopathy cost billions of dollars in America every year [21]. Common treatments for tendinopathy include physical therapy, administration of NSAIDs, and more recently platelet-rich plasma (PRP).

Because the precise pathogenic mechanisms of tendinopathy remain elusive, most of the current treatment options are directed at alleviating the symptoms such as pain and swelling without treating underlying cause and therefore they are less effective. Moreover, a single treatment option is almost out of question because it is increasingly recognized that tendinopathy represents a spectrum of disorders that may arise from a wide range of etiological factors such as mechanical, neurologic, genetic, or a combination of these factors [22–24]. Therefore, a better understanding of the precise mechanisms for the pathology of tendinopathy is essential to improve treatment efficacy. This chapter focuses on reviewing the current advances in understanding the pathogenic mechanisms for the development of tendinopathy.

Biological Changes in Tendinopathic Tendons

Clinically, tendinopathy is presented with focal pain, stiffness, and tenderness to palpation [25]. The pain in tendinopathic conditions may be caused by a multitude of factors including neuropeptides (SP, CGRP) and neurotransmitters such as glutamate [26–28]. SP can cause vasodilation and increase cell metabolism, cell viability, and cell proliferation in tenocytes. Both SP and CGRP are released by nociceptors, and SP is known to be released by tenocytes [29]. Moreover, SP and CGRP have been identified in nerve fascicles in large and small blood vessels in tendinopathy [30]. Additionally, high intra-tendinous levels of glutamate and its receptor N-methyl-D-aspartate (NMDA) have been demonstrated in tendinopathy [31, 32]. The neurotransmitter acetylcholine (AcH) that is produced by activated tenocytes is also implicated as a causative factor of pain [33]. Finally, various ion channels in tenocytes that mediate calcium signaling have also been implicated in pain generation in tendinopathy [28].

Tendinopathic tendons undergo substantial changes in structural and mechanical properties, and these changes can be detected by macro-

scopic, microscopic, and sonographic methods [34, 35]. Normal tendons are brilliant white in appearance with a viscoelastic structure and low cellularity. The collagen is highly organized parallel bundles with densely packed collagen fibers that are quite uniform in diameter and orientation. The spindle-shaped tenocyte nuclei are aligned parallel to collagen bundles. In contrast, tendinopathic tendons look gray or brown with a soft, fragile, and disorganized tissue of loose texture [36]. The collagen bundles are disorganized, and the fibers vary in diameter and orientation [37]. The composition of tendon matrix undergoes substantial changes including a decrease in collagen type I and increase in collagen type III, proteoglycans, and GAG [38]. Increased vascularity, lipid deposits, proteoglycan accumulation and calcification, either alone or in combination, can be seen at late-stage tendinopathy [39, 40] (Fig. 2.1).

At the cellular level, tendinopathic tendons contain cells that lose their normal parallel alignment and their spindle shape. Their long thin cytoplasmic projections also shorten. These cells may enlarge in size, increase in cell number, and become apoptotic or necrotic [41]. In some instances, cells also round up and exhibit a chondrocytic appearance [42], which may indicate aberrant differentiation of TSCs into chondrocytes in response to excessive mechanical loading [43]. Such aberrant differentiation has been demonstrated in isolated TSCs under high mechanical loading that differentiated into non-tenocyte phenotypes such as chondrocytes and osteocytes [44]. Moreover, increased production of PGE_2 in Achilles and patellar tendon tissues in mice subjected to intense treadmill running decreased the proliferation and induced differentiation of TSCs into non-tenocyte phenotypes which are indications of degenerative changes in tendon [45].

Hence, the change in tendon cell function may bring a plethora of structural and functional changes to ECM. As a consequence of such pathologic changes in tendon matrix, tendon weakens in its mechanical strength and becomes prone to injury. The changes in the gene expression levels of major matrix molecules are consis-

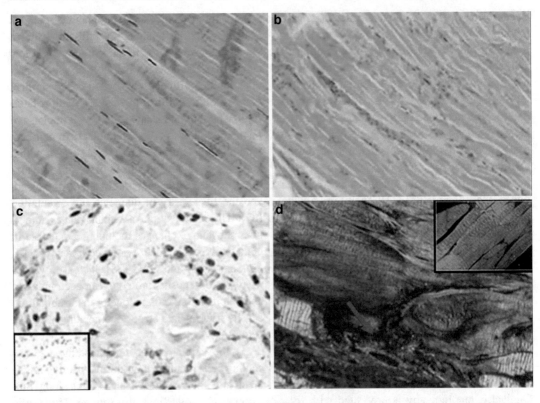

Fig. 2.1 Late-stage tendinopathy shows increased vascularity, lipid deposits, proteoglycan accumulation, and calcification (alone or in combination)

tently observed in tendinopathic tendons of humans and in animal models of tendinopathy [46, 47]. For instance, in pathologic human tendon matrix, increased mRNA levels of collagen type I (without increase in protein levels though) and type III and increased levels of collagen type III protein are observed [48]. Type III collagen is thinner and less capable of forming organized fibrils and therefore results in rapid collagen disorganization. High levels of gene expression of other matrix components such as biglycan, fibromodulin, aggrecan, fibronectin, and tenascin-C also occur in tendinopathic tendons. In addition, matrix metalloproteinases (MMPs, ADAMTS) and their inhibitors (TIMPs) are disproportionately expressed in tendinopathic tendons [49]. The changes in the matrix components, collagen cross-links, and matrix degradative enzymes explain the matrix disturbances, whereas the expression of various inflammatory cytokines and alarmins, excessive apoptosis, and

hypoxia account for the deregulation of cellular activities [36]. In summary, the clinical manifestation of tendinopathy as pain and disability has several underlying structural, cellular, and molecular changes in tendon tissues that are involved in degeneration of tendons. Moreover, tendinopathy represents a spectrum of disorders with multiple etiological factors of which mechanical loading is suggested to be the major one in active populations such as athletes.

Development of Tendinopathy

Several risk factors that fall into intrinsic and extrinsic categories have been identified that predispose both active and sedentary populations to tendinopathy. The intrinsic factors include advancing age, sex, and obesity, and ailments such as diabetes and rheumatologic diseases [15, 50]. Changes in cellular activity and matrix composition, which in turn lead to changes in the tendon's structural and mechanical properties, may explain the increased incidence of tendinopathy in older population due to aging [51]. Sex differences and hormonal background may contribute to tendon injuries with the female more susceptible to repetitive trauma [52]. The poor adaptation response of tendon matrix to loading due to the inhibitory effect of estrogen on collagen synthesis and fibroblast proliferation and lower increase in collagen synthesis in response to loading may explain why women are more susceptible to tendon overuse injuries [53]. Obesity is also linked to tendinopathy development [54]. Several genetic variants of matrix components including tenascin-C, MMP-3, and VEGF that are regulated by mechanical loading are also associated with the risk of developing Achilles tendinopathy [55–57].

The main extrinsic factor for acute and chronic injury is "abnormal/excessive" mechanical loading on tendon. Abnormal loading is linked to exercise, sports-related activities, and specific work settings. While acute tendon injury ensues after one-time overloading, tendinopathy mainly occurs from repetitive mechanical loading placed on the tendon [1]. Such a "fatigue-loading" may lead to tendon micro-tears [58]. Evidence of tendon micro-tears due to cyclic mechanical loading has been observed in rabbits [59]. Tendinopathy may start with fatigue loading, which results in the accumulation of micro-damage to the tendon over the course of many loading cycles [60]. It is speculated that this fatigue-induced tendon injury occurs when the rate of tendon damage exceeds the rate of repair over time [48].

Although the exact cellular and molecular processes that drive changes in tendon physiology are yet to be determined, there has been a considerable progress to delineate the pathways in the recent years by gene and protein analyses. Excess mechanical load causes perturbation to cells that initiates various signaling pathways, a process known as mechanotransduction [61]. A number of gene pathways are altered in tendinopathies such as those of ECM, vasculature, and intracellular signaling mechanisms [1, 22]. As a result, several biological factors are produced

including MMPs, growth factors, cytokines, and prostaglandins, which will lead to defective ECM remodeling [62].

A few theoretical models have been proposed to explain the pathogenesis of tendinopathy. Both the continuum model that proposes a chronic degenerative disorder without involving an inflammatory process and a "failed healing" response theory have been proposed [25, 63]. The continuum model suggests that the progression of tendon pathology is a three-stage process in sequence: reactive tendinopathy, tendon disrepair, and tendon degeneration. The early stages of reactive tendinopathy, according to this model, may present a non-inflammatory, proliferative tissue reaction, usually in response to acute tensile overload. The tendon thickens due to the accumulation of large amounts of proteoglycans and an increase in bound water, with minimal collagen damage or separation. The next stage is dis-repair which is characterized by greater tissue matrix breakdown, with collagen separation, proliferation of abnormal tenocytes, and some increase in tendon neo-vascularity. The final stage of tendinopathy sees a further disruption of collagen, widespread cell death, and extensive ingrowth of neovessels and nerves into the tendon substance, leading to an essentially irreversible stage of degenerative tendon pathology [63].

It is clear that this theory of tendinopathy development mechanism disregards the role of tendon inflammation in the development of tendinopathy. This may reflect the fact that due to lack of available tissues from early-stage tendinopathy, and later presentation of tendon conditions by human patients, possible inflammatory events in the early stages of tendinopathy may have been subdued or cleared. Moreover, a majority of clinical studies rely on histological analysis, and very few studies have assessed inflammatory cells such as monocytes and macrophages in tendinopathic specimens using immunohistochemical techniques to detect inflammatory mediators. This situation may explain why clinical signs of inflammation and invading inflammatory cells were rarely observed in early studies [27, 64].

Moreover, the pro-inflammatory role of potent inflammatory mediator, PGE_2, in tendinopathy has been well established through numerous in vitro and in vivo studies [65–68]. Prostaglandins are produced constitutively for normal remodeling and repair and also in response to injury. In vivo levels of PGE_2 were elevated in Achilles tendon after acute exercise estimated by microdialysis in trained runners. PGE_2 concentration increased in blood during running and returned to baseline in the recovery period, whereas interstitial PGE_2 concentration was elevated in the early recovery phase [69]. High levels of PGE_2 depress collagen synthesis in tendon cells and upregulate degradative enzyme activity [70]. Moreover, in mice subjected to intense treadmill running, PGE_2 production in Achilles and patellar tendon tissues increases, which may decrease the proliferation and induce differentiation of TSCs into non-tenocyte; thus, high levels of PGE_2 produced by large mechanical loading may contribute to the development of degenerative tendinopathy [45].

Other studies in tendinopathic specimens support the role of inflammation in tendinopathy. In tendons obtained from symptomatic patellar tendinopathy patients, the mast cell density was three times higher than in control tendons, and $CD3^+$ lymphocytes and $CD68^+$ macrophages were present in low level but not quantifiable enough [71]. In Achilles tendinopathy patients, the number of B cells, T cells, and macrophages were significantly greater compared to those from patients with ruptured Achilles tendon [72]. In a recent study, immunohistochemical evaluation of biopsy specimens from non-ruptured chronic tendinopathic Achilles tendons showed presence of macrophages, T lymphocytes, and mast cells [73]. CD68-$KP1^+$ macrophages and $CD34^+$ endothelial cells were significantly more numerous in tendinopathic tendons compared with healthy tendons.

Another study in human supraspinatus tendons from rotator cuff tendinopathy patients shows the significantly increased presence of inflammatory $CD14^+$ monocyte/macrophages in early, intermediate, and advanced stages of diseased tendons compared to healthy tendon samples [74]. Furthermore, several studies have demonstrated increased expression of various inflammatory cytokines including TNF-α, IL-1β, and IL-6 from tendon tissues in animal models of tendinopathy [42, 75, 76]. Thus, recent evidence suggests that inflammation and degeneration are closely interrelated in the development of tendinopathy [45, 77, 78].

Recently, a new theory on the role of inflammation in tendinopathy development has been proposed [20]. According to the theory, inflammation in tendinopathy mainly involves three cellular compartments: stromal, immune-sensing, and infiltrating compartments. The stromal compartment is populated with tenocytes that are responsible for tissue remodeling and repair. The immune-sensing compartment consists of macrophages and mast cells. They may respond to tissue damage by eliciting pro-inflammatory and anti-inflammatory mediators. The infiltrating compartment consists of immune cells that are recruited through tenocytes. The three compartments act in a coordinated fashion to elicit interactions between inflammatory response and ECM remodeling, the consequences of which affect tendon homeostasis. Once activated by various inflammatory mediators, resident tenocytes and immune cells recruit T cells, mast cells, and macrophages. The influx of such immune cells is a normal healing and remodeling response; however, in tendinopathic tendons, this pathway may turn pathologic. Tenocytes respond by secreting various inflammatory cytokines and chemokines such as IL-1β, IL-17, IL-33, and TNF-α [20].

Additionally, excessive apoptosis has been associated with tendinopathy, although the precise mechanism is unclear [79, 80]. Several factors including mechanical overuse, hypoxia and oxidative stress, and inflammation are thought to contribute to the regulation of apoptosis in tendinopathy [80, 81]. The increased number of apoptotic tendon cells in degenerative tendons could affect the rate of collagen synthesis and repair of compromised tendon matrix [41].

Several molecules collectively called alarmins have been implicated in the development of tendinopathy [36]. Alarmins such as heat shock proteins (HSPs) and hypoxia-inducible factor-1α (HIF-1α) which are thought to initiate and perpetuate sterile inflammatory response are elevated in human tendinopathy models. Cyclic stretching significantly increased HSP72 expression in human tenocytes, and significant upregulation of HSPs was observed in early tendinopathy in rat supraspinatus tendinopathy models and in human torn supraspinatus tendon tissue [82, 83]. Hypoxic cell injury as a critical regulator of pathophysiologic mechanism of early human tendinopathy also has been suggested based on the results from a recent study that showed increased expression of HIF-1α in tendinopathy specimens by immunostaining [84]. In addition, marked increase in inflammatory cells such as macrophages and mast cells was observed by immunostaining in tendinopathy samples. They also observed that hypoxia induces apoptosis in primary human tenocytes by overexpression of HSP70 and apoptotic markers such as Bcl-2 and clusterin. In addition, hypoxia altered collagen matrix regulation (increase in collagen III and decrease in collagen I mRNA expression) and promoted cytokine (IL-6), chemokine (IL-8), and MCP-1 production, supporting the notion that hypoxic tenocytes could initiate leukocyte recruitment. A previous in vitro study also showed increased expression of HIF-1α in cyclically stretched rat Achilles tendon fibroblasts [85].

In tendinopathic tendons, tissue metaplasia as a histological change has been often reported [39, 86, 87]. The expression of cartilage markers such as aggrecan and Sox-9 have been linked to tendon overuse [88, 89]. The presence of chondrogenic, osteogenic, and adipogenic phenotypes in tendinopathic tendons [39] suggests the role of newly discovered TSCs in the development and persistence of tendinopathy. Using an in vitro model system that can apply various stretching magnitudes to cells to mimic in vivo repetitive mechanical loading of tendons, small mechanical loading was shown to induce TSC differentiation into tenocytes, while large loading induced both tenocyte and non-tenocyte differentiation [44]. The in vitro findings match with the in vivo observations. In an animal model of repetitive mechanical loading via treadmill running, moderate treadmill running increased TSC proliferation and collagen production, but intensive treadmill running induced the expression of those genes related to fatty, cartilage, and bony tissues (LPL, Sox-9, Runx-2, and Osterix), and tendon-related genes (Coll. I and tenomodulin) in the mouse patellar and Achilles tendons [43]. Hence, aberrant differentiation of TSCs into non-tenocytes in response to excessive mechanical loading conditions placed on the tendons may be a causative factor for the development of degenerative tendinopathy.

Concluding Remarks

Tendinopathy affects millions of Americans every year. The current treatments are inadequate since they are largely palliative. This situation stems from the fact that tendinopathy is a spectrum of tendon disorders that develop due to multi-etiologic factors. The major one among those causal factors is the abnormal mechanical loading placed on the tendons such as in the athletic setting. It is clear that to improve the treatment of tendinopathy, basic science studies are required so that one can define the cellular and molecular mechanisms that are responsible for a particular type of tendinopathy such as the one caused by mechanical overloading.

Conventionally, the development of tendinopathy is thought to involve overuse-induced microdamage to tendons and subsequent apoptosis and production of MMPs in the tendon matrix by tenocytes, the dominant cells that are responsible for the homeostasis and repair of tendon once injured. However, the recent discovery of TSCs has offered different perspectives on the causative mechanisms of tendinopathy. The latest studies suggested that TSCs may be responsible for the development of degenerative tendinopathy by undergoing non-tenocyte differentiation in response to excessive mechanical loading placed on tendons. Future studies may investigate whether blocking aberrant differentiation of TSCs can prevent the development of tendinopathy.

It is known that in response to mechanical overloading, tendon inflammation ensues, which is characterized by an abnormal increase in the levels of COX-2 and PGE_2. Such high PGE_2 levels may induce aberrant differentiation of TSCs into non-tenocytes such as adipocytes, chondrocytes, and osteocytes that produce fat-, cartilage- and bone-like tissues in tendons and consequently compromise tendon structure and function. However, the upstream molecular events through which mechanical overloading triggers inflammatory responses in tendons/tendon cells and eventual tendon degeneration are unknown. In this regard, alarmin molecules may play an important role in the initiation of early-stage tendinopathy, and this is a research area that should be actively explored in future.

References

1. Kjaer M. Role of extracellular matrix in adaptation of tendon and skeletal muscle to mechanical loading. Physiol Rev. 2004;84(2):649–98.
2. Kannus P. Structure of the tendon connective tissue. Scand J Med Sci Sports. 2000;10(6):312–20.
3. Nourissat G, Berenbaum F, Duprez D. Tendon injury: from biology to tendon repair. Nat Rev Rheumatol. 2015;11(4):223–33.
4. Elliott DH. Structure and function of mammalian tendon. Biol Rev Camb Philos Soc. 1965;40:392–421.
5. Birk DE, Southern JF, Zycband EI, Fallon JT, Trelstad RL. Collagen fibril bundles: a branching assembly unit in tendon morphogenesis. Development. 1989;107(3):437–43.
6. Benjamin M, Ralphs JR. Tendons and ligaments – an overview. Histol Histopathol. 1997;12(4):1135–44.
7. Birch HL, Thorpe CT, Rumian AP. Specialisation of extracellular matrix for function in tendons and ligaments. Muscles Ligaments Tendons J. 2013;3(1):12–22.
8. Komi PV, Fukashiro S, Jarvinen M. Biomechanical loading of Achilles tendon during normal locomotion. Clin Sports Med. 1992;11(3):521–31.
9. Birch HL. Tendon matrix composition and turnover in relation to functional requirements. Int J Exp Pathol. 2007;88(4):241–8.
10. Benjamin M, Ralphs JR. The cell and developmental biology of tendons and ligaments. Int Rev Cytol. 2000;196:85–130.
11. Benjamin M, Kaiser E, Milz S. Structure-function relationships in tendons: a review. J Anat. 2008;212(3):211–28.
12. Bi Y, Ehirchiou D, Kilts TM, Inkson CA, Embree MC, Sonoyama W, et al. Identification of tendon stem/progenitor cells and the role of the extracellular matrix in their niche. Nat Med. 2007;13(10):1219–27.
13. Zhang J, Wang JH. Characterization of differential properties of rabbit tendon stem cells and tenocytes. BMC Musculoskelet Disord. 2010;11:10.
14. Clayton RA, Court-Brown CM. The epidemiology of musculoskeletal tendinous and ligamentous injuries. Injury. 2008;39(12):1338–44.
15. O'Neill S, Watson PJ, Barry S. A Delphi study of risk factors for Achilles tendinopathy – opinions of world tendon experts. Int J Sports Phys Ther. 2016;11(5):684–97.
16. Maffulli N, Khan KM, Puddu G. Overuse tendon conditions: time to change a confusing terminology. Arthroscopy. 1998;14(8):840–3.
17. Wang JH, Iosifidis MI, Fu FH. Biomechanical basis for tendinopathy. Clin Orthop Relat Res. 2006;443:320–32.
18. Sharma P, Maffulli N. Tendon injury and tendinopathy: healing and repair. J Bone Joint Surg Am. 2005;87(1):187–202.
19. Dean BJF, Dakin SG, Millar NL, Carr AJ. Review: emerging concepts in the pathogenesis of tendinopathy. Surgeon. 2017;15(6):349–54.
20. Millar NL, Murrell GA, McInnes IB. Inflammatory mechanisms in tendinopathy – towards translation. Nat Rev Rheumatol. 2017;13(2):110–22.
21. McGonagle D, Marzo-Ortega H, Benjamin M, Emery P. Report on the second international Enthesitis Workshop. Arthritis Rheum. 2003;48(4):896–905.
22. Riley G. Chronic tendon pathology: molecular basis and therapeutic implications. Expert Rev Mol Med. 2005;7(5):1–25.
23. Wang JH. Mechanobiology of tendon. J Biomech. 2006;39(9):1563–82.
24. Kaux JF, Forthomme B, Goff CL, Crielaard JM, Croisier JL. Current opinions on tendinopathy. J Sports Sci Med. 2011;10(2):238–53.
25. Fu SC, Rolf C, Cheuk YC, Lui PP, Chan KM. Deciphering the pathogenesis of tendinopathy: a three-stages process. Sports Med Arthrosc Rehabil Ther Technol. 2010;2:30.
26. Gotoh M, Hamada K, Yamakawa H, Inoue A, Fukuda H. Increased substance P in subacromial bursa and shoulder pain in rotator cuff diseases. J Orthop Res. 1998;16(5):618–21.
27. Alfredson H, Thorsen K, Lorentzon R. In situ microdialysis in tendon tissue: high levels of glutamate, but not prostaglandin E2 in chronic Achilles tendon pain. Knee Surg Sports Traumatol Arthrosc. 1999;7(6):378–81.
28. Rio E, Moseley L, Purdam C, Samiric T, Kidgell D, Pearce AJ, et al. The pain of tendinopathy: physiological or pathophysiological? Sports Med. 2014;44(1):9–23.
29. Bjur D, Alfredson H, Forsgren S. The innervation pattern of the human Achilles tendon: studies of the normal and tendinosis tendon with markers for general and sensory innervation. Cell Tissue Res. 2005;320(1):201–6.
30. Alfredson H, Lorentzon R. Sclerosing polidocanol injections of small vessels to treat the chronic pain-

ful tendon. Cardiovasc Hematol Agents Med Chem. 2007;5(2):97–100.

31. Scott A, Alfredson H, Forsgren S. VGluT2 expression in painful Achilles and patellar tendinosis: evidence of local glutamate release by tenocytes. J Orthop Res. 2008;26(5):685–92.

32. Schizas N, Weiss R, Lian O, Frihagen F, Bahr R, Ackermann PW. Glutamate receptors in tendinopathic patients. J Orthop Res. 2012;30(9):1447–52.

33. Forsgren S, Grimsholm O, Jonsson M, Alfredson H, Danielson P. New insight into the non-neuronal cholinergic system via studies on chronically painful tendons and inflammatory situations. Life Sci. 2009;84(25–26):865–70.

34. Khan KM, Cook JL, Bonar F, Harcourt P, Astrom M. Histopathology of common tendinopathies. Update and implications for clinical management. Sports Med. 1999;27(6):393–408.

35. Riley GP. Gene expression and matrix turnover in overused and damaged tendons. Scand J Med Sci Sports. 2005;15(4):241–51.

36. Millar NL, Murrell GA, McInnes IB. Alarmins in tendinopathy: unravelling new mechanisms in a common disease. Rheumatology (Oxford). 2013;52(5):769–79.

37. Kader D, Saxena A, Movin T, Maffulli N. Achilles tendinopathy: some aspects of basic science and clinical management. Br J Sports Med. 2002;36(4):239–49.

38. Rees SG, Dent CM, Caterson B. Metabolism of proteoglycans in tendon. Scand J Med Sci Sports. 2009;19(4):470–8.

39. Kannus P, Jozsa L. Histopathological changes preceding spontaneous rupture of a tendon. A controlled study of 891 patients. J Bone Joint Surg Am. 1991;73(10):1507–25.

40. Lui PP, Chan LS, Lee YW, Fu SC, Chan KM. Sustained expression of proteoglycans and collagen type III/type I ratio in a calcified tendinopathy model. Rheumatology (Oxford). 2010;49(2):231–9.

41. Yuan J, Wang MX, Murrell GA. Cell death and tendinopathy. Clin Sports Med. 2003;22(4):693–701.

42. Thorpe CT, Chaudhry S, Lei II, Varone A, Riley GP, Birch HL, et al. Tendon overload results in alterations in cell shape and increased markers of inflammation and matrix degradation. Scand J Med Sci Sports. 2015;25(4):e381–91.

43. Zhang J, Wang JH. The effects of mechanical loading on tendons – an in vivo and in vitro model study. PLoS One. 2013;8(8):e71740.

44. Zhang J, Wang JH. Mechanobiological response of tendon stem cells: implications of tendon homeostasis and pathogenesis of tendinopathy. J Orthop Res. 2010;28(5):639–43.

45. Zhang J, Wang JH. Production of PGE(2) increases in tendons subjected to repetitive mechanical loading and induces differentiation of tendon stem cells into non-tenocytes. J Orthop Res. 2010;28(2):198–203.

46. Chaudhury S, Carr AJ. Lessons we can learn from gene expression patterns in rotator cuff tears and tendinopathies. J Shoulder Elbow Surg. 2012;21(2):191–9.

47. Jelinsky SA, Rodeo SA, Li J, Gulotta LV, Archambault JM, Seeherman HJ. Regulation of gene expression in human tendinopathy. BMC Musculoskelet Disord. 2011;12:86.

48. Riley G. The pathogenesis of tendinopathy. A molecular perspective. Rheumatology (Oxford). 2004;43(2):131–42.

49. Jones GC, Corps AN, Pennington CJ, Clark IM, Edwards DR, Bradley MM, et al. Expression profiling of metalloproteinases and tissue inhibitors of metalloproteinases in normal and degenerate human Achilles tendon. Arthritis Rheum. 2006;54(3):832–42.

50. Magnan B, Bondi M, Pierantoni S, Samaila E. The pathogenesis of Achilles tendinopathy: a systematic review. Foot Ankle Surg. 2014;20(3):154–9.

51. Zhou B, Zhou Y, Tang K. An overview of structure, mechanical properties, and treatment for age-related tendinopathy. J Nutr Health Aging. 2014;18(4):441–8.

52. Hansen M, Kjaer M. Sex hormones and tendon. Adv Exp Med Biol. 2016;920:139–49.

53. Liu SH, Al-Shaikh RA, Panossian V, Finerman GA, Lane JM. Estrogen affects the cellular metabolism of the anterior cruciate ligament. A potential explanation for female athletic injury. Am J Sports Med. 1997;25(5):704–9.

54. Gaida JE, Cook JL, Bass SL. Adiposity and tendinopathy. Disabil Rehabil. 2008;30(20–22):1555–62.

55. Mokone GG, Gajjar M, September AV, Schwellnus MP, Greenberg J, Noakes TD, et al. The guanine-thymine dinucleotide repeat polymorphism within the tenascin-C gene is associated with achilles tendon injuries. Am J Sports Med. 2005;33(7):1016–21.

56. Raleigh SM, van der Merwe L, Ribbans WJ, Smith RK, Schwellnus MP, Collins M. Variants within the MMP3 gene are associated with Achilles tendinopathy: possible interaction with the COL5A1 gene. Br J Sports Med. 2009;43(7):514–20.

57. Rahim M, El Khoury LY, Raleigh SM, Ribbans WJ, Posthumus M, Collins M, et al. Human genetic variation, sport and exercise medicine, and Achilles tendinopathy: role for angiogenesis-associated genes. OMICS. 2016;20(9):520–7.

58. Magnusson SP, Langberg H, Kjaer M. The pathogenesis of tendinopathy: balancing the response to loading. Nat Rev Rheumatol. 2010;6(5):262–8.

59. Nakama LH, King KB, Abrahamsson S, Rempel DM. Evidence of tendon microtears due to cyclical loading in an in vivo tendinopathy model. J Orthop Res. 2005;23(5):1199–205.

60. Fung DT, Wang VM, Andarawis-Puri N, Basta-Pljakic J, Li Y, Laudier DM, et al. Early response to tendon fatigue damage accumulation in a novel in vivo model. J Biomech. 2010;43(2):274–9.

61. Ingber DE. Cellular mechanotransduction: putting all the pieces together again. FASEB J. 2006;20(7):811–27.

62. Kjaer M, Langberg H, Heinemeier K, Bayer ML, Hansen M, Holm L, et al. From mechanical loading to collagen synthesis, structural changes and

function in human tendon. Scand J Med Sci Sports. 2009;19(4):500–10.

63. Cook JL, Purdam CR. Is tendon pathology a continuum? A pathology model to explain the clinical presentation of load-induced tendinopathy. Br J Sports Med. 2009;43(6):409–16.

64. Alfredson H, Lorentzon R. Chronic tendon pain: no signs of chemical inflammation but high concentrations of the neurotransmitter glutamate. Implications for treatment? Curr Drug Targets. 2002;3(1):43–54.

65. Langberg H, Skovgaard D, Karamouzis M, Bulow J, Kjaer M. Metabolism and inflammatory mediators in the peritendinous space measured by microdialysis during intermittent isometric exercise in humans. J Physiol. 1999;515(Pt 3):919–27.

66. Wang JH, Jia F, Yang G, Yang S, Campbell BH, Stone D, et al. Cyclic mechanical stretching of human tendon fibroblasts increases the production of prostaglandin E2 and levels of cyclooxygenase expression: a novel in vitro model study. Connect Tissue Res. 2003;44(3–4):128–33.

67. Cilli F, Khan M, Fu F, Wang JH. Prostaglandin E2 affects proliferation and collagen synthesis by human patellar tendon fibroblasts. Clin J Sport Med. 2004;14(4):232–6.

68. Khan MH, Li Z, Wang JH. Repeated exposure of tendon to prostaglandin-E2 leads to localized tendon degeneration. Clin J Sport Med. 2005;15(1):27–33.

69. Langberg H, Skovgaard D, Petersen LJ, Bulow J, Kjaer M. Type I collagen synthesis and degradation in peritendinous tissue after exercise determined by microdialysis in humans. J Physiol. 1999;521 Pt 1:299–306.

70. Riquet FB, Lai WF, Birkhead JR, Suen LF, Karsenty G, Goldring MB. Suppression of type I collagen gene expression by prostaglandins in fibroblasts is mediated at the transcriptional level. Mol Med. 2000;6(8):705–19.

71. Scott A, Lian O, Bahr R, Hart DA, Duronio V, Khan KM. Increased mast cell numbers in human patellar tendinosis: correlation with symptom duration and vascular hyperplasia. Br J Sports Med. 2008;42(9):753–7.

72. Schubert TE, Weidler C, Lerch K, Hofstadter F, Straub RH. Achilles tendinosis is associated with sprouting of substance P positive nerve fibres. Ann Rheum Dis. 2005;64(7):1083–6.

73. Kragsnaes MS, Fredberg U, Stribolt K, Kjaer SG, Bendix K, Ellingsen T. Stereological quantification of immune-competent cells in baseline biopsy specimens from Achilles tendons: results from patients with chronic tendinopathy followed for more than 4 years. Am J Sports Med. 2014;42(10):2435–45.

74. Dakin SG, Martinez FO, Yapp C, Wells G, Oppermann U, Dean BJ, et al. Inflammation activation and resolution in human tendon disease. Sci Transl Med. 2015;7(311):311ra173.

75. Millar NL, Wei AQ, Molloy TJ, Bonar F, Murrell GA. Cytokines and apoptosis in supraspinatus tendinopathy. J Bone Joint Surg Br. 2009;91(3):417–24.

76. Rees JD, Stride M, Scott A. Tendons – time to revisit inflammation. Br J Sports Med. 2014;48(21):1553–7.

77. Fredberg U, Stengaard-Pedersen K. Chronic tendinopathy tissue pathology, pain mechanisms, and etiology with a special focus on inflammation. Scand J Med Sci Sports. 2008;18(1):3–15.

78. Battery L, Maffulli N. Inflammation in overuse tendon injuries. Sports Med Arthrosc. 2011;19(3):213–7.

79. Lian O, Scott A, Engebretsen L, Bahr R, Duronio V, Khan K. Excessive apoptosis in patellar tendinopathy in athletes. Am J Sports Med. 2007;35(4):605–11.

80. Benson RT, McDonnell SM, Knowles HJ, Rees JL, Carr AJ, Hulley PA. Tendinopathy and tears of the rotator cuff are associated with hypoxia and apoptosis. J Bone Joint Surg Br. 2010;92(3):448–53.

81. Egerbacher M, Arnoczky SP, Caballero O, Lavagnino M, Gardner KL. Loss of homeostatic tension induces apoptosis in tendon cells: an in vitro study. Clin Orthop Relat Res. 2008;466(7):1562–8.

82. Barkhausen T, van Griensven M, Zeichen J, Bosch U. Modulation of cell functions of human tendon fibroblasts by different repetitive cyclic mechanical stress patterns. Exp Toxicol Pathol. 2003;55(2–3):153–8.

83. Millar NL, Murrell GA. Heat shock proteins in tendinopathy: novel molecular regulators. Mediators Inflamm. 2012;2012:436203.

84. Millar NL, Reilly JH, Kerr SC, Campbell AL, Little KJ, Leach WJ, et al. Hypoxia: a critical regulator of early human tendinopathy. Ann Rheum Dis. 2012;71(2):302–10.

85. Petersen W, Varoga D, Zantop T, Hassenpflug J, Mentlein R, Pufe T. Cyclic strain influences the expression of the vascular endothelial growth factor (VEGF) and the hypoxia inducible factor 1 alpha (HIF-1alpha) in tendon fibroblasts. J Orthop Res. 2004;22(4):847–53.

86. Lagier R, Gerster JC. Disabling ossification of the patellar tendon. Ann Rheum Dis. 1991;50(5):338–9.

87. Maffulli N, Reaper J, Ewen SW, Waterston SW, Barrass V. Chondral metaplasia in calcific insertional tendinopathy of the Achilles tendon. Clin J Sport Med. 2006;16(4):329–34.

88. Archambault JM, Jelinsky SA, Lake SP, Hill AA, Glaser DL, Soslowsky LJ. Rat supraspinatus tendon expresses cartilage markers with overuse. J Orthop Res. 2007;25(5):617–24.

89. Reuther KE, Thomas SJ, Evans EF, Tucker JJ, Sarver JJ, Ilkhani-Pour S, et al. Returning to overuse activity following a supraspinatus and infraspinatus tear leads to joint damage in a rat model. J Biomech. 2013;46(11):1818–24.

Rotator Cuff Tendons

3

Jonathan S. Kirschner, Lawrence V. Gulotta,
and Terrence Thomas

Abbreviations

SLAP   Superior labrum anterior and posterior

Introduction

Symptomatic rotator cuff tendinopathy affects approximately 16–34% of the population [2] and can be a source of significant functional disability. Rotator cuff tendinopathies are seen as a natural part of aging, with a marked increase in incidence in patients over 50 years of age [3]. The supraspinatus is the most commonly affected tendon in rotator cuff tendinopathies. Milgrom et al. found that in the seventh decade, over 50% of dominant shoulders had a rotator cuff tear, and this increased to 80% in those over 80, although not all of these radiographic tendinopathies are symptomatic. Much work needs to be done to determine why some aging-related cuff tendinopathy patients have anatomic abnormalities but no

J. S. Kirschner (✉) · T. Thomas
Department of Physiatry, Hospital for Special
Surgery, New York, NY, USA
e-mail: kirschnerj@hss.edu

L. V. Gulotta
Shoulder and Elbow Division, Sports Medicine
Institute, Hospital for Special Surgery,
New York, NY, USA
e-mail: gulottal@hss.edu

pain, while others are symptomatic. Besides advancing age, overuse cuff tendinopathies are common in manual and repetitive labor, especially those occupations that require overhead activity. Smoking, hyperlipidemia, diabetes, and obesity are well-known risk factors as well [4].

Anatomy

The shoulder has exceptional multiplanar mobility at the sacrifice of static stability. Proper coordination of the scapula and periscapular muscles is essential for normal glenohumeral range of motion, with the clavicle acting as a strut and allowing the scapula to protract and retract, elevate, or depress [5]. In order for full forward flexion to occur, the scapula upwardly rotates and tilts posteriorly while the clavicle elevates, posteriorly rotates, and retracts. This occurs through articulations at the acromioclavicular and sternoclavicular joints and at the scapulothoracic articulation.

The static stabilizers are the glenoid labrum, the glenohumeral joint capsule, the bones – the scapula, humerus, and the clavicle—and the ligaments – the superior and inferior glenohumeral, coracoacromial, coracohumeral, and acromioclavicular ligaments (See Fig. 3.1). The dynamic stabilizers are mainly the muscles that act upon the scapula. The rotator cuff muscles rotate the humerus about the scapula. Their function is maximized when the scapula is retracted and

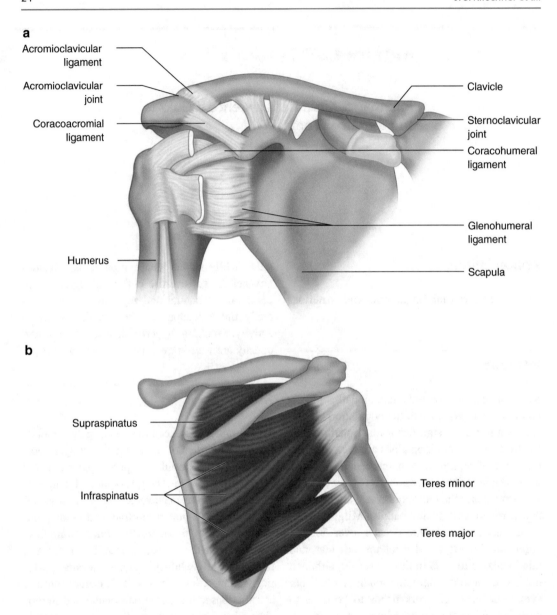

Fig. 3.1 Bony and ligamentous anatomy of the shoulder

depressed. Retraction is accomplished by the rhomboid and middle trapezius, while depression is accomplished by the lower trapezius and latissimus dorsi. Scapular elevation is achieved initially through activation of the serratus anterior, which not only keeps the scapula stabilized on the thoracic wall but also posteriorly tilts and elevates the scapula. The lower trapezius and rhomboids also play a large role in upward

scapular rotation, humeral elevation, and maintenance of overall dynamic stability (See Fig. 3.2).

The rotator cuff is made up of the supraspinatus, infraspinatus, teres minor, and subscapularis (see Fig. 3.3). The rotator cuff helps to keep the humeral head stabilized in the glenoid fossa, as the shoulder abducts and elevates, thus minimizing premature humeral elevation which could lead to subacromial impingement. The shallow glenoid

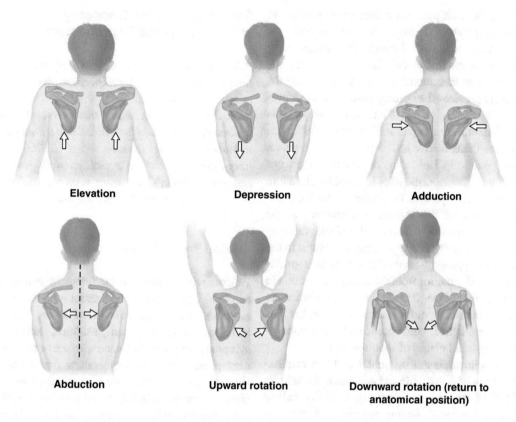

Fig. 3.2 Scapular motion

Fig. 3.3 Rotator cuff
muscles

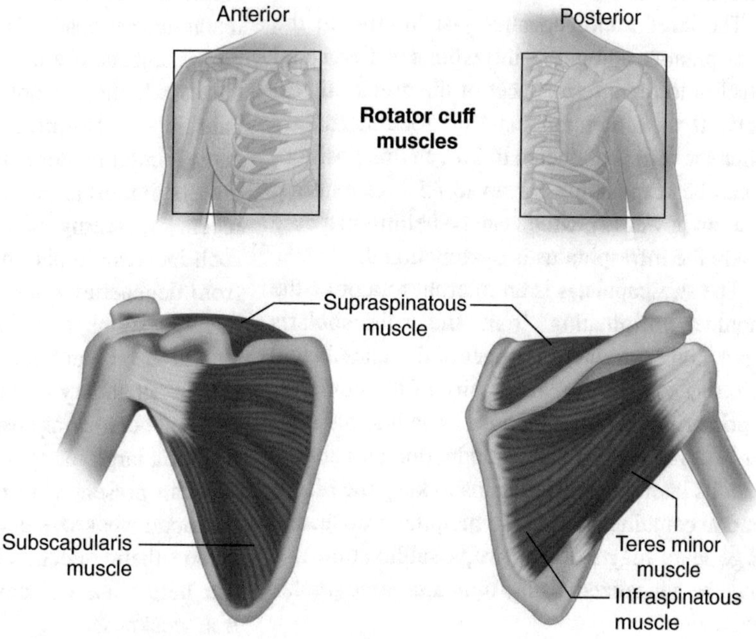

cavity by itself does not confer much stability to the glenohumeral joint. Instead, stability is achieved primarily through the compressive effects of the rotator cuff that serve to keep the humeral head centered in the glenoid while the deltoid provides the primary power for arm elevation. Because of its line of action, the deltoid pulls the humeral head superior. The rotator cuff counteracts these forces and depresses the humeral head inferiorly. Hence, the deltoid and the rotator cuff serve antagonistic roles in shoulder elevation.

The supraspinatus originates at the supraspinous fossa of the scapula and attaches at the superior and middle facets of the greater tuberosity [6]. It mainly acts as a humeral elevator in the scapular plane ("scaption"), which is approximately 30° anterior from the anatomic position in the coronal plane. It is difficult to purely isolate any of the rotator cuff muscles, however, because many are active, both eccentrically and concentrically, in all planes of shoulder motion.

The infraspinatus originates in the infraspinatus fossa of the scapula and attaches to the middle facet of the greater tuberosity. It is not only a humeral external rotator, mainly with the arm adducted at the side, but it also participates in abduction. It is typically tested with the arm against the trunk, elbow flexed at 90°, with the hand in a neutral position.

The teres minor attaches just inferior to the infraspinatus along the infraspinatus fossa and attaches to the inferior facet of the greater tuberosity. It is a humeral external rotator, mainly when the arm is abducted to 90°. In this position, it can be responsible for up to 45% of external rotation power [7], which can be helpful in a case where the infraspinatus is dysfunctional.

The subscapularis is an internal rotator of the shoulder, originating from the subscapularis fossa along the anterior aspect of the scapula and inserting to the lesser tuberosity of the humerus. It primarily not only functions as an internal rotator but also plays a part in adduction and abduction. Its lateral extension helps to keep the biceps tendon contained within the bicipital groove, and large tears may lead to biceps subluxation that may be visualized using dynamic sonographic evaluation.

Supraspinatus Tendinopathy with Subacromial Impingement

A 36-year-old female presents with right anterolateral shoulder pain due to overuse from swimming. While her pain has progressed and is occasionally sharp in nature, there was no initial trauma that instigated her pain. Exam shows glenohumeral internal rotation deficit (GIRD) and pain-limited rotator cuff muscle strength. Neer's test and Hawkin's test were positive, and the Jobe's maneuver (empty can test) was painful.

Clinical Presentation

Patients with rotator cuff tendinopathy and subacromial impingement can present with acute or acute on chronic pain localized to the lateral shoulder. Onset is often insidious, although symptoms may wax and wane with use or patients may present with an acute onset. Acute onset shoulder pain without prior history raises suspicion for tear as well. Nocturnal symptoms typically involve pain when lying on the side of pathology at night. Following an impingement episode, patients might report sensitivity to even subtle rotator cuff muscle activation. The most commonly described painful movements involve reaching overhead, behind the back, or carrying heavy objects. Acuity of the injury typically discloses whether or not the majority of patients' pain is due to chronic degeneration, or more acute, inflammatory process. Therefore, it is always important to ask whether there was a recent worsening of chronic shoulder pain, as such increase in pain might signify a conversion from degenerative tendinopathy to acute tendon tear. Questions related to arm/shoulder weakness should also be entertained carefully as weakness can be secondary to nerve pathologies such as a cervical nerve compression, brachial plexus injuries, or a large rotator cuff tear. Rotator cuff injuries can present with pain-related weakness but profound weakness is usually absent. A diagnostic anesthetic injection into the subacromial bursa can help tease out pain-limited weakness from true weakness.

Intrinsic factors of tendinopathy have been discussed in Chaps. 1 and 2. Extrinsic factors specific to rotator cuff tendons are believed to be mostly mechanical. Subacromial impingement has been described as one of such mechanical causes of rotator cuff tendinopathy. As initially described by Neer in 1972, subacromial impingement causes compressive loads on the tendon [8]. Anything narrowing the subacromial space can cause subacromial impingement. Subacromial impingement is most commonly believed to result from subacromial bony spurs, acromial morphology type II or III (curved or hooked) acromion, coracoacromial ligament thickening, and acromioclavicular joint hypertrophy. Spurs are seen as part of advancing age on plain radiograph, and spurs 5 mm or larger are associated with bursal-sided partial tears, with a potential progression to full tears [9]. While acromial index is not associated with rotator cuff tendinopathy, the acromial angle in which the acromion is laterally downsloped is another important radiographic finding that has been associated with rotator cuff tendon tears [10, 11] (see Fig. 3.4). Acromial angles do correlate with acromial morphology. For example, C shape is often related to type 1 morphology and L shape related to type II [12]. Functional narrowing can also occur through several mechanisms. Scapular dyskinesis and winging can result in narrowing of the subacromial space. Glenohumeral capsular tightness or contractures can result in humeral head elevation that narrows the subacromial space [13]. Lastly, muscular imbalance may narrow the subacromial space and contribute to impingement [14].

Physical Examination

The purpose of the shoulder examination is to rule out other coexisting injuries while establishing the diagnosis of rotator cuff tendinopathy. Intra-articular pathology is often associated with mechanical symptoms like locking, catching or grinding, warmth, swelling, or crepitus, and history may be vague with multiple positive exam maneuvers. Rotator cuff pathology typically does not have those mechanical symptoms and is usually elicited with cuff testing maneuvers. A careful examination allows for an assessment of the degree of injury and should identify any biomechanical risk factors that can be targeted during rehabilitation such as scapular dyskinesis and subacromial impingement syndrome. Often the basic parts of the shoulder examination are more helpful than special maneuvers. The components of basic shoulder examination include an inspection for alignment and asymmetry, passive and active shoulder range of motion, a cervical spine assessment, an upper extremity neurovascular exam, rotator cuff strength, shoulder and chest flexibility, scapular positioning at rest and with dynamic maneuvers, and palpation for tenderness, swelling, warmth, and crepitation.

Inspection should assess for muscle bulk, posture, alignment, and asymmetry in a resting shoulder and in different scapular positions. It requires proper exposure with a gown open to the back, a sports bra for women, or shirtless for men. During range of motion assessment, one should assess for asymmetric scapular movement known as scapular dyskinesis. This is defined as alterations in the normal position of the scapula

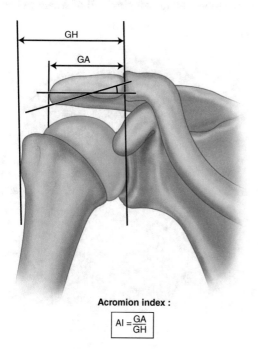

Acromion index :

$$AI = \frac{GA}{GH}$$

Fig. 3.4 Acromial index

during coupled scapulohumeral movements, generally assessed with progressive shoulder abduction. Scapular motion should be assessed for degree of elevation, protraction, and rotation and for the presence of winging. An association has been shown between abnormal scapular muscle activity and a higher risk of rotator cuff tendinopathy. In particular, weakness and delayed firing of the serratus anterior [15] and lower trapezius are well-known risk factors for cuff tendinopathy [16]. Weakness and delayed firing of these two muscles create abnormal scapular positioning, which narrows the supraspinatus outlet and leads to tendon impingement. Impingement syndrome secondary to scapular dyskinesis is typically associated with a type III dyskinesis pattern [17], with prominence of the superomedial scapular border, or a type II pattern, with prominence of the entire medial border [18] (see Fig. 3.5). This is often associated with levator scapula tenderness with forward head posture and is indicative of insufficient scapular upward rotation.

Excessive protraction also narrows the supraspinatus outlet and causes impingement [19].

The dominant throwing shoulder in athletes is typically depressed and protracted at rest. With abduction to 90°, look for premature elevation of the scapula ("positive shrug sign") [20]. This is believed to be secondary to excessive upper trapezius tone or inhibition of the lower trapezius. Observe for excessive scapular protraction, winging, and loss of scapulohumeral rhythm (see Fig. 3.6). Use the contralateral shoulder as a reference, and have the patient use a light weight if necessary to tease out any subtle asymmetries. Have the patient put their hands on their hips, put the arms "out like an airplane," and then have them touch above their head. Have them lower their arms in the frontal plane to accentuate any medial winging. Repeat several times, if necessary, including with the arms in a coronal or scapular plane. To assess for serratus anterior muscle strength and to elicit accentuated medial winging, have the patient perform a wall push-up or "pushup with a plus" (see Fig. 3.7). Abnormalities may be due to functional weakness or to lesions of the long thoracic nerve (medial winging), spinal accessory nerve, dorsal scapular nerve, or C5 nerve roots (lateral winging), all of which can be

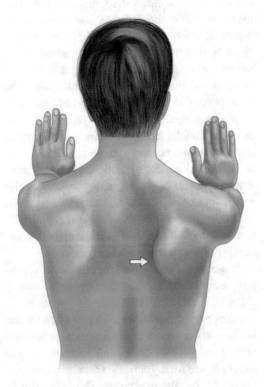

Fig. 3.5 An example of scapular dyskinesis, type II pattern

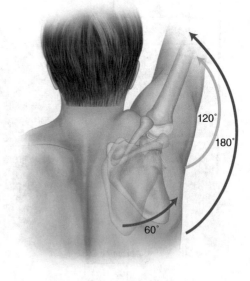

Fig. 3.6 Scapulohumeral rhythm

a

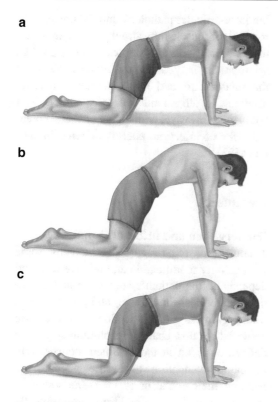

b

c

Fig. 3.7 "Push-up with a plus"

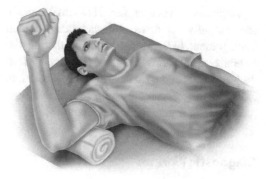

Fig. 3.8 Evaluation of internal and external rotation

assessed with an electrodiagnostic evaluation (nerve conduction studies/electromyography). A thorough cervical spine and neuromuscular examination of the upper limbs should be performed to rule out other sources of pain or weakness such as radiculopathy, facet joint arthrosis, or brachial plexus or other nerve disorders such as suprascapular neuropathy.

A passive assessment of "true" glenohumeral internal and external rotation is important and needs to be done with the scapula stabilized. An effective way to stabilize the scapula is to have patients lie on their back on the examining table so that the scapula is stabilized against the hard table. Then internal and external rotations can be evaluated (see Fig. 3.8). This is more reliable than combined assessment of abduction/external rotation (asking the patient to reach overhead and scratch their back) or combined internal rotation/adduction (to reach underneath and scratch your back). These assess compound movements and patients can "cheat" with excessive scapular winging or thoracic mobility and

demonstrate a falsely normal range of motion [21, 22]. As discussed for internal shoulder impingement, elite overhead athletes tend to have increased external and decreased internal rotation [23]. When total arc of motion is preserved, this is considered normal adaptation. When internal rotation is limited and the total arc of motion is decreased by more than 20°, this is not normal and called a glenohumeral internal rotation deficit (GIRD). This is associated with posterior capsule tightness and excessive strain on the rotator cuff and frequently occurs in patients with rotator cuff tendinopathy [17].

Several examination maneuvers have been developed to assess for subacromial impingement and supraspinatus tendinopathy. With the Neer's maneuver, the arm is passively elevated and internally rotated in the frontal plane to assess for subacromial impingement. It has been shown to be very sensitive but not specific for rotator cuff disease [24]. The Hawkins-Kennedy maneuver places the patient in 90° of shoulder abduction and elbow flexion in the scapular plane, and then provides an internal rotation force while keeping the scapula stabilized. This also has a high sensitivity and low specificity for rotator cuff tendinopathy [25] but not for full thickness tears [26]. The Jobe test, also known as the empty can test, is performed with the patient's arm in the scapular plane, arm elevated to 90° with a resistive downward force applied. This is a way to activate the supraspinatus and elicit pain from tendinosis or partial tear. According to a biomechanical study performed at Mayo Clinic, the Neer maneuver tests impingement of the supraspinatus, whereas the Hawkins-Kennedy test actually assesses subscapularis tendon impingement [27]. In one study analyzing the Neer's test, Hawkins-Kennedy test, Jobe's test, drop arm sign, and weakness in external rotation, 3/5 positive tests ruled in subacromial impingement and fewer than that ruled it out [28].

Diagnostic Workup

X-Ray

First-line imaging studies typically include plain radiographs to assess for congenital anomalies that may predispose a patient to impingement such as os acromiale (unfused accessory ossification center), hooked acromial morphology, and subacromial spurs. Indirect signs of rotator cuff disease may be cortical irregularity or enthesopathy of the greater tuberosity, calcific deposition. Plain radiographs may also be helpful to rule out other pathologies that can cause shoulder pain such as glenohumeral or acromioclavicular arthritis or tumors.

Ultrasound

Ultrasound has excellent spatial resolution, is readily available, is cost-effective, and is at least as accurate as MRI for detecting both partial and full-thickness rotator cuff tendon tears [29]. A systematic review found ultrasound to have a sensitivity of 0.79 and a specificity of 0.94 for diagnosing tendinosis without tear [30]. As it is typically available in the examination room, ultrasound can give clinicians the ability to differentiate between tendinopathies with and without a tear, thereby improving their ability to decide on proper treatment options [31]. For example, if a fairly large tear (>50%) is seen when the clinical picture was that of tendonitis, that might significantly change patient management toward earlier surgical intervention.

MRI

Modern MRI at 1.5 Tesla and above has excellent sensitivity and specificity for detecting rotator cuff tendinopathy, including the assessment of tears. In addition, MRI can assess for co-existing intra-articular pathology and the presence of rotator cuff muscle fatty atrophy, which may predict poorer response to surgical repair [32]. MR arthrography is typically not indicated to assess the rotator cuff and has a similar diagnostic accuracy to ultrasound and conventional MRI but is more invasive, with higher cost and potential risks of infection, allergy, or renal impairment [33].

Treatments

Conservative and Interventional

Treatment of rotator cuff tendinopathy starts with activity modification and relative rest, and depends on the patient's vocational and avocational activities, time frame, and goals. This is true regardless of the tendon involved (see Table 3.1 for flow chart) Expectations should be defined early on in the treatment course, with regular re-evaluation to ensure patients are meeting their goals, or to intervene sooner if they are not. These conditions are typically treated in a conservative manner [34], with injections reserved for refractory cases. The nature of the pathology helps guide treatment as well. For tendinopathy deemed mostly driven by extrinsic factors, posture, biomechanics, scapular motions, subacromial impingement, and posterior capsule tightness are addressed. For intrinsic rotator cuff disease not responsive to physical therapy, treatments targeted to injured parts of tendons such as percutaneous needle or ultrasonic tenotomy, dextrose hyperosmolar injection, and platelet rich plasma may be helpful in an attempt to alter abnormal tendon biology. However, while safe, evidence for these treatments are limited.

Rehabilitation of rotator cuff tendon injuries follows four key phases. The first phase is aimed at decreasing pain and inflammation and restoring a normal range of motion. The second phase is aimed at normalizing strength, initially using isometric and then concentric strengthening programs, and graduating patients to eccentric strengthening programs. The third phase focuses on maximizing dynamic stability and the fourth

Table 3.1 Algorithm for treatment of rotator cuff tendinopathy

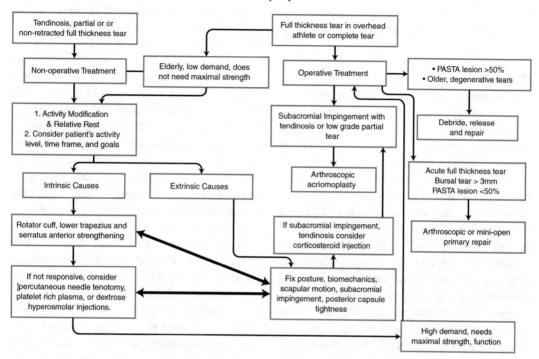

phase is to help patients return to sport-specific or other usual activities. If pain is limiting rehabilitation participation, pain control using ice, non-steroidal anti-inflammatory drugs, or corticosteroid injections is practiced. Although successful in addressing pain, corticosteroids have been shown to impair tendon healing and reparative processes [35, 36]. Thus, there has been a recent movement away from the use of corticosteroids for rotator cuff injuries. When used, however, subacromial corticosteroid injection may provide short-term relief for up to 9 months [37, 38].

Other injection options include hyaluronic acid, platelet-rich plasma (PRP), bone marrow aspirates, and prolotherapy. One study showed that autologous conditioned plasma – a low concentration form of PRP – was a good alternative to corticosteroid and reduced pain sooner in patients with partial rotator cuff tears but without a longer-term difference [39]. However, Kesikburun in 2013 found no significant difference in outcomes of patients with rotator cuff tendinopathy and partial tears receiving PRP injections compared to an exercise program [40]. There were several differences in the two studies,

however. In the first (positive) study they performed aggressive needle tenotomy and injection was intra-tendinous while in the second (negative) study they performed injection into the subacromial space. Besides, the PRP formulation was not well characterized, making it difficult to draw any meaningful conclusions. It is the authors experience (JK) that once pain is under control and intrinsic factors are optimized, extrinsic factors, which include movements of the scapula and humerus, can be comfortably addressed. The goal is to achieve optimal scapular retraction, posterior tilt, external rotation and upward elevation, and good clearance of the proximal humerus in the subacromial space with overhead motion [41]. It is also important to maximize core and trunk control, especially trunk extension, hip extension, and external rotation to maximize scapular function.

Patients should perform exercises that promote firing of the middle and lower trapezii, while minimizing firing of the upper trapezius and levator scapulae. These exercises include side-lying external rotation, side-lying forward flexion, prone horizontal abduction with external rotation, and prone extension [42]. It is important to strengthen the periscapular muscles and serratus anterior and then progress to rotator cuff strengthening [43].

Operative

For refractory cases that are not responsive to physical therapy and non-operative treatments, surgical treatment can be considered. Surgical intervention should largely be reserved for patients with clear evidence of an extrinsic mechanism for their impingement – such as a large acromial bone spur, a laterally downsloping acromion, or AC joint arthritis resulting in inferior bone spurring. The vast majority of patients that present with rotator cuff tendinopathy have either intrinsic tendinopathy due to tendon degeneration or a concomitant problem such as capsular contracture or scapular dyskinesis. In this setting, surgery should be avoided and alternative treatment options such as injections and/or physical therapy should be continued. Therefore, surgery indicated solely to treat rotator cuff tendinopathy is rarely indicated.

Historically, surgeons have performed open anterior acromioplasty along with resection of the coracoacromial ligament and subacromial bursa to treat subacromial impingement syndrome [44]. Although the open procedure achieved good results in terms of pain relief, an arthroscopic approach has become the standard of care due to its minimally invasive nature. The purpose of the subacromial decompression procedure is to decompress the narrow space by which the rotator cuff tendon must pass and/or to remove the inflamed subacromial bursa. By smoothening and resecting the hypertrophied anterolateral undersurface of the acromion, the friction between the rotator cuff tendon and the acromion is diminished. This arthroscopic procedure also allows the surgeon to assess any damage to the glenohumeral joint, biceps tendon, and/or rotator cuff, which can be addressed in the same operation [44]. If the impingement is thought to be due to hypertrophic osteoarthritis at the AC joint, then a concomitant distal clavicle resection should also be performed.

Three portals are typically made: a posterior viewing portal, a lateral working portal, and an anterior outflow portal. A shaver or a burr is typically used to shave the anterior portion of the acromion such that it is level with the remaining acromion. An extensive subacromial bursectomy is also performed. It is important to inspect the articular and bursal sides of the rotator cuff and debride or repair the cuff as necessary. In cases of calcific tendonitis, calcium is identified as a blistering of the bursal surface of the rotator cuff. This is incised and the calcium deposit is debrided. There is typically a small tear in the rotator cuff following removal of the calcium, which may be repaired with a suture anchor.

Partial thickness rotator cuff tears are often found at the time of an acromioplasty surgery. These can be on either the bursal or the articular side. Articular-sided tears can be debrided, partially repaired, or taken down and then fully repaired. The final decision on which of these treatments is indicated depends on the integrity of the remaining rotator cuff tissue. Tears involving less than 50% of width of the footprint should be debrided while those larger than that should undergo partial repair.

Bursal-sided partial thickness tears are typically more painful and warrant more aggressive treatment through repair when compared to articular-sided partial tears [1]. The bursal surface is relatively hypervascular and its collagen bundles are thicker than that of the articular surface; favorable blood supply to the region promotes more successful tendon healing [1].

The procedure is performed in the outpatient setting, and patients are instructed to wear a sling for comfort only for the first 24–48 hours if there are no repairs performed (please see following sections for rehabilitation after rotator cuff repair). They are then allowed to use their shoulder as tolerated. Physical therapy concentrating on maintaining range of motion early, and strengthening the rotator cuff and periscapular muscles later, is usually performed for 3 months.

In a clinical study done by Odenbring et al. [45], outcomes of 29 open and 31 arthroscopic acromioplasties were compared. The findings showed that excellent or good results were obtained in 77% of shoulders done arthroscopically and that good results lasted for up to 12–14 years after the procedure. The long-term results of procedures performed arthroscopically were significantly greater than those associated with an open procedure. In another study by Norlin and Adolfsson [46], 162 patients underwent arthroscopic subacromial decompression without rotator cuff repair. During the 10- to 13-year follow-up period, patients' isolated full thickness supraspinatus tears did not show signs of clinical progression, which suggests that arthroscopic subacromial decompression treatment for impingement syndrome shows promising long-term results.

Infraspinatus Tendinopathy with Internal Impingement

A 29-year-old male baseball player presents with a seven-month history of progressive right posterolateral shoulder pain. There is no specific history of trauma or injury. His discomfort is associated with overhead activity when his arm is cocked and fully externally rotated while throwing. Exam shows painful range of motion with hyperabduction and external rotation and asymmetric ROM between his dominant and non-dominant shoulders. His dominant shoulder has 110° of external rotation and 20° of internal rotation. His non-dominant shoulder has 90° of external rotation and 60° of internal rotation. He has focal tenderness to palpation at the posterior shoulder just inferior to the acromion. Rotator cuff strength is normal but the serratus anterior is weak, as assessed by medial scapular winging with a wall push-up.

Clinical Presentation

It is also important to note that other types of shoulder impingement have been described. Jobe [47] and others describe an impingement where the supra- or infraspinatus tendon gets impinged between the humeral head and the posterior glenoid rim in overhead athletes, a phenomenon commonly referred to as "internal shoulder impingement." Humeral instability and posterior capsule tightness are believed to be the cause of internal shoulder impingement [48]. Posterior capsule tightness occurs from maladaptions to throwing including increased external rotation and glenohumeral internal rotation deficit (GIRD). The posterior capsule remodels and tightens causing the humerus to translate superoposteriorly. This causes impingement of the humerus against the superoposterior labrum and articular side of the supra and infraspinatus, placing excessive stress on the biceps tendon and superior anterior labrum, often leading to tears of one or more of these structures as well [49]. Internal shoulder impingement typically results in episodic pain in the posterior shoulder, rather than lateral or anterior shoulder pain, which is more common with subacromial impingement or with biceps-labral pathology in more severe cases.

Physical Examination

On physical examination, patients typically have pain in the cocking phase of throwing or in the flexed, abducted externally rotated position. There may be tenderness just inferolateral to the acromion or along the infraspinatus tendon or posterior-superior glenohumeral joint. It is important to evaluate internal and external range of motion to ensure that they are symmetric to the contralateral side. Careful observation of the scapula is also necessary since throwing athletes can develop scapular dyskinesis that is best addressed with physical therapy. Concomitant pathology must also be considered and a Speed's test for biceps tendinopathy, and O'Brien's Active Compression Test should be performed to evaluate for superior labral tears (SLAP tears).

Imaging

Radiographs may be helpful to rule out Bankart injuries, Hill-Sachs deformities, calcific tendinopathy, or signs of glenohumeral osteoarthritis.

Axillary radiographs may show a Bennett lesion, an exostosis of the posterior glenoid due to traction of the posterior capsule that occurs with the throwing motion [50]. These may be better characterized on CT or MRI arthrography, which has the advantage of evaluating the infraspinatus and posterior labrum. MR without arthrography may make it difficult to differentiate labrum from the Bennett lesion [51].

Treatment

Conservative

Because GIRD is believed to predispose one to infraspinatus tendinopathy, and is especially prevalent in overhead athletes [52], internal rotation stretching using maneuvers like the "sleeper stretch" is important and should be considered. Often patients have pain and tenderness at the coracoid process, associated with a tight pectoralis minor. This muscle should be stretched as well [53], especially for patients with subcoracoid impingement. Full range of motion may be facilitated with manual therapies such as scapular glides or other soft tissue techniques. Those with internal impingement may also benefit from the cross-body stretch, where one moves the arm into horizontal adduction to increase the internal range of motion.

Interventional

Injections have a limited role in the treatment of internal impingement syndrome. Anesthetic injections targeting Bennett lesions [54] at the posteroinferior glenohumeral joint have been described to aid in diagnosis, and corticosteroid injections may be performed for symptomatic relief, targeting the glenohumeral joint or infraspinatus tendon [49].

Operative

Most throwing athletes with internal impingement can successfully be treated with non-operative measures. Indications for surgery include persistent symptoms that limit a patient's return to play, despite adequate rest, rehabilitation, and attempt at a phased return to competition. Surgical patients should have a symmetric arc of rotational motion compared to the contralateral shoulder.

At the time of surgery, a so-called "kissing lesion" with fraying or tearing of the posterior-superior labrum and fraying of the posterior-superior rotator cuff is seen. All labral and/or biceps pathology should be identified and addressed with repair. Bennett lesions can be exposed through a posterior capsulotomy and excised with a motorized shaver.

While all identified pathology should be addressed at the time of surgery, care must be taken when considering the treatment of the rotator cuff. The pathology in the rotator cuff is often seen as an articular-sided partial tear of the infraspinatus which occurred due to impingement on the posterior glenoid. This occurs during the late cocking phase of throwing and is thought to allow throwers to generate the torque needed to compete at high levels. Aggressive repair of these rotator cuff tears can prevent the athlete from achieving that motion post-op, thereby limiting their ability to return to play. For this reason, partial tears that include up to 80% of the width of the footprint should be treated with debridement. For tears that include greater than 80% of the footprint, repair should be performed using a single row, lateralized technique. In a case series, Dines et al. [55] reported that five of six Major League Baseball pitchers were able to return to their previous level of competition using this technique. This is in comparison to a study by Mazoue and Andrews which showed that only 1 of 12 professional pitchers was able to return following a formal mini-open repair with transosseous bone tunnels [56].

Postoperatively, patients are treated in a sling for 4–6 weeks following by physical therapy to restore the range of motion. Strengthening begins at 3 months and patients can begin an interval throwing program around 4–6 months out from surgery. A full return to competitive throwing sports typically takes up to 12 months.

Complete Rotator Cuff Tear

A 70-year-old avid tennis player slips while hiking and reaches for a branch to prevent herself from falling. She feels severe pain in the anterolateral shoulder and notes an inability to fully abduct or flex her arm without pain. Bruising develops along her upper arm until she can see you in the office several days later. On examination there is full passive glenohumeral motion but active elevation is limited and painful. When the patient's arm is passively elevated, she is unable to prevent it from falling to her side, a positive "drop-arm sign."

Clinical Presentation

Patients with an acute painful forced eccentric abduction followed by the inability to raise their arm are likely to have suffered a large rotator cuff tear. A full thickness tear by definition extends from the bursal surface to the articular surface, but it may be confined to a small area and not require operative repair. A massive or complete rotator cuff tear has been defined as a tear involving >67% of greater tuberosity exposure [57]. Others define it as two or three tendons being completely torn and retraced at least to the level of the glenoid. These have a more guarded prognosis and may require surgical intervention depending on the activity level and demands of the patient.

Physical Examination

Patients with rotator cuff tendinosis may have pain-limited weakness, but if there is marked weakness, this should raise the suspicion for complete tear. This can be assessed with the drop arm test, where the patient is asked to fully abduct their arm and then lower it down slowly. While this may be pain limited, failure to slowly control the arm suggests complete cuff tear. Weakness in external rotation, a positive drop arm sign, and a

painful arc during abduction from 60 to 120° have been shown to predict a 91% chance of full thickness rotator cuff tear [58]. Other maneuvers to test rotator cuff strength are the hornblower's sign for infraspinatus and teres minor, and the belly press test or lift off sign for subscapularis integrity. Each of these maneuvers has low sensitivity and specificity by itself to diagnose or differentiate cuff tear from tendinosis, although subscapularis tests may be more specific [59].

Diagnostic Workup

Imaging
Radiographs are the initial study of choice to assess for a high riding humeral head which is suggestive of a complete or massive rotator cuff tear, particularly when the acromiohumeral distance is <6 mm [60]. Ultrasound or MRI may be used to confirm the diagnosis. Ultrasound has a sensitivity of 92.3% and specificity of 94.4% for diagnosing full thickness rotator cuff tears [61]. MRI has a sensitivity of 92.1% and a specificity of 92.9% to diagnose full thickness tears [62]. Sensitivity increases to 95.4% and specificity 98.9% when intraarticular gadolinium is added.

Treatment

Interventional
Injections into the subacromial bursa or glenohumeral joint (they will be contiguous if the tear is complete) may be performed for symptomatic pain relief but will not heal the tendon. Treatment is primarily non-operative or surgical depending on the patient's age, functional demands, degree of fatty infiltration of the tendon, and presence of concomitant osteoarthritis.

Operative
Patients with acute, traumatic rotator cuff tears are best treated with surgical fixation. Factors such as the presence of arthritis or humeral head elevation of the X-ray, or significant tendon

retraction or fatty infiltration of the rotator cuff musculature on the MRI suggest a chronic tear and can be treated with an initial trial of non-operative care.

Repair of full thickness rotator cuff tears is most commonly performed arthroscopically. The long head of the biceps tendon should also be assessed and its pathology addressed through either a tenodesis or tenotomy if present.

An acromioplasty is typically performed first if there is an impingement lesion, or fraying, of the undersurface of the coracoacromial ligament associated with a type III acromial spur. Gartsman et al. have shown that there are no benefits to performing an acromioplasty in patients with type I or II acriomions in terms of functional outcomes or radiographic rotator cuff healing rates.

A thorough bursectomy is also performed to aid in visualization. The tear configuration should then be determined as well as the ease to which the tendon can be mobilized to the footprint of the tuberosity. The goal is a tension-free repair of the tendon to the bone. For larger or more chronic tears, releases may need to be performed in order to untether the tendon from surrounding structures to facilitate repair.

Once the tendon is mobilized to the footprint, tuberosity is then abraded down to bleeding bone. It is important not to be overly aggressive as this can jeopardize the pullout strength of the suture anchors. Suture anchors are then placed into the bone of the greater tuberosity. A transosseous-equivalent repair should be performed when possible. This requires the first row of suture anchors to be placed at the medial aspect of the footprint, by the articular margin. The sutures from those medial row anchors are then placed through the torn rotator cuff tendon. Arthroscopic knots are then tied and loaded into two lateral row, knotless anchors. Those tails of sutures going to the lateral row anchors serve to compress the lateral portion of the repaired tendon to the bone and improve the overall surface area available for healing [63].

Postoperatively, patients are immobilized in a sling for 4–6 weeks to allow for rotator cuff healing. This is followed by protected range of motion with the goal to achieve approximately 90% of normal range of motion by 3 months.

Strengthening is initiated at 3 months and patients are allowed a gradual return to recreational activities. Patients are counseled that full return to activities can take 6–9 months.

Conclusion

Rotator cuff tendinopathy is a common cause of shoulder pain, whether due to intrinsic or extrinsic overload, resulting in tendon degeneration, inflammation, and/or tears of various degrees. The condition typically improves with rehabilitation focused on proper scapular mechanics and stability, rotator cuff strengthening, and posterior capsule stretching. Injections of corticosteroid, dextrose, or orthobiologics such as platelet-rich plasma are often performed, but long-term efficacy has been unproven. Surgical options can be good for refractory cases or when patients have less-than-optimal strength due to a sizable tear.

References

1. Seitz AL, McClure PW, Finucane SI, Boardman ND, Michener LA. Mechanisms of rotator cuff tendinopathy: intrinsic, extrinsic or both? Clin Biomech. 2011;26:1–12.
2. Silverstein BA, Viikari-Juntura E, Fan ZJ, Bonauto DK, Bao S, Smith C. Natural course of nontraumatic rotator cuff tendinitis and shoulder symptoms in a working population. Scand J Work Environ Health. 2006;32(2):99–108.
3. Milgrom C, Schaffler M, Gilbert S, van Holsbeeck M. Rotator-cuff changes in asymptomatic adults. The effect of age, hand dominance and gender. J Bone Joint Surg Br. 1995;77:296–8.
4. Rechardt M, Shiri R, Karppinen J, Jula A, Heliövaara M, Viikari-Juntura E. Lifestyle and metabolic factors in relation to shoulder pain and rotator cuff tendinitis: a population-based study. BMC Musculoskelet Disord. 2010;11:165. https://doi.org/10.1186/1471-2474-11-165.
5. Kibler BW, Sciasia A. Current concepts: scapular dyskinesis. Br J Sports Med. 2010;44:300–5.
6. Jacobson JA. Fundamentals of musculoskeletal ultrasound. 2nd ed. Philadelphia: Saunders; 2012. (U. Michigan).
7. Khan KM, Cook JL, Bonar F, Harcourt P, Astrom M. Histopathology of common tendinopathies. Update and implications for clinical management. Sports Med. 1999;27(6):393–408.

8. Neer CS. Anterior acromioplasty for the chronic impingement syndrome in the shoulder: a preliminary report. J Bone Joint Surg Am. 1972;54:41–50.

9. Ogawa K, Yoshida A, Inokuchi W, Naniwa T. Acromial spur: relationship to aging and morphologic changes in the rotator cuff. J Shoulder Elbow Surg. 2005;14(6):591–8.

10. Toivonen DA, Tuite MJ, Orwin JF. Acromial structure and tears of the rotator cuff. J Shoulder Elbow Surg. 1995;4(5):376–83.

11. Hamid N, Omid R, Yamaguchi K, Steger-May K, Stobbs G, Keener JD. Relationship of radiographic acromial characteristics and rotator cuff disease: a prospective investigation of clinical, radiographic, and sonographic findings. J Shoulder Elbow Surg. 2012;21(10):1289–98.

12. Guo X, Ou M, Yi G, et al. Correction between the morphology of acromion and acromial angle in Chinese population: a study on 292 scapulas. Biomed Res Int. 2018;2018:3125715. Published 2018 Nov 11. https://doi.org/10.1155/2018/3125715.

13. Lin JJ, Lim HK, Yang JL. Effect of shoulder tightness on glenohumeral translation, scapular kinematics, and scapulohumeral rhythm in subjects with stiff shoulders. J Orthop Res. 2006;24(5):1044–51. https://doi.org/10.1002/jor.20126.

14. Reddy AS, Mohr KJ, Pink MM, Jobe FW. Electromyographic analysis of the deltoid and rotator cuff muscles in persons with subacromial impingement. J Shoulder Elbow Surg. 2000;9(6):519–23. https://doi.org/10.1067/mse.2000.109410.

15. Diederichsen LP, Norregaard J, Dyhre-Poulsen P, Winther A, Tufekovic G, Bandholm T, et al. The activity pattern of shoulder muscles in subjects with and without subacromial impingement. J Electromyogr Kinesiol. 2008;19:789–99.

16. Cools AM, Witvrouw EE, Declercq GA, et al. Scapular muscle recruitment patterns: trapezius muscle latency with and without impingement symptoms. Am J Sports Med. 2003;31:542–9.

17. Burkhart SS, Morgan CD, Kibler WB. The disabled throwing shoulder: spectrum of pathology part I: pathoanatomy and biomechanics. Arthroscopy. 2003;19:404–20.

18. Ludewig PM, Cook TM. Alterations in shoulder kinematics and associated muscle activity in people with symptoms of shoulder impingement. Phys Ther. 2000;80:276–91.

19. Solem-Bertoft E, Thuomas K, Westerberg C. The influence of scapular retraction and protraction on the width of the subacromial space. An MRI study. Clin Orthop. 1993;296:99–103.

20. Jia X, Ji JH, Petersen SA, et al. Clinical evaluation of the shoulder shrug sign. Clin Orthop Relat Res. 2008;466:2813–9.

21. Mallon WJ, Herring CL, Sallay PI, et al. Use of vertebral levels to measure presumed internal rotation at the shoulder: a radiographic analysis. J Shoulder Elbow Surg. 1996;5:299–306.

22. Kebatse M, McClure P, Pratt N. Thoracic position effect on shoulder range of motion, strength, and three dimensional scapular kinetics. Arch Phys Med Rehabil. 1999;80:945–50.

23. Ellenbecker TS, Roetert EP, Bailie DS, et al. Glenohumeral joint total rotation range of motion in elite tennis players and baseball pitchers. Med Sci Sports Exerc. 2002;34:2052–6.

24. Leroux JL, Thomas E, Bonnel F, Blotman F. Diagnostic value of clinical tests for shoulder impingement syndrome. Rev Rhum Engl Ed. 1995;62:423–8.

25. MacDonald PB, Clark P, Sutherland K. An analysis of the diagnostic accuracy of the Hawkins and Neer subacromial impingement signs. J Shoulder Elbow Surg. 2000;9:299–301.

26. Park HB, Yokota A, Gill HS, El Rassi G, McFarland EG. Diagnostic accuracy of clinical tests for the different degrees of subacromial impingement syndrome. J Bone Joint Surg Am. 2005;87:1446–55.

27. Yamamoto N, Muraki T, Sperling JW, Steinmann SP, Itoi E, Cofield RH, An KN. Impingement mechanisms of the Neer and Hawkins signs. J Shoulder Elbow Surg. 2009;18:942–7.

28. Michener LA, Walsworth MK, Doukas WC, Murphy KP. Reliability and diagnostic accuracy of 5 physical examination tests and combination of tests for subacromial impingement. Arch Phys Med Rehabil. 2009;90:1898–903.

29. Yablon CM, Jacobson JA. Rotator cuff and subacromial pathology. Semin Musculoskelet Radiol. 2015;19(3):231–42.

30. Roy JS, Braën C, Leblond J, et al. Diagnostic accuracy of ultrasonography, MRI and MR arthrography in the characterisation of rotator cuff disorders: a systematic review and meta-analysis. Br J Sports Med. 2015;49(20):1316–28. https://doi.org/10.1136/bjsports-2014-094148.

31. Lee SU, Joo SY, Kim SK, Lee SH, Park SR, Jeong C. Real-time sonoelastography in the diagnosis of rotator cuff tendinopathy. J Shoulder Elbow Surg. 2016;25(5):723–9.

32. Kuzel BR, Grindel S, Papandrea R, Ziegler D. Fatty infiltration and rotator cuff atrophy. J Am Acad Orthop Surg. 2013;21(10):613–23.

33. Roy J, Braën C, Leblond J, Desmeules F, Dionne CE, MacDermid JC, Bureau NJ, Frémont P. Diagnostic accuracy of ultrasonography, MRI and MR arthrography in the characterisation of rotator cuff disorders: a systematic review and meta-analysis. Br J Sports Med. 2015;49:1316–28.

34. Morrison DS, Frogameni AD, Woodworth P. Nonoperative treatment of subacromial impingement syndrome. J Bone Joint Surg Am. 1997;79(5):732–7.

35. Scutt N, Rolf CG, Scutt A. Glucocorticoids inhibit teknocyte proliferation and tendon progenitor cell recruitment. J Orthop Res. 2006;24:173–82.

36. Lee HJ, Kim YS, Ok JH, Lee YK, Ha MY. Effect of a single subacromial prednisolone injection in acute rotator cuff tears in a rat model. Knee Surg Sports Traumatol Arthrosc. 2015;23(2):555–61.

37. Mohamadi A, Chan JJ, Claessen FM, Ring D, Chen NC. Corticosteroid injections give small and transient pain relief in rotator cuff tendinosis: a meta-analysis. Clin Orthop Relat Res. 2017;475(1):232–43.

38. Arroll B, Goodyear-Smith F. Corticosteroid injections for painful shoulder: a meta-analysis. Br J Gen Pract. 2005;55(512):224–8.

39. von Wehren L, Blanke F, Todorov A, Heisterbach P, Sailer J, Majewski M. The effect of subacromial injections of autologous conditioned plasma versus cortisone for the treatment of symptomatic partial rotator cuff tears. Knee Surg Sports Traumatol Arthrosc. 2016;24(12):3787–92.

40. Kesikburun S, Tan AK, Yilmaz B, Yaşar E, Yazicioğlu K. Platelet-rich plasma injections in the treatment of chronic rotator cuff tendinopathy: a randomized controlled trial with 1-year follow-up. Am J Sports Med. 2013;41(11):2609–16.

41. Kibler WB. Shoulder rehabilitation: principles and practice. Med Sci Sports Exerc. 1998;30(4 Suppl):S40–50.

42. Cools A, Dewitte V, Lansweert F, Notebaert D, Roets A, Soetens B, Cagnie B, Witvrouw EE. Rehabilitation of scapular muscle balance: which exercises to prescribe? Am J Sports Med. 2007;35(10):1744–51.

43. Ellenbecker TS, Cools A. Rehabilitation of shoulder impingement syndrome and rotator cuff injuries: an evidence-based review. Br J Sports Med. 2010;44(5):319–27.

44. Koester MC, George MD, Kuhn JE. Shoulder impingement syndrome. Am J Med. 2005;118(5):452–5.

45. Odenbring S, Wagner P, Atroshi I. Longterm outcomes of arthroscopic acromioplasty for chronic shoulder impingement syndrome: a prospective cohort study with a minimum of 12 years' follow-up. Arthroscopy. 2008;24(10):1092–8.

46. Norlin R, Adolfsson L. Small full thickness tears do well ten to thirteen years after arthroscopic subacromial decompression. J Shoulder Elbow Surg. 2008;17(1 suppl):12S–6S.

47. Jobe CM. Superior glenoid impingement. Orthop Clin North Am. 1997;28(2):137–43. https://doi.org/10.1016/s0030-5898(05)70274-1.

48. Kvitne RS, Jobe FW. The diagnosis and treatment of anterior instability in the throwing athlete. Clin Orthop Relat Res. 1993:107–23.

49. Corpus KT, Camp CL, Dines DM, Altchek DA, Dines JS. Evaluation and treatment of internal impingement of the shoulder in overhead athletes. World J Orthop. 2016;7(12):776–84.

50. Ferrari JD, Ferrari DA, Coumas J, Pappas AM. Posterior ossification of the shoulder: the Bennett lesion: etiology, diagnosis, and treatment. Am J Sports Med. 1994;22(2):171–6. https://doi.org/10.1177/036354659402200204.

51. Freehill MT, Mannava S, Higgins LD, Lädermann A, Stone AV. Thrower's exostosis of the shoulder: a systematic review with a novel classification. Orthop J Sports Med. 2020;8(7):2325967120932101. Published 2020 Jul 14. https://doi.org/10.1177/2325967120932101.

52. Wilk KE, Macrina LC, Arrigo C. Passive range of motion characteristics in the overhead baseball pitcher and their implications for rehabilitation. Clin Orthop Relat Res. 2012;470(6):1586–94.

53. Turgut E, Duzgun I, Baltaci G. Stretching exercises for shoulder impingement syndrome: effects of 6-week program on shoulder tightness, pain and disability status. J Sport Rehabil. 2017;17:1–20.

54. Nakagawa S, Yoneda M, Hayashida K, Mizuno N, Yamada S. Posterior shoulder pain in throwing athletes with a Bennett lesion: factors that influence throwing pain. J Shoulder Elbow Surg. 2006;15(1):72–7.

55. Dines JS, Jones K, Maher P, Altchek D. Arthroscopic management of full-thickness rotator cuff tears in major league baseball pitchers: the lateralized footprint repair technique. Am J Orthop (Belle Mead NJ). 2016;45(3):128–33.

56. Mazoue C, Andrews J. Repair of full-thickness rotator cuff tears in professional baseball players. Am J Sports Med. 2006;34(2):182–9. https://doi.org/10.1177/0363546505279916. Epub 2005 Oct 31

57. Schumaier A, Kovacevic D, Schmidt C, Green A, Rokito A, Jobin C, Yian E, Cuomo F, Koh J, Gilotra M, Ramirez M, Williams M, Burks R, Stanley R, Hasan S, Paxton S, Hasan S, Nottage W, Levine W, Srikumaran U, Grawe B. Defining massive rotator cuff tears: a Delphi consensus study. J Shoulder Elbow Surg. 2020;29(4):674–80. https://doi.org/10.1016/j.jse.2019.10.024. PMID: 32197762; PMCID: PMC7100923.

58. Jia X, Petersen SA, Khosravi AH, Almareddi V, Pannirselvam V, McFarland EG. Examination of the shoulder: the past, the present, and the future. J Bone Joint Surg Am. 2009;91(Suppl 6):10–8.

59. Somerville LE, Willits K, Johnson AM, Litchfield R, LeBel ME, Moro J, Bryant D. Clinical assessment of physical examination maneuvers for rotator cuff lesions. Am J Sports Med. 2014;42(8):1911–9. https://doi.org/10.1177/0363546514538390. Epub 2014 Jun 16

60. Goutallier D, Le Guilloux P, Postel JM, Radier C, Bernageau J, Zilber S. Acromio humeral distance less than six millimeters: its meaning in full-thickness rotator cuff tear. Orthop Traumatol Surg Res. 2011;97(3):246–51.

61. Nazarian LN, Jacobson JA, Benson CB, et al. Imaging algorithms for evaluating suspected rotator cuff disease: Society of Radiologists in Ultrasound consensus conference statement. Radiology. 2013;267(2):589–95. https://doi.org/10.1148/radiol.13121947.

62. de Jesus JO, Parker L, Frangos AJ, Nazarian LN. Accuracy of MRI, MR arthrography, and ultrasound in the diagnosis of rotator cuff tears: a meta-analysis. AJR Am J Roentgenol. 2009;192(6):1701–7.

63. Miyazaki AN, et al. Evaluation of the functional results after rotator cuff arthroscopic repair with the suture bridge technique. Rev Bras Ortop (English Edition). 2017;52(2):164–8. https://doi.org/10.1016/j.rboe.2016.05.008.

Biceps Tendon

4

Alyssa Neph, Michael O'Connell, Jason J. Shin, Albert Lin, and Eric R. Helm

Abbreviations

CSI	Ccorticosteroid injection
ESWT	Extracorporeal shock wave therapy
FABS	Flexed Aabducted Ssupinated
NSAID	Nnon-steroidal anti-inflammatory drug
SLAP	Superior Llabrum Aanterior and Pposterior

Introduction

Tendinopathy of the long head of the biceps is one of the leading causes of shoulder pain [1]. While epidemiologic studies vary, one systematic review reported that the incidence of biceps tendinopathy in the painful shoulder ranges anywhere from 22% to 78% [2]. Proximal tendi-

Electronic Supplementary Material The online version of this chapter (https://doi.org/10.1007/978-3-030-65335-4_4) contains supplementary material, which is available to authorized users.

A. Neph · M. O'Connell · E. R. Helm (✉)
Department of Physical Medicine and Rehabilitation, University of Pittsburgh, Pittsburgh, PA, USA
e-mail: nepham@upmc.edu; oconnellm5@upmc.edu; helmer@upmc.edu

J. J. Shin · A. Lin
Department of Orthopedic Surgery, University of Pittsburgh, Pittsburgh, PA, USA
e-mail: lina2@upmc.edu

nopathy is more likely to occur in the elderly or in highly active individuals, especially overhead athletes or those whose occupation requires rigorous manual activity [1, 3]. Distal tendinopathy is rare, representing only 3% of all biceps injuries and occurring in 1.2 of 100,000 people per year [4, 5]. Distal injuries are most commonly complete ruptures and can be seen in bodybuilders, weightlifters, and football players [3]. Males account for 80% of distal ruptures, typically involving the dominant arm [6]. The incidence of distal biceps tendinosis is thought to be even less common than ruptures, but these are likely underdiagnosed [7]. There have been only a few reported cases of proximal short head ruptures [6].

While not linked specifically to the biceps tendon, both intrinsic and extrinsic factors have been implicated in tendinopathy. Intrinsic factors within the tendon can result in degeneration and chronic tendinosis structural changes, including excessive overload from eccentric contraction, age, smoking, and comorbid conditions such as inflammatory arthropathy, obesity, and diabetes mellitus [5]. Medications contributing to tendon degeneration include anabolic and oral steroids, statins, and flouroquinolones [8, 9]. Extrinsic factors include physical forces on the tendon and the surrounding environment. The close proximity of the proximal long head within the rotator interval and other glenohumeral structures inevitably results in biceps tendon lesions being closely connected with other shoulder pathology.

Anatomy

The long head of the biceps tendon originates within the glenohumeral joint at the supraglenoid tubercle and superior glenoid labrum. It then passes anteriorly and laterally over the humeral head into the rotator interval, which is a triangular space defined superiorly by the anterior border of the supraspinatus, inferiorly by the superior border of the subscapularis, and with the coracoid process acting as the base [10] (See Fig. 4.1). Within this interval, fibers from the coracohumeral ligament and superior glenohumeral ligament form the biceps pulley, which is a sling-like band of tissue that surrounds and stabilizes the long head of the biceps as it enters the bicipital groove [11]. Within this groove, the long head travels between the greater and lesser tuberosities

and then exits the joint deep to the transverse humeral ligament. The long head of the biceps tendon is surrounded by a reflection of synovial sheath that is continuous with the glenohumeral joint. The short head of the biceps tendon, which originates medial to the long head at the coracoid process, joins with the coracobrachialis to form the conjoint tendon [5]. The conjoint tendon then merges with the long head of the biceps at the level of the deltoid insertion to form the common muscle belly of the biceps brachii [4].

The distal biceps tendon is a flat extra-synovial structure. The tendon crosses the antecubital fossa, rotating 90° externally, to insert on the posterior ulnar aspect of the radial tuberosity (see Fig. 4.2). This twisting fiber arrangement allows the biceps to act as the most powerful forearm supinator. There is a bifid distal biceps tendon in

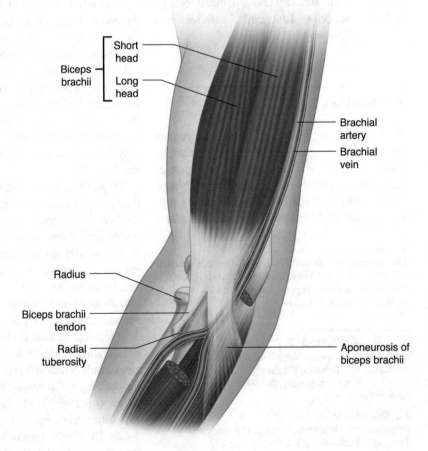

Fig. 4.1 Proximal long head of biceps (short head not shown). Coracoacromial (CAL), coracohumeral (CHL), conoid (CoL), superior glenohumeral (SGHL), transverse humeral (TL), and trapezoid (TrL) ligaments are labeled

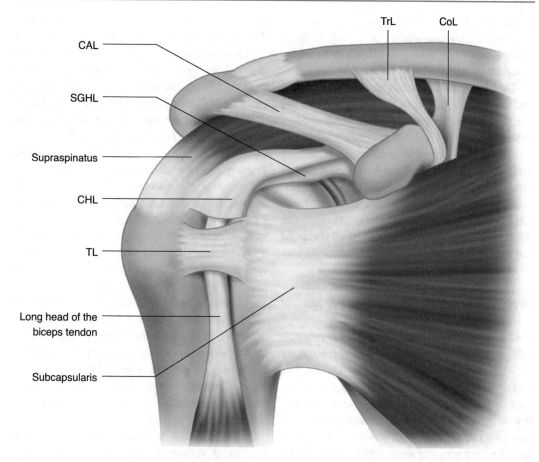

Fig. 4.2 Distal biceps tendon inserting on posterior ulnar aspect of the radial tuberosity with overlying aponeurosis/lacertus fibrosis of the biceps brachii

25–48% of the population. In these individuals, the long head inserts farther from the axis of rotation, and more proximal than the short head, suggesting that it is the dominant supinator, while the short head acts as a more powerful forearm flexor [12]. The bicipital aponeurosis or lacertus fibrosis arises from the medial aspect of the muscle belly and crosses the antecubital fossa medially. It merges with the proximal forearm flexor fascia and inserts on the border of the ulna. This fascia protects the median nerve, brachial artery, and brachial vein, which lie medial to the biceps tendon. If the lacertus fibrosis remains intact, it can help prevent retraction of a ruptured tendon, which is an important factor in the timing and treatment of ruptures [13]. There is a bicipi-toradial bursa between the tendon and radial tuberosity that acts to reduce friction during pronation and supination; this is the most common region of distal tendinopathy [5].

The musculocutaneous nerve (C5, 6, 7) innervates the biceps and runs between the biceps brachii and brachialis muscles. It terminates as the lateral antebrachial cutaneous nerve, which supplies sensation to the lateral forearm. The lateral antebrachial cutaneous nerve lies superficially making it vulnerable to injury during operative treatment of distal biceps tears [12]. The ascending branches of the anterior humeral circumflex artery supply the proximal biceps. Distal branches of the brachial artery and the posterior interosseous recurrent artery supply the distal biceps. There is a 2-cm zone of hypo-vascularity just proximal to the distal biceps insertion that may predispose it to degeneration and rupture, although most tendinopathies occur more distally at the insertion on the radial tuberosity as previously mentioned [12].

The biceps tendon serves as a powerful flexor and the main supinator of the forearm when the elbow is at least partially flexed. Many studies have supported the role of the long head of the biceps tendon in maintaining glenohumeral joint stability, and analysis has shown that it provides anterior stabilization of the glenohumeral joint by increasing resistance to torsional forces on the humeral head, especially when the shoulder is in an externally rotated and abducted position [14, 15].

Proximal Long Head Tendinopathy

A 44-year-old male construction worker presents with a five-month history of progressive right anterior shoulder pain. There is no specific history of trauma or injury. His discomfort is associated with weakness and a "snapping sensation" that is typically worse with overhead activities and lifting heavy objects. Exam shows weakness and impaired range of motion of his right shoulder. He has focal tenderness on palpation in his right bicipital groove. There is a positive Speed's and Yergason's test, reproducing his presenting anterior shoulder pain.

Clinical Presentation

Tendinopathy of the proximal long head rarely presents as an isolated condition, typically developing as a secondary process from underlying shoulder dysfunction in 90–95% of cases [16]. Rotator cuff tendinopathy, impingement syndrome, glenohumeral osteoarthritis or instability, and biomechanical dysfunction from scapular dyskinesias force the long head to compensate for increasing instability of the shoulder joint. Tenosynovitis develops as the synovial sheath becomes irritated and inflamed from repetitive mechanical overloading and microtrauma.

Eventually, this leads to both inflammatory and degenerative processes that work synergistically in the pathogenesis of tendinopathy, thus resulting in a thickened, hypertrophied, and fibrotic tendon [17]. As the hour glassed-shaped tendon moves within the groove, shear forces and traction cause it to become fixed by adhesions and scar tissues [18]. The degenerated, entrapped tendon leads to progressive clinical symptoms. Primary biceps tendinopathy, which can be presumed after co-existing shoulder pathology is excluded, has been attributed to congenital variants in osseous anatomy [19].

The most common presenting complaint is anterior shoulder pain with radiation distally over the biceps muscle belly [20]. Typical rotator cuff tendinopathy symptoms, including generalized shoulder pain with overhead activity and discomfort while lying on the affected side, are common as studies report biceps pathology in 76–85% of rotator cuff tears [8]. In overhead athletes, pain may be especially worse during follow-through motion as the humeral head translates anteriorly, increasing impingement of the biceps tendon [21].

Long-standing tendinosis may result in a weakened tendon, increasing the risk of rupture [18]. Ruptures most commonly result from sudden or forceful eccentric contraction of the long head, such as when a patient catches an object that falls unexpectedly or shovels heavy snow [22]. However, many ruptures are spontaneous because they take place in degenerated tendons [18]. Patients may present with a sudden "pop" accompanied with acute pain, swelling, and ecchymosis. Proximal ruptures often have a classic "Popeye deformity," which can be seen as a focal bulge as the muscle mass moves distally. The most common sites of rupture include the tendon origin and the musculotendinous junction [19]. Proximal long head instability, ranging from subluxation to dislocation, can result in clinical symptoms of anterior shoulder pain, catching, popping, or an audible and palpable "snap" during movement. The long head most frequently subluxes medially and superficially toward the subscapularis insertion on the lesser tuberosity [23]. It is extremely uncommon for instability to occur in the absence of rotator cuff abnormalities, and the subscapularis is the most commonly involved muscle [24]. The biceps pulley, responsible for securing the long head within the groove, must also be disrupted for the tendon to become unstable [25].

Tendinopathy of the biceps can also occur near its origin at the biceps anchor. Snyder et al. described a specific group of lesions, termed SLAP (superior labrum anterior and posterior) lesions, involving the superior aspect of the labrum and origin of the biceps tendon [26]. Eccentric contraction of the long head when the arm is abducted and externally rotated results in excessive stress on the biceps tendon, gradually detaching the superior labrum and biceps origin from the glenoid tissue [27]. Most commonly seen in overhead athletes, symptomology is vague and nonspecific, but the most common complaints include anterior shoulder pain, sensations of instability, and episodic clicking when the arm is in a throwing position [28].

Physical Examination

When examining for proximal biceps tendinopathy, it is imperative to perform a complete shoulder exam due to the high rate of concomitant shoulder pathology. Inspection, palpation, range of motion, manual muscle testing, special testing for rotator cuff pathology, and neurovascular assessment of the entire upper extremity should be performed before focusing on the proximal biceps. A cervical spine examination should also be conducted, as cervical radiculopathy can contribute to shoulder girdle pain/weakness. In the majority of patients with biceps lesions, inspection is unremarkable with the notable exception of biceps tendon ruptures. In this scenario, edema and bruising may be present along with an obvious muscle mass, representing the detached muscle belly [20]. Palpation over the proximal long head within the bicipital groove should elicit point tenderness (see Table 4.1).

The two most commonly performed special tests for biceps tendinopathy are Yergason's and Speed's tests (see Table 4.1 and Figs. 4.3 and 4.4) [29, 30]. The modest sensitivity and specificity of these maneuvers reflect the challenge that clinicians face in distinguishing biceps tendinopathy from other causes of anterior shoulder pain.

Given the high association of biceps tendinopathy with SLAP lesions, maneuvers must be performed to evaluate the pathology at the superior labrum complex. Two common exam maneuvers include O'Brien's active compression test and the biceps load test II (see Table 4.1). No exam maneuver has proven superior over the other in accurately and consistently diagnosing a SLAP lesion, nor has a set of clinical maneuvers proven more efficacious than individual stand-alone testing [31–33].

Diagnostic Workup

Ultrasound

Musculoskeletal ultrasound is an important tool that can be utilized in the assessment and confirmation of proximal long head tendon pathology (see Table 4.2a). Studies have shown that it has superior efficacy in detecting normal tendons, full-thickness and partial-thickness tears, and non-tear abnormalities of the biceps tendon when compared to MRI [34–36].

The exam begins proximally within the groove at the rotator interval, and scanning continues distally in both long and short axes until ending at the myotendinous junction. The normal appearance of the long head will reflect the typical sonographic appearance of most tendons, described as hyperechoic with a linear, fibrillar pattern of echotexture [23]. Because the biceps tendon sheath communicates directly with the glenohumeral joint, any inflammatory or degenerative process of the shoulder can result in fluid accumulation within this sheath (see Fig. 4.5) [37]. Dynamically assessing the proximal tendon with internal and external rotation of the shoulder should be performed as abnormal positioning of the tendon may only

Table 4.1 Descriptions of the most common physical exam maneuvers and corresponding positive findings

Physical exam maneuvers				
Test	Exam maneuver	Positive finding	Sensitivity	Specificity
Palpation of biceps tendon	To identify the tendon, palpate the greater tubercle of the humerus, and move medially into the groove. Flex the patient's elbow to 90° while internally and externally rotating the arm until the long head can be palpated under the examiner's fingers [77]	Pain along the biceps tendon	98%	70%
Speed's test	Patient flexes their supinated and extended arm against the examiner's isometric resistance while the examiner palpates the long head within the bicipital groove (see Fig. 4.4)	Pain along the biceps tendon	63–68%	55%
Yergason's test	Patient's arm should be pronated and elbow flexed to 90° along their torso (see Fig. 4.3). The patient then attempts to supinate their arm against the examiner's isometric resistance while the examiner palpates the long head within the bicipital groove	Pain along the biceps tendon	32–37%	86%
O'Briens test (active compression test)	Patient flexes their extended arm 90°, adducts 10°, and internally rotates the arm until the thumb is pointing downward. The examiner then pushes down on the patient's arm and assesses for pain or a clicking sensation in the shoulder. Next, the patient supinates their forearm and the examiner again pushes downward	If the click or pain is less prominent on with supination, the test is considered positive for a SLAP lesion	28–73%	63–94%
Biceps load test II	Patient is placed in the supine position with the shoulder externally rotated and placed in 120° of abduction, the elbow is flexed to 90°, and the forearm is supinated. The examiner then provides resistance as the patient is asked to flex the elbow	Pain in the shoulder region indicates a positive test for SLAP lesion	90%	97%
Hook test	Patient flexes elbow to 90° and fully supinates the forearm. Examiner uses index finger to "hook" distal biceps tendon from the lateral edge of the antecubital fossa and pulls anteriorly	Unable to "hook" a cord like structure = distal rupture If intact but painful = partial tear or tendinosis	100%	100%
Biceps squeeze test	Similar to Thompson test for Achilles-patient's arm rests in slight pronation with elbow flexed between 60 and 80° and examiner squeezes biceps muscle belly with both hands, observing for forearm supination	Lack of forearm supination = distal rupture	96%	100%
Biceps crease interval	Measure the distance between the antecubital crease and the cusp of the distal biceps descent (where biceps turns most sharply toward the fossa)	>6 cm or ratio of >1.2 from side to side = distal rupture	92–96%	80–100%

occur during these movements. If a subluxation or dislocation is present, a painful click or snap is often seen during dynamic assessment, with medial displacement over the top of the lesser tuberosity.

Additional Imaging

Plain films play little role in diagnosing biceps tendinopathy. However, if underlying impingement or osteoarthritis of the acromioclavicular or glenohumeral joint is suspected, radiographs serve a useful tool in detecting arthritic changes that may be contributing to shoulder pain. Studies have demonstrated that the sensitivity and specificity of MRI and MRA may be insufficient in detecting proximal biceps pathology, especially tendinosis [38, 39]. Advanced imaging should be reserved for cases where labral pathology is suspected or when conservative management has failed and the clinical course is leading

toward surgery. MRA is preferred over MRI in diagnosing SLAP tears [40]. Proximal biceps tendon subluxation can be associated with

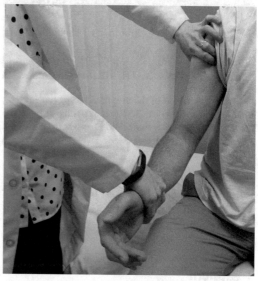

Fig. 4.4 During Yergason's test, the patient flexes their elbow to 90° and attempts to supinate their forearm against resistance while the examiner palpates the tendon of the long head within the bicipital groove

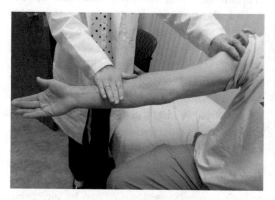

Fig. 4.3 During Speed's test, the patient flexes and supinates their extended arm against the examiner's isometric resistance

Table 4.2a   Findings on ultrasound exam of proximal biceps tendon

Ultrasound examination		
Sonographic finding	Differential	Distinguishing factors
Increased fluid surrounding proximal sheath	Joint effusion, tenosynovitis	Joint effusion: symmetric distention around the sheath, possibly with accumulation of fluid in other joint recesses, such as the subscapular recess or subacromial bursa Tenosynovitis: focal distention of sheath, pain with transducer pressure, hyperemia on Doppler assessment[23]
Absence of proximal long head	Subluxation/dislocation, full-thickness tear/rupture	Subluxation/dislocation: long head commonly found medial and superficial toward the subscapularis insertion on the lesser tuberosity [23] Rupture: long head stump typically found when scanning distally
Increased blood flow on Doppler	Acute inflammatory state (tendinitis, tenosynovitis, infection), tendinosis	Acute inflammation: due to hyperemia Tendinosis: due to neovascularization[a]
Loss of linear, hyperechoic tendon pattern	Partial thickness tear, tendinosis	Partial-thickness tear: well-defined anechoic/hypoechoic abnormality Tendinosis: tendon thickening, heterogeneous hypoechoic enlargement, calcifications, neovascularization [23]
Posterior acoustic shadowing	Partial thickness tear (less likely), complete tear	If seen, it likely signifies the presence of hemorrhage from a complete rupture (or less likely partial tear). The dense hyperechoic fluid causes acoustic shadowing and may obscure the detailed evaluation of deeper structures

When correlated clinically, imaging serves as a valuable tool for the clinician in determining diagnosis and direction of treatment

[a]In a study analyzing patients clinically diagnosed with tendinopathy of the long head of the biceps tendon, 22/28 patients were found to have neovascularization via immunohistochemical staining [78]

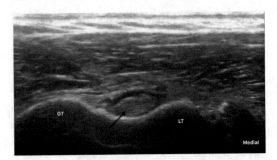

Fig. 4.5 Ultrasound of the proximal biceps brachii long head tendon (*arrow*) in short axis coursing through the bicipital groove. Hypoechoic fluid is seen surrounding the tendon. Greater (GT) and lesser (LT) tuberosities are labeled

full-thickness subscapularis tears and further imaging with ultrasound or MRI may be indicated for confirmation.

Treatment

Conservative

Nonoperative management involves a combination of physical therapy, oral medications, and interventional techniques. Treatment should be focused on both the biceps and any underlying shoulder dysfunction. Initial management should allow for relative rest, activity modification, and pain control.

Non-steroidal Anti-inflammatory Drug (NSAID)

A systematic review of the literature suggests that both oral and topical non-steroidal anti-inflammatory drugs (NSAIDs) are effective in the management of pain associated with tendinopathy in the short term, but no evidence has proven that chronic use of NSAIDs provides any long-term benefit [41, 42]. If there is no contraindication to oral NSAID use, ibuprofen 600–800 mg QID (maximum daily dose of 3200 mg) or naproxen 250–500 mg BID (maximum daily dose of 1000 mg) can be recommended for 7–14 days [43]. If the side effect profile of NSAIDs precludes its use, acetaminophen 1000 mg TID is a reasonable alternative.

Physical Therapy

Physical therapy is similar to that of rotator cuff tendinopathy as previously discussed in Chap. 3. This is because at the time of physical therapy enrollment, diagnosis is typically not etiological and also because concomitant pathologies within rotator cuff tendons are common. The biceps tendon therapy program should focus on the entire kinetic chain of the upper extremity, including the scapular stabilizers. After pain is adequately controlled, the first step involves restoring passive range of motion with progression to active range of motion. Next, gradual strengthening of the scapular stabilizers and individual rotator cuff muscles should follow. Initial training should focus on isometric exercises, which allows for muscle strengthening without adding any stress to the tendon. As the muscle becomes stronger, concentric and eccentric training is implemented, which increases tensile load as the muscle changes in length. Eccentric contraction has been to shown to both normalize tendon structure by increasing collagen synthesis and to halt the degenerative cascade by decreasing neovascularization and tendon swelling [44]. After strengthening, progression to dynamic stability exercises and specific return-to-activity movements are implemented.

Iontophoresis, phonophoresis, and therapeutic ultrasound have been studied in various tendinopathies with modest data showing their efficacy in improving outcomes [45, 46]. Extracorporeal shock wave therapy (ESWT) and diathermy have shown promising results in several large studies involving various tendinopathies, but none have specifically examined the biceps tendon [47].

Interventional

Corticosteroid injections (CSIs) continue to be a common practice in biceps tendinopathy. Most authors recommend injection if the patient's pain is unrelieved by an initial trial of oral analgesics or if further pain relief is needed to initiate and tolerate a rehab program [48]. Injections may target the concomitant shoulder pathologies by injecting into the subacromial or glenohumeral joint space, or by directly injecting into the tendon sheath of the long head. Multiple studies

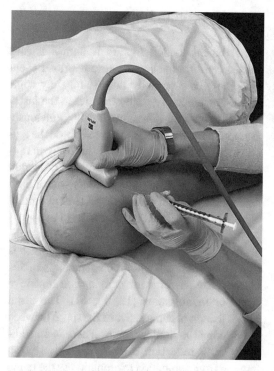

Fig. 4.6 Recommended positioning for injection into the sheath of the proximal tendon of the long head of the biceps. Patient is supine with arm in neutral position and palm facing upward. The transducer is placed in an anatomic transverse plane over the bicipital groove

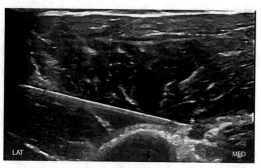

Fig. 4.7 Proximal right biceps tendon sheath viewed in short axis (asterisk). The needle is visualized approaching the target in a lateral to medial, in plane approach

have proven that CSIs improve pain and outcomes in the short term, but this effect is reversed in the intermediate and long term as steroids inhibit collagen synthesis and increase risk of tendon rupture [49, 50]. If indicated, most clinicians recommend a single injection into the sheath of the proximal long head, preferably under ultrasound guidance to minimize risk of intra-tendinous injection [51]. If ultrasound were to be used, the literature indicates that the most technique is to use lateral to medial, in plane approach, with the biceps tendon viewed in short axis (see Figs. 4.6 and 4.7; Video 4.1) [52, 53]. Injectate volumes typically consist of 1 mL of corticosteroid in combination with 0.5–2.0 mL of anesthetic [54]. Utilizing sonographic guidance is recommended as one randomized controlled trial demonstrated significantly greater accuracy when comparing ultrasound-guided versus unguided injections into the proximal

long head tendon sheath [51]. Regenerative injection techniques, including platelet-rich plasma (PRP) and prolotherapy, are increasingly being studied in the treatment of various chronic tendinopathies. Several case reports of biceps tendinopathy successfully treated with PRP have been reported [55]. One study comparing PRP and prolotherapy in patients with biceps tendinopathy found both treatments to be effective, but leukocyte-rich PRP showed a significant better response in long term [56].

Operative

Surgical treatment of the long head of biceps tendon is reserved for patients who have failed nonsurgical management in setting of anterior shoulder pain and positive exam findings consistent with biceps tendinopathy. Surgically treated conditions include, but are not limited to, partial tendon tears, tenosynovitis, tendon instability, select types of SLAP tears (see Fig. 4.8). There are no set guidelines for duration of nonsurgical management. Instead, recommending surgical intervention is individualized for each patient. Biceps tenotomy and tenodesis are two of the most common surgical procedures for treating long head of biceps pathology. In appropriately indicated patients, both options can provide reliable symptomatic relief and patient satisfaction.

Biceps tenotomy has advantages that include decreased surgical time, technical ease of the procedure, no implant cost, and no postopera-

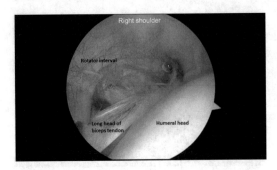

Fig. 4.8 Arthroscopic view of the right shoulder visualized from the posterior portal. The long head of the biceps tendon is inflamed and mildly frayed as it is coursing toward the bicipital groove

tive immobilization. Reported disadvantages include decreased supination strength, biceps fatigue, and cosmetic Popeye deformity (70% of patients) [57, 58].

Biceps tenodesis involves cutting the tendon from its anchor site and reattaching it onto the humerus. It is indicated in younger or active patients, laborers, and overhead athletes, as well as in those who would deem cosmetic deformity to be unacceptable. Tenodesis can be performed arthroscopically or using an open technique. Described complications include infection, musculocutaneous nerve neuropathy, humeral fracture, and hardware failure. In a study of 350 patients treated with open subpectoral biceps tenodesis, the reported rate of complications was 0.7% [59]. Despite much debate and controversy surrounding the optimal location for tenodesis and the fixation method, overall, biceps tenodesis is a successful procedure with low rates of complication [58].

Distal Biceps Tendon Rupture

A 55-year-old man presents with sudden onset of sharp, tearing pain in his anterior elbow after hearing a "pop" while performing heavy bicep curls. He endorses weakness and pain with activities requiring elbow flexion and has had difficulty turning doorknobs [60]. On inspection, he has swelling and ecchymosis over the antecubital fossa but it is difficult to appreciate any change in muscle contour.

Clinical Presentation

Distal biceps tendon rupture is almost always caused by a traumatic eccentric overload event with the elbow partially flexed and fully supinated. The tendon typically ruptures at the insertion site on the radial tuberosity. Previously asymptomatic tendinosis may predispose the tendon to rupture [13]. The lacertus fibrosis can rupture with the tendon, allowing for tendon retraction. Occasionally, in patients with a bifid tendon, there is an isolated single tendon rupture of either the long head or short head [5].

Apart from distal biceps tendon rupture, tendinosis can be symptomatic without a tear, which is caused by friction, bony impingement as radius clears ulnar on forearm rotation, and repetitive stress or microtrauma [12, 13, 61]. The distal biceps tendon occupies 85% of the space between the proximal radioulnar joints. There is an additional 50% reduction in the joint space when moving from supination to pronation as the radial tuberosity moves posteriorly. Irregularity of the radial tuberosity may lead to increased impingement of the tendon and thus causing tendinosis or degeneration [12]. As distal biceps tendinopathy can present with lateral elbow pain and mimic common extensor tendinopathy (CET), physicians should elicit history pertaining to CET (see Chap. 5).

Physical Examination

A "reverse Popeye" sign may be challenging to appreciate due to swelling and difficulty contracting the biceps muscle [62]. General ecchymosis and swelling in the antecubital fossa will be seen in biceps tendon tears. In both tendinosis and tears, forearm supination weakness is usually more prominent than weakness in elbow flexion [61]. The most common examination maneuvers to evaluate distal biceps rupture include the hook test, biceps squeeze test, and biceps crease interval (see Table 4.1) [63, 64]. The hook test is the most sensitive test; however, the examiner must be careful to not mistake the biceps tendon for the lacterus fibrosis, which will feel like a flat sheet-like material when palpated from the medial aspect [62]. Pain provocation tests in which the examiner provides resistance during elbow flexion and forearm supination may elicit pain in distal biceps tendinosis or rupture [5, 13]. Distal rupture may also be diagnosed with the passive pronation and supination test in which the biceps muscle belly does not move distally with passive pronation or proximally with supination with the elbow in 90° of flexion [4].

Diagnostic Workup

MRI

The gold standard imaging modality for the diagnosis of tendinosis versus tear of the distal biceps tendon remains the MRI. Optimal positioning is in the "FABS view" in which the patient lays prone with their elbow flexed, shoulder abducted overhead, and forearm supinated so the thumb is pointed upward. This position allows for accurate visualization of the full length of the distal biceps tendon [65]. A complete tear may be demonstrated as fiber discontinuity or absence of the tendon attachment on the radial tuberosity with hyperintense soft tissue edema/hematoma [66]. MRI can be used to evaluate lacertus fibrosis rupture and tendon retraction, which will help with surgical planning. Focal marrow edema in the radial tuberosity may also be seen in complete or partial tendon tears [7]. Signs of a partial tear and tendinosis include alteration of intra-tendinous

signal, altered tendon thickness, paralleling fluid, and fluid filled bursa [65, 66].

X-Ray

Plain films are not typically useful except in evaluating avulsion fracture or osseous reaction of the radial tuberosity seen with some complete ruptures. Enlargement or irregularity of the radial tuberosity may be seen, which leaves the tendon susceptible to injury [13].

Ultrasound

As previously discussed, ultrasound examination offers many advantages over other imaging modalities. During evaluation of the distal biceps, ultrasound shows 95% sensitivity and 71% specificity in diagnosing complete versus partial tears [67]. Altered echogenicity with either tendon thickening or thinning and contour irregularities are typically seen with partial tears, while tendon hypertrophy and heterogeneous hypoechoic changes due to edema are seen with tendinosis [66]. A complete tear is visualized as an anechoic or hypoechoic discontinuity of the tendon with or without retraction. There may also be hyperechoic peritendinous fluid, which usually signifies hemorrhage and may be a very sensitive sign of complete tendon rupture. The presence of hyperechoic fluid casts a shadow on ultrasound image, in an artifact called "posterior acoustic shadowing," making it difficult to evaluate deeper structural details (see Table 4.2b) [66]. While shadowing has a poor sensitivity for diagnosing

Table 4.2b Findings on ultrasound exam of distal biceps tendon

Ultrasound examination		
Sonographic finding	Differential	Distinguishing factors
Increased blood flow on Doppler	Acute inflammatory state (tendinitis, tenosynovitis, infection), tendinosis	Acute inflammation: due to hyperemia Tendinosis: due to neovascularization
Loss of linear, hyperechoic tendon pattern	Partial thickness tear, tendinosis	Partial-thickness tear: well-defined anechoic/hypoechoic abnormality Tendinosis: tendon thickening, heterogeneous hypoechoic enlargement, calcifications, neovascularization [23]
Posterior acoustic shadowing	Partial thickness tear, complete tear	If seen, it likely signifies the presence of hemorrhage from a complete rupture (or less likely partial tear). The dense hyperechoic fluid causes acoustic shadowing and may obscure the detailed evaluation of deeper structures

When correlated clinically, imaging serves as a valuable tool for the clinician in determining diagnosis and direction of treatment partial tears, studies suggest that the lack of shadowing can exclude a complete tear [67].

Treatment

Conservative

Non-operative treatment is considered for tendonitis, partial tears, and tendinosis of distal biceps tendon. The general principle is similar to other enthesopathies using a combination of relative rest, activity modification, physical therapy, and both pharmacologic and non-pharmacologic modalities as described in the proximal biceps tendon section. Physical therapy programs typically involve the combination of stretching and strengthening with progression from isometric to concentric to eccentric exercises as suggested for proximal tendinopathy. Use of NSAIDs has been tried in acute phases for the above-stated indications but without a long-term benefit. Nitroglycerin topical patches can be used over the tendon to promote local vasodilation for tendinosis, increasing the blood supply and thus improving tendon repair [68].

Interventional

Corticosteroid injections may be trialed for tendonitis, partial tear, and sometimes for tendinosis, but it may not improve the long-term outcome for distal tendinopathy [68]. Regenerative medications such as platelet-rich plasma (PRP) may be recommended for refractory cases of biceps tendinopathy. There have been reports of positive outcomes after only one to two leukocyte-rich PRP (type 1B per Mishra classification) injections for distal biceps tendinopathy [69]. The safest recommended approach for distal biceps tendon sheath injection is a posterior approach in order to avoid injuries to the brachial artery, which lies just medial to the tendon. For this approach, the patient is positioned in supine with their arm flexed at the elbow and forearm hyperpronated. The transducer is oriented in short axis on the posterior forearm about 3–4 cm distal to the olecranon (see Fig. 4.9). The needle is then advanced in plane to the transducer in a radial to ulnar direction, targeting the superficial surface

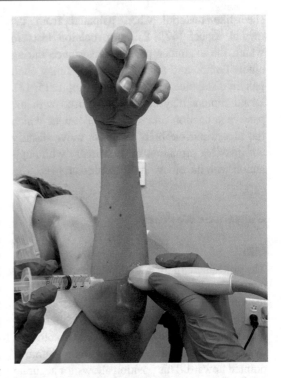

Fig. 4.9 Recommended positioning for peritendinous injection of the distal biceps using a posterior approach. Patient is in supine with elbow flexed and forearm hyperpronated. The transducer is placed in a short axis plane over the posterior forearm, distal to the olecranon. The needle is guided in an in-plane radial to ulnar approach

of the biceps tendon at the distal attachment to the radius [54]. Injectate volumes for CSI are similar to that mentioned for proximal bicep tendon sheath injection and PRP protocols widely vary.

Radial extracorporeal shock wave therapy (rESWT) may also stimulate cell proliferation, angiogenesis, and collagen synthesis, and many trials have shown improvement in pain and functional limitations over placebo or other alternative therapies [70]. A recent study found that a single session of rESWT using 2000 shock waves with energy flux density of 0.18 mJ/mm was safe and effective in decreasing pain in chronic distal biceps tendinopathy [61].

Operative

There is no definitive data on when to refer to surgery for distal biceps tendinosis and partial tears but most studies recommend trialing conservative treatment for at least 6–12 months [65]. Complete tears can result in up to 40% loss of supination strength, 79% loss of supination endurance, 30% loss of flexion strength, and 30% loss of flexion endurance [71, 72]. To restore strength and function, surgical repair is favored in the young and active population, while non-operative treatment can be considered for older patients who are able to tolerate flexion and supination strength deficits.

When planning for surgical treatment, time from injury is a critical factor, as longer delays result in a retracted tendon that may be adhered to the surrounding tissue. Consequently, more dissection is involved to mobilize the tissue, which can increase the complexity of the case and the complications associated with repair [73].

Surgical repair of distal biceps tendon rupture can be performed through either single or dual incision approach, using various fixation techniques and implants. Regardless of the chosen surgical method, the published studies report good to excellent outcomes with respect to recovery of strength and endurance with low rates of complications. A classic article by Morrey et al. demonstrated recovery of 97% of elbow flexion and 95% supination strength compared to the contralateral extremity, following surgical repair [72]. Most commonly described complications after surgery include injury to the lateral antebrachial cutaneous nerve. Other less common complications include heterotopic ossification, stiffness, re-rupture, and persistent pain [74].

Proximal Short Head

While tendinopathy of the proximal short head of the biceps is rare, it should still be considered in patients presenting with shoulder pain. Much like impingement of the long head tendon, there may be impingement at the coracoid process when the lesser tuberosity infringes on this region during flexion and internal rotation of the arm. Patients will present with anterior shoulder pain that may radiate down the arm; however, typical shoulder impingement exam maneuvers, such as Neer's

and Hawkins', will be negative. The tendon origin at the coracoid process may be tender to palpation and worse with passive flexion at the shoulder. Diagnosis may be confirmed with injection of 3–4 mL of local anesthetic between the coracoid process and the humeral head [75]. Following the anesthetic injection with a CSI, typically consisting of 2–3 mL anesthetic and 1 mL of 40 mg/mL DepoMedrol, can result in decreased pain and increased function.

There are very few case reports of isolated proximal short head tendon rupture. The mechanism of injury is described as an abrupt flexion and adduction of the arm with the elbow in extension, which places the short head under the greatest strain. Patients will present with sudden onset of anterior shoulder pain, a "popping" sensation, ecchymosis, swelling, and a mini-"Popeye" sign with a hollow site medial to the biceps brachii long head, where the short head muscle belly normally lies. Shoulder flexion will be weak and there will be tenderness at the coracoid process without a palpable tendon. Histological examinations have revealed degenerative changes in the tendon that were severe enough to cause failure. Surgical repair involves reattachment of the tendon either to the coracobrachialis tendon or partially to the coracoid process and partially to the long head biceps tendon [76].

References

1. Singaraju VM, Kang RW, Yanke AB, McNickle AG, Lewis PB, Wang VM, et al. Biceps tendinitis in chronic rotator cuff tears: a histologic perspective. J Shoulder Elb Surg. 2008;17(6):898–904.
2. Redondo-Alonso L, Chamorro-Moriana G, Jimenez-Rejano JJ, Lopez-Tarrida P, Ridao-Fernandez C. Relationship between chronic pathologies of the supraspinatus tendon and the long head of the biceps tendon: systematic review. BMC Musculoskelet Disord. 2014;15:377.
3. Brown DP, Freeman ED, Cuccurullo SJ, Ng U, Maitin IB. Musculoskeletal Medicine. In: Cuccurullo SJ, editor. Physical medicine and rehabilitation board review. 3rd ed. New York: Demos Medical Publishing; 2014. p. 171–3.
4. McDonald LS, Dewing CB, Shupe PG, Provencher MT. Disorders of the proximal and distal aspects of the biceps muscle. J Bone Joint Surg Am. 2013;95(13):1235–45.

5. Stevens K, Kwak A, Poplawski S. The biceps muscle from shoulder to elbow. Semin Musculoskelet Radiol. 2012;16(4):296–315.

6. Ward JP, Shreve MC, Youm T, Strauss EJ. Ruptures of the distal biceps tendon. Bull Hosp Jt Dis. 2014;72(1):110–9.

7. Donaldson O, Vannet N, Gosens T, Kulkarni R. Tendinopathies around the elbow part 2: medial elbow, distal biceps and triceps tendinopathies. Shoulder Elbow. 2014;6(1):47–56.

8. Gill HS, El Rassi G, Bahk MS, Castillo RC, McFarland EG. Physical examination for partial tears of the biceps tendon. Am J Sports Med. 2007;35(8):1334–40.

9. Bass E. Tendinopathy: why the difference between tendinitis and tendinosis matters. Int J Ther Massage Bodywork. 2012;5(1):14–7.

10. Zappia M, Reginelli A, Russo A, D'Agosto GF, Di Pietto F, Genovese EA, et al. Long head of the biceps tendon and rotator interval. Musculoskelet Surg. 2013;97(Suppl 2):S99–108.

11. Nakata W, Katou S, Fujita A, Nakata M, Lefor AT, Sugimoto H. Biceps pulley: normal anatomy and associated lesions at MR arthrography. Radiographics. 2011;31(3):791–810.

12. Quach T, Jazayeri R, Sherman OH, Rosen JE. Distal biceps tendon injuries – current treatment options. Bull NYU Hosp Jt Dis. 2010;68(2):103–11.

13. Ramsey ML. Distal biceps tendon injuries: diagnosis and management. J Am Acad Orthop Surg. 1999;7(3):199–207.

14. Kumar VP, Satku K, Balasubramaniam P. The role of the long head of biceps brachii in the stabilization of the head of the humerus. Clin Orthop Relat Res. 1989;244:172–5.

15. Warner JJ, McMahon PJ. The role of the long head of the biceps brachii in superior stability of the glenohumeral joint. J Bone Joint Surg Am. 1995;77(3):366–72.

16. Beall DP, Williamson EE, Ly JQ, Adkins MC, Emery RL, Jones TP, et al. Association of biceps tendon tears with rotator cuff abnormalities: degree of correlation with tears of the anterior and superior portions of the rotator cuff. AJR Am J Roentgenol. 2003;180(3):633–9.

17. Abate M, Silbernagel KG, Siljeholm C, Di Iorio A, De Amicis D, Salini V, et al. Pathogenesis of tendinopathies: inflammation or degeneration? Arthritis Res Ther. 2009;11(3):235.

18. Longo UG, Loppini M, Marineo G, Khan WS, Maffulli N, Denaro V. Tendinopathy of the tendon of the long head of the biceps. Sports Med Arthrosc. 2011;19(4):321–32.

19. Curtis AS, Snyder SJ. Evaluation and treatment of biceps tendon pathology. Orthop Clin North Am. 1993;24(1):33–43.

20. Virk MS, Cole BJ. Proximal biceps tendon and rotator cuff tears. Clin Sports Med. 2016;35(1):153–61.

21. Abrams JS. Special shoulder problems in the throwing athlete: pathology, diagnosis, and nonoperative management. Clin Sports Med. 1991;10(4):839–61.

22. Simons S. DB. Biceps tendiopathy and tendon rupture 2017. Available from: http://www.uptodate.com/contents/biceps-tendinopathy-and-tendon-rupture.

23. Jacobson JA. Fundamentals of musculoskeletal ultrasound. 2nd ed. Philadelphia: Elsevier Saunders; 2012.

24. Eakin CL, Faber KJ, Hawkins RJ, Hovis WD. Biceps tendon disorders in athletes. J Am Acad Orthop Surg. 1999;7(5):300–10.

25. Krupp RJ, Kevern MA, Gaines MD, Kotara S, Singleton SB. Long head of the biceps tendon pain: differential diagnosis and treatment. J Orthop Sports Phys Ther. 2009;39(2):55–70.

26. Snyder SJ, Karzel RP, Pizzo WD, Ferkel RD, Friedman MJ. Arthroscopy classics. SLAP lesions of the shoulder. Arthroscopy. 2010;26(8):1117.

27. Burkhart SS, Morgan CD. The peel-back mechanism: its role in producing and extending posterior type II SLAP lesions and its effect on SLAP repair rehabilitation. Arthroscopy. 1998;14(6):637–40.

28. Bedi A, Allen AA. Superior labral lesions anterior to posterior-evaluation and arthroscopic management. Clin Sports Med. 2008;27(4):607–30.

29. Calis M, Akgun K, Birtane M, Karacan I, Calis H, Tuzun F. Diagnostic values of clinical diagnostic tests in subacromial impingement syndrome. Ann Rheum Dis. 2000;59(1):44–7.

30. Chen HS, Lin SH, Hsu YH, Chen SC, Kang JH. A comparison of physical examinations with musculoskeletal ultrasound in the diagnosis of biceps long head tendinitis. Ultrasound Med Biol. 2011;37(9):1392–8.

31. Hegedus EJ, Goode AP, Cook CE, Michener L, Myer CA, Myer DM, et al. Which physical examination tests provide clinicians with the most value when examining the shoulder? Update of a systematic review with meta-analysis of individual tests. Br J Sports Med. 2012;46(14):964–78.

32. Guanche CA, Jones DC. Clinical testing for tears of the glenoid labrum. Arthroscopy. 2003;19(5):517–23.

33. Kim SH, Ha KI, Ahn JH, Kim SH, Choi HJ. Biceps load test II: a clinical test for SLAP lesions of the shoulder. Arthroscopy. 2001;17(2):160–4.

34. Dubrow SA, Streit JJ, Shishani Y, Robbin MR, Gobezie R. Diagnostic accuracy in detecting tears in the proximal biceps tendon using standard nonenhancing shoulder MRI. Open Access J Sports Med. 2014;5:81–7.

35. Rodeo SA, Nguyen JT, Cavanaugh JT, Patel Y, Adler RS. Clinical and ultrasonographic evaluations of the shoulders of elite swimmers. Am J Sports Med. 2016;44(12):3214–21.

36. Skendzel JG, Jacobson JA, Carpenter JE, Miller BS. Long head of biceps brachii tendon evaluation: accuracy of preoperative ultrasound. AJR Am J Roentgenol. 2011;197(4):942–8.

37. Bianchi S. Shoulder. In: Bianchi S, Martinoli C, editors. Ultrasound of the musculoskeletal system. Berlin/Heidelberg/New York: Springer; 2009. p. 189–332.

38. Carr RM, Shishani Y, Gobezie R. How accurate are we in detecting biceps tendinopathy? Clin Sports Med. 2016;35(1):47–55.

39. Malavolta EA, Assuncao JH, Guglielmetti CL, de Souza FF, Gracitelli ME, Ferreira Neto AA. Accuracy of preoperative MRI in the diagnosis of disorders of the long head of the biceps tendon. Eur J Radiol. 2015;84(11):2250–4.

40. Smith TO, Drew BT, Toms AP. A meta-analysis of the diagnostic test accuracy of MRA and MRI for the detection of glenoid labral injury. Arch Orthop Trauma Surg. 2012;132(7):905–19.

41. Burnham R, Gregg R, Healy P, Steadward R. The effectiveness of topical diclofenac for lateral epicondylitis. Clin J Sport Med. 1998;8(2):78–81.

42. Petri M, Dobrow R, Neiman R, Whiting-O'Keefe Q, Seaman WE. Randomized, double-blind, placebo-controlled study of the treatment of the painful shoulder. Arthritis Rheum. 1987;30(9):1040–5.

43. Andres BM, Murrell GA. Treatment of tendinopathy: what works, what does not, and what is on the horizon. Clin Orthop Relat Res. 2008;466(7):1539–54.

44. Woodley BL, Newsham-West RJ, Baxter GD. Chronic tendinopathy: effectiveness of eccentric exercise. Br J Sports Med. 2007;41(4):188–98; discussion 99

45. Klaiman MD, Shrader JA, Danoff JV, Hicks JE, Pesce WJ, Ferland J. Phonophoresis versus ultrasound in the treatment of common musculoskeletal conditions. Med Sci Sports Exerc. 1998;30(9):1349–55.

46. Nirschl RP, Rodin DM, Ochiai DH, Maartmann-Moe C, Group D-A-S. Iontophoretic administration of dexamethasone sodium phosphate for acute epicondylitis. A randomized, double-blinded, placebo-controlled study. Am J Sports Med. 2003;31(2):189–95.

47. Albert MB, Fromm H. Extracorporeal shock-wave lithotripsy of gallstones with the adjuvant use of cholelitholytic bile acids. Semin Liver Dis. 1990;10(3):197–204.

48. Schickendantz M, King D. Nonoperative management (including ultrasound-guided injections) of proximal biceps disorders. Clin Sports Med. 2016;35(1):57–73.

49. Blair B, Rokito AS, Cuomo F, Jarolem K, Zuckerman JD. Efficacy of injections of corticosteroids for subacromial impingement syndrome. J Bone Joint Surg Am. 1996;78(11):1685–9.

50. Chechick A, Amit Y, Israeli A, Horoszowski H. Recurrent rupture of the achilles tendon induced by corticosteroid injection. Br J Sports Med. 1982;16(2):89–90.

51. Hashiuchi T, Sakurai G, Morimoto M, Komei T, Takakura Y, Tanaka Y. Accuracy of the biceps tendon sheath injection: ultrasound-guided or unguided injection? A randomized controlled trial. J Shoulder Elb Surg. 2011;20(7):1069–73.

52. Zhang J, Ebraheim N, Lause GE. Ultrasound-guided injection for the biceps brachii tendinitis: results and experience. Ultrasound Med Biol. 2011;37(5):729–33.

53. Stone TJ, Adler RS. Ultrasound-guided biceps peritendinous injections in the absence of a distended tendon sheath: a novel rotator interval approach. J Ultrasound Med. 2015;34(12):2287–92.

54. Atlas of ultrasound-guided musculoskeletal injections. McGraw-Hill Education; 2014. 455 p.

55. Ibrahim VM, Groah SL, Libin A, Ljungberg IH. Use of platelet rich plasma for the treatment of bicipital tendinopathy in spinal cord injury: a pilot study. Top Spinal Cord Inj Rehabil. 2012;18(1):77–8.

56. Moon Y. Comparative studies of PRP and prolotherapy for proximal biceps tendinitis. Clin Shoulder Elbow. 2011;14:153–8.

57. Klonz A, Loitz D, Reilmann H. Proximal and distal ruptures of the biceps brachii tendon. Unfallchirurg. 2003;106(9):755–63.

58. Mellano CR, Shin JJ, Yanke AB, Verma NN. Disorders of the long head of the biceps tendon. Instr Course Lect. 2015;64:567–76.

59. Nho SJ, Reiff SN, Verma NN, Slabaugh MA, Mazzocca AD, Romeo AA. Complications associated with subpectoral biceps tenodesis: low rates of incidence following surgery. J Shoulder Elb Surg. 2010;19(5):764–8.

60. Thompson JC. Netter's concise orthopaedic anatomy. 2nd ed. Philadelphia: Saunders Elsevier; 2010.

61. Furia JP, Rompe JD, Maffulli N, Cacchio A, Schmitz C. Radial extracorporeal shock wave therapy is effective and safe in chronic distal biceps tendinopathy. Clin J Sport Med. 2016;

62. O'Driscoll SW, Goncalves LB, Dietz P. The hook test for distal biceps tendon avulsion. Am J Sports Med. 2007;35(11):1865–9.

63. ElMaraghy A, Devereaux M, Tsoi K. The biceps crease interval for diagnosing complete distal biceps tendon ruptures. Clin Orthop Relat Res. 2008;466(9):2255–62.

64. Ruland RT, Dunbar RP, Bowen JD. The biceps squeeze test for diagnosis of distal biceps tendon ruptures. Clin Orthop Relat Res. 2005;437:128–31.

65. Hobbs MC, Koch J, Bamberger HB. Distal biceps tendinosis: evidence-based review. J Hand Surg Am. 2009;34(6):1124–6.

66. Champlin J, Porrino J, Dahiya N, Taljanovic M. A visualization of the distal biceps tendon. PM R. 2017;9(2):210–5.

67. Lobo Lda G, Fessell DP, Miller BS, Kelly A, Lee JY, Brandon C, et al. The role of sonography in differentiating full versus partial distal biceps tendon tears: correlation with surgical findings. AJR Am J Roentgenol. 2013;200(1):158–62.

68. Rees JD, Wilson AM, Wolman RL. Current concepts in the management of tendon disorders. Rheumatology (Oxford). 2006;45(5):508–21.

69. Barker SL, Bell SN, Connell D, Coghlan JA. Ultrasound-guided platelet-rich plasma injection for distal biceps tendinopathy. Shoulder Elbow. 2015;7(2):110–4.

70. Visco V, Vulpiani MC, Torrisi MR, Ferretti A, Pavan A, Vetrano M. Experimental studies on the biological effects of extracorporeal shock wave therapy on

tendon models. A review of the literature. Muscles Ligaments Tendons J. 2014;4(3):357–61.

71. Baker BE, Bierwagen D. Rupture of the distal tendon of the biceps brachii. Operative versus non-operative treatment. J Bone Joint Surg Am. 1985;67(3):414–7.

72. Morrey BF, Askew LJ, An KN, Dobyns JH. Rupture of the distal tendon of the biceps brachii. A biomechanical study. J Bone Joint Surg Am. 1985;67(3):418–21.

73. Kelly EW, Morrey BF, O'Driscoll SW. Complications of repair of the distal biceps tendon with the modified two-incision technique. J Bone Joint Surg Am. 2000;82-A(11):1575–81.

74. Haverstock J, Athwal GS, Grewal R. Distal Biceps Injuries. Hand Clin. 2015;31(4):631–40.

75. Karim MR, Fann AV, Gray RP, Neale DF, Escarda JD. Enthesitis of biceps brachii short head and coracobrachialis at the coracoid process: a generator of shoulder and neck pain. Am J Phys Med Rehabil. 2005;84(5):376–80.

76. Postacchini F, Ricciardi-Pollini PT. Rupture of the short head tendon of the biceps brachii. Clin Orthop Relat Res. 1977;124:229–32.

77. McFarland EG. Examination of the biceps tendon and superior labrum anterior and posterior (SLAP) lesions. In: Kim T, Park H, editors. Examination of the shoulder: the complete guide. New York: Thieme; 2006. p. 213–43.

78. Zabrzynski J, Paczesny L, Lapaj L, Grzanka D, Szukalski J. Process of neovascularisation compared with pain intensity in tendinopathy of the long head of the biceps brachii tendon associated with concomitant shoulder disorders, after arthroscopic treatment. Microscopic evaluation supported by immunohistochemical. Folia Morphol (Warsz). 2018;77(2):378–85.

Common Extensor Tendon/ Common Flexor Tendon

5

Allison Schroeder, Kentaro Onishi, and Scott Joshua Szabo

Abbreviations

ABI	Autologous blood injection
CET	Common extensor tendon
CFPT	Common flexor-pronator tendon
CSI	Corticosteroid injection
ESWT	Extracorporeal shock wave therapy
NSAID	Non-steroidal anti-inflammatory drug
PIN	Posterior interosseous nerve
PNE	Percutaneous needle electrolysis
PNT	Percutaneous needle tenotomy
PRP	Platelet-rich plasma
PrT	Prolotherapy
PUT	Percutaneous ultrasonic tenotomy
RTL	Radiofrequency thermal lesioning

A. Schroeder (✉)
Department of Physical Medicine and Rehabilitation, University of Pittsburgh, Pittsburgh, PA, USA
e-mail: schroederan@upmc.edu

K. Onishi
Department of Physical Medicine and Rehabilitation, Department of Orthopedic Surgery, University of Pittsburgh, Pittsburgh, PA, USA

Department of Orthopedic Surgery, University of Pittsburgh, Pittsburgh, PA, USA
e-mail: onishik2@upmc.edu

S. Joshua Szabo
Department of Orthopedic Surgery, University of Pittsburgh, Pittsburgh, PA, USA

Introduction

Common extensor tendon (CET) tendinopathy was initially described in 1873 and is commonly referred to as tennis elbow or lateral epicondylitis [1]. However, the most pathophysiologically accurate terminology, CET tendinopathy, will be used in this chapter [2, 3]. CET tendinopathy is the second most frequent orthopedic diagnosis of the upper limb and affects 1–3% of the general population [3, 4]. CET tendinopathy affects both genders equally and it is most common in the fourth to fifth decades of life [4]. The dominant extremity is more commonly affected, and it is far more common to have an insidious onset, although traumatic cases have also been reported [5, 6]. CET ruptures are reported rarely in case reports in the literature [7, 8].

Common flexor-pronator tendon (CFPT) tendinopathy is commonly referred to as "golfer's elbow," medial epicondylitis, and medial epicondylosis. CFPT tendinopathy has a prevalence of 0.4% in the general population with CET tendinopathy being diagnosed four to ten times more often [4, 9, 10]. Like CET tendinopathy, it is also a disease of the middle aged with repetitive stress presumed to be the major cause [9, 11]. Rupture of the CFPT is also extremely rare [12, 13].

© Springer Nature Switzerland AG 2021
K. Onishi et al. (eds.), *Tendinopathy*, https://doi.org/10.1007/978-3-030-65335-4_5

Anatomy

CET tendinopathy is most commonly caused by repetitive contraction and microtearing of the wrist extensors that originate from the lateral epicondyle [2, 14, 15]. Because of the unique anatomic location of the tendons and proximity to the capitellum, the extensor carpi radialis brevis (ECRB) and extensor digitorium communius (EDC) are believed to be the most commonly affected tendons, as they are subject to additional stress when compressed by the contracting extensor carpi radialis longus and they rub across the capitellum with elbow extension [2, 14, 15]. CET tendinopathy is histologically associated with angiofibroblastic changes and characterized by granulation tissue formation [16]. (See Chapters 1 and 2 on the pathophysiology of overuse tendon injuries.)

For CFPT tendinopathy, the pronator teres and flexor carpi radialis attach to the anterior aspect of the medial epicondyle and are most commonly injured [17] (Fig. 5.6). Histological change most commonly associated with CFPT tendinopathy is similar to that of CET tendinopathy. The flexor-pronator group is an important dynamic stabilizer at the medial elbow [18, 19].

Common Extensor Tendon (CET) Tendinopathy

A 37-year-old male construction worker with diabetes and a 15 pack year history of smoking presents with 4 months of progressive, focal left lateral elbow pain over the lateral epicondyle. He does not recall trauma or injury and he denies any sensory alteration. His discomfort is exacerbated by turning door knobs and opening jars. He has focal tenderness on palpation at the lateral epicondyle. Exam was positive for Cozen's, Maudsley's, and Chair tests. There is no reproduction of pain with resisted biceps activation.

Clinical Presentation

CET tendinopathy presents with focal pain over the lateral epicondyle, 1–2 cm distal to the lateral epicondyle (Fig. 5.1) [20, 21]. Pain is usually atraumatic, of insidious onset, and aggravated by resisted wrist extension and passive wrist flexion [22]. CET tendinopathy can be rarely due to traumatic blows to the tendon, resulting in either partial or complete tear and has a worse presentation, often requiring surgery.

A thorough, but focused, history should be conducted based on Table 5.1. Clinical assessment of severity is important, as a more aggressive management plan may be employed if symptoms are interfering with function and activities of daily living. The clinician must also elicit information to evaluate other possible causes of lateral elbow pain that can mimic CET tendinopathy (Table 5.2). Typically, neurological deficits, elbow instability/laxity, and mechanical symptoms such as popping or clicking argue against a primary diagnosis of CET tendinopathy [23, 24].

Those who engage in manual labor are at a particularly high risk, particularly those who perform over 1 hour per day of repetitive wrist extension and flexion [20]. In butchers and fish processing

Fig. 5.1 Anatomy of the extensor muscles of the forearm. Note origin on or near the lateral epicondyle of the humerus, the site of pain in common extensor tendinopathy at the elbow

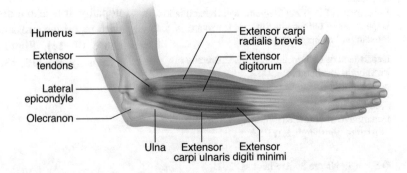

Table 5.1 History and physical exam for tendinopathy at the elbow

History: OPQRST mnemonic		Physical Exam: I PROMISE mnemonic	
O: Onset Occupation	"When did the pain start?" "What were you doing when you first noticed the pain?" "What do you do for work? (Unique movements? Ergonomics? Equipment used?)" "Has there been a change in your work or hobbies in the few months prior to onset of pain?" "Which is your dominant hand?"	**I:** Inspection	Swelling Ecchymosis Scars Carrying angle (normal is ~7° for males and ~13° for females)
P: Palliative factors Provocative factors	"What makes the pain better?" "What makes the pain worse?"	**P:** Palpation	Lateral epicondyle Medial epicondyle Olecranon process/triceps tendon Radial tuberosity/biceps tendon
Q: Quality of pain	"How would you describe the pain?" "Is there locking, popping, or clicking?"	**ROM:** Range of motion	Active and passive ROM at the elbow, neck, shoulder, wrist Normal elbow ROM: −0–150° extension/flexion −50° supination −50° pronation Compare to contralateral side
R: Radiation	"Does the pain move or radiate?"	**I:** Innervation (neurological exam)	Myotomal strength exam of upper extremity Dermatomal sensory exam of upper extremity Cervical spine exam
S: Severity Sports-related history	"What is the pain on a scale of 1/10 now and at its worst?" "Do you have pain with daily activities?" "What do you do for fun/exercise/sport?"	**SE:** Special exam	Cozen's test Maudsley's test Chair test Mill's test
T: Timing Treatments previously rendered? Tobacco use	"When do you feel the pain?" "At what time of day is the pain worst?" "Is the pain constant?" "What treatments have you tried? Were they helpful?" "Do you currently use tobacco products?"		Valgus and varus stress O'Driscol test Resisted wrist pronation/supination and flexion Tinel's test over cubital tunnel Milking test

workers the incidence rate is as high as 15% [25]. With increasing use of computers in recent years, typing has also been reported as a risk factor [26]. Both smoking and chronic hyperglycemia have been implicated as risk factors for CET tendinopathy [26, 27]. In racquet sports, such as tennis, the incidence of CET tendinopathy is significantly higher in novice players and those who use a one-handed backhand stroke, likely resulting from poor technique/conditioning and increased tendon loading with prolonged eccentric contraction, respectively [28, 29]. Wrist-neutral hits are believed to be safer than wrist-driven movements.

Off-center hits with the racquet, a strong grip strength, and high string tension are some of the factors that predispose racquet sports players to CET [30, 31]. Common belief is that proper grip size and use of a string vibration damper the risk for CET in racquet sports players, but this has not been completely established [32, 33].

Physical Examination

CET tendinopathy examination should be conducted in a systematic fashion as outlined in

Table 5.2 Differential diagnosis of atraumatic CET

Differential diagnosis	Key facts
Radial tunnel syndrome/posterior interosseous neuritis	Compression of the posterior interosseous nerve (usually in the Arcade of Frosche).
	Diffuse aching pain over wrist extensor muscles and positive Maudsley's test. Pain may radiate to the dorsal hand or may be sharp and shooting along the dorsal forearm and may be increased by resisted supination or nerve palpation. Rarely has associated sensory/motor changes.
	Pain worsened by wearing a counterforce brace of the forearm.
	Radial nerve lidocaine injection can be diagnostic if it results in pain relief.
	Electromyography is often inconclusive. Ultrasound may show thickening of the nerve.
Distal biceps tendinopathy	Tendinopathy of the biceps tendon just proximal to or at its insertion on the radial tuberosity.
	Pain in the antecubital region that is exacerbated by resisted supination.
	Tenderness tends to be more medial and anterior to that experienced in CET.
	X-rays are often inconclusive. MRI is preferred.
Osteochondritis dissecans	Osteochondritis of subchondral bone at a localized lesion (most common site in the elbow is the capitellium).
	Pain is often dull and poorly localized to the lateral elbow. May be associated with decreased ROM and locking/catching in more advanced disease.
	More frequently seen in adolescents and is often without point tenderness compared to CET.
	Diagnosed with plain radiographs followed by MRI if necessary.
Lateral ulnar collateral ligament instability (posterior lateral elbow rotary instability)	Injury to the lateral ulnar collateral ligament (most commonly traumatic).
	Pain in terminal elbow extension (i.e., when pushing up out of a chair). Mechanical symptoms are present. Patient often has difficulty performing ADLs.
	Pain is only in terminal elbow extension and pain is not worsened with resisted wrist extension as in CET, but these injuries may coexist.
	X-rays are often inconclusive; MRI with arthrogram is preferable.
Posterior lateral elbow plica (lateral synovial fringe)	Plica are hypertrophic synovial folds
	Symptoms include aching, stiffness, intermittent loss of motion, and catching at the elbow, but it often presents as CET that fails conservative management.
	Site of tenderness is posterior to the lateral epicondyle and centered at the posterior radiocapitellar joint (as seen in CET).
	Diagnosis is made with arthroscopy as these lesions are often missed on MRI.
Radiocapitellar osteoarthrosis	Loss of cartilage, thickening of subchondral bone, and synovitis.
	Resting joint pain and stiffness that feels deep with restricted ROM with pronation/supination.
	Tenderness may be vague and often elicited with radiocapitellar compression testing.
	X-ray is diagnostic.
Cervical radiculopathy	Compression of the nerve root as it exits the spinal canal (C5/C6 lesions are commonly mistaken for CET).
	Radiation of pain from the cervical spine that is reproduced by palpation of the cervical spine or Spurling's maneuver. Focal motor, reflex, or sensory changes associated with the affected nerve will be seen.
	Sensory changes and neuropathic pain may also be present (which are absent in CET).
	Diagnosis is clinical and MRI is the imaging study of choice.

CET common extensor tendinopathy; *ROM* range of motion; *MRI* magnetic resonance imaging

Table 5.1. In typical CET tendinopathy, one will not notice swelling or ecchymosis, and inspection is usually unremarkable. With palpation, tenderness is elicited at the lateral epicondyle or within 1–2 cm distal to it. Elbow range of motion is normal; however, end-range wrist flexion may elicit pain at the lateral epicondyle. Neurological examination should begin at the neck and should include assessment of alteration in myotomal strength and dermatomal sensation.

• Special examination should include resisted wrist extension with the elbow in full extension and the forearm in pronation with radial deviation of the wrist (Cozen's test; Fig. 5.2). The amount of pain and/or weakness can provide insight into the extent of tendinopathy. Chair test is performed by asking patients to attempt to lift a chair by using a three-finger pinch (Fig. 5.3). Resisted middle-finger test (Maudsley's test) is also used to assess CET

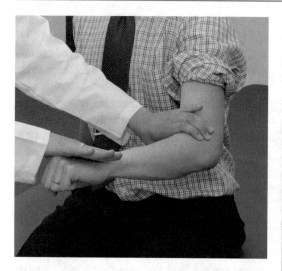

Fig. 5.2 Cozen's test. Cozen's test is performed by having the patient place the elbow in full extension with the forearm in pronation and the wrist radially deviated; the examiner then resists wrist extension

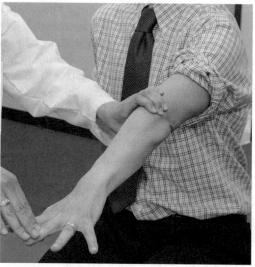

Fig. 5.4 Maudsley's test. Maudsley's test is also known as the resisted middle finger test where the patient attempts to extend the middle finger against the resistance of the examiner. Of note, this is also often positive in radial tunnel syndrome and additional tests must be performed to ensure accurate diagnosis

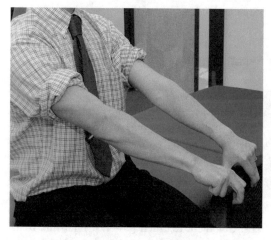

Fig. 5.3 Chair test. Chair test is performed by asking patients to attempt to lift a chair by using a three-finger pincher grasp

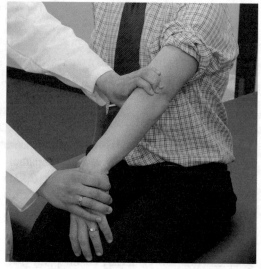

Fig. 5.5 Mill's test. Mill's test is a passive test during which the examiner palpates the lateral epicondyle while passively extending the elbow, pronating the forearm, and fully flexing the wrist

tendinopathy (Fig. 5.4). Mill's test is a passive test during which the examiner palpates the lateral epicondyle while passively extending the elbow, pronating the forearm, and fully flexing the wrist (Fig. 5.5). Physicians should keep in mind that both Maudsley's test and Mills test are often (and sometimes more commonly) positive in radial tunnel syndrome or posterior interosseous nerve (PIN) irritation

[34]. Varus stress tests should be performed to assess underlying ligamentous laxity not only to rule out radial collateral ligament complex

(radial collateral ligament, lateral ulnar collateral ligament, and annular ligament) injury but also to prognosticate CET tendinopathy, as radial collateral ligament complex injury has been associated with poor response to conservative management in patients diagnosed with CET tendinopathy [35]. This ligament can be assessed using the lateral pivot-shift test (also known as O'Driscoll test, and usually performed under anesthesia) where patients are supine with the affected arm overhead; the forearm is supinated and valgus stress is applied while flexing the elbow. The radiocapitellar compression test is used to assess osteoarthritis of the elbow radiocapitellar articulation by loading through the wrist across the elbow and supinating/pronating the forearm through various degrees of flexion. The distal biceps tendon is examined by palpation and resisted supination, and injury to this tendon can present with similar subjective complaints and may be mistaken for CET.

Diagnostic Workup

CET tendinopathy is considered a clinical diagnosis and initial imaging is not recommended but can be obtained in confounding or refractory cases.

X-Ray and MRI

X-rays can be useful if onset is traumatic or acute in order to rule out osseous and articular pathology [36]. Magnetic resonance imaging (MRI) should be reserved for patients who fail to improve or when another diagnosis is suspected based on thorough clinical evaluation. When employed, MRI has been found to have high sensitivity and specificity (83–100%) for CET tendinopathy [37]. MRI should always be interpreted in a clinical context, correlating MRI findings with patient symptoms as normal age-related degenerative changes occur in asymptomatic patients [38].

Ultrasound

Musculoskeletal ultrasound can be an affordable and accessible alternative to MRI to image soft tissue of the elbow [39]. The contralateral elbow can be imaged simultaneously to provide a control [40]. Sonographic findings indicative of CET tendinopathy include outward bowing of the tendon, presence of hypoechoic fluid adjacent to the tendon, tendon thickening, decreased tendon echogenicity, ill-defined margins of the tendon, intra-tendinous calcifications, bony irregularity at the tendon insertion site, and increased vascularity within the tendon [37, 40]. Ultrasound is operator dependent and reported sensitivity and specificity are variable. However, when used as an extension of history and physical examinations, diagnostic ultrasound can be helpful. As technology continues to advance, different ultrasound modes are aiding in diagnostic accuracy. A recent study found that real-time sonoelastography, which measures the stiffness of a target tissue, was superior to traditional 2D grayscale (i.e., "black and white" mode) or color Doppler ultrasound in discriminating tendons with CET tendinopathy [41].

Treatment

Conservative

CET tendinopathy is typically self-limiting and up to 90% of patients will recover by 1 year [42, 43]. The goal of conservative management is pain relief and progressive rehabilitation with return to previous activities. In most patients with CET tendinopathy, treatment should be multimodal and there is currently no consensus on the best treatment regimen [44–47]. First-line treatments typically include a trial of physical therapy and use of counterforce brace [44, 45]. Treatments are summarized in Table 5.3.

Physical Therapy

Physical therapy, including strengthening and stretching exercises, is a widely accepted initial treatment measure for CET tendinopathy. Modalities such as friction massage, manipulation, cryotherapy, electrical stimulation, ultrasound, and iontophoresis are frequently used to complement stretching and strengthening. While there is no consensus on proper dosage (type of exercise and volume) of physical therapy, an

Table 5.3 Treatment of tendinopathy at the elbow

First line	Second line	"New horizon" and third line
Physical therapy: Stretching[a] Strengthening[a] Modalities:[b] Friction massage Manipulation Cryotherapy Electrical stimulation Deep heat ultrasound Iontophoresis Low-level laser therapy Counterforce brace[a] Wrist brace[c] Kinesio taping[b] Non-steroidal anti-inflammatory drugs[b]	Corticosteroid injections[d] Platelet-rich plasma[a] Prolotherapy[a] Percutaneous needle tenotomy[b] Topical nitroglycerin[c] Extracorporeal shock wave therapy[b]	Botulinum toxin injections[b] Radiofrequency thermal lesioning[b] Percutaneous ultrasonic tenotomy[c] Surgery[f]

[a]Strong evidence
[b]Weak evidence
[c]Fair evidence
[d]Limited efficacy
[e]Good evidence
[f]If symptoms persist for more than 6–12 months or tendon rupture has occurred

ideal program should include use of modalities for pain control, stretching, and ROM exercises, as well as a progressive strengthening program [48–50]. The strengthening component of the program should include eccentric strengthening exercises [48–50]. Ultimately, simulated movements, particularly for athletes, should be practiced before he/she returns to sport or occupation [48–50]. In general, supervised physical therapy sessions are more effective than a home exercise program (HEP), but a HEP can still be considered in motivated patients if a busy schedule makes it difficult to attend office-based therapies [51]. Physicians are responsible for monitoring physical therapy progression at follow-up visits and details of exercise sessions should be elicited.

Elbow Bracing and Taping
A counterforce brace worn correctly (i.e., just distal to the lateral epicondyle) pretensions the common extensor tendon and is effective in the management of symptoms from CET tendinopathy [52, 53]. Extensor wrist splints have also been shown to decrease the pain associated with CET tendinopathy [54]. Kinesio taping resulted in improvement in pain, grip strength, and functional measures in patients with common flexor/pronator tendinopathy and can be used in CET tendinopathy as well [55].

Non-steroidal Anti-inflammatory Drugs (NSAIDs)
Both oral and topical non-steroidal anti-inflammatory drugs (NSAIDs) have been studied for the treatment of CET tendinopathy with inconclusive results. A short 10- to 14-day course of oral NSAIDs in the absence of contraindications such as cardiac or renal abnormalities or history of gastrointestinal bleed can be considered if pain is the patient's primary concern [56]. Topical NSAIDs, however, may be a more attractive option as they have fewer gastrointestinal side effects [57].

Topical Nitroglycerin
The use of nitroglycerin patches has been shown to significantly reduce activity-induced elbow pain with activity, reduce epicondylar tenderness, and improve functional measures and outcomes in the long term [58, 59]. However, nitroglycerin patches do have several adverse effects including headaches (which may be severe), facial flushing, and dermatitis at the contact site and their use should not be combined with phosphodiesterase inhibitors [58].

Interventional
If patients with CET tendinopathy fail to improve with first-line treatment, many clinicians will next offer non-surgical interventional treatments.

Corticosteroid Injection (CSI)
Despite recent gains in the understanding of pathophysiology of the degenerative nature of tendinopathy, corticosteroid injections (CSIs) are still commonly used to address pain associated with CET tendinopathy [60]. While CSI is known to result in reliable short-term pain and functional improvements, a randomized control investiga-

tion performed by Coombs et al. showed that CSI-treated groups fare poorly compared to the physical therapy group in the long term [25, 61–64]. Additionally, administration of greater than three CSIs at the elbow is associated with poor surgical outcomes if surgery is eventually required [65].

Platelet Rich-Plasma Injection (PRP) and Autologous Blood Injection (ABI)

Platelet-rich plasma injection (PRP) aims to restore normal mechanical properties of the injured tendon by promoting normal collagen synthesis [60] (see Chap. 20 for details on PRP). Studies have compared leukocyte-rich PRP to both corticosteroid injection and percutaneous needle tenotomy for the lateral elbow, and PRP injection appears to be superior in long-term pain control and functional improvements [66–68]. A recent retrospective investigation also shows better outcome with PRP when compared to surgical debridement [69]. Autologous blood injection (ABI) has also been tried, but it was found to be inferior to PRP in pain control and resulted in more procedure-related adverse reactions [70].

Prolotherapy Injection (PrT)

Prolotherapy injection (PrT) is an injectable treatment that involves use of irritants, most frequently dextrose, to create local inflammation. Such chemical irritation is theorized to attract inflammatory mediators and improve blood supply to the diseased tendon, resulting in remodeling of tendon and improved function and pain [71] (see Chap. 21 for details on PrT). When compared to placebo, PrT has been shown to improve both pain and function without adverse side effects for up to 4 months [72, 73]. While both PrT and PRP are currently not covered by insurance, PrT is frequently priced lower than PRP, and PrT can be considered for recalcitrant CET cases. There are no studies that identify algorithms correlating to adverse effects of PrT followed by CSIs or PRP and vice versa.

Percutaneous Needle Tenotomy (PNT)

Percutaneous needle tenotomy (PNT) is an office-based procedure where a needle is used to repeatedly fenestrate the diseased portions of tendon under sonographic guidance [74]. In a case series study, 58 subjects were treated using PNT and 80% of these subjects reported good to excellent result at an average follow-up duration of 28 months, and a subsequent corticosteroid injection was not necessary [75] (see Chap. 18 for details on PNT).

Extracorporeal Shock Wave Therapy (ESWT)

ESWT is performed using a generator that transmits sound waves that theoretically injure the disease tendon as a means of restarting the healing cascade, but results have been mixed with regards to its efficacy [76–78]. ESWT also has concerning reported side effects, including reddening of the skin, pain at the site of treatment, hematomas, migraines, and syncope [79].

Percutaneous Mechanical Procedures and Botulinum Toxin Injection

New horizon treatments for recalcitrant CET tendinopathy that can be tried prior to surgery include percutaneous ultrasonic tenotomy (PUT), ultrasound-guided radiofrequency thermal lesioning (RTL), ultrasound-guided percutaneous needle electrolysis (PNE), and botulinum toxin injections. PUT is an office-based ultrasound-guided procedure that uses ultrasonic energy to remove diseased tissue under local anesthesia. This procedure has been FDA-approved for tendinopathies including CET tendinopathy and studies show some clinical benefit as well as improvement of tendon appearance on follow-up imaging [80] (see Chap. 18 for details on PUT.) RTL works by means of heat dissipation and is a proposed treatment for recalcitrant symptoms from CET tendinopathy lasting greater than 6 months, showing improvement in both pain and function [81]. PNE consists of the application of a galvanic current through an acupuncture needle and has been shown to reduce the symptoms and degenerative structural changes of CET tendinopathy evident on ultrasound [82]. Botulinum toxin injections for CET tendinopathy have shown to improve pain, likely working by both (1) a direct analgesic effect and by (2) an induction of paralysis of muscles injected that allows for rest of the tendon [83, 84].

Operative

Surgery is typically reserved for those who do not improve with conservative therapy and have continued symptoms and disability at 6–12 months. Several surgical techniques (open, arthroscopic, and percutaneous microtenotomy) have been described for the treatment of CET tendinopathy with no differences in postoperative pain, recurrences, or failures among the different surgical techniques [85, 86]. The general surgical principle consists of first identifying the affected portion of the tendon which is excised to further facilitate a biologic response and is then usually repaired. Those undergoing arthroscopic treatment (repair/debridement) have greater functional outcomes and more rapid return to work with utilization of less postoperative physical therapy compared to those undergoing an open procedure [87, 88]. In most patients, surgery achieved "excellent" results when rated by patients or defined as return to full activity with no pain [2, 89]. Those more likely to have residual symptoms after surgery are those with a high level of baseline symptoms, acute occurrence of symptoms, or long duration of symptoms [90]. Patients typically recover in 4–12 weeks with 95% achieving good to excellent results and only about 1.5% of patients requiring surgical revision surgery, which is usually successful [65].

Common Flexor/Pronator Tendon (CFPT) Tendinopathy

A 42-year-old right-handed female avid golfer presents with a 7-month history of progressive, focal medial right elbow pain that worsens in the peak of golf season. She does not recall trauma or injury. She denies neck pain and numbness and tingling of the right upper extremity. There is tenderness to palpation over the pronator teres and flexor carpi radialis origin near the medial epicondyle and pain with resisted wrist flexion and pronation. Tinel's sign is negative over the course of the ulnar nerve.

Clinical Presentation

CFPT tendinopathy is often insidious in onset along the medial elbow and worsened by resisted forearm pronation and wrist flexion; acute trauma rarely precipitates symptoms [91]. A thorough, but focused, history should be conducted, like that for CET tendinopathy (Table 5.1). Information to evaluate other possible causes of medial elbow pain especially ulnar neuritis and ulnar collateral ligament (UCL) pathology that can mimic or coexist with CFPT tendinopathy must be elicited (Table 5.4). Twenty to twenty four percent of refractory cases of CFPT tendinopathy have been cited to have associated ulnar neuropathy and require a concomitant ulnar nerve release, with the most common site for ulnar nerve compression being found just distal to the medial epicondyle where the ulnar nerve penetrates the flexor carpi ulnaris arcade [92]. CFPT tendinopathy has been found to be associated with C6 and C7 radiculopathy since weakness of the flexor carpi radialis and pronator teres resulting from the radiculopathy allows for easy onset of CFPT tendinopathy [93].

Repetitive overloading and microtearing of the flexor-pronator mass and excessive valgus stress at the elbow are presumed to lead to CFPT. Smoking, obesity, repetitive movements, forceful activities, and concomitant upper extremity musculoskeletal disorders are associated with CFPT [4, 94]. CFPT seems to be more common among athletes, including golfers and athletes performing repetitive overhead movements (such as baseball players, tennis players, and swimmers) [95, 96].

Physical Examination

CFPT tendinopathy is associated with tenderness to palpation over the pronator teres and/or flexor carpi radialis origin at or within 5 mm of the medial epicondyle (Fig. 5.6) [97]. Resisted pronation and/or resisted wrist flexion will reproduce symptoms in most patients, with the elbow in extension. Grip strength is decreased in patients with CFPT tendinopathy, but the

Table 5.4 Differential diagnosis of CFPT

Differential diagnosis	Key features
Cubital tunnel syndrome/ulnar neuritis/ulnar nerve subluxation	Compression of the ulnar nerve just distal to the medial epicondyle where it penetrates the flexor carpi ulnaris arcade.
	Numbness and tingling of the fourth (medial side) and fifth digits and possible weakness/atrophy of interosseous muscles. Symptoms exacerbated with arm in extreme flexion. Positive Tinel test.
	Presence of neuropathic symptoms distinguishes it from CFPT.
	Diagnosed by EMG/NCS or ultrasound.
UCL insufficiency (on spectrum of little league elbow)	Sprain or tear of the ulnar collateral ligament.
	Commonly occurs in the overhead throwing athlete. Pain and mechanical symptoms are present with the elbow in terminal extension.
	Pain with valgus stress of the elbow distinguishes it from CFPT.
	Plain radiographs are often inconclusive and MRI is necessary for diagnosis.
Cervical radiculopathy	Compression of the nerve root as it exits the spinal canal (C6/C7 lesions allow for easy onset of CFPT).
	Radiation of pain from the cervical spine, reproduced by palpation of the cervical spine or Spurling's maneuver. Focal motor, reflex, or sensory changes associated with the affected nerve will be seen.
	Sensory changes and neuropathic pain in the presence of neck pain distinguish it from CFPT.
	Diagnosis is clinical and MRI is the imaging study of choice.
Osteoarthrosis	Loss of cartilage, thickening of subchondral bone, and synovitis.
	Resting joint pain and stiffness that feels deep with restricted ROM at the extremes of flexion/extension.
	It is more common in the elderly or those with prior injury to the joint.
	Tenderness will be within the joint rather than just distal to the medial epicondyle like in CFPT.
	X-ray is diagnostic.

CFPT common flexor/pronator tendinopathy, *ROM* range of motion, *MRI* magnetic resonance imaging, *EMG/NCS* electromyography/nerve conduction studies

decrease is less when compared to those with CET tendinopathy [98]. One must also evaluate the shoulder for concomitant pathologies and the neck for cervical radiculopathy and spinal stenosis. Ulnar nerve compression can mimic CFPT tendinopathy and a thorough neurological examination is imperative. Ulnar neuritis can be identified by a positive Tinel sign along the course of the ulnar nerve or a positive elbow Phalen's text. One should also evaluate the subluxation of the nerve, which occurs in 16% of the population, but is often asymptomatic [99]. Ulnar collateral ligament (UCL) injury is identified by pain with valgus stress when the elbow is in 60, 90, or 120 degrees of flexion or a positive milking test (pull on the thumb with the elbow flexed to 90 degrees and the forearm supinated) [99]. Tenderness of the medial UCL is usually found more posterior than the insertion of the flexor-pronator mass.

Diagnostic Workup

X-Ray and MRI

As with CET tendinopathy, in CFPT tendinopathy, initial imaging is not indicated but can be obtained in confounding or refractory cases. Radiographs often appear negative, but they may show calcification adjacent to the medial epicondyle with traction spurs [100]. On MRI, tendinosis is indicated by tendon thickening and increased signal intensity on any sequence [37, 101]. The presence of high T2 signal intensity within the common flexor tendon and the presence of soft tissue edema were found to be the most specific findings of CFPT tendinopathy on MRI [102]. MRI can be used to evaluate surrounding structures including ulnar neuritis (thickened nerve with increased signal on T2-weighted images just distal to the cubital tunnel) and UCL sprain (high signal intensity in

Fig. 5.6 Anatomy of
the flexor muscles of the
forearm. Note origin on
or near the medial
epicondyle of the
humerus, the site of pain
in common flexor
tendinopathy at the
elbow

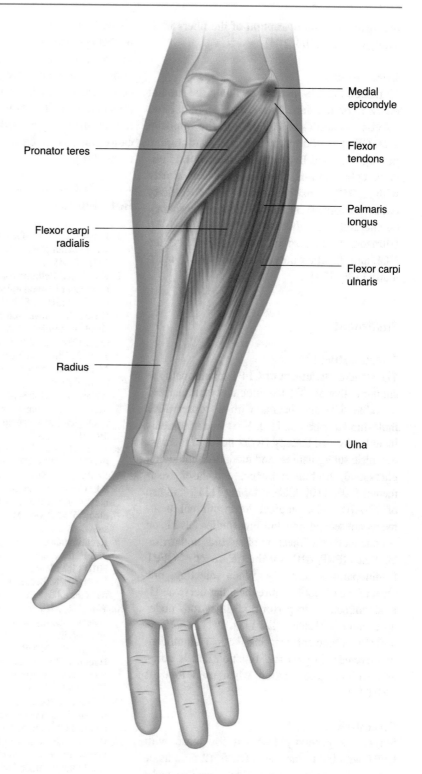

the ligament, with disruption of the fibers indicating rupture) [103, 104].

Ultrasound

Ultrasound can be used to evaluate the medial elbow in both a static and dynamic manner and affords the ability to compare to the opposite side. CFPT tendinopathy displays sonographic findings of focal hypoechoic areas, intratendinous calcifications, and cortical irregularity with a 95% sensitivity and 92% specificity (when performed by an experienced operator), comparable to that of MRI [37, 105]. Ultrasound can also be used to evaluate the UCL and the ulnar nerve statically and dynamically [106–108].

Treatment

Conservative

The standard treatment of CFPT tendinopathy is similar to that of CET tendinopathy (summarized in Table 5.3) and begins with a conservative multi-modal approach [17]. First-line treatments include physical therapy (wrist flexor stretching, eccentric strengthening, and modalities including ultrasound, friction massage, and laser treatments) [109, 110], kinesio taping [111], and use of NSAIDs. Non-surgical interventional treatments are second line, but few studies have been conducted on the injection of steroids and orthobiologics (PRP, ABI) for the treatment of CFPT tendinopathy specifically. When injecting, one must take care not to injure the ulnar nerve and it is recommended to perform all injections under ultrasound guidance [112, 113]. PUT is a "new horizon" treatment that has shown significant improvement in pain and function and is quick and without complication when used to treat CFPT [114].

Operative

Surgery is generally reserved for those with CFPT who fail to improve after 6–12 months of conservative management. Open surgical technique is preferred, with excision and debridement of affected tissue, decortication of the medial epicondyle, and repair of the tendon back to the medial epicondyle [115]. Arthroscopic technique has been historically avoided due to the risk of injury to the ulnar nerve [17]. Recently, percutaneous radiofrequency-based microtenotomy to treat chronic CFPT showed significant long-term improvement in pain without significant complications and is an emerging, less invasive treatment [116].

References

1. Runge F. Zur Gênese and behandlung des schreibekrampfes. Berliner Klin Wchnschr. 1873;10:245–8.
2. Nirschl RP, Pettrone FA. Tennis elbow. The surgical treatment of lateral epicondylitis. J Bone Joint Surg Am. 1979;61(6a):832–9.
3. Nirschl RP. Prevention and treatment of elbow and shoulder injuries in the tennis player. Clin Sports Med. 1988;7(2):289–308.
4. Shiri R, Viikari-Juntura E, Varonen H, Heliovaara M. Prevalence and determinants of lateral and medial epicondylitis: a population study. Am J Epidemiol. 2006;164(11):1065–74.
5. Verhaar JA. Tennis elbow. Anatomical, epidemiological and therapeutic aspects. Int Orthop. 1994;18(5):263–7.
6. Scher DL, Wolf JM, Owens BD. Lateral epicondylitis. Orthopedics. 2009;32(4):0147–7447.
7. Smith AG, Kosygan K, Williams H, Newman RJ. Common extensor tendon rupture following corticosteroid injection for lateral tendinosis of the elbow. Br J Sports Med. 1999;33(6):423–4; discussion 4–5.
8. Kachrimanis G, Papadopoulou O. Acute partial rupture of the common extensor tendon. J Ultrasound. 2010;13(2):74–5.
9. Leach RE, Miller JK. Lateral and medial epicondylitis of the elbow. Clin Sports Med. 1987;6(2):259–72.
10. Wolf JM, Mountcastle S, Burks R, Sturdivant RX, Owens BD. Epidemiology of lateral and medial epicondylitis in a military population. Mil Med. 2010;175(5):336–9.
11. Hamilton PG. The prevalence of humeral epicondylitis: a survey in general practice. J R Coll Gen Pract. 1986;36(291):464–5.
12. Allred DW, Rayan GM. Flexor carpi radialis tendon rupture following chronic wrist osteoarthritis: a case report. J Okla State Med Assoc. 2003;96(5):211–2.
13. Polatsch DB, Foster LG, Posner MA. An unusual rupture of the flexor carpi radialis tendon: a case report. Am J Orthop (Belle Mead NJ). 2006;35(3):141–3.
14. Bunata RE, Brown DS, Capelo R. Anatomic factors related to the cause of tennis elbow. J Bone Joint Surg Am. 2007;89(9):1955–63.

15. Kraushaar BS, Nirschl RP. Tendinosis of the elbow (tennis elbow). Clinical features and findings of histological, immunohistochemical, and electron microscopy studies. J Bone Joint Surg Am. 1999;81(2):259–78.

16. Goldie I. Epicondylitis lateralis humeri (epicondylalgia or tennis elbow). A pathogenetical study. Acta Chir Scand Suppl. 1964;57(Suppl 339):1+.

17. Ciccotti MG, Ramani MN. Medial epicondylitis. Tech Hand Up Extrem Surg. 2003;7(4):190–6.

18. Seiber K, Gupta R, McGarry MH, Safran MR, Lee TQ. The role of the elbow musculature, forearm rotation, and elbow flexion in elbow stability: an in vitro study. J Shoulder Elb Surg. 2009;18(2):260–8.

19. Glousman RE, Barron J, Jobe FW, Perry J, Pink M. An electromyographic analysis of the elbow in normal and injured pitchers with medial collateral ligament insufficiency. Am J Sports Med. 1992;20(3):311–7.

20. Fernandez-Carnero J, Binderup AT, Ge HY, Fernandez-de-las-Penas C, Arendt-Nielsen L, Madeleine P. Pressure pain sensitivity mapping in experimentally induced lateral epicondylalgia. Med Sci Sports Exerc. 2010;42(5):922–7.

21. Ruiz-Ruiz B, Fernandez-de-Las-Penas C, Ortega-Santiago R, Arendt-Nielsen L, Madeleine P. Topographical pressure and thermal pain sensitivity mapping in patients with unilateral lateral epicondylalgia. J Pain. 2011;12(10):1040–8.

22. Orchard J, Kountouris A. The management of tennis elbow. BMJ. 2011;342:d2687.

23. Naam NH, Nemani S. Radial tunnel syndrome. Orthop Clin North Am. 2012;43(4):529–36.

24. Ferdinand BD, Rosenberg ZS, Schweitzer ME, Stuchin SA, Jazrawi LM, Lenzo SR, et al. MR imaging features of radial tunnel syndrome: initial experience. Radiology. 2006;240(1):161–8.

25. Bisset L, Beller E, Jull G, Brooks P, Darnell R, Vicenzino B. Mobilisation with movement and exercise, corticosteroid injection, or wait and see for tennis elbow: randomised trial. BMJ. 2006;333(7575):939.

26. Shiri R, Viikari-Juntura E. Lateral and medial epicondylitis: role of occupational factors. Best Pract Res Clin Rheumatol. 2011;25(1):43–57.

27. Otoshi K, Takegami M, Sekiguchi M, Onishi Y, Yamazaki S, Otani K, et al. Chronic hyperglycemia increases the risk of lateral epicondylitis: the Locomotive Syndrome and Health Outcome in Aizu Cohort Study (LOHAS). Springerplus. 2015;4:407.

28. De Smedt T, de Jong A, Van Leemput W, Lieven D, Van Glabbeek F. Lateral epicondylitis in tennis: update on aetiology, biomechanics and treatment. Br J Sports Med. 2007;41(11):816–9.

29. Giangarra CE, Conroy B, Jobe FW, Pink M, Perry J. Electromyographic and cinematographic analysis of elbow function in tennis players using single- and double-handed backhand strokes. Am J Sports Med. 1993;21(3):394–9.

30. King MA, Kentel BB, Mitchell SR. The effects of ball impact location and grip tightness on the arm, racquet and ball for one-handed tennis backhand groundstrokes. J Biomech. 2012;45(6):1048–52.

31. Mohandhas BR, Makaram N, Drew TS, Wang W, Arnold GP, Abboud RJ. Racquet string tension directly affects force experienced at the elbow: implications for the development of lateral epicondylitis in tennis players. Shoulder Elbow. 2016;8(3):184–91.

32. Hatch GF 3rd, Pink MM, Mohr KJ, Sethi PM, Jobe FW. The effect of tennis racket grip size on forearm muscle firing patterns. Am J Sports Med. 2006;34(12):1977–83.

33. Hatze H. The effectiveness of grip bands in reducing racquet vibration transfer and slipping. Med Sci Sports Exerc. 1992;24(2):226–30.

34. Mills GP. The treatment of "tennis elbow.". Br Med J. 1928;1(3496):12–3.

35. Clarke AW, Ahmad M, Curtis M, Connell DA. Lateral elbow tendinopathy: correlation of ultrasound findings with pain and functional disability. Am J Sports Med. 2010;38(6):1209–14.

36. Pomerance J. Radiographic analysis of lateral epicondylitis. J Shoulder Elb Surg. 2002;11(2):156–7.

37. Miller TT, Shapiro MA, Schultz E, Kalish PE. Comparison of sonography and MRI for diagnosing epicondylitis. J Clin Ultrasound. 2002;30(4):193–202.

38. Milz S, Tischer T, Buettner A, Schieker M, Maier M, Redman S, et al. Molecular composition and pathology of entheses on the medial and lateral epicondyles of the humerus: a structural basis for epicondylitis. Ann Rheum Dis. 2004;63(9):1015–21.

39. Levin D, Nazarian LN, Miller TT, O'Kane PL, Feld RI, Parker L, et al. Lateral epicondylitis of the elbow: US findings. Radiology. 2005;237(1):230–4.

40. Konin GP, Nazarian LN, Walz DM. US of the elbow: indications, technique, normal anatomy, and pathologic conditions. Radiographics. 2013;33(4):E125–47.

41. Kocyigit F, Kuyucu E, Kocyigit A, Herek DT, Savkin R, Aslan UB, et al. Association of real-time sonoelastography findings with clinical parameters in lateral epicondylitis. Rheumatol Int. 2016;36(1):91–100.

42. Binder AI, Hazleman BL. Lateral humeral epicondylitis--a study of natural history and the effect of conservative therapy. Br J Rheumatol. 1983;22(2):73–6.

43. Coonrad RW, Hooper WR. Tennis elbow: its course, natural history, conservative and surgical management. J Bone Joint Surg Am. 1973;55(6):1177–82.

44. Sims SE, Miller K, Elfar JC, Hammert WC. Nonsurgical treatment of lateral epicondylitis: a systematic review of randomized controlled trials. Hand (N Y). 2014;9(4):419–46.

45. Bisset L, Paungmali A, Vicenzino B, Beller E. A systematic review and meta-analysis of clinical trials on physical interventions for lateral epicondylalgia. Br J Sports Med. 2005;39(7):411–22; discussion –22.

46. Struijs PA, Kerkhoffs GM, Assendelft WJ, Van Dijk CN. Conservative treatment of lateral epicondylitis: brace versus physical therapy or a combination of both-a randomized clinical trial. Am J Sports Med. 2004;32(2):462–9.

47. Luginbuhl R, Brunner F, Schneeberger AG. No effect of forearm band and extensor strengthening exercises for the treatment of tennis elbow: a prospective randomised study. Chir Organi Mov. 2008;91(1):35–40.

48. Martinez-Silvestrini JA, Newcomer KL, Gay RE, Schaefer MP, Kortebein P, Arendt KW. Chronic lateral epicondylitis: comparative effectiveness of a home exercise program including stretching alone versus stretching supplemented with eccentric or concentric strengthening. J Hand Ther. 2005;18(4):411–9. quiz 20

49. Tyler TF, Thomas GC, Nicholas SJ, McHugh MP. Addition of isolated wrist extensor eccentric exercise to standard treatment for chronic lateral epicondylosis: a prospective randomized trial. J Shoulder Elb Surg. 2010;19(6):917–22.

50. Svernlov B, Adolfsson L. Non-operative treatment regime including eccentric training for lateral humeral epicondylalgia. Scand J Med Sci Sports. 2001;11(6):328–34.

51. Stasinopoulos D, Stasinopoulos I, Pantelis M, Stasinopoulou K. Comparison of effects of a home exercise programme and a supervised exercise programme for the management of lateral elbow tendinopathy. Br J Sports Med. 2010;44(8):579–83.

52. Jafarian FS, Demneh ES, Tyson SF. The immediate effect of orthotic management on grip strength of patients with lateral epicondylosis. J Orthop Sports Phys Ther. 2009;39(6):484–9.

53. Snyder-Mackler L, Epler M. Effect of standard and Aircast tennis elbow bands on integrated electromyography of forearm extensor musculature proximal to the bands. Am J Sports Med. 1989;17(2):278–81.

54. Garg R, Adamson GJ, Dawson PA, Shankwiler JA, Pink MM. A prospective randomized study comparing a forearm strap brace versus a wrist splint for the treatment of lateral epicondylitis. J Shoulder Elb Surg. 2010;19(4):508–12.

55. Dilek B, Batmaz I, Sariyildiz MA, Sahin E, Ilter L, Gulbahar S, et al. Kinesio taping in patients with lateral epicondylitis. J Back Musculoskelet Rehabil. 2016;29(4):853–8.

56. Labelle H, Guibert R, Joncas J, Newman N, Fallaha M, Rivard CH. Lack of scientific evidence for the treatment of lateral epicondylitis of the elbow. An attempted meta-analysis. J Bone Joint Surg. 1992;74(5):646–51.

57. Burnham R, Gregg R, Healy P, Steadward R. The effectiveness of topical diclofenac for lateral epicondylitis. Clin J Sport Med. 1998;8(2):78–81.

58. Paoloni JA, Appleyard RC, Nelson J, Murrell GA. Topical nitric oxide application in the treatment of chronic extensor tendinosis at the elbow: a ran-

59. McCallum SD, Paoloni JA, Murrell GA. Five-year prospective comparison study of topical glyceryl trinitrate treatment of chronic lateral epicondylosis at the elbow. Br J Sports Med. 2011;45(5):416–20.

60. Chen J, Wang A, Xu J, Zheng M. In chronic lateral epicondylitis, apoptosis and autophagic cell death occur in the extensor carpi radialis brevis tendon. J Shoulder Elb Surg. 2010;19(3):355–62.

61. Tonks JH, Pai SK, Murali SR. Steroid injection therapy is the best conservative treatment for lateral epicondylitis: a prospective randomised controlled trial. Int J Clin Pract. 2007;61(2):240–6.

62. Smidt N, van der Windt DA, Assendelft WJ, Deville WL, Korthals-de Bos IB, Bouter LM. Corticosteroid injections, physiotherapy, or a wait-and-see policy for lateral epicondylitis: a randomised controlled trial. Lancet. 2002;359(9307):657–62.

63. Claessen FM, Heesters BA, Chan JJ, Kachooei AR, Ring D. A meta-analysis of the effect of corticosteroid injection for enthesopathy of the extensor carpi radialis brevis origin. J Hand Surg. 2016;41(10):988–98.e2.

64. Coombes BK, Bisset L, Brooks P, Khan A, Vicenzino B. Effect of corticosteroid injection, physiotherapy, or both on clinical outcomes in patients with unilateral lateral epicondylalgia: a randomized controlled trial. JAMA. 2013;309(5):461–9.

65. Degen RM, Cancienne JM, Camp CL, Altchek DW, Dines JS, Werner BC. Three or more preoperative injections is the most significant risk factor for revision surgery after operative treatment of lateral epicondylitis: an analysis of 3863 patients. J Shoulder Elb Surg. 2017;26(4):704–9.

66. Mishra AK, Skrepnik NV, Edwards SG, Jones GL, Sampson S, Vermillion DA, et al. Efficacy of platelet-rich plasma for chronic tennis elbow: a double-blind, prospective, multicenter, randomized controlled trial of 230 patients. Am J Sports Med. 2014;42(2):463–71.

67. Thanasas C, Papadimitriou G, Charalambidis C, Paraskevopoulos I, Papanikolaou A. Platelet-rich plasma versus autologous whole blood for the treatment of chronic lateral elbow epicondylitis: a randomized controlled clinical trial. Am J Sports Med. 2011;39(10):2130–4.

68. Gosens T, Peerbooms JC, van Laar W, den Oudsten BL. Ongoing positive effect of platelet-rich plasma versus corticosteroid injection in lateral epicondylitis: a double-blind randomized controlled trial with 2-year follow-up. Am J Sports Med. 2011;39(6):1200–8.

69. Karaduman M, Okkaoglu MC, Sesen H, Taskesen A, Ozdemir M, Altay M. Platelet-rich plasma versus open surgical release in chronic tennis elbow: a retrospective comparative study. J Orthop. 2016;13(1):10–4.

70. Arirachakaran A, Sukthuayat A, Sisayanarane T, Laoratanavoraphong S, Kanchanatawan W, Kongtharvonskul J. Platelet-rich plasma versus autologous blood versus steroid injection in lateral epicondylitis: systematic review and network meta-analysis. J Orthop Traumatol. 2016;17(2):101–12.

71. Rabago D, Slattengren A, Zgierska A. Prolotherapy in primary care practice. Prim Care. 2010;37(1):65–80.

72. Scarpone M, Rabago DP, Zgierska A, Arbogast G, Snell E. The efficacy of prolotherapy for lateral epicondylosis: a pilot study. Clin J Sport Med. 2008;18(3):248–54.

73. Rabago D, Lee KS, Ryan M, Chourasia AO, Sesto ME, Zgierska A, et al. Hypertonic dextrose and morrhuate sodium injections (prolotherapy) for lateral epicondylosis (tennis elbow): results of a single-blind, pilot-level, randomized controlled trial. Am J Phys Med Rehabil. 2013;92(7):587–96.

74. McShane JM, Nazarian LN, Harwood MI. Sonographically guided percutaneous needle tenotomy for treatment of common extensor tendinosis in the elbow. J Ultrasound Med. 2006;25(10):1281–9.

75. McShane JM, Shah VN, Nazarian LN. Sonographically guided percutaneous needle tenotomy for treatment of common extensor tendinosis in the elbow: is a corticosteroid necessary? J Ultrasound Med. 2008;27(8):1137–44.

76. Pettrone FA, McCall BR. Extracorporeal shock wave therapy without local anesthesia for chronic lateral epicondylitis. J Bone Joint Surg Am. 2005;87(6):1297–304.

77. Rompe JD, Decking J, Schoellner C, Theis C. Repetitive low-energy shock wave treatment for chronic lateral epicondylitis in tennis players. Am J Sports Med. 2004;32(3):734–43.

78. Melegati G, Tornese D, Bandi M, Rubini M. Comparison of two ultrasonographic localization techniques for the treatment of lateral epicondylitis with extracorporeal shock wave therapy: a randomized study. Clin Rehabil. 2004;18(4):366–70.

79. Haake M, Boddeker IR, Decker T, Buch M, Vogel M, Labek G, et al. Side-effects of extracorporeal shock wave therapy (ESWT) in the treatment of tennis elbow. Arch Orthop Trauma Surg. 2002;122(4):222–8.

80. Barnes DE. Ultrasonic energy in tendon treatment. Oper Tech Orthop. 2013;23:78–83.

81. Lin CL, Lee JS, Su WR, Kuo LC, Tai TW, Jou IM. Clinical and ultrasonographic results of ultrasonographically guided percutaneous radiofrequency lesioning in the treatment of recalcitrant lateral epicondylitis. Am J Sports Med. 2011;39(11):2429–35.

82. Valera-Garrido F, Minaya-Munoz F, Medina-Mirapeix F. Ultrasound-guided percutaneous needle electrolysis in chronic lateral epicondylitis: short-term and long-term results. Acupunct Med. 2014;32(6):446–54.

83. Kalichman L, Bannuru RR, Severin M, Harvey W. Injection of botulinum toxin for treatment of chronic lateral epicondylitis: systematic review and meta-analysis. Semin Arthritis Rheum. 2011;40(6):532–8.

84. Placzek R, Drescher W, Deuretzbacher G, Hempfing A, Meiss AL. Treatment of chronic radial epicondylitis with botulinum toxin A. A double-blind, placebo-controlled, randomized multicenter study. J Bone Joint Surg Am. 2007;89(2):255–60.

85. Szabo SJ, Savoie FH 3rd, Field LD, Ramsey JR, Hosemann CD. Tendinosis of the extensor carpi radialis brevis: an evaluation of three methods of operative treatment. J Shoulder Elb Surg. 2006;15(6):721–7.

86. Gregory BP, Wysocki RW, Cohen MS. Controversies in surgical management of recalcitrant enthesopathy of the extensor carpi radialis brevis. J Hand Surg Am. 2016;41(8):856–9.

87. Solheim E, Hegna J, Oyen J. Arthroscopic versus open tennis elbow release: 3- to 6-year results of a case-control series of 305 elbows. Arthroscopy. 2013;29(5):854–9.

88. Peart RE, Strickler SS, Schweitzer KM Jr. Lateral epicondylitis: a comparative study of open and arthroscopic lateral release. Am J Orthop. 2004;33(11):565–7.

89. Coleman B, Quinlan JF, Matheson JA. Surgical treatment for lateral epicondylitis: a long-term follow-up of results. J Shoulder Elb Surg. 2010;19(3):363–7.

90. Solheim E, Hegna J, Oyen J. Extensor tendon release in tennis elbow: results and prognostic factors in 80 elbows. Knee Surg Sports Traumatol Arthrosco. 2011;19(6):1023–7.

91. Ciccotti MG, Charlton WP. Epicondylitis in the athlete. Clin Sports Med. 2001;20(1):77–93.

92. Vangsness CT Jr, Jobe FW. Surgical treatment of medial epicondylitis. Results in 35 elbows. J Bone Joint Surg. 1991;73(3):409–11.

93. Lee AT, Lee-Robinson AL. The prevalence of medial epicondylitis among patients with c6 and c7 radiculopathy. Sports Health. 2010;2(4):334–6.

94. Descatha A, Leclerc A, Chastang JF, Roquelaure Y. Medial epicondylitis in occupational settings: prevalence, incidence and associated risk factors. J Occup Environ Med. 2003;45(9):993–1001.

95. Grana W. Medial epicondylitis and cubital tunnel syndrome in the throwing athlete. Clin Sports Med. 2001;20(3):541–8.

96. Chen FS, Rokito AS, Jobe FW. Medial elbow problems in the overhead-throwing athlete. J Am Acad Orthop Surg. 2001;9(2):99–113.

97. Bennett JB. Lateral and medial epicondylitis. Hand Clin. 1994;10(1):157–63.

98. Pienimaki TT, Siira PT, Vanharanta H. Chronic medial and lateral epicondylitis: a comparison of pain, disability, and function. Arch Phys Med Rehabil. 2002;83(3):317–21.

99. Safran M, Ahmad CS, Elattrache NS. Ulnar collateral ligament of the elbow. Arthroscopy. 2005;21(11):1381–95.

100. Ciccotti MC, Schwartz MA, Ciccotti MG. Diagnosis and treatment of medial epicondylitis of the elbow. Clin Sports Med. 2004;23(4):693–705. xi

101. Martin CE, Schweitzer ME. MR imaging of epicondylitis. Skelet Radiol. 1998;27(3):133–8.

102. Kijowski R, De Smet AA. Magnetic resonance imaging findings in patients with medial epicondylitis. Skelet Radiol. 2005;34(4):196–202.

103. Andreisek G, Crook DW, Burg D, Marincek B, Weishaupt D. Peripheral neuropathies of the median, radial, and ulnar nerves: MR imaging features. Radiographics. 2006;26(5):1267–87.

104. Walz DM, Newman JS, Konin GP, Ross G. Epicondylitis: pathogenesis, imaging, and treatment. Radiographics. 2010;30(1):167–84.

105. Park GY, Lee SM, Lee MY. Diagnostic value of ultrasonography for clinical medial epicondylitis. Arch Phys Med Rehabil. 2008;89(4):738–42.

106. Miller TT, Adler RS, Friedman L. Sonography of injury of the ulnar collateral ligament of the elbow-initial experience. Skelet Radiol. 2004;33(7):386–91.

107. Beekman R, Schoemaker MC, Van Der Plas JP, Van Den Berg LH, Franssen H, Wokke JH, et al. Diagnostic value of high-resolution sonography in ulnar neuropathy at the elbow. Neurology. 2004;62(5):767–73.

108. Van Den Berg PJ, Pompe SM, Beekman R, Visser LH. Sonographic incidence of ulnar nerve (sub)luxation and its associated clinical and electrodiagnostic characteristics. Muscle Nerve. 2013;47(6):849–55.

109. Dingemanse R, Randsdorp M, Koes BW, Huisstede BM. Evidence for the effectiveness of electrophysical modalities for treatment of medial and lateral epicondylitis: a systematic review. Br J Sports Med. 2014;48(12):957–65.

110. Tyler TF, Nicholas SJ, Schmitt BM, Mullaney M, Hogan DE. Clinical outcomes of the addition of eccentrics for rehabilitation of previously failed treatments of golfers elbow. Int J Sports Phys Ther. 2014;9(3):365–70.

111. Chang HY, Wang CH, Chou KY, Cheng SC. Could forearm Kinesio taping improve strength, force sense, and pain in baseball pitchers with medial epicondylitis? Clin J Sport Med. 2012;22(4):327–33.

112. Stahl S, Kaufman T. Ulnar nerve injury at the elbow after steroid injection for medial epicondylitis. J Hand Surg. 1997;22(1):69–70.

113. Huang Z, Du S, Qi Y, Chen G, Yan W. Effectiveness of ultrasound guidance on intraarticular and periarticular joint injections: systematic review and meta-analysis of randomized trials. Am J Phys Med Rehabil. 2015;94(10):775–83.

114. Barnes DE, Beckley JM, Smith J. Percutaneous ultrasonic tenotomy for chronic elbow tendinosis: a prospective study. J Shoulder Elb Surg. 2015;24(1):67–73.

115. Vinod AV, Ross G. An effective approach to diagnosis and surgical repair of refractory medial epicondylitis. J Shoulder Elb Surg. 2015;24(8):1172–7.

116. Tasto JP, Richmond JM, Cummings JR, Hardesty R, Amiel D. Radiofrequency microtenotomy for elbow epicondylitis: midterm results. Am J Orthop. 2016;45(1):29–33.

Wrist and Hand Tendons

6

David Impastato, Brian C. Liem, Jerry Huang, and Mark A. Harrast

Abbreviations

A1 pulley	Annular 1 pulley
APL	Abductor pollicis longus
CMC	Carpometacarpal
DIP	Distal interphalangeal joint
ECRB	Extensor carpi radialis brevis
ECRL	Extensor carpi radialis longus
ECU	Extensor carpi ulnaris
EDC	Extensor digitorum communis
EDM	Extensor digiti minimi
EIP	Extensor indicis proprius
EPB	Extensor pollicis brevis
EPL	Extensor pollicis longus
FCR	Flexor carpi radialis
FCU	Flexor carpi ulnaris
FDP	Flexor digitorum profundus
FDS	Flexor digitorum superficialis
FPL	Flexor pollicis longus
MCP	Metacarpophalangeal
NSAID	Non-steroidal anti-inflammatory drug
PIP	Proximal interphalangeal joint
TFCC	Triangular fibrocartilaginous complex

D. Impastato · B. C. Liem
UW Medicine Sports Medicine Center at Husky Stadium, University of Washington, Seattle, WA, USA
e-mail: dimpas@uw.edu; bliem@uw.edu

J. Huang
Department of Orthopaedics and Sports Medicine, University of Washington, Seattle, WA, USA
e-mail: jihuang@uw.edu

M. A. Harrast (✉)
Department of Rehabilitation Medicine, University of Washington, Seattle, WA, USA
e-mail: mharrast@uw.edu

Introduction

The wrist and hand are among the most common sites for tendinopathy to develop and can be very challenging to accurately diagnose and, thus, appropriately treat. A wide range of 5–25% of all athletic injuries involves the wrist and hand. Tendinopathy, specifically, of this region is often due to repetitive movements involved in one's daily work, hobbies, or daily activities, and it can have a large socioeconomic and quality of life impact [1, 2]. Overuse injuries are common in both sports and occupational medicine. The most common overuse tendinopathy of the wrist and hand, De Quervain tenosynovitis, is seen in racquet sport and rowing athletes and involves the first dorsal compartment. Stenosing tenosynovitis at the A1 pulley, or trigger finger, is the next most common tendinopathy of the wrist and hand and is more frequently seen in the non-athletic population. Traumatic tendon ruptures and tears occur most typically in sports. Mallet finger is a terminal extensor tendon rupture of any finger and is the most common closed tendon injury of the wrist and hand in athletes. Jersey finger, another common traumatic tendon injury in sports, affects the opposite side of the digit and is an avulsion of the flexor digitorum profundus from its insertion. It involves the ring finger over 75% of the time.

This chapter highlights tendinopathies of the wrist and hand with a focus on comparing and contrasting various tendinopathies in close proximity in order to assist the reader in accurate diagnosis and treatment. This chapter is anatomically organized as follows:

I. Volar compartment
    (a) Flexor carpi radialis
    (b) Flexor carpi ulnaris
    (c) Flexor digitorum profundus
        (i) Trigger finger
        (ii) Jersey finger
    (d) Flexor digitorum superficialis
        (i) Trigger finger
    (e) Flexor pollicis longus + flexor digitorum profundus ➔ Linburg–Comstock syndrome
II. Dorsal compartment
    (a) Abductor pollicis longus + extensor pollicis brevis ➔ de Quervain's
    (b) Extensor carpi radialis longus + extensor carpi radialis brevis ➔ intersection syndrome
    (c) Extensor pollicis longus
    (d) Extensor indicis proprius + extensor digitorum
        (i) Mallet finger
        (ii) Boutonniere deformity
    (e) Extensor digiti minimi
        (i) Vaughn-Jackson syndrome
    (f) Extensor carpi ulnaris

Volar Compartment

Flexor Carpi Radialis Tendinopathy

A 28-year-old female with remote history of scaphoid fracture and history of rheumatoid arthritis presents with a five-month history of atraumatic palmar hand pain at the ulnar aspect of trapezium bone. Pain is worse with resisted radial deviation of the wrist and with passive ulnar deviation and extension of the wrist.

Anatomy

The FCR tendon acts to flex and radially deviate the wrist. The distal tendon of the flexor carpi radialis (FCR) forms in the mid-forearm and inserts primarily on to the base of the second metacarpal, with a lesser attachment to the base of the third metacarpal [2, 3]. The tendon lies in a sheath from the distal aspect of the forearm to the distal aspect of the trapezium. This sheath forms a tunnel at the level of the trapezium, composed of the medial groove of the trapezium and two fibers of the flexor retinaculum – the superficial lamina, which is attached to the scaphoid and trapezium, and the deep lamina which is attached to the trapezium [3]. At the level of this tunnel, 90% of the sheath is occupied by the tendon. It is this narrow tunnel in combination with underlying anatomical changes (e.g., tendon thickening) that can cause tendon compression, resulting in further pathology, also known as stenosing tenosynovitis [4, 5]. Thus, FCR pathology is most commonly in this narrow tunnel at the level of the trapezium.

Clinical Presentation

Although not a common injury, FCR tendinopathy can be functionally limiting. The patient will typically present with pain over the tunnel encasing the FCR tendon, located at the volar radial wrist over the distal wrist crease. The pain is insidious in nature, worsening with resisted flexion of the wrist or radial deviation. There may be associated swelling at the site of tenderness [2, 4, 6]. Tendinopathy of the FCR is often associated with previous scaphoid fracture, distal radius fracture, wrist ganglion, repetitive wrist flexion movements, rheumatoid arthritis, or blunt trauma [4, 7, 8].

Physical Examination

In addition to inspection, palpating over the distal FCR tendon can determine if there is swelling around the tendon versus presence of a ganglion cyst in the aforementioned fibro-osseous tunnel that the FCR tendon courses through at the level of the trapezium. Provocative maneuvers consist largely of resisted wrist flexion while in radial deviation. Stretching the tendon through passive wrist extension can also reproduce pain [2, 6].

Fig. 6.1 Ganglion cyst in direct contact with FCR tendon

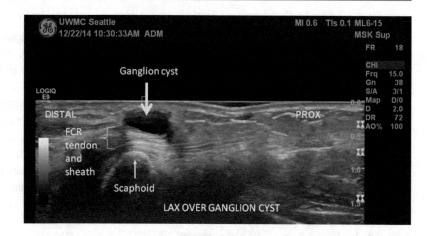

Diagnostic Workup

Diagnostic workup for FCR tendinopathy is minimal. A basic X-ray screen (PA, lateral, and oblique) of the wrist can be obtained to evaluate for thumb carpometacarpal (CMC) osteoarthritis, scaphotrapeziotrapezoid (STT) osteoarthritis, previous scaphoid fracture, or previous distal radius fracture leading to irritation or compression of the tendon. More specifically, an osteophyte from a degenerative STT joint can, overtime, result in fraying and tendinopathy of the FCR. In addition, ultrasound may be useful as a ganglion cyst can be visualized or inflammation around the tendon can be assessed with power Doppler (see Fig. 6.1) [4, 9]. MRI is rarely indicated, but it can evaluate tendinitis with increased T2 signal around the tendon. Lastly, local anesthetic has been injected into the location of tenderness and around the tendon to help confirm FCR tendinopathy as a pain generator [2].

Treatments

Initially, occupational therapy focusing on stretching and progressive strengthening, NSAIDs, and icing the wrist can be prescribed [4]. This treatment option should be performed in the setting of relative rest. If appropriate rest is difficult, a wrist orthosis can be provided with wrist flexion set at approximately 25 degrees (see Table 6.1) [6, 10]. Injection of the FCR tendon sheath using an anesthetic with corticosteroid can be considered for severely symptomatic cases. Injecting corticosteroid into the tendon sheath should be performed with ultrasound imaging

Table 6.1 Splinting position for common wrist/hand tendinopathies

Tendon	Splint position
FCR tendinopathy	Wrist hand orthosis – wrist flexion at 25°
FCU tendinopathy	Wrist hand orthosis – Wrist flexion at 25°
Trigger finger	MCP10-15° flexion with free interphalangeal joint
De Quervain's	Thumb spica splint
Intersection syndrome	Wrist hand orthosis – wrist extension at 15°
Extensor tendinopathy	Wrist hand orthosis – wrist extension at 15°
Mallet finger	DIP splinted in extension with PIP free
Boutonniere deformity	PIP splinted in extension with DIP free
EDM tendinopathy	Wrist hand orthosis – wrist extension at 15°
ECU tendinopathy	Wrist hand orthosis – wrist extension at 15°

guidance to ensure accuracy of needle placement and, thus, limiting the risk of intra-tendinous injection which carries a risk of tendon rupture. If the tendon were to rupture, the patient typically has symptom relief with little functional deficit. This is due to compensation from the other wrist flexor, the flexor carpi ulnaris (FCU) tendon, as well as other tendons compensating for radial deviation of the wrist (the extensor radialis longus/brevis) [4].

Finally, if conservative measures fail and the diagnosis is continuing to limit the patient and cause discomfort, surgical management can be considered. The surgical approach is through the volar aspect of the wrist, proximal to the wrist crease. The palmar cutaneous branch of the median nerve, the lateral antebrachial cutaneous nerve, and the superficial radial nerve run near this incision and precise dissection should be used to avoid injury of these sensory nerves, which can lead to numbness over the region or painful hyperesthesia. Once the surgeon dissects down to the FCR tendon, the tunnel, more specifically, the flexor retinaculum at the level of the trapezium, is released followed by tendon sheath decompression. FCR tendon sheath decompression is performed with debridement of the tendon back to healthy fibers. Complete release is obtained when the tendon mobilizes from the trapezial groove. If arthritic changes or compression by a ganglion is present, complete removal of the osteophyte or the cyst should be obtained to prevent refractory tendinopathy. Surgical outcomes tend to relieve symptoms and have low recurrence rates [2, 4, 7, 11]. In cases of a high-grade partial FCR tendon rupture, surgical debridement of the distal tendon and completion of the rupture provide pain relief.

Flexor Carpi Ulnaris Tendinopathy

A 45-year-old manual laborer reports a few week history of pain and swelling over the distal volar wrist on the ulnar side. It is worsened with repetitive movements such as using a screwdriver. Pain is recreated with palpation over the volar pisiform bone and with resisted wrist flexion.

Anatomy

The flexor carpi ulnaris (FCU) tendon inserts onto the pisiform, hook of hamate, and base of fifth metacarpal, but it does not pass through an enclosed sheath like most other hand and wrist tendons [11]. The FCU tendon acts to flex and ulnar deviate the wrist. Repetitive wrist flexion and ulnar deviation can cause irritation of the tendon as it inserts and runs over the pisiform bone, and hence tendinopathy is typically located at the insertion site of the tendon [3]. Activities such as golf and tennis utilize this repetitive movement causing microtrauma to the tendon, often causing longitudinal tears of the tendon [2, 6].

Clinical Presentation

The patient usually reports insidious onset of pain located where the tendon runs over the pisiform bone, proximal to its insertion. The pain is worsened with resisted flexion and ulnar deviation. The differential diagnosis includes pisotriquetral osteoarthrosis, triangular fibrocartilage complex (TFCC) tears, fractures of the hook of the hamate and pisiform, and lunotriquetral ligament injury [6]. FCU tendinitis tends to present with development of pain over a more acute time frame followed by inflammation, swelling, and decreased range of motion [11–13].

Physical Examination

Tenderness to palpation is usually present where the tendon continues over the pisiform bone, proximal to its insertion on the base of the fifth metacarpal [14]. Pain is also present with resisted wrist flexion in ulnar deviation and swelling can be seen around the location of pain [6, 14]. Often times, pisotriquetral osteoarthrosis will also have pain with resisted wrist flexion; however, crepitus is usually appreciated with this condition with hypermobility of the pisiform. Tendinopathy of the FCU can often mimic the physical exam for septic joint, with warmth, erythema, and tenderness being the primary findings on exam [13].

Diagnostic Workup

Plain radiographs and ultrasound can aid in diagnosis. X-ray can be useful to rule out pisotriquetral osteoarthrosis and to evaluate for calcifications located in the FCU. However, calcifications will not always be seen on x-ray. It is recommended to obtain a lateral wrist radiograph with the wrist in slight supination and extension to better visualize the pisotriquetral articulation [2, 6]. In addition, ultrasound examination could be beneficial in identifying calcific deposits in and around the tendon as well as associated neovascularization, signifying an inflammatory condition [15]. However, a small case series reported difficulty in distinguishing between FCU tendinopathy and other rheumatologic conditions [16]. This study demonstrated US evidence of the following in all patients who had an underlying inflammatory rheumatologic disorder and pain at the pisiform (i.e., insertion of the FCU tendon): peritendinous effusion, pisiform erosive cortical irregularities, and peritendinous soft tissue thickening. These sonographic findings were not demonstrated in the cohort that did not have an underlying rheumatologic condition. Thus, besides the typical clinical hallmarks of rheumatologic disease, US imaging may be helpful to enhance the diagnostic sensitivity.

Finally, calcification of the FCU tendon is the most common form of calcific tendinitis of the wrist and hand. Due to the severity and rapid onset of pain with acute calcific tendonitis, it is commonly mistaken for a septic joint (most commonly the pisotriquetral joint), gout, or a fracture. Basic X-rays (AP and oblique views of the wrist) and negative joint aspiration can be diagnostic [13].

Treatments

Initial treatment can be started with anti-inflammatories (NSAIDs), rest, and splinting. A wrist orthosis positioned in 25 degrees of wrist flexion is commonly used to facilitate rest of the wrist flexor tendons [2, 6]. McAuliffe et al. found that many patients demonstrated degeneration of the tendon fibers and were better treated with progressive stretching and strengthening as opposed to NSAIDs [11]. Most commonly, eccentric wrist flexion in both supination and pronation is performed [15].

When these conservative therapies do not provide relief, corticosteroid injection is the next step in management. In cases of calcific tendinitis, patients demonstrated up to 60% relief with corticosteroid injection [11]. One case report demonstrated 50% pain reduction using sclerosing therapy with polidocanol under power and laser Doppler guidance in combination with eccentric exercises to treat FCU tendinopathy [15]. In addition, it has been proposed that mechanical disruption of existing calcium deposits and removal, such as seen in percutaneous needle tenotomy and calcific lavage, can be beneficial [13].

If the patient's symptoms are refractory to the above treatment, surgery can be performed to remove calcific deposits, adhesions, and potential removal of the pisiform [6]. Surgery is performed

with a small incision over the hypothenar eminence with care to protect the ulnar nerve. Once the dissection reaches the pisiform, dissection around the pisiform and removal is complete. A Z-plasty can be performed to lengthen the FCU tendon to reduce tension without concern for reduced wrist function [17].

Trigger Finger: Flexor Digitorum Profundus and Flexor Digitorum Superficialis Tendinopathy

A 33-year-old recreational softball player with history of hypothyroidism treated with levothyroxine presents with pain over her ring finger for 5 months with more recent onset of "triggering" where her finger occasionally "catches" while trying to extend the ring finger from a fully flexed position.

Anatomy

Trigger finger is one of the most common tendinopathies of the hand. Both the flexor digitorum profundus (FDP) and the flexor digitorum superficialis (FDS) pass through the annular 1 (A1) pulley, a fibrous flexor sheath [11]. The prime action of the FDS tendon is flexion of the proximal interphalangeal joint (PIP), while the FDP tendon flexes the distal interphalangeal (DIP) joint. Pathology occurs most commonly at the A1 pulley, which is located over the metacarpophalangeal joint on the volar aspect of the palm, with thickening of the pulley, and can also occur from focal swelling of the flexor tendons, with FDP being more commonly involved than the FDS tendon [4]. Inflammation may cause nodular enlargement of the tendon distal to the pulley, to the flexor tendon sheath, or thickening of the A1 pulley causing stenosis. The mechanism of the triggering is entrapment of the flexor tendon at the level of the A1 pulley, causing the finger to be blocked from flexion or extension due to difficulty of flexor tendon gliding through the fibrous tunnel [3].

Clinical Presentation

Patients routinely present with pain and "triggering" of their finger or the finger getting "stuck" with movements. The patient may report a mass in the volar palm where the pain is located. If present for a prolonged period, flexion contracture of the proximal interphalangeal joint can develop [4, 11]. Trigger finger is more common in females and patients with diabetes, thyroid disease, rheumatoid arthritis, amyloidosis, and those who participate in weight lifting, baseball, or gymnastics. The most commonly affected digits are the ring and middle fingers [2]. Patients often complain of the pain and triggering being worse in the morning and the finger loosening through the course of the day, as the tendon sheath is stretched out.

Physical Examination

The classic physical exam finding is painful locking of the digit due to the inflamed tendon becoming trapped at the constricted tendon sheath, as it is being moved through the range of motion. In some instances, it may be difficult to passively range the finger if significant thickening exists. In addition, a tender nodule may be felt outside the A1 pulley, which is the flexor tendon folding due to inability to pass through the pulley with finger flexion and extension [2, 4]. In patients with chronic trigger finger, flexion contracture of the proximal interphalangeal joint may develop, with inability to passively extend the joint fully.

Diagnostic Workup

Diagnostic tests are not required in patients with trigger finger as it is a clinical diagnosis. However, both the FDS and FDP tendons along with the A1 pulley can be easily assessed on ultrasound (see Fig. 6.2). Dynamic ultrasound can be used to visualize the restriction of the tendons through the A1 pulley. In some instances, folding of the tendon may be seen as it attempts to pass through the pulley [9]. The differential diagnosis for trigger finger includes a subluxed extensor tendon over the MCP joint from a sagittal band rupture, lateral band subluxation over the PIP joint, a partial flexor tendon injury, or a tendon tumor. Essentially any focal enlargement of these flexor tendons can create a triggering, or catching, sensation at the A1 pulley.

Treatments

The first-line treatment for a trigger finger is splinting and NSAIDs. Patients can be placed in a splint that stabilizes the metacarpophalangeal (MCP) joint in full extension or mild flexion of 10–15 degrees, while allowing movements at the interphalangeal joints. Splinting can provide relief in 40–87% of patients [18, 19]. Therapy, directed at gliding of the FDP and FDS tendons, is often used in combination with a splint, but it has not been demonstrated to be a reliable treatment option. However, there is evidence that if a response is obtained using hand therapy patients have a lower rate of recurrence [4]. Corticosteroid injections are often used early after diagnosis because of the high success rate and decreased rate of recurrence (see Fig. 6.3) [20, 21]. One study demonstrated no difference whether injection was performed intra-sheath or extra-sheath using ultrasound guidance [22]. Another study demonstrated 57% relief at 6 months without ultrasound guidance versus 90% relief at 6 months with ultrasound guidance [23]. Preliminary results have demonstrated improvement in pain scores and function with radial extracorporeal shockwave therapy [24]. Poor outcomes are associated with chronic triggering, inflammatory conditions, diabetes, and having multiple trigger fingers [2].

If non-surgical measures fail, patients are typically referred for surgery. Open or percutaneous releases are commonly performed releases of the A1 pulley. This is often performed with the patient awake with local anesthesia to allow the patient to move the finger during the procedure and confirm resolution of locking and triggering after release of the A1 pulley [11]. If a flexion contracture is present prior to surgery, additional intervention is usually required to release the checkrein ligaments and possibly volar plate [4]. Surgical success rates of up to 97% have been reported, with minimal difference between percutaneous and open release [2, 25]. Lastly, ultrasound-guided A1 pulley release has been described but there is a lack of randomized and comparative trials [26]. A recent prospective trial showed 81% symptomatic relief with ultrasound-guided pulley release and minimal complications [27].

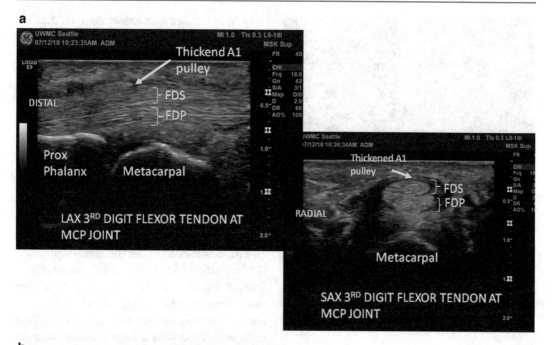

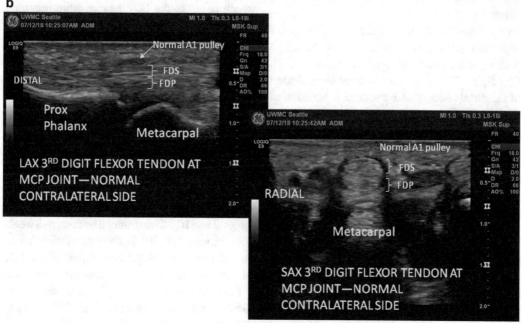

Fig. 6.2 (**a**) Trigger finger third digit: thickened flexor tendon and pulley in LAX and SAX. (**b**) Normal contralateral third digit flexor tendon and pulley in LAX and SAX

Jersey Finger: Flexor Digitorum Profundus Tendon Rupture

A 16-year-old high-school linebacker has acute onset of ring finger pain that occurred after *attempting to make a tackle. The DIP of the ring finger is held in extension and a small nodule is appreciated in the palm. No active DIP flexion is present on exam.*

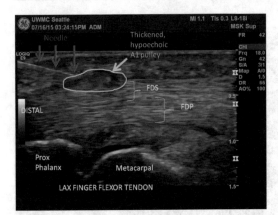

Fig. 6.3 Sonographically guided A1-flexor tendon inter-space corticosteroid injection using anatomic longitudinal view. Needle is aimed underneath A1 pulley, superficial to flexor tendons. Medications used: 1 cc of 10 mg/cc triamcinolone and 0.5 cc of 1% lidocaine, 30-G, 1-inch needle. For more information, see Bodor M. Ultrasound-Guided First Annular Pulley Injection for Trigger Finger." AIUM 2009

Anatomy

Jersey finger results from a rupture of the flexor digitorum profundus' attachment to the distal phalanx on the volar surface of the second through fifth digits. FDP is mainly responsible for flexion of the distal phalanx with minimal production of flexion at the proximal interphalangeal joint and metacarpal phalangeal joint [3]. This injury is typically due to forceful hyperextension of the distal interphalangeal joint with the FDP in maximal contraction [6]. Interestingly, studies have shown that the FDP to the ring finger has a lower tensile strength, making it the most prone to rupture. It is involved in 75% of the cases [28].

Clinical Presentation

The patient usually will recall a specific incident with or without an audible pop that produced the deformity. The finger is usually held with the DIP extended from unopposed terminal extensor tendon pull. Patients often present with pain over the DIP joint. However, patients also commonly complain of pain in the palm with a soft tissue mass from the retracted tendon [6].

Physical Examination

On examination, the patient typically is unable to flex the DIP actively, but the examiner will be able to flex it passively. The deformity will typi-

cally be associated with tenderness over the FDP attachment site as well as tenderness more proximally at the level of the retracted tendon [6]. There is often a palpable mass in the distal palm corresponding to the proximal stump of the tendon.

Diagnostic Workup

As in other tendon ruptures, X-rays should be taken to rule out avulsion fracture [6]. Case reports demonstrate ultrasound's ability to see cortical irregularity, diagnose avulsion fracture, and see tendon disruption [29]. FDP ruptures are classified by the Leddy and Packer classification system, which is based on the level of proximal FDP retraction after it is avulsed and whether a fracture coexists. In type 1, the FDP tendon retracts into the palm. In type II, it retracts to the level of the proximal interphalangeal joint. Type III is associated with a large fracture fragment which prevents the FDP tendon from retracting beyond the distal interphalangeal joint. Finally, type IV includes both a fracture and an avulsion of the tendon from the fractured fragment with retraction of the tendon to the palm [30].

Treatments

Treatment for FDP rupture is almost always surgical and timing depends on the classification of the injury (see Table 6.2) [10, 31]. If the tendon retracts below the PIP joint (types I and IV), surgery should be performed within a week of the injury. If it has not retracted beyond the PIP joint (types II and III), the repair can be done 6–8 weeks after the injury [6, 30]. In chronic injuries that are missed or neglected, primary repair of the FDP tendon is sometimes not possible. Treatment options include a two-stage flexor tendon reconstruction versus accepting having a "FDS finger" that does not bend at the DIP joint.

Table 6.2 Tendon injuries of the wrist and hand requiring early surgical referral

Jersey finger (FDP)
Linburg-Comstock syndrome (FPL & FDP)
Extensor pollicis longus rupture
Mallet finger with instability or subluxation (EIP/EDC)
Boutonniere deformity with open injury or avulsion (EIP/EDC)

Linburg-Comstock Syndrome

A 29-year-old male who recently began playing the piano reports insidious onset of pain at the volar wrist and occasional thumb cramping. On exam, the patient is unable to flex the DIP of the thumb and index finger separately. Pain is provoked with extension of the index finger's DIP when the thumb DIP is flexed.

Anatomy

Linburg-Comstock syndrome consists of an anomalous connection between the flexor pollicis longus (FPL) and the flexor digitorum profundus to the index finger. It has been reported in up to 31% of the general population [32]. However, it is unclear as to the percent of individuals who have the congenital version versus those who have an acquired form from adhesions [2].

Clinical Presentation

Most patients will not have symptoms, though they notice simultaneous flexion of index finger DIP while flexing the thumb IP joint. Some patients will report insidious onset of activity-related vague pain on the volar, radial surface of their wrist and may report cramping of the thumb [2].

Physical Examination

The main physical exam finding is simultaneous flexion of the DIP of the index finger when attempting to flex the thumb. Pain can be produced with passive extension of the DIP of the index finger with active thumb flexion [2].

Diagnostic Workup

MRI and dynamic ultrasound can reveal the anomalous connection. The ultrasound can be placed distally in the palm to obtain a view of the FPL and index FDP tendons. The patient is then asked to alternate flexing the thumb and index finger, resulting in simultaneous movement of both tendons on ultrasound imaging [33].

Treatments

If the patient is symptomatic, surgical intervention is the mainstay of treatment and usually consists of release of the tendon interconnec-

tions at the level of the distal forearm. The approach is near the FCR tendon and radial artery, with care being taken to protect the artery [34].

Dorsal Compartment (See Fig. 6.4 and Table 6.3)

De Quervain's Tenosynovitis: Abductor Pollicis Longus and Extensor Pollicis Brevis Tendinopathy

A 31-year-old female who has been nursing her newborn for the past 4 months presents with insidious onset of pain over the right dorsal radial aspect of the wrist that radiates proximally to the forearm. Slight swelling and erythema are present along with tenderness to palpation over the XsiteX. sight. In addition, Finkelstein's test is positive.

Anatomy

De Quervain's tenosynovitis is a common tendinopathy affecting the first dorsal compartment of

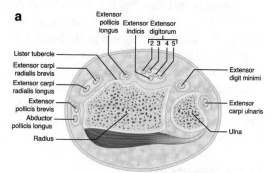

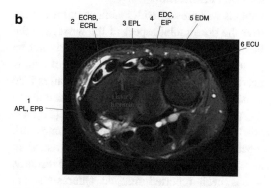

Fig. 6.4 (**a, b**) Dorsal compartment of the wrist at the level of Lister's tubercle. (**a**). Illustration. (**b**). Axial T2 MRI

Table 6.3 Dorsal wrist compartments and associated pathology

Compartment	Tendon	Common pathology
1	EPB, APL	De Quervain's, Texter's thumb
2	ECRL, ECRB	Intersection syndrome
3	EPL	Drummer's wrist
4	EIP, EDC	Extensor tenosynovitis, Mallet finger
		Tenosynovitis, Mallet finger, Boutonniere deformity
5	EDM	Vaughn-Jackson syndrome
6	ECU	Snapping ECU

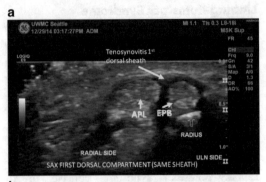

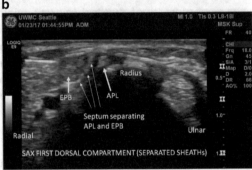

Fig. 6.5 (**a**). First dorsal compartment (NOT separated). (**b**). First dorsal compartment (separated)

the wrist, which includes the tendon sheath of the abductor pollicis longus (APL) and extensor pollicis brevis (EPB) tendons. Much is still unknown about the pathophysiology of de Quervain's; however, it is thought that the EPB is commonly more affected than the APL [4, 11, 35, 36]. The sheath lies just radial to the radial styloid and can be palpated at this location [3]. In over 60% of the population, these two tendons lie in a common extensor sheath, where in others the two tendons are separated (see Fig. 6.5) [4]. It has been reported that separate compartments with the EPB tendon in its own subsheath are present in up to 71% of patients with de Quervain's versus only 20% without de Quervain's [35]. It is thought that having a separate compartment more commonly increases the gliding resistance of the EPB tendon with a tighter tunnel, predisposing to pathology [37].

Clinical Presentation

Patients will present with insidious onset of pain over the dorsoradial aspect of the wrist near the base of the thumb. Swelling may or may not be present, but tenderness over this compartment is nearly always present [4]. Tenderness can radiate proximally along the distal forearm or distally to the thumb metacarpophalangeal joint [10]. De Quervain's tenosynovitis commonly occurs with repeated abduction/adduction of the wrist, such as lifting a baby or hammering [4]. More recently, it has been reported that de Quervain's can develop from repetitive text messaging, thus it is also known as texter's thumb [38]. Other com-

mon but less described tendinopathies associated with texting are of the adductor pollicis, first dorsal interossei, extensor pollicis longus, and extensor digitorum communis tendons [39].

Physical Examination

Palpation over the first dorsal compartment usually elicits pain [4]. Finkelstein's test is a common provocative maneuver and is positive in the majority of cases. This test consists of placing the patient's thumb in the palm of the hand and grasping the thumb with the other fingers of the hand. The patient then adducts the hand (ulnarly deviates) and if pain is produced along the course of the first dorsal compartment, the test is considered positive [4]. This test should always be compared bilaterally because it is sometimes positive in asymptomatic individuals and sometimes is negative if only the EPB is affected [2, 4]. The diagnosis can be made more specific by determining if the tendons exist in a common sheath or a separate sheath. One physical exam maneuver described to elucidate if the two tendons are in separate sheaths is performing resisted thumb extension and then resisted abduction of the thumb. If extension is more painful, then it is likely there are two separate compartments and the EPB is primarily affected. If pain is present with both, then it is unclear if one tendon is contributing to pathology more than the other. This would not provide clarification if two separate compartments exist, since the EPB also contributes to thumb abduction [36]. This can assist the clinician to perform tailored therapy in these individuals.

Diagnostic Workup

Typically, X-rays are not indicated except to evaluate for thumb carpometacarpal joint arthritis as the source of symptoms [4]. Ultrasound can demonstrate increased Doppler signal around the tendon sheath and has been reported as a reliable method for diagnosing de Quervain's disease and determining if one or two compartments exist [40].

Treatments

Common conservative options consist of NSAIDs, immobilization in a forearm based thumb spica splint, hand therapy, and corticosteroid injections [4]. Corticosteroid injections are particularly gratifying with a short-term success rate of 62–100% [4, 41]. However, the intermediate- and long-term duration of benefit is truly unknown as most studies demonstrate follow-up anywhere between 1 month and rarely to 2 years [11]. One theory for the wide range of benefit with corticosteroid injection may be the presence of septum separation of the two tendons. If patients have this septum, they are more likely to fail corticosteroid injection, unless both sheaths or the tendon demonstrating pathology is injected [42]. Ultrasound guidance can be utilized to direct the needle into the correct tendon sheath when an intracompartmental septum is present [23]. A recent systematic review demonstrated that splint immobilization combined with corticosteroid injection improves the success rate over either intervention alone [43]. Nonsurgical treatment can be effective for the majority of cases, but it is much less effective if the APL and EPB

tendons are in separate compartments [4]. There is one case report describing refractory de Quervain's in which needle tenotomy and platelet-rich plasma injection were performed to both the APL and EPB tendons. After the procedure, the patient was given a thumb spica splint for 2 weeks and underwent hand therapy from week 2 to week 10. The patient reported a 74% pain reduction after 3 months and a 63% pain reduction after 6 months [44].

Surgical approach consists of a small incision over the first dorsal compartment with careful dissection to avoid injury to the superficial radial nerve. Once the tendon sheath is located, the sheath is released longitudinally to decompress the tendons [4]. Care is taken to incise the sheath as dorsally as possible to leave a volar retinacular flap which helps prevent subluxation of the tendons. The surgeon should evaluate for the existence of two separate tendon sheaths, and if present, a release of both should be performed [2, 4]. The EPB tendon is identified intraoperatively by isolated passive flexion-extension of the thumb MCP joint as the APL tendons do not cross the MCP joint.

Proximal Intersection Syndrome/ Oarsmen's Wrist: Extensor Carpi Radialis Longus and Brevis Tendinopathy

An 18-year-old rower presents with insidious onset of pain over the dorsal forearm about five centimeters proximal to the wrist. The patient reports feeling a scraping sensation with restricted wrist extension and thumb extension.

Anatomy

Intersection syndrome is a tendinopathy involving the crossover point of the first and second dorsal compartments of the wrist, approximately five centimeters proximal to the wrist crease (see Fig. 6.6) [2, 6]. Extensor carpi radialis longus (ECRL) and extensor carpi radialis brevis (ECRB) tendons make up the second dorsal compartment and insert onto the base of the second and third metacarpals on the dorsal surface, respectively. They both are responsible for wrist

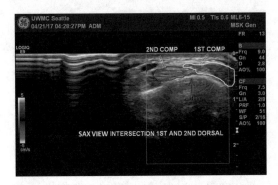

Fig. 6.6 US SAX image of intersection point of first and second dorsal compartments

extension and abduction of the hand [3]. The mechanism of this tendinopathy is thought to be due to rubbing of the two compartments at this location [4, 11]. Intersection syndrome is often called "oarsmen's wrist." [10]

Clinical Presentation
The patient will report tenderness located over the intersection of these two compartments proximal to Lister's tubercle and proximal to the location of de Quervain's tenosynovitis [4]. It is commonly associated with repetitive wrist extension and is seen often in rowers, weight lifters, and racquet sport athletes [4, 6].

Physical Examination
Physical examination is limited in intersection syndrome. Tenderness on the dorsoradial distal forearm approximately 4-5 cm proximal to the wrist with palpation is important. A "wet leather" crepitus can be palpable or produced with wrist flexion-extension [2, 4]. Pain is often reproduced with resisted wrist extension and thumb extension/abduction [45]. Pain may be provoked by Finkelstein's test; however, the pain is experienced more proximal than what is typical in de Quervain's, which is the most common competing diagnosis.

Diagnostic Workup
Imaging does not tend to be helpful in this condition, as it is a clinical diagnosis [4]. Ultrasound could be used to demonstrate hypoechoic tendon, increased vascular signal near the tendon, and edema around the tendon at the point where the second and first compartments cross [46, 47]. MRI may show peritendinous edema surrounding the tendons of the first and second dorsal compartments centered at the point of crossover. An injection of anesthetic can be placed near the intersection point, and if pain is relieved, one can more confidently diagnose the patient with intersection syndrome [4].

Treatments
Conservative management is the treatment of choice. The patient is advised to rest from activities causing discomfort and utilize a splint placing the wrist in 15 degrees of extension. If the patient demonstrated a good response to anesthetic injection, or the clinical and sonographic presentations are classic, corticosteroid injection could be used [4]. Conservative care is usually beneficial in up to 60% of patients [48]. No study has been published on use of platelet-rich plasma or viscosupplementation for this indication.

If conservative measures fail, the patient can undergo surgical interventions. A few different surgical options are available. The first consists of incision over the location of pain and dissection to the tendon sheaths, at which point the fascia of ECRL and ECRB are released. The second intervention entails releasing the second compartment at a more distal site. Both approaches have reported excellent relief of symptoms [48, 49]. Finally, there is a technique in which both the first and second dorsal compartments are released [2].

Drummer's Wrist: Extensor Pollicis Longus Tendinopathy/Rupture
A 17-year-old male drummer presents with acute onset of dorsal distal thumb pain after a marathon session with the band. There is an inability to fully extend the distal thumb phalanx and swelling can be seen around the tendon.

Anatomy
The third dorsal compartment consists of the extensor pollicis longus (EPL), which runs just medial to Lister's tubercle, and is associated with

extensor pollicis longus tenosynovitis which can lead to rupture of the tendon from its attachment on the dorsal distal phalanx, otherwise known as Drummer's wrist [3]. The tendon turns acutely around Lister's tubercle, which serves as a pulley to the EPL tendon, making it prone to injury with repeated movement [4]. The EPL tendon acts to both extend the thumb IP joint and adduct the thumb through its pivot on Lister's tubercle. It is thought that swelling in this compartment alters blood flow to the tendon making the tendon more prone to rupture from local trauma to the wrist (see Fig. 6.7) [50].

Clinical Presentation

This condition is most common in patients with rheumatoid arthritis, an associated distal radius fracture, or those who have fallen on an extended wrist. It has been proposed that drummers are at risk due to the repeated force applied to thumb extension during drumming. Patients typically present with pain and swelling just ulnar to Lister's tubercle [4].

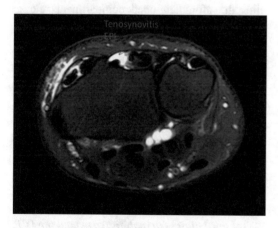

Fig. 6.7 EPL tenosynovitis: Axial T2 MR image of the wrist of a 25 y/o PhD physics and mathematics student with a six month history of gradual onset of dorsal wrist pain without a history of trauma. The symptoms worsened with studying (significant writing of equations). Exam showed mild swelling at the dorsal wrist, ulnar to the area of Lister's tubercle. Pain with active thumb extension. X-rays did not show any bony abnormality. MRI demonstrated swelling of the fourth dorsal tendon sheath. Treatment: Immobilization with thumb spica splint × 4 weeks followed by home exercises and return to normal activities at 6 weeks posttreatment

Physical Examination

Patients report prolonged symptoms, usually at least a few months [2]. Thumb flexion or extension typically reproduces the pain, which is worsened with resisted motion. As in most tendinopathies, crepitus may be appreciated but more commonly the patient will report a snapping of the tendon with movements [4]. Swelling can also be appreciated around the tendon. In the case of tendon rupture, the patient may not be able to fully extend the distal phalanx of their thumb [2].

Diagnostic Workup

Plain films are obtained to rule out a coexisting distal radial fracture [4]. Ultrasound can be utilized to evaluate for disorganization of tendon fibers or neovascularization around the tendon sheath and to evaluate for tendon rupture.

Treatments

Conservative treatment generally consists of activity modification and splinting for non-ruptured tendinopathy. Corticosteroid injections in this location should be used more cautiously given the concern that an increase in local tissue pressure from the volume of injectate may contribute to tendon rupture at the friction site of Lister's tubercle [4, 11]. Surgical management is considered for recalcitrant tendinosis symptoms and all cases of ruptured tendon and consists of an incision over Lister's tubercle with dissection to the third compartment. The tendon sheath is then released and the extensor pollicis longus is externalized outside the sheath in order to prevent further rubbing against the bony prominence [4]. If the tendon appears to be significantly weakened or if the tendon is ruptured, a tendon transfer (typically with the extensor indicis proprius) may be performed to improve thumb function [2].

Extensor Indicis and Extensor Digitorum Communis Tendinopathy

A 38-year-old female with history of psoriatic arthritis presents with a 3-month history of intermittent swelling and pain over the distal dorsal forearm. On palpation, a fullness is appreciated

over the painful area. Resisted extension of the index finger reproduces the pain.

Anatomy

The fourth dorsal compartment of the wrist includes the extensor indicis proprius (EIP) and extensor digitorum communis (EDC). The extensor indicis inserts into the extensor expansion of the index finger, while the extensor digitorum inserts into the extensor expansion of the index, middle, ring, and small fingers. The extensor expansion is a fibrous sheath that holds the tendon over the dorsal surface of the joints. These tendons gradually integrate with the extensor expansion to its attachment on the dorsal distal phalanx [3]. The prime action of extensor indicis is to independently extend the index finger and help extend the hand. The action of the extensor digitorum communis is extension of the respective digits at the metacarpophalangeal joints and of the hand at the wrist.

Clinical Presentation

The presenting symptom is most commonly pain and swelling over the location of the fourth compartment. Occasionally, a mass may be present due to inflammation and hypertrophy of the tenosynovium [51]. This condition is usually seen in those with rheumatoid arthritis or other inflammatory conditions, and can also develop in the setting of distal radial fractures [4].

Physical Examination

There is often fullness over the dorsum of the hand and wrist. The pain can be worsened by extension of the wrist causing an impingement of the swollen tendons against the extensor retinaculum [4, 11]. If the extensor indicis is more involved, then resisted extension of the index finger is more painful than extension of the other digits [2]. When a mass is present, it can be seen moving distally as the fingers are brought into a clenched fist [51].

Diagnostic Workup

Extensor tenosynovitis of the EIP and EDC is a clinical diagnosis. Ultrasound could be utilized to evaluate for fluid or increased vascularization around the tendons of the fourth dorsal compartment [46]. Radiographs should be obtained to rule out radiocarpal and midcarpal arthritis or Kienbock's disease as causes of dorsal wrist pain and swelling. In cases of extensive tenosynovitis, the differential diagnosis should include rheumatoid arthritis and other inflammatory arthropathies as well as atypical mycobacterial infections [52].

Treatments

Treatment begins with nonoperative management which consists of rest, splinting the wrist in 15 degrees of extension and fingers in full extension, NSAIDs, and corticosteroid injections [2]. Conservative management is usually successful.

If the patient is not improving, surgical management is performed to release pressure in the fourth dorsal compartment [4]. In these cases, an incision is made over the compartment to release it. Debridement of the pathologic tendon is then performed. A retrospective review of 11 patients, who failed conservative measures, underwent surgery with 10 of 11 becoming asymptomatic after the aforementioned compartment release and tendon debridement [51]. In some situations, an accessory muscle, extensor digitorum brevis, lies on the compartment creating increased pressure [4, 11]. If this is found, the accessory muscle is commonly removed to alleviate the pressure [2, 4].

Mallet Finger: Terminal Extensor Tendon Rupture

A 17-year-old boy who enjoys playing basketball presents with a painful third digit. He attempted to grab a rebound and felt acute pain at the distal dorsal third digit with inability to extend the DIP. On exam, the DIP of the middle finger is held in flexion. The joint passively extends but does not extend on active attempts.

Anatomy

Mallet finger is an injury of the terminal extensor tendon distal to the DIP joint of any digit. It can be caused by an avulsion facture of the distal phalanx at the insertion of the extensor tendon or rupture of the extensor expansion itself (see

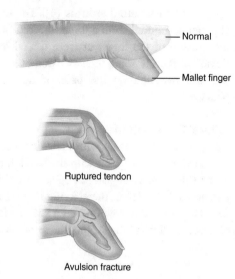

Fig. 6.8 Mallet finger: normal, mallet finger (ruptured tendon and avulsion fracture)

Fig. 6.8). It is one of the most common tendon injuries in athletes [3, 45]. A hyperflexion force to the extended DIP joint typically results in tendon rupture [6].

Clinical Presentation

The patient may recall an incident consistent with hyperflexion of the DIP joint after which the finger is held in a flexed position at the DIP joint. Post injury, patients usually lose the ability to extend at the DIP joint [2]. In addition, the loss of function is accompanied with significant edema around the DIP [10, 31, 45]. Mallet finger most commonly presents in the middle, ring, and little fingers [45].

Physical Examination

Physical exam may demonstrate the distal phalanx held in a flexed position due to unopposed action of FDP, tenderness over the dorsal distal phalanx, and inability of the patient to actively extend at the DIP joint. However, the examiner routinely is able to passively extend the DIP joint unless injury occurred several weeks prior due to development of a contracture [6]. There may also be hyperextension of the PIP joint, resulting in a swan-neck deformity of the injured digit.

Diagnostic Workup

X-rays are performed to evaluate for a bony mallet with an associated avulsion fracture and can best be visualized on lateral views [6, 45]. Ultrasound has recently been in use for mallet finger evaluation. A classic finding includes a soft tissue mass that is irregular in appearance near the proximal interphalangeal joint, signifying retracted tendon. If an avulsion is present, one might also see the fractured bone fragment as a hyperechoic mass [53].

Treatments

The digit should initially be treated with the DIP joint splinted in extension for at least 6 weeks and kept extended for 24 hours per day even during low-impact activities. Following the first 6 weeks, a nighttime splint is used for 2–6 more weeks. The PIP joint is left free [6, 45, 54]. A 2004 Cochrane review did not find significant difference between the use of different types of splints [55]. After this period, the patient should begin flexion-based exercises in attempts to remove joint stiffness and regain flexor strength [6]. Indications for surgical intervention include open injuries (i.e., laceration of the extensor tendon), chronic injuries (>12 weeks), and instability of the DIP joint (commonly seen with large avulsion fractures) with volar subluxation of the distal phalanx [6, 45]. Common techniques include Kirschner wire, pull through wiring, and figure of eight wiring [54]. Splinting can be considered in avulsion fractures if the fragment involves less than 30 percent of the articular surface without joint subluxation. If subluxation of the DIP joint is present, the patient should undergo surgical treatment of the bony mallet to reduce the DIP joint and bring the avulsion fragment in closer approximation to the distal phalanx [10, 31].

Boutonniere Deformity: Extensor Tendon Central Slip Defect

A 42-year-old female with a history of uncontrolled rheumatoid arthritis presents with a painful finger. Her middle finger is held in hyperextension at the DIP joint and flexion at the PIP joint. She reports she was making dinner and heard a "pop" with development of the deformity. The patient cannot extend the PIP but the examiner can.

Anatomy

Boutonniere deformity is an appearance of the finger in hyperextension at the DIP joint and flexion at the PIP joint [3]. This results from a defect in the central slip of the extensor tendon, causing the lateral bands to sublux to the volar side of the finger placing the PIP in flexion while placing tension on the extensor attachment to the distal phalanx causing hyperextension at the DIP joint (see Fig. 6.9) [3, 4]. Boutonniere deformity can occur from a traumatic injury or develop as a

sequela of rheumatoid arthritis [4]. The central slip can be injured from a direct laceration over the dorsum of the finger or from forced hyperflexion of the PIP joint, with avulsion of the central slip insertion on the base of the middle phalanx [6].

Clinical Presentation

The patient will present with their finger hyperextended at the DIP joint with flexion deformity at the PIP joint. They will not be able to actively extend the PIP joint of the affected finger [6, 10, 31]. They sometimes will report a specific injury that occurred resulting in the above positioning

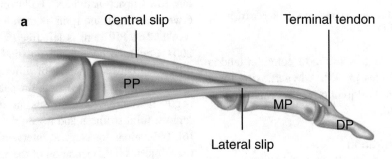

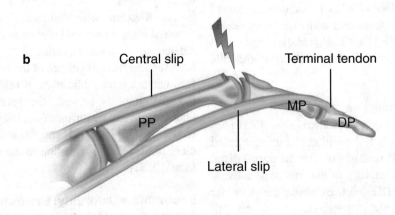

Fig. 6.9 (a, b) Boutonniere deformity: (a) normal alignment and (b) boutonniere deformity caused by a central slip extensor tendon injury

of the finger [6]. There also will be edema near the time of injury, but the patient usually has little to no pain when they are evaluated [45].

Physical Examination

Physical exam will demonstrate the finger in the aforementioned position and sometimes is accompanied by tenderness over the PIP joint. The patient will be unable to extend the PIP joint, but the examiner can passively extend this joint [6]. The Elson test is often performed which consists of flexing the PIP to 90 degrees and asking the patient to extend the PIP against resistance to the middle phalanx. The test is positive if the DIP joint is rigid with weak PIP extension as the finger is extended from the terminal extension of the lateral bands over the DIP joint. If the DIP joint is supple and floppy, the central slip is intact. This test is important as patients with acute central slip injuries may not present initially with obvious flexion deformity at the PIP joint, but rather just weak PIP extension [45].

Diagnostic Workup

Limited diagnostic evaluation is typically performed; however, X-ray can be beneficial if the examiner is worried about an associated avulsion fracture [6]. Ultrasound can show a lack of tendon inserting onto the middle phalanx on the dorsal surface but intact lateral bands inserting onto the distal phalanx [53].

Treatments

Treatment consists of splinting of the PIP joint in extension for 6 weeks. During this time, the DIP joint should be left free to undergo flexion exercises to prevent contracture formation and development of DIP hyperextension. If the PIP joint cannot be passively extended, then the patient should undergo serial casting [6]. Indications for surgical interventions include open injuries and acute avulsion fracture when greater than a third of the cortical surface is present with an articular step off or when conservative management fails [6, 10, 31]. The central slip is either directly repaired with nonabsorbable sutures or repaired back down to its insertion with a suture anchor or small screw in cases of an avulsion fracture at the

insertion. Multiple surgical approaches exist for chronic central slip injuries with boutonniere deformities including central slip reconstruction with lateral band augmentation and distal extensor tenotomy [45].

Vaughn-Jackson Syndrome: Extensor Digiti Minimi Tendinopathy/Rupture

A 68-year-old female with rheumatoid arthritis presents with gradual onset of pain at the distal dorsal ulna. She reports increased pain with gripping objects. On exam, the patient has radial deviation of the wrist and ulnar deviation of the fingers. Gripping and resisted fifth digit extension reproduce the pain.

Anatomy

The extensor digiti minimi (EDM) is in the fifth dorsal compartment of the wrist. EDM originates on the lateral epicondyle of the humerus, lies on the dorsal surface between the radius and ulna, and inserts into the extensor expansion of the fifth digit [3]. The main function of extensor digiti minimi is to extend the fifth digit at the metacarpophalangeal and interphalangeal joint.

Vaughn-Jackson syndrome, seen in patients with rheumatoid arthritis, occurs when the wrist begins to deviate radially bringing the ulnar-sided extensor tendons over the ulna. Repeated subluxation results in extensor tendon rupture beginning with the most ulnar tendons first. EDM ruptures first, but rupture may go unnoticed because EDC extends all four digits simultaneously. Similarly, in caput ulna, defined as instability of the distal radioulnar joint with dorsal ulna head prominence, the EDM tendon can rupture. Caput ulna is normally associated with destruction of the joint secondary to rheumatoid arthritis [56].

Clinical Presentation

Vaughn-Jackson syndrome is seen commonly in individuals with rheumatologic conditions and is associated with disruption or rupture of the tendons to extensor digiti minimi and extensor digitorum [57]. Pain and swelling are typically present over this compartment at the distal head of the ulna [2, 4]. The patient may report repetitive hand use, especially writing, as the cause of the pain [2].

Physical Examination

Pain is typically induced by finger flexion while making a fist and sometimes with resisted fifth digit extension [2]. In EDM rupture, patients are unable to selectively extend the small finger in isolation with the other digits held in flexion.

Diagnostic Workup

This is a clinical diagnosis. As mentioned with other tendinopathies, ultrasound can demonstrate hypervascularity, edema, or loss of tendon visualization at the attachment site. The workup should include radiographs of the wrist to rule out caput ulna with ulnar head prominence or a large dorsal osteophyte causing attritional rupture of the EDM tendon. It is important to rule out ruptures of other tendons including extensor carpi ulnaris (ECU) pathology.

Treatments

As in previous diagnoses, conservative care consisting of rest, splinting, NSAIDs, and corticosteroid injection can be trialed [2]. If this is ineffective, surgical release of the compartment and tenosynovectomy can be performed in cases of tenosynovitis [2, 58]. In this case, caution must be taken to avoid the dorsal cutaneous branches of the ulnar nerve [2]. In the case of EDM rupture, tendon transfers from the adjacent EDC tendons are performed. However, concomitant correction of the underlying cause, radial deviation of the wrist (caput ulnae syndrome) or distal radial ulnar joint instability, must be addressed to prevent future tendon ruptures [56].

Extensor Carpi Ulnaris Tendinopathy

A 32-year-old female tennis player presents with a painful snapping sensation over the dorsal ulnar aspect of the wrist during her tennis practice. When wrist extension is tested with the wrist in supination, the patient reports pain. In addition, the ECU synergy test reproduces the pain.

Introduction

Extensor carpi ulnaris tendinopathy is the second most common tendinopathy of the wrist [6]. The ECU tendon runs between the head and styloid of the ulna in the sixth dorsal compartment and inserts on the dorsal base of the fifth metacarpal [3]. It passes through a groove on the ulnar side of the distal ulna and is covered by a ligament, which can lead to compression and inflammation. A unique feature of this tendon is that it has a separate tendon sheath that assists in stabilizing the ulnar carpal bones and the distal radioulnar joint [59]. The extensor carpi ulnaris tendon typically becomes painful with tendinopathy or subluxation of the tendon [4]. The snapping extensor carpi ulnaris is a unique condition in which the tendon of ECU snaps over the ulna styloid with extension or adduction of the hand [3]. ECU subluxation is more commonly reported in athletes, in particular tennis players, after an injury to the wrist with disruption of the ECU subsheath. The ECU lies in close proximity to the TFCC making it difficult to distinguish between the pathologies of the two [4].

Clinical Presentation

Pain in ECU tendinopathy may be difficult to localize, but it is commonly over the ECU tendon on the dorsal ulnar aspect of the wrist and is worsened with wrist supination, flexion, and ulnar deviation [4]. The patient commonly reports insidious onset of pain with worsening of pain during gripping combined with extension and ulnar deviation as seen in racquet sports and rowing [4, 6]. Those with ECU subluxation may not only have a similar history of pain but also experience a pop when performing ulnar deviation with extension [6].

Physical Examination

The extensor carpi ulnaris is a unique muscle in that it causes ulnar deviation of the hand when the arm is pronated but contributes to extension of the wrist when the arm is in supination [4]. Due to this, the examiner can attempt resisted motion in both of the above settings to illicit pain [4, 45]. Sensory disturbance may be present in the distribution of the dorsal ulnar cutaneous nerve due to its location over the tendon sheath [4]. Another commonly used test is the ECU synergy test (Fig. 6.10), which can help distinguish between ECU tendinopathy and TFCC injury. This test is performed by placing the patient's elbow on the table and supinating the forearm. The digits are extended and the examiner grasps the first two digits of the hand. The patient then attempts to abduct the thumb while the examiner is palpating the ECU tendon. If pain is present, it is likely ECU pathology rather than TFCC pathology [60]. Lastly, to evaluate for snapping of the ECU, the patient's hand is moved from supination and wrist extension to wrist flexion and ulnar deviation. The test is positive if a snap is heard or the tendon is visualized moving out of the groove with forearm rotation [4].

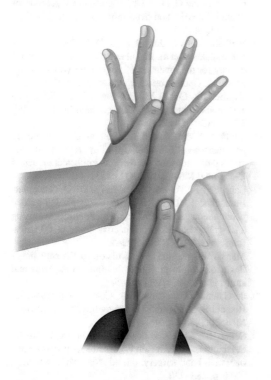

Fig. 6.10 ECU synergy test. The examiner grasps the patient's thumb and long finger with one hand and palpates the ECU tendon with the other. The examiner then has the patient radially deviate the thumb against resistance. The test is considered positive if pain is induced along the dorsal ulnar aspect of the wrist by this procedure

Diagnostic Workup

Ultrasound or MRI can be used to assess for tendinopathic changes [4, 59]. Ultrasound would demonstrate tendon thickening, hypervascularity, and edema around the tendon [46]. In addition, dynamic ultrasound can be utilized in attempts to visualize tendon subluxation with provocative maneuvers [4]. MRI can help rule out TFCC injury if the examiner is unsure which may be contributing to the patient's pain [6]. Plain films can also be obtained to view the position of the distal ulna, as a positive variance increases the incidence of TFCC injuries. Finally local anesthetic injections sometimes are used to differentiate between ECU pathology versus intra-articular pathology in the ulnar wrist [4]. The differential diagnosis includes ECU subluxation, EDM tendinopathy, pisotriquetral arthritis, and triangular fibrocartilage complex injury.

Treatments

Initial treatment consists of conservative measures as surgery is not commonly necessary. The patient can be placed in a wrist splint with 15 degrees of extension and given anti-inflammatory medications [4]. Patients are instructed to avoid active ulnar deviation of the wrist. Often an ulnar-based thermoplast splint is more helpful than a standard short-arm thermoplast splint. Corticosteroid injection into the ECU tendon sheath with ultrasound guidance can be performed [59]. In the case of recurrent ECU subluxation, the patient can be placed in cast immobilization with the wrist in a pronated and dorsiflexed position for 6 weeks [6].

Surgery can be attempted if conservative measures have failed. Traditionally, an incision is placed over the ECU tendon with careful dissection to avoid the dorsal cutaneous branch of the ulnar nerve. The tendon sheath is released with tenosynovectomy in cases of ECU tenosynovitis. A longitudinal tear of the ECU tendon can be treated with debridement back to healthy tissue and suturing of the defect. After surgery, the wrist is immobilized in 15–20 degrees of extension for 2 weeks. In cases of ECU tendon subluxation, the subsheath is repaired or reconstructed using the extensor retinaculum [4, 11, 59, 61]. Postoperatively, the arm is placed in a long arm cast at 90 degrees of elbow flexion, neutral forearm rotation, and 30 degrees of wrist extension for 4–6 weeks [2, 59].

References

1. Armstron T, Fine L, Goldstein S, Lifshitz Y, Silverstein B. Ergonomic considerations in hand and wrist tendinitis. The Journal of Hand Surgery. 1987;12(5 Pt 2):830–7.
2. Elder G, Harvey E. Chapter 15: Hand and Wrist Tendinopathies. In: Maffulli MD, PhD N, Renstrom MD, PhD P, Leadbetter MDW, editors. Tendon injuries: basic science and clinical medicine. 1st ed. London: Springer; 2005;137–49.
3. Standring S. Chapter 50 Wrist and Hand. In: Gray's anatomy: the anatomical basis of clinical practice. 41st ed. New York: Elsevier; 2016:862–94.
4. Adams JE, Habbu R. Tendinopathies of the hand and wrist. J Am Acad Orthop Surg. 2015;23(12):741–50.
5. Bishop AT, Gabel G, Carmichael SW. Flexor carpi radialis tendinitis. Part I: operative anatomy. J Bone Joint Surg Am. 1994;76(7):1009–14.
6. Finnoff J. Chapter 35: Upper Limb Pain and Dysfunction. In: Cifu D, editor. Braddom's: physical medicine and rehabilitation. 5th ed. Philadelphia: Elsevier; 2016:769–80.
7. Gabel G, Bishop AT, Wood MB. Flexor carpi radialis tendinitis. Part II: results of operative treatment. J Bone Joint Surg Am. 1994;76(7):1015–8.
8. Eshed I, Feist E, Althoff CE, Hamm B, Konen E, Burmester GR, et al. Tenosynovitis of the flexor tendons of the hand detected by MRI: an early indicator of rheumatoid arthritis. Rheumatology (Oxford). 2009;48(8):887–91.
9. Jacobson J. Chapter 5 Wrist and Hand Ultrasound. In: Fundamentals of musculoskeletal ultrasound. 2nd ed. Philadelphia: Elsevier; 2013;110–61.
10. Garnham A, Ashe M, Gropper P, Race D. Chapter 24 Hand and finger injuries. In: Brukner P, Kahn K, editors. Brukner and Kahn's clinical sports medicine. 4th ed. Sydney: McGraw-Hill; 2012. p. 435–48.
11. McAuliffe JA. Tendon disorders of the hand and wrist. J Hand Surg Am. 2010;35(5):846–53; quiz 53
12. Ryan WG. Calcific tendinitis of flexor carpi ulnaris: an easy misdiagnosis. Arch Emerg Med. 1993;10(4):321–3.
13. Torbati SS, Bral D, Geiderman JM. Acute calcific tendinitis of the wrist. J Emerg Med. 2013;44(2):352–4.
14. Budoff JE, Kraushaar BS, Ayala G. Flexor carpi ulnaris tendinopathy. J Hand Surg Am. 2005;30(1):125–9.
15. Knobloch K, Gohritz A, Spies M, Vogt PM. Neovascularisation in flexor carpi ulnaris tendinopathy: novel combined sclerosing therapy and eccentric training of the forearms in athletics' wrist pain. BMJ Case Rep. 2009;2009:bcr08.2008.0714.
16. Wick MC, Weiss RJ, Arora R, Gabl M, Gruber J, Jaschke W, et al. Enthesiopathy of the flexor carpi ulnaris at the pisiform: findings of high-frequency sonography. Eur J Radiol. 2011;77(2):240–4.
17. Palmieri TJ. Pisiform area pain treatment by pisiform excision. J Hand Surg Am. 1982;7(5):477–80.
18. Valdes K. A retrospective review to determine the long-term efficacy of orthotic devices for trigger finger. J Hand Ther. 2012;25(1):89–95; quiz 6
19. Quinnell RC. Conservative management of trigger finger. Practitioner. 1980;224(1340):187–90.
20. Castellanos J, Muñoz-Mahamud E, Domínguez E, Del Amo P, Izquierdo O, Fillat P. Long-term effectiveness of corticosteroid injections for trigger finger and thumb. J Hand Surg Am. 2015;40(1):121–6.
21. Dala-Ali BM, Nakhdjevani A, Lloyd MA, Schreuder FB. The efficacy of steroid injection in the treatment of trigger finger. Clin Orthop Surg. 2012;4(4):263–8.
22. Shinomiya R, Sunagawa T, Nakashima Y, Yoshizuka M, Adachi N. Impact of corticosteroid injection site on the treatment success rate of trigger finger: a prospective study comparing ultrasound-guided true intra-sheath and true extra-sheath injections. Ultrasound Med Biol. 2016;42(9):2203–8.
23. Orlandi D, Corazza A, Silvestri E, Serafini G, Savarino EV, Garlaschi G, et al. Ultrasound-guided procedures around the wrist and hand: how to do. Eur J Radiol. 2014;83(7):1231–8.
24. Malliaropoulos N, Jury R, Pyne D, Padhiar N, Turner J, Korakakis V, et al. Radial extracorporeal shockwave therapy for the treatment of finger tenosynovitis (trigger digit). Open Access J Sports Med. 2016;7:143–51.
25. Werthel JD, Cortez M, Elhassan BT. Modified percutaneous trigger finger release. Hand Surg Rehabil. 2016;35(3):179–82.
26. Smith J, Rizzo M, Lai JK. Sonographically guided percutaneous first annular pulley release: cadaveric safety study of needle and knife techniques. J Ultrasound Med. 2010;29(11):1531–42.
27. Lapègue F, André A, Meyrignac O, Pasquier-Bernachot E, Dupré P, Brun C, et al. US-guided percutaneous release of the trigger finger by using a 21-gauge needle: a prospective study of 60 cases. Radiology. 2016;280(2):493–9.
28. Manske PR, Lesker PA. Avulsion of the ring finger flexor digitorum profundus tendon: an experimental study. Hand. 1978;10(1):52–5.
29. de Gautard G, de Gautard R, Celi J, Jacquemoud G, Bianchi S. Sonography of Jersey finger. J Ultrasound Med. 2009;28(3):389–92.
30. Seiler IIIJ. Chapter 6 flexor tendon injury. In: Wolfe S, Hotchkiss R, Pederson W, Kozin S, editors. Green's operative hand surgery. 6th ed. New York: Elsevier; 2011. p. 183–230.
31. Garnham A, Ashe M, Gropper P, Race D. Brukner & Khan, editors. Brukner & Khan's clinical sports medicine (4th ed.). Sydney; New York: McGraw-Hill; 2012.
32. Linburg RM, Comstock BE. Anomalous tendon slips from the flexor pollicis longus to the flexor digitorum profundus. J Hand Surg Am. 1979;4(1):79–83.

33. Furukawa K, Menuki K, Sakai A, Oshige T, Nakamura T. Linburg-Comstock syndrome: a case report. Hand Surg. 2012;17(2):217–20.

34. Rennie WR, Muller H. Linburg syndrome. Can J Surg. 1998;41(4):306–8.

35. Alemohammad AM, Yazaki N, Morris RP, Buford WL, Viegas SF. Thumb interphalangeal joint extension by the extensor pollicis brevis: association with a subcompartment and de Quervain's disease. J Hand Surg Am. 2009;34(4):719–23.

36. Alexander RD, Catalano LW, Barron OA, Glickel SZ. The extensor pollicis brevis entrapment test in the treatment of de Quervain's disease. J Hand Surg Am. 2002;27(5):813–6.

37. Ilyas AM, Ilyas A, Ast M, Schaffer AA, Thoder J. De quervain tenosynovitis of the wrist. J Am Acad Orthop Surg. 2007;15(12):757–64.

38. Ashurst JV, Turco DA, Lieb BE. Tenosynovitis caused by texting: an emerging.disease. J Am Osteopath Assoc. 2010;110(5):294–6.

39. Sharan D, Ajeesh PS. Risk factors and clinical features of text message injuries. Work. 2012;41(Suppl 1):1145–8.

40. Lee KH, Kang CN, Lee BG, Jung WS, Kim DY, Lee CH. Ultrasonographic evaluation of the first extensor compartment of the wrist in de Quervain's disease. J Orthop Sci. 2014;19(1):49–54.

41. Rowland P, Phelan N, Gardiner S, Linton K, Galvin R. The effectiveness of corticosteroid injection for de Quervain's stenosing tenosynovitis (DQST): a systematic review and meta-analysis. J Orthop Sci. 2015;9:437–44.

42. De Keating-Hart E, Touchais S, Kerjean Y, Ardouin L, Le Goff B. Presence of an intracompartmental septum detected by ultrasound is associated with the failure of ultrasound-guided steroid injection in de Quervain's syndrome. J Hand Surg Eur Vol. 2016;41(2):212–9.

43. Cavaleri R, Schabrun SM, Te M, Chipchase LS. Hand therapy versus corticosteroid injections in the treatment of de Quervain's disease: a systematic review and meta-analysis. J Hand Ther. 2016;29(1):3–11.

44. Peck E, Ely E. Successful treatment of de Quervain tenosynovitis with ultrasound-guided percutaneous needle tenotomy and platelet-rich plasma injection: a case presentation. PM R. 2013;5(5):438–41.

45. Chauhan A, Jacobs B, Andoga A, Baratz ME. Extensor tendon injuries in athletes. Sports Med Arthrosc. 2014;22(1):45–55.

46. Plotkin B, Sampath SC, Motamedi K. MR imaging and US of the wrist tendons. Radiographics. 2016;36(6):1688–700.

47. Giovagnorio F, Miozzi F. Ultrasound findings in intersection syndrome. J Med Ultrason (2001). 2012;39(4):217–20.

48. Grundberg AB, Reagan DS. Pathologic anatomy of the forearm: intersection syndrome. J Hand Surg Am. 1985;10(2):299–302.

49. Williams JG. Surgical management of traumatic non-infective tenosynovitis of the wrist extensors. J Bone Joint Surg Br. 1977;59-B(4):408–10.

50. Kardashian G, Vara AD, Miller SJ, Miki RA, Jose J. Stenosing synovitis of the extensor pollicis longus tendon. J Hand Surg Am. 2011;36(6):1035–8.

51. Cooper HJ, Shevchuk MM, Li X, Yang SS. Proliferative extensor tenosynovitis of the wrist in the absence of rheumatoid arthritis. J Hand Surg Am. 2009;34(10):1827–31.

52. Hogan JI, Hurtado RM, Nelson SB. Mycobacterial musculoskeletal infections. Infect Dis Clin N Am. 2017;31(2):369–82.

53. Lee SA, Kim BH, Kim SJ, Kim JN, Park SY, Choi K. Current status of ultrasonography of the finger. Ultrasonography. 2016;35(2):110–23.

54. Smit JM, Beets MR, Zeebregts CJ, Rood A, Welters CF. Treatment options for mallet finger: a review. Plast Reconstr Surg. 2010;126(5):1624–9.

55. Handoll HH, Vaghela MV. Intervention for treating mallet finger injuries. Cochrane Database Syst Rev. 2004;3:CD004574.

56. Strauch R. Chapter 5 extensor tendon injury. In: Wolfe S, Hotchkiss R, Pederson W, Kozin S, editors. Green's operative hand surgery. 6th ed. Philadelphia: Elsevier; 2011. p. 152–82.

57. Mazhar T, Rambani R. Vaughan-Jackson-like syndrome as an unusual presentation of Kienböck's disease: a case report. J Med Case Rep. 2011;5:325.

58. Hooper G, McMaster MJ. Stenosing tenovaginitis affecting the tendon of extensor digiti minimi at the wrist. Hand. 1979;11(3):299–301.

59. Garcia-Elias M. Tendinopathies of the extensor carpi ulnaris. Handchir Mikrochir Plast Chir. 2015;47(5):281–9.

60. Ruland RT, Hogan CJ. The ECU synergy test: an aid to diagnose ECU tendonitis. J Hand Surg Am. 2008;33(10):1777–82.

61. Kollitz KM, Iorio ML, Huang JI. Assessment and treatment of extensor carpi ulnaris tendon pathology: a critical analysis review. JBJS Rev. 2015;3(6):01874474.

Rectus Abdominis and Hip Adductor Tendons ("Athletic Pubalgia/Sports Hernia")

7

Gerardo Miranda-Comas, Eliana Cardozo, Svetlana Abrams, and Joseph E. Herrera

Abbreviations

FAI   Femoroacetabular impingement
NSAID   Non-steroidal anti-inflammatory drug
ROM   Range of motion

Introduction

Athletic pubalgia, also known as sports(man's) hernia, Gilmore's groin, or simply core muscle injury, refers to an overuse disorder of pain in the groin and/or peripubic region associated with activities that involve trunk extension, running, kicking, and cutting movements [1]. The pathophysiology of this disorder may involve multiple etiologies and anatomic structures. In this chapter, we will focus on rectus abdominis aponeurosis injury and adductor longus tendinopathy.

The original version of this chapter was revised. The correction to this chapter can be found at https://doi.org/10.1007/978-3-030-65335-4_22

G. Miranda-Comas (✉) · E. Cardozo · S. Abrams
J. E. Herrera
Department of Rehabilitation and Human Performance, Icahn School of Medicine at Mount Sinai, New York, NY, USA
e-mail: Gerardo.miranda-comas@mountsinai.org;
Eliana.cardozo@mountsinai.org;
Joseph.herrera@mountsinai.org

Anatomy

A review of the relevant anatomy includes the rectus sheath which contains the rectus abdominis muscle, originating at the pubic symphysis and iliac crests and inserting on the xiphoid process and costal cartilages. Additionally, the rectus sheath houses the superior and inferior epigastric vessels, the lymphatics, and the ventral rami of the T7-L1 nerves, which enter the sheath laterally. The superior part of the rectus abdominis is totally enveloped within the rectus sheath, while the inferior one-quarter is supported posteriorly only by the transversalis fascia and the peritoneum [4]. The relevant medial thigh musculature includes the adductor longus muscle which originates at the body of the pubis, inferior to the pubic crest, and inserts in the middle third of the linea aspera of the femur, and the adductor brevis muscle which originates on the body and inferior ramus of the pubis and attaches on the pectineal line and proximal femur. The adductor magnus muscle lies medial, originating at the inferior ramus of the pubis, ramus of the ischium, and ischial tuberosity and inserting on the femur. Lastly, the gracilis muscle has its origin at the body and inferior ramus of the pubis and inserts on the femur (see Fig. 7.1) [4].

One of the most important anatomic characteristics that contribute to this pathology is the confluent sheath anterior to the pubis formed by the rectus abdominis and adductor longus tendons. The pubic aponeurosis which is formed by the rectus abdominis, the conjoint tendon (internal oblique and transverse abdominis) and the external oblique muscles, is also confluent with the adductor longus and gracilis muscles [5]. The pubic symphysis is the common denominator in the different movements that occur in the anterior pelvis, making this area susceptible to injury.

Mechanism of Injury

In the past, several terms have been used to describe groin pain in the athlete including sportsman's hernia, athletic hernia, Gilmore's groin. Athletic pubalgia is considered the more appropriate and most recent term used to describe groin overuse injury with or without hernia. Groin pain accounts for only approximately 5% of all visits to a musculoskeletal clinic, but it is common in specific sports requiring twisting, cutting, pivoting, and kicking including soccer, ice hockey, field hockey, American football, ballet, and martial arts [1–3].

The etiology of athletic pubalgia is multifactorial. Injury risk factors include muscle imbalances at the pubic symphysis, decreased hip abduction range of motion, and prior groin muscle strains [1, 5]. Specifically, the pubic symphysis is the center and acts as a fulcrum where large opposing forces occur between the rectus abdominis and the adductor longus. When there is an imbalance, and the abdominal musculature is weak in relation to the adductor musculature, injury may occur (see Fig. 7.2) [5].

The injury may involve the abdominal musculature (rectus abdominis, transverse fascia at the posterior inguinal wall, external oblique aponeurosis, conjoint tendon) or the tendons of the medial thigh muscles (more commonly the adductor longus) [1, 3, 5]. Meyers et al. coined the term "pubic joint" to describe the rotational joint which encompasses both pubic bones, the pubic symphysis, and all the anterior pelvic musculature around these bones (Fig. 7.2) [6]. A commonly described mechanism of injury involves hyperextension of the trunk, with or without hip abduction, adduction, flexion-extension.

Athletic Pubalgia/Sports Hernia/ Rectus Abdominis-Adductor Longus Tendinopathy

Case Presentation

A 21-year-old collegiate soccer player presents with 2-month history of worsening right-sided groin area pain. Pain is focal at the pubic symphysis area, and this started shortly after a match. He reports exacerbation with kicking, better with rest. Three years earlier, he was evaluated for right hip pain and found with evidence of acetabular femoral head over coverage on bilateral hip plain X-rays. This previous episode was treated with relative rest and physical therapy with complete resolution of symptoms.

Clinical Presentation

The athlete will usually present with insidious unilateral groin and lower abdominal and/or adductor area pain of gradual progression. Some patients may report acute tearing sensation. Symptoms are usually absent at rest, exacerbated by activities such as kicking and running, although lower level activities or sneezing and coughing may provoke pain [3, 7].

Physical Examination

The physical exam should be performed systematically to rule out associated pathologies since many patients will have numerous abnormal findings related to other causes of groin pain. Initial evaluation includes observation for anatomic asymmetry or tissue deformities, followed by direct palpation to the pubic bones, pubic symphysis, medial inguinal floor, distal rectus abdominis, and the adductor musculature. Patients may also have pain with resisted hip adduction and with maneuvers that increase abdominal pressure, such as resisted sit-ups or Valsalva maneuver [5, 7, 8]. Additionally, there may be concomitant intra-articular hip pathology, such as femoral acetabular impingement, symptomatic acetabular labral tears, or hip osteoarthritis. This may become apparent with findings such as limited hip range of motion and pain with internal rotation; therefore, a thorough hip examination should be included. The athlete should also have a standard inguinal hernia exam [8]. Functional evaluation includes single leg stance; although it is not specific for medial hip/groin

Fig. 7.1 Thigh muscle origins and insertions

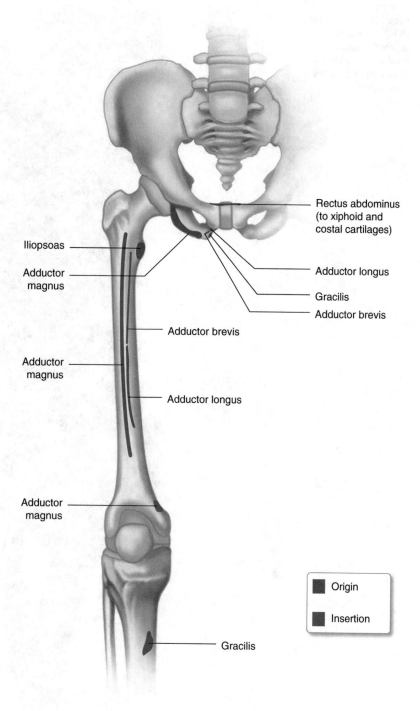

Anterior view

Iliopsoas

Adductor magnus

Rectus abdominus (to xiphoid and costal cartilages)

Adductor longus

Gracilis

Adductor brevis

Adductor brevis

Adductor magnus

Adductor longus

Adductor magnus

Gracilis

Origin

Insertion

Fig. 7.2 Opposite
vector forces at the
pubic symphysis: rectus
abdominis exerts a
superior directional
force and the adductor
longus exerts an inferior
directional force

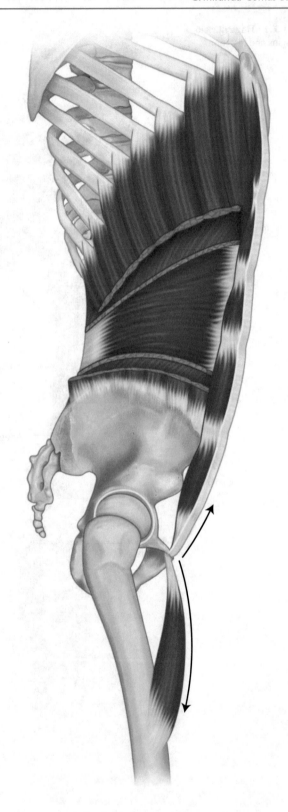

pain, it is useful in identifying symptomatic hip pathology. Gait analysis evaluates for Trendelenburg sign in muscle tear or neurologic injury, as well as dynamic leg-length discrepancy. Lastly, it should be noted that there may be no abnormal findings on physical exam in some athletes with athletic pubalgia [3, 7].

Athletic Pubalgia and Femoral Acetabular Impingement

Athletic pubalgia may be associated with other hip/groin pathologies, including femoral acetabular impingement (FAI). There are three types of FAI: cam, pincer, and mixed (Fig. 7.3). In the pincer type, there is usually acetabular over coverage of the femoral head causing impingement. In the cam type, hip impingement is caused by a deformity of the femoral head-neck junction with a bony bump which impinges on the rim of the acetabulum [9]. Decreased internal rotation of the hip in FAI leads to altered biomechanics in the hip joint, including increased stress on the public symphysis, which may predispose patients to injury. Birmingham et al. studied the effect of FAI on rotational motion at the pubic symphysis on cadavers. The results showed increased rotation motion at the pubic symphysis with FAI-cam impingement [10]. Clinically, it is important to diagnose and treat both conditions to ensure better patient outcomes.

Diagnostic Workup

Imaging studies are useful when evaluating groin pain.

X-Ray

Plain X-rays, including AP pelvis and frog leg lateral views, are used to evaluate bony alignment, avulsion fractures, and signs of FAI.

MRI

For suspected athletic pubalgia, the recommended imaging modality is a pelvic MRI. There are specific MRI protocols used to evaluate athletic pubalgia. These MRIs include the typical large field of view bony pelvis sequences and smaller field of view sequences centered around the pubic symphysis [11]. The MRI should be of high resolution and include sagittal pelvic sequences as well as oblique, transverse, T2, and fat-suppressed sequences if adductor pathology is suspected [8]. Palisch et al. described five categories of athletic pubalgia injury patterns that can be found on MRI, which include (1) unilateral or bilateral rectus abdominis/adductor aponeurosis injury (most common), (2) midline rectus abdominis/adductor aponeurosis plate injury (pubic plate injury), (3) osteitis pubis, (4) adductor tendon origin injury, and (5) other core muscle injury. [11] Of note, osteitis pubis is not commonly included under athletic pubalgia and is considered its own entity. The first and second injury patterns will be identified as a cleft of fluid-equivalent signal at the aponeurosis or under the midline pubic plate. MRI findings of the other injury patterns include bone marrow edema in the pubic bodies representing osteitis pubis, adductor longus tendinosis, proximal adductor, and/or distal rectus abdominis myotendinous strains or atrophy [12, 13].

Ultrasound

Ultrasound (US) may also be used in further evaluating suspected cases of athletic pubalgia. US provides high-resolution imaging of the muscles and tendons, the ability to obtain dynamic images and the real time location of symptoms [14]. Sonographic evaluation includes assessment of the rectus abdominis aponeurosis and the adductor tendon at their respective attachments to the pubic symphysis for evidence of tendinosis, tendon tear, or aponeurosis tear. Sono-palpation over the peripubic myotendinous attachments is helpful in identifying the main pain generator. US can be used to evaluate the inguinal canal to assess for inguinal or femoral hernia at rest and during Valsalva maneuver, specifically evaluating the posterior wall of the inguinal canal [14]. Additionally, US can be used to guide procedures for diagnosis and treatment. Evaluation of the pubic symphysis for osteitis pubis is limited by the lack of penetration of US through bone, but in addition to secondary findings that may suggest the diagnosis, a sono-guided injection is often

Fig. 7.3 Types of
femoroacetabular
impingement (FAI):
Pincer FAI and CAM
FAI

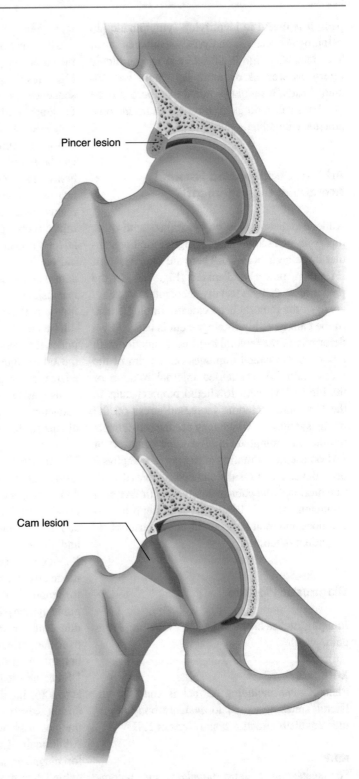

diagnostic and therapeutic. Other procedures can be performed with the aid of ultrasound, including percutaneous tenotomy and platelet-rich plasma infiltration.

Treatment

Conservative

The first line of treatment in athletic pubalgia is nonoperative. Management should be approached in a stepwise fashion to ensure safe return to activity. Just as is the case for other tendon injuries discussed in other chapters, rehabilitation of the athletic pubalgia can be divided into acute, recovery, functional, and return-to-play phases. Rehabilitation protocols vary, but all are designed to alleviate pain and improve range of motion and strength with a focus on return to function. During the acute phase of rehabilitation, the main goals are relative rest of injured area and treatment of the symptom complex. Cryotherapy, transcutaneous nerve or high-voltage galvanic electrical stimulation, and analgesics or a short course of anti-inflammatory medication (NSAIDs) are used to alleviate pain and decrease edema. To avoid contractures, education regarding posture and neutral spine is provided, and ROM is improved through hip and lumbar spine mobilization. Active stretching and isometric strengthening exercises of the hip musculature are implemented during this phase as well. Exercises focusing on transverse abdominis strengthening are crucial for successful rehabilitation since delayed onset and poor transversus abdominis muscle activation has been shown to be associated with longstanding groin pain [15, 16]. The focus of rehabilitation during the recovery phase is to continue to correct biomechanical deficits, improve muscle control and balance, retrain proprioception, and start sports specific activity. Improving functional ROM of the hips and the lumbar spine is essential and should be worked in a pain-free range. The individual may progress static core strengthening and increase recruitment of hip and pelvic stabilization with continued focus on transversus abdominis strengthening with introduction of double leg functional exercises. Standing stabilization may be challenged with resistance or balance disturbance, and functional activity may progress from double leg to single leg exercises. The functional phase of rehabilitation should focus on increasing power and endurance while improving neuromuscular control. Rehabilitation at this stage should work on the entire kinematic chain addressing specific functional deficits. During this stage, functional ROM deficits should be corrected in the lumbopelvic area and hips. Dynamic core training is accomplished with the use of neutral spine during activity on stable and unstable surfaces. Strengthening may now include concentric and eccentric exercises, as well as plyometric training. The patient may now progress into sports-specific drills [15]. Factors to consider in the return-to-play decision include absence of symptoms at rest and with sports activity, normal flexibility, strength and neuromuscular control, and psychologic readiness. Although the recovery varies by individual and injury severity, an approximate timeline for conservative treatment trial is 6–8 weeks [15].

Interventional

When symptoms fail to improve with a targeted rehabilitation program, non-surgical interventions have been shown to help treat this condition. Although corticosteroid use in tendinous areas has fallen in disuse, there is some evidence that suggests its use in patients with athletic pubalgia. Jose and colleagues reviewed the outcome of ultrasonography-guided corticosteroid injections for 12 patients with athletic pubalgia [17]. These patients were evaluated with ultrasound and were found to have partial or complete tears around the insertion of the rectus abdominis and/or the adductor longus origin. These individuals returned to their preinjury activity levels 6 weeks following successful ultrasonography-guided steroid injection. Furthermore, none of the patients opted for surgical repair during their follow-up (ranging from 6 to 19 months) [17]. On the other hand, US-guided needle tenotomy and treatment with platelet rich plasma (PRP) may be a more promising option for the treatment of athletic pubalgia, but this requires further research.

[18–20]. Although studies regarding the role of PRP in athletic pubalgia are limited, a case report of athletic pubalgia due to distal rectus abdominis tendinopathy that was treated with targeted ultrasound-guided PRP injection and tenotomy resulted in complete resolution of symptoms in a lacrosse player [21].

Operative

If conservative management fails to improve symptoms associated with athletic pubalgia or affects athletic performance, surgical intervention may be indicated. In fact, one study showed better outcomes in soccer players with chronic groin pain who selected to undergo surgical intervention as opposed to conservative management [22]. Surgical techniques employed for hernia management in an athlete can be classified into three broad categories: (1) open primary tissue repair, (2) open tension-free mesh repair, and (3) laparoscopic posterior mesh repair [8]. There is no consensus as to the optimal approach, and success of the surgery is largely dependent on surgeon expertise. Of note, a newer technique described by Harr and Brody combined a suture repair of the inguinal floor and a rectus and adductor longus tenotomy. Utilizing this technique allowed 22 athletes to return to their respective sports and regain their ability to perform at a high level without further surgery returning to full activity in 6–8 weeks. According to the authors, this may be the optimal surgical management option since this combination technique addresses both vector forces on the pubic bone and the inguinal floor weakness [23].

Other Proximal Adductor Tendons Injuries

Other proximal adductor tendon injuries must be considered in the setting of chronic groin pain, although exact prevalence is unknown for these other tendons. The adductor magnus (AM) is located on the medial side of the thigh and consists of two parts. The pubofemoral portion or adductor portion arises from the ischiopubic ramus, while the ischiocondylar portion or extensor portion arises from the tuberosity of the ischium. The lateral part of the AM muscle is called the adductor minimus. Avulsions may occur at the origin of the AM muscle commonly seen in activities that require opposing lower limb flexion-extension or abduction motions like "the splits" in cheerleading [24]. A wide variation in the dimensional characteristics of the ischiocondylar portion of the AM tendon among cadaver specimens suggests that injury to this tendon may mimic symptoms of other proximal tendons such as the hamstring [25].

The gracilis tendon-muscle construct is the most superficial construct on the medial aspect of the thigh, crossing the hip and knee joint making it susceptible to injury. Its function is to adduct the thigh, flex the knee, and internally rotate the tibia [4]. There is limited data regarding isolated gracilis construct injuries, but most injuries occur in the proximal-middle third of the thigh, at the musculotendinous junction [26]. The described mechanism of injury is related to an eccentric muscle contraction where the hip is placed in internal rotation and maximum flexion, with a fully extended knee.

References

1. Oliveira A, Andreoli C, Ejnisman B, Queiroz R, Pires O, Falótico G. Epidemiological profile of patients diagnosed with athletic pubalgia. Rev Bras Ortop (English Edition). 2016;51(6):692–6.
2. Nam A, Brody F. Management and therapy for sports hernia. J Am Coll Surg. 2008 Jan;206(1):154–64.
3. Elattar O, Choi H-R, Dills VD, Busconi B. Groin injuries (athletic pubalgia) and return to play. Sports Health. 2016;8(4):313–23.
4. Hansen JT, Netter FH. Netter's clinical anatomy. 1st ed. Philadelphia, PA: Saunders/Elsevier; 2014. Print.
5. Cohen B, Kleinhenz D, Schiller J, Tabaddor R. Understanding athletic pubalgia: a review. R I Med J. 2016;99(10):31–5.
6. Meyers WC, Yoo E, Devon ON, et al. Understanding "sports hernia" (athletic pubalgia): the anatomic and pathophysiologic basis for abdominal and groin pain in athletes. Oper Tech Sports Med. 2007;15:165–77.
7. Anderson K, Strickland SM, Warren R. Hip and groin injuries in athletes. Am J Sports Med. 2001;29:521–7.
8. Brunt LM. Hernia management in the athlete. Adv Surg. 2016;50(1):187–202.

9. Jaberi FM, Parvizi J. Hip pain in young adults: femoroacetabular impingement. J Arthroplasty. 2007;22(7 Suppl 3):37–42.

10. Birmingham PM, Kelly BT, Jacobs R, Mcgrady L, Wang M. The effect of dynamic femoroacetabular impingement on pubic symphysis motion: a cadaveric study. Am J Sports Med. 2012;40(5):1113–8.

11. Palisch A, Zoga AC, Meyers WC. Imaging of athletic pubalgia and core muscle injuries. Clin Sports Med. 2013;32(3):427–47.

12. Larbi A, Pesquer L, Reboul G, Omoumi P, Perozziello A, Abadie P, et al. MRI in patients with chronic pubalgia: is precise useful information provided to the surgeon? A case-control study. Orthop Traumatol Surg Res. 2016;102(6):747–54.

13. Hegazi TM, Belair JA, Mccarthy EJ, Roedl JB, Morrison WB. Sports injuries about the hip: what the radiologist should know. Radiographics. 2016;36(6):1717–45.

14. Morley N, Grant T, Blount K, Omar I. Sonographic evaluation of athletic pubalgia. Skeletal Radiol. 2016;45(5):689–99.

15. Ellsworth AA, Zoland MP, Tyler TF. Athletic pubalgia and associated rehabilitation. Int J Sports Phys Ther. 2014;9(6):774–84.

16. Cowan SM, Schache AG, Brunker P, et al. Delayed onset of transversus abdominis in long-standing groin pain. Med Sci Sports Exerc. 2004:2040–5.

17. Jose J, Buller LT, Fokin A, et al. Ultrasound-guided corticosteroid injection for the treatment of athletic pubalgia: a series of 12 cases. J Med Ultrasound. 2015;23:71–5.

18. Tahririan MA, Moezi M, Motififard M, Nemati M, Nemati A. Ultrasound guided platelet-rich plasma injection for the treatment of rotator cuff tendinopathy. Adv Biomed Res. 2016;5:200. https://doi.org/10.4103/2277-9175.190939.

19. James SLJ, Ali K, Pocock C, et al. Ultrasound guided dry needling and autologous blood injection for patellar tendinosis. Br J Sports Med. 2007;41:518–21; discussion 522.

20. Ferrero G, Fabbro E, Orlandi D, et al. Ultrasound-guided injection of platelet-rich plasma in chronic Achilles and patellar tendinopathy. J Ultrasound. 2012;15(4):260–6. https://doi.org/10.1016/j.jus.2012.09.006.

21. Scholten PM, Massimi S, Dahmen N, Diamond J, Wyss J. Successful treatment of athletic pubalgia in a lacrosse player with ultrasound-guided needle tenotomy and platelet-rich plasma injection: a case report. PMR. 2015;7(1):79–83.

22. Ekstrand J, Ringbog S. Surgery versus conservative treatment in soccer players with chronic groin pain: a prospective, randomized study in soccer players. Eur J Sports Traumatol Rel Res. 2001;23:141–5.

23. Harr JN, Brody F. Sports hernia repair with adductor tenotomy. Hernia. 2017;21(1):139–47.

24. Anderson K, Strickland SM, Warren R. Hip and groin injuries in athletes. Am J Sports Med. 2001;29(4):521–33.

25. Obey MR, Broski SM, Spinner RJ, Collins MS, Krych AJ. Anatomy of the adductor magnus origin: implications for proximal hamstring injuries. Orthop J Sports Med. 2016;4(1):23–5.

26. Pedret C, Balius R, Barceló P, Miguel M, Lluís A, Valle X, Gougoulias N, Malliaropoulos N, Maffulli N. Isolated tears of the gracilis muscle. Am J Sports Med. 2011;39(5):1077–80.

Proximal Hamstring Tendons

Lindsay Ramey Argo, Ryan S. Selley,
Vehniah K. Tjong, and Joseph Ihm

Abbreviations

ESWT extracorporeal shock wave therapy
MRI   magnetic resonance imaging
PHT   proximal hamstring tendinopathy
US   ultrasound

Introduction

The hamstrings are one of the most commonly injured structures among athletes. Injuries to the hamstrings can be seen in a variety of physical activities, including contact and non-contact sports, as well as in inactive individuals. Hamstring injuries may involve tendons, muscles, or both and are cited as the most common injury in Australian rules football, the second most common injury in American rules football [1, 2], and have reported prevalence rates as high as 51% (34% acute, 17% chronic) among dancers [3].

The most common injury involves an injury to muscle (i.e., a muscle strain), typically occurring at the proximal hamstring myotendinous junction [4]. However, other regions of the muscle-tendon unit can be involved, including the proximal tendons, the tendon substance side of the myotendinous junction, or the growth plate adjacent to the proximal tendon attachment in adolescents [4–6]. These injuries may require a different treatment approach and have different prognoses.

Two types of hamstring injury mechanisms have been described in the literature. Type 1 injuries are more common and involve acute injuries to the myotendinous junction, most commonly affecting the long head of the biceps femoris proximally. They are typically seen in sprinters and occur during the terminal swing phase of the gait cycle when the hamstring muscles eccentrically contracts to decelerate the swinging limb and prepare for foot strike [7, 8]. Type 2 injuries are less common and occur during active stretching, similar to a slow eccentric load, with the hip moving into flexion with the knee in extension. These are caused by excessive lengthening of the hamstrings and are seen frequently in dancing, slide tackling, and high kicking [4, 9, 10]. Type 2 injuries typically affect the proximal free tendons, most commonly the semimembranosus, without involvement of the adjacent muscle [4]. For this reason, type 2 hamstring strains may be more accurately classified as a form of proximal

L. R. Argo (✉)
Department of Physical Medicine and Rehabilitation,
University of Texas Southwestern, Dallas, TX, USA
e-mail: lnr8t@virginia.edu

R. S. Selley · V. K. Tjong
Department of Orthopedic Surgery, Northwestern
University, Chicago, IL, USA

J. Ihm
Shirley Ryan Ability Lab, Northwestern University,
Chicago, IL, USA
e-mail: jihm1@sralab.org

© Springer Nature Switzerland AG 2021
K. Onishi et al. (eds.), *Tendinopathy*, https://doi.org/10.1007/978-3-030-65335-4_8

hamstring tendinopathy (PHT) rather than a traditional muscle strain, as detailed below.

For consistency in this chapter, a hamstring strain will refer to injury of one or more of the hamstrings at the proximal myotendinous junction, with or without concomitant injury to the adjacent proximal hamstring tendon substance. Injury affecting only the proximal free tendon will not be classified as a strain, but rather as a form of PHT. When an acute, complete tendon tear or osseus avulsion is discussed, the term avulsion injury will be used. When the site of injury is not specified, as is common in older literature, the more generic term "hamstring muscle-complex injury" will be used. When possible, the injuries described in previous studies will be named according to this categorization.

PHT, independent of and proximal to the myotendinous junction, refers to a pathologic process that occurs within one or more of the proximal hamstring tendons resulting in lower buttock and/or posterior thigh pain. Tendinopathy is a process that can include intratendinous collagen disorganization, partial or complete tendon tearing of various sizes from micro- to macro-sized tears, and intratendinous calcifications with or without peritendinous inflammation [11, 12]. Some suggest that it occurs as a result of overuse and mechanical overload, though studies on tendinosis show evidence of intrasubstance abnormalities among inactive individuals, with or without symptoms [13, 14]. Tendinopathy is also known to predispose athletes to future worsening of injuries, partly attributable to a declining tendon quality due to accumulative changes as stated above [15].

PHT was first described in 1988 under the name "hamstring syndrome" [16] and various case reports and research studies have led to growing knowledge over the years. The prevalence of PHT has not been studied formally and is unknown. It can affect athletes in various sports and at all levels of participation but has been reported most frequently in sprinters, hurdlers, mid-to-long-distance runners, dancers, and endurance athletes [4, 11, 16, 17]. The semimembranosus tendon is most commonly affected, though any tendon can be involved [18]. Sciatic nerve involvement has been reported in a number of PHT cases [18], with subsequent symptoms related to this, such as pain or numbness in the distribution of the sciatic nerve. Given the proximity of the sciatic nerve to the semimembranosus tendon [19], this is not surprising; however, the rate of involvement of the sciatic nerve has not been well described.

In its most severe form, hamstring injury can include avulsion at the proximal hamstring origin. Avulsion has been used to describe a variety of acute tears of the proximal hamstring tendons, including complete tear of one or more tendons from the ischial tuberosity and osseous avulsion at the apophysis of the ischial tuberosity in skeletally immature athletes [6, 20, 21]. In a retrospective review of 72 avulsion injuries, complete tears of the tendon from the ischial tuberosity were most common (87.5%) and most demonstrated some degree of tendon end retraction [21]. The sciatic nerve was found to be involved, as demonstrated by tethering of the nerve to the tendon edge by magnetic resonance imaging (MRI), in 28.6% of cases with complete tears, more commonly when there was a greater degree of tendon end retraction and/or a longer duration from symptom onset to treatment [21]. Avulsion of the proximal hamstring origin results in severe, acute lower buttock and/or posterior thigh pain with associated weakness. These typically happen when a sudden forced eccentric contraction of the hamstring muscles occurs against resistance. This can be due to direct or indirect forces on the lower limb [6]. This injury has been reported in water skiers, dancers, and gymnasts [6, 21, 22], but this can also occur in inactive individuals when someone slips or falls and the hips are forced into a split position. The prevalence of avulsion injuries is currently unknown.

In this chapter, we discuss the anatomy, clinical presentation, diagnosis, and treatment of injuries to the proximal hamstring tendons, including myotendinous strain, PHT, and avulsion injury.

Anatomy

The hamstrings are composed of three muscles: the semitendinosus and semimembranosus medially and the biceps femoris and short and long heads laterally. The semimembranosus and the conjoint tendon of semitendinosus and long head of biceps femoris originate from the ischial tuberosity, in close proximity to the sciatic nerve and the origin of the quadratus femoris. The short head of biceps femoris originates along the shaft of the femur at the linea aspera. The semimembranosus and semitendinosus extend along the posteromedial thigh to insert at the medial tibial condyle or the pes anserinus of the medial tibia, respectively. The biceps femoris extends along the posterolateral thigh to the lateral side of the fibular head. As a myotendinous structure where three of the four muscles cross two joints, contributing to both knee flexion and hip extension, it is at high risk of injury, particularly during eccentric contractions [22, 23].

Proximal Hamstring Tendon Injury

A 21-year-old collegiate football player presents with acute on chronic gluteal pain after the first day of practice back from his summer time off. Pain worsened during a sprinting drill, and is associated with regional ecchymosis in proximal posterior thigh. He was previously diagnosed with proximal hamstring tendinopathy with two discreet episodes of recurrence leading up to this episode. He was managed conservatively both previous times. For the first time, this time, he reports some tingling down the posterior thigh to the level of calf. On exam, activation of hamstring results in exquisite pain at proximal hamstring area. Though ecchymosis is present, there was no palpable defect on palpation at proximal posterior thigh region.

Clinical Presentation

Proximal hamstring injuries typically present with unilateral posterior thigh and/or lower buttock pain. If the sciatic nerve is involved, pain or other neuropathic symptoms may radiate below the knee [18, 21]. Pain is often worsened with activities that require repetitive contraction of the hamstring (e.g., running, fast walking) or direct pressure (e.g., sitting) [11, 16–18].

Proximal hamstring strains and avulsion injuries commonly present with acute, sharp, stabbing pain after direct or indirect trauma. The individual may recall an audible "pop" at the time of injury [5, 9, 10]. If the injury occurs during sport, the athlete typically is unable to return to play [9, 10]. There may be significant bruising and swelling with a palpable defect in the muscle or tendon [21]. The patient may demonstrate a stiff-legged gait to avoid hip and knee flexion [24]. With a complete avulsion, weakness is expected.

In contrast, PHT commonly presents with gradual onset of pain without trauma or inciting event [17, 18]. A subset of patients with a previously described type 2 injury may report acute onset of pain during stretching. Details regarding any pre-existing symptoms should be elicited, as previous hamstring pain has been more commonly reported in this population [4, 5]. These individuals are often able to continue participating in their athletic activity and walk without gait alteration [5]. Bruising, swelling, muscle defect, and weakness are uncommon complaints in patients with PHT unless a significant acute partial or complete tear is present as part of the chronic tendinopathic process.

The most commonly cited risk factor for proximal hamstring muscle-complex injury is prior hamstring injury [23]. Recurrence rates as high as 30% have been reported following hamstring strain [25]. Many theorize that injuries of the hamstring muscle and tendon cause an architectural change at the cellular level, where scar tissue replaces normal muscle or tendon fibers, predisposing this region to further injury. When assessing risk factors for avulsion injuries, studies have shown that a primary risk factor is underlying pathology within the tendon that existed prior to the avulsion. As early as 1933, McMaster et al. found that disease processes predispose to myotendinous rupture, and tendon ruptures do not occur if the tendon is healthy [26]. In 1991, a study assessing the histologic features of 891 spontaneously ruptured tendons versus 443 healthy, recently deceased controls found that 67% of the control group demonstrated normal, healthy tendons whereas none of the ruptured group was found to have normal, healthy tendons

[27]. Two prior studies, discussed in detail later, have demonstrated a high rate of proximal hamstring tendon changes among asymptomatic individuals [13, 14].

Additional risk factors for hamstring tendon or myotendinous injury include older age [28–31], suboptimal hamstring and quadriceps flexibility [28, 32], impaired lumbopelvic control [11], and hamstring muscle weakness [28, 32–34]. A particular area of focus has been on assessing hamstring strength compared to quadriceps strength. A prospective study found that a strength imbalance between the eccentric hamstrings and concentric quadriceps resulted in a fourfold increase in risk ratio of hamstring muscle-complex injuries (risk ratio, 4.66; 95% confidence interval [CI], 2.01–10.8) compared to a more balanced strength profile [33]. The authors suggested that the relatively limited eccentric strength of the hamstrings could not offset the stronger concentric action of the quadriceps, particularly during terminal swing phase of walking or running, resulting in the increased risk of injury [33]. However, subsequent studies in elite soccer players have shown limited association between strength testing and subsequent hamstring injury, with only isokinetic quadriceps concentric strength having any association, challenging the clinical value of strength testing in predicting future injury [35].

A number of additional risk factors for tendinopathy has been described at other sites, including the Achilles and patellar tendons. While these risk factors have not been studied in relation to the proximal hamstring tendon, it is reasonable to advise an individual to minimize the contribution of modifiable risk factors to reduce future problems until formal data can be collected. Systemic risk factors for tendinopathy at other sites include obesity [36], central adiposity [37], diabetes [38, 39], hypertension [36], dyslipidemia [40, 41], and genetic predisposition [42]. As discussed above, abnormal biomechanics [43–47], muscle inflexibility [48], and decreased muscle strength [40, 42, 49] are primary non-systemic intrinsic risk factors associated with tendinopathy at various sites. Extrinsic risk factors include mechanical overload [50, 51], training errors [47, 50],

improper equipment [51], and, likely, smoking [51]. Specific medications may also predispose to tendon pathology, including fluoroquinolones [52, 53], corticosteroids [36], hormones [36], nonsteroidal anti-inflammatory drugs (NSAIDs) [54, 55], and retinoids [56].

The differential diagnosis for proximal hamstring tendon injury should remain broad and include potential causes for local or referred pain to the lower buttock and posterior thigh, including lumbar radicular pain, peripheral neuropathy such as an injury to posterior cutaneous nerve of the thigh, hip or sacroiliac joint pathology, injury to the deep external rotator muscles of the hip, ischial bursitis, vascular claudication, or pelvic stress fracture. It is important to determine the type of proximal hamstring tendon injury as this affects treatment and recovery. Many prior reports of avulsion injuries of the proximal hamstring origin describe a significant delay in diagnosis and treatment, with individuals often receiving a diagnosis of hamstring strain based on clinical evaluation [6, 21]. If significant weakness, ecchymosis, and/or palpable defect are appreciated on examination, advanced imaging, such as magnetic resonance imaging (MRI) or ultrasound (US), should be considered [23].

Physical Examination

Physical examination should begin with inspection, to look for any bruising, swelling, or asymmetry to suggest a hamstring strain or avulsion injury [23]. Next, the examiner should palpate over the ischial tuberosity and proximal hamstring tendon to assess for a palpable defect suggestive of an avulsion injury [9, 23], asymmetry in the girth of the tendon suggestive of chronic tendinopathy with a partial tear, or focal tenderness, which can be seen in all types of injury. Range of motion (ROM) testing, or measurement of the popliteal angle, should include passive straight leg raise and active knee extension in the supine position with the hip flexed at 90 degrees, to assess for inflexibility and pain provocation [9].

Strength testing of the hamstring muscles should assess knee flexion and hip extension in multiple length-tension positions given their biarticular function [9]. Knee flexion strength should be tested with the patient lying prone, with maximal resistance against knee flexion being applied at 15 and 90 degrees of knee flexion [9]. Hip extension strength should be tested with the patient lying prone, with resistance applied against hip extension with the knee in both 0 and 90 degrees of flexion [9]. While provocation of pain can occur with all types of injuries, weakness is more commonly seen following avulsion injuries or complete tears at the myotendinous junction; weakness is uncommon with low-grade strain or tendinopathy without a tear [57].

Additional special tests have been described to assess hamstring injuries, including the Puranen-Orava test, the bent-knee stretch test, and the modified bent-knee stretch test. The Puranen-Orava test is performed by stretching the hamstring muscles in the standing position with one hip flexed at 90 degrees, the knee fully extended, and the foot on a support [16] (Fig. 8.1). The bent-knee stretch test is performed with the patient lying supine; the hip and knee of the symptomatic lower limb are maximally flexed, then the examiner slowly extends the knee passively [11] (Fig. 8.2). The modified bent-knee stretch test is performed with the patient lying in supine with the hip and knee of the symptomatic leg fully extended; the examiner maximally flexes the hip and knee and then rapidly straightens the knee passively [17] (Fig. 8.2). All three tests are considered positive if the patient's typical pain is reproduced at the hamstring origin on the symptomatic side [11, 16, 17]. In a recent study, the modified bent-knee stretch test was found to be most sensitive and specific for PHT, though all three tests were found to have similar degrees of sensitivity (0.76–0.89) and specificity (0.82–0.91) [17]. A test to further assess strength is the supine plank test [11]. In this test, the patient is positioned supine resting on his/her elbows with hips and knees extended and is instructed to elevate the pelvis and then alternately lift each leg in a straight leg raise (Fig. 8.3). Pelvic collapse or rotation of planted leg indicates hamstring weakness while reproduction of typical pain suggests the hamstring to be the pain generator.

When a proximal hamstring tendon injury is suspected, a thorough physical exam is warranted to exclude other diagnoses. This should include a full assessment of the hips, sacroiliac joints, and lumbar spine. Diffuse pain that is difficult to localize may suggest referred pain, while a more focal pain and an unchanging pain distribution may suggest a local pain generator, such as the proximal hamstring tendon [11]. A complete neurologic examination of the lower extremities should be performed to look for evidence of a lumbosacral radiculopathy. Neural tension tests, such as the seated slump test, should be used to help identify sciatic nerve or lumbosacral nerve root involvement [9]. A vascular exam of the lower extremities should also be completed.

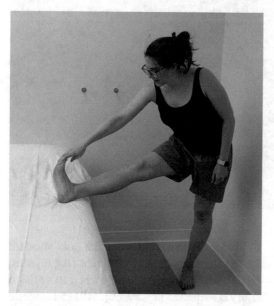

Fig. 8.1 Puranen-Orava test: stretching the hamstring muscles in the standing position with the hip flexed at 90 degrees, the knee fully extended, and the foot on a support

Imaging

Use of plain films of the pelvis with an anteroposterior (AP) view for the evaluation of proximal

Fig. 8.2 Bent-knee stretch and modified bent-knee stretch test: (**a**) the patient lying supine with the hip and knee of the symptomatic lower limb maximally flexed. (**b**) Then the examiner *slowly* (bent-knee stretch) or *rapidly* (modified bent-knee stretch) extends the knee passively

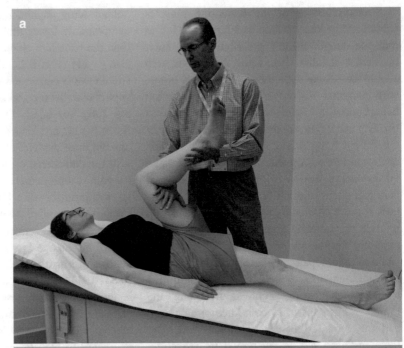

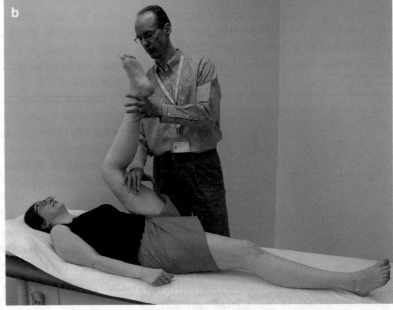

hamstring strain, tendinopathy, or avulsion is of limited benefit unless an osseous avulsion, typically an apophyseal injury at the ischial tuberosity in a skeletally immature athlete, is suspected [21, 58]. Similarly, bone scans are of no value in evaluating for tendon pathology. MRI and US are currently the preferred imaging modalities.

MRI is often described as the gold standard for the diagnosis of proximal hamstring injuries, particularly in the acute setting when an avulsion injury is suspected [23, 59, 60]. MRI can evaluate the location of tissue injury (myotendinous vs. free tendon), help determine the chronicity of injury, identify the number of muscles or tendons

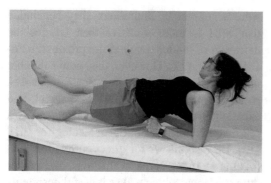

Fig. 8.3 Supine Plank Test: The patient is positioned supine resting on his/her elbows with hips and knees extended and is instructed to elevate the pelvis and then alternately lift each leg in a straight leg raise. Pelvic collapse, rotation, or pain at the hamstring origin when the contralateral leg is lifted indicates weakness

Table 8.1 Grading system for hamstring strain injuries

Grade	Pathophysiology/Imaging features	Clinical presentation
I	Tear of only a few muscle fibers of the myotendinous unit	Mild pain with or without minor swelling, no significant weakness
II	Partial tear of the musculotendinous unit, with some fibers remaining intact	Moderate pain with some degree of weakness
III	Complete tear of the musculotendinous unit	Pain, loss of strength, and complete loss of muscle function

Table modified from Kilcoyne et al. [151]

involved, determine the degree of retraction, if any, and quantify the size of injury [61].

Hamstring strains appear as increased intramuscular signal on T2-weighted images, representing fluid at the myotendinous junction. Hamstring strains are graded based on symptom severity and/or loss of structural integrity on imaging [23, 62]. Grade I strains are mild, presenting with minor discomfort and no significant loss of strength, with minimal or no loss of the structural integrity on imaging. Grade II strains demonstrate increased discomfort and mild deficits in strength, with evidence of a partial, or incomplete, tear on imaging. Grade III strains are severe and demonstrate significant loss of muscle strength and function, with evidence of a complete tear at the myotendinous unit on imaging (Table 8.1) [21, 62]. The paradigm for grading hamstring strains is typically based on imaging findings in conjunction with clinical findings. There is evidence to suggest that clinical findings alone may be as good a predictor of recovery as imaging findings for hamstring strains [63]. For this reason, we advocate for the use of imaging along with clinical findings to determine grade or extent of soft tissue injury given that the physical exam can prognosticate independent of grade.

In contrast, avulsion injuries appear as complete loss of fiber continuity at the hamstring origin. In cases of avulsion of the free tendon from the ischial tuberosity, the degree of retraction of the free tendon edge should be determined as this may affect treatment. Chronic avulsions are indicated by absence of a fluid at the margins of the tendon, fatty infiltration with atrophy of the involved muscles, and scarring of the tendon to adjacent structures [21]. In comparison to strains and avulsions, PHT is suggested on MRI by increased intratendinous T2 signal and increased tendon thickness [12]. Supportive MRI findings include peritendinitis, partial tendon tears, and reactive edema within the ischial tuberosity [11–13, 25, 60, 64]. Of note, these findings have been reported among asymptomatic individuals, so they should always be interpreted in the context of clinical symptoms and physical exam findings [13, 14]. In all injuries, the sciatic nerve should be assessed for evidence of compression or tethering [21].

In recent years, US has become a reliable method for evaluating the proximal hamstrings. Studies have shown US to be an effective way to identify and assess the extent of acute hamstring injuries [25, 59, 65]. Hypoechogenicity within the muscle at the myotendinous junction is suggestive of a hamstring strain [64]. US findings consistent with PHT include hypoechoic thickening of the proximal hamstring tendon, loss of the normal fibrillar pattern of the tendon, hypoechoic or anechoic areas within the tendon indicating a partial tear, cortical irregularity of the adjacent bone representing enthesopathy, peritendinous fluid, and hyperechogenic foci in the tendon representing calcifications [12, 59, 65]. Power doppler can be used to assess for neovascularization, which is suggestive of a more chronic process. Hypoechogenicity of the tendon with complete discontinuity of fibers, with or without retraction, is consistent with an avulsion injury.

Direct comparisons of the sensitivity and specificity of MRI versus US for detection of both acute and chronic proximal hamstring injuries are limited. In the acute period, US has been shown to have similar sensitivity to MRI with the following exceptions: for avulsion injuries, for deep muscle injuries, for cases with pre-existing scar tissue, or for injury follow-up [9, 25, 59]. In one prospective study comparing MRI and US findings of 60 male professional Australian-rules football players with clinically suspected hamstring strains, US was found to have a similar sensitivity to MRI (75% vs. 70%, respectively) in the acute period; however, MRI had a higher sensitivity than US at follow-up (59.2% vs. 51.0% at 2 weeks and 35.7% and 22.2% at 6 weeks, respectively). MRI was also found to have increased sensitivity for detecting subtle edema and deep muscle injuries [25]. For this reason, measuring the size of injury with MRI may be more accurate than with US in the acute period [9]. In another retrospective review of 170 patients with clinically suspected hamstring muscle-complex injuries, 16 individuals were found to have a proximal hamstring avulsion during surgical exploration. Among these individuals, 100% of the avulsions were identified on prior MRIs, whereas only 50% were identified on prior US [59]. Few studies have compared MRI and US sensitivities directly for evaluation of more chronic PHT. In one retrospective review of 65 patients with a mean age of 37.4 (range 19–65) years undergoing US-guided injection for chronic PHT, 35 were found to have prior MRI images. When US and MRI findings were compared among these 35 patients, MRI was able to detect peritendinous edema and bone marrow edema more accurately, while US was better able to detect tendinous calcifications in this study. While there were a number of limitations, they concluded that MRI is more sensitive than US for the detection of tendinopathy at the proximal hamstring origin [12]. However, they note a number of benefits of US, including decreased costs, real-time evaluation, dynamic assessment, and excellent spatial resolution, which make US a reasonable choice for initial screening for PHT [12]. US also allows for direct correlation with focal tenderness, serial evaluations, and procedure guidance, which makes it useful despite its potentially lower sensitivity.

Similar to other sites of tendinosis, studies have found a high rate of MRI findings suggestive of PHT among asymptomatic individuals. In a 2006 retrospective review of 259 asymptomatic patients with a median age of 60 (range 13–89), 65% demonstrated MRI findings consistent with PHT, including tendinosis (39%), partial tear (40%), or complete tear (5%) of the proximal hamstring tendons [14]. In a more recent retrospective study of 118 consecutive patients with a mean age of 41 (4–87 years) receiving a pelvis MRI, more than 90% had increased T1 or T2 signal within the proximal hamstring tendons, despite less than 18% having symptoms or physical exam findings to suggest the diagnosis of PHT [13]. In this study, findings associated with symptomatic tendinosis included increased tendon thickness, increased peritendinous T2 signal with distal feathery appearance, and ischial tuberosity edema [13]. Thus, the importance of interpreting imaging findings in the clinical context cannot be overemphasized.

Treatment

The primary goals in the treatment of proximal hamstring injury include returning the athlete to prior activity level and minimizing the risk of recurrent pain or reinjury [9]. The majority of individuals with hamstring injuries can achieve these goals with a conservative approach, while rare cases require more aggressive treatment, including injections or surgery.

Conservative

A three-phase approach to rehabilitation of acute proximal hamstring muscle-complex injuries has been well described in the literature and is detailed in Table 8.2 [9, 10]. Briefly, phase I focuses on decreasing pain and swelling, minimizing scar formation, and initiating low-intensity neuromuscular control exercises without resistance. Phase II involves increasing the intensity and range of exercises, initiating eccentric training within a limited range of motion (Fig. 8.4a), and progressing the neuromuscular exercises [9, 10]. Phase III involves progressing the eccentric exercise program, advancing the neuromuscular exercises, and incorporating sport-specific exercises with the goal of returning to unrestricted activity. Cited return-to-sport criteria include full concentric and eccentric strength and full functional abilities with sport-specific movements at maximum speed and intensity, all done without pain [9]. A recent systematic review assessing criteria for rehabilitation progression and return to play across 9 studies with 601 acute

Table 8.2 Rehabilitation protocol for hamstring muscle-complex injuries [9, 10]

Phase	Phase 1	Phase 2	Phase 3
Goals:	Decrease pain and swelling Prevent scar formation Improve neuromuscular control	Increase ROM to full Begin eccentric training Progress neuromuscular training	Progress eccentric training Advanced neuromuscular training Sport-specific exercises Return to full activity
Symptom management:	Brief period of RICE: Rest, Ice, Compression, Elevation NAIDS for pain management: No clear benefit and may hinder healing [152, 153]	Symptom-free at rest	Symptom-free at rest
Walking/ running:	Crutches and shorten stride-length for pain Progress to pain-free, unrestricted gait	Normal walking	Normal walking Pain-free jogging at submaximal speed, progress to full speed
Exercise protocol			
ROM:	Limit by pain tolerance Excessive stretch may promote scar formation [154]	Progress to full passive and active ROM	Full, pain-free active and passive ROM
Neuromuscular control:	Low-intensity lumbopelvic stabilization: single-limb balance, frontal stepping drills	Increase intensity and speed of neuromuscular control, agility, and trunk stabilization exercises	Progressive agility and trunk stabilization exercises Incorporate functional, dynamic, sport-specific drills
Resistance training:	None	Introduce eccentric strengthening slowly without reaching end ROM Example: Supine bent-knee bridge walk-out (Fig. 8.4a)	Eccentric strengthening exercises progressed to full ROM: Supine single-limb chair bridges (Fig. 8.4b) Single-limb balance windmill touches with dumbbells (Fig. 8.4c)
Ready to progress:	Pain-free walking Pain-free very slow jog Pain-free, submaximal isometric hamstring contraction: 90° knee flexion	Full, pain-free ROM Pain-free jogging, forward and backward, at 50% maximum speed	Pain-free palpation Full, pain-free concentric and eccentric strength Absence of kinesiophobia Pain-free, full sport-specific movements at maximum speed and intensity

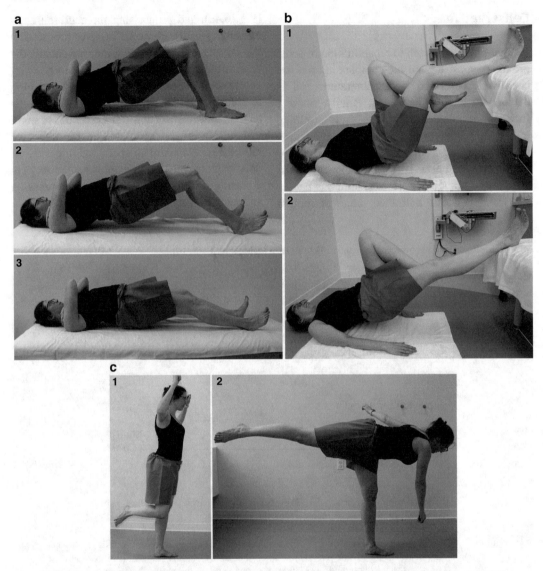

Fig. 8.4 Examples of eccentric exercises for the hamstring muscles. (**a**) Supine bent-knee bridge walk-out: Start in supine bridge position [1] and gradually walk the feet away from hips while maintaining bridge position (2- > 3). (**b**) Supine single-limb chair bridges: With one leg on a station object [1], raise hips and pelvis off the ground into a bridge position [2]. (**c**) Single-limb balance windmill touches with or without dumbbells: begin in single-limb stance position with arms/dumbbells overhead [1] and perform windmill motion under control with end position of touching hand/dumbbell to the floor [2]

hamstring muscle-complex injuries reported that subjective pain is the most commonly used criteria for rehabilitation progression, while clinical assessment and performance tests were used for return to play decisions. They emphasized the need for more objective and clinically practical criteria when making exercise progression and return to play decisions [66].

While this rehabilitation approach has been well described, no trials directly compared this protocol to other rehabilitation approaches or to natural recovery with progression of activity guided by pain. A Cochrane review done in 2012 identified only two randomized controlled trials (RCTs) assessing specific rehabilitation approaches for hamstring injuries [67]. The first study compared once daily versus four times daily stretching exercises among 80 athletes, mean age 20.5 years, with a clinically diagnosed grade II hamstring muscle-complex injury; more frequent stretching was associated with earlier return to activity [68]. In the other RCT, 24 athletes were assigned to either an agility and trunk stabilization program or an isolated hamstring stretching and strengthening program. Those in the progressive agility and trunk stabilization program demonstrated an earlier return to play (22.2 ± 8.3 vs. 37.4 ± 27.6 days) and lower reinjury rate (7.7% vs. 70%) [69]. Based on this review, the authors found limited evidence that recovery time for elite athletes can be reduced with more frequent daily stretching, and preliminary evidence that exercise to correct movement dysfunction can reduce recovery time and reinjury rate among mixed-level athletes [67]. Since the publication of this review, another RCT of 29 athletes did not find a difference in return to sport time when comparing a progressive agility and trunk stabilization program with a progressive running and eccentric strengthening program, with both approaches showing benefit [70]. An additional RCT by Askling et al. compared two rehabilitation protocols, one emphasizing eccentric strengthening and the other concentric. In this study, 56 elite sprinters and jumpers with MRI-confirmed acute hamstring injury involving the myotendinous junction (57%) and/or proximal tendon (43%) were randomly assigned to either a lengthening protocol emphasizing eccentric strengthening and range of motion or a conventional rehabilitation protocol emphasizing concentric strengthening. The lengthening group had a significantly shorter return to activity time (49 vs. 86 days), supporting the use of eccentric exercises in the treatment of acute hamstring injuries [71]. This held true for injuries with and without involvement of the proximal tendon, though injuries involving the proximal tendon

required a longer recovery time regardless of treatment [71]. Similar results were seen in another RCT by the same authors using the same study protocol among 75 Swedish elite football players with MRI-confirmed acute hamstring injuries [72]. A recent meta-analysis of the two aforementioned RCTs by Askling et al. found a significantly reduced time to return to play with use of a strengthening protocol emphasizing eccentric strengthening as compared to a conventional program (hazard ratio [HR], 3.22; 95% confidence interval, 2.17–4.77; $p = 0.0001$) though there was no change in reinjury rate [73]. Aside from this study by Askling et al., the aforementioned studies did not specify the location of injury to the myotendinous junction or the proximal free tendon. For this reason, it is unclear if the protocols used in these studies are best suited for myotendinous strains, proximal tendinosis, or both.

Few studies have focused on the optimal rehabilitation of isolated proximal hamstring tendon injuries. Based on studies of tendinosis at other sites, rehabilitation typically focuses on eccentric strengthening [74–76]. A number of prior studies have shown the benefit of eccentric exercises in the treatment of Achilles and patellar tendinosis [77–81]. However, the mechanism of benefit from performing eccentric exercises is not well understood; it has been attributed to the greater tendon load generated when compared to concentric exercises [82], increased collagen synthesis [83], decreased neovascularization [84–86], or force fluctuations from tendon loading and unloading [87]. In addition to the exercises depicted in Fig. 8.4, eccentric exercises can be performed with a hamstring curl machine, reverse planks, ball curls, kneeling "Norwegian" or "Nordic" leg curls, and standing single- or double-leg dead lifts [9]. Exercises should be performed at a level that produces mild discomfort, since this has been the goal in many studies that have evaluated the effectiveness of eccentric exercises on pain in tendinosis. Of note, a recent RCT suggests that heavy, slow resistance training is as effective as eccentric exercises in the treatment of Achilles tendinosis with increased short-term patient satisfaction [88]. While further research is needed, these results suggest this to be a potentially effective alternative treatment option to eccentric training for hamstring tendinosis. Similar to hamstring strain, prior case reports have described good recovery when lumbopelvic stabilization is incorporated with eccentric strengthening [89].

Resources describing and assessing conservative management of proximal hamstring avulsion injuries are limited but have shown promising outcomes [23, 62, 90, 91]. One study, by Sallay et al., trialed non-operative management of proximal hamstring rupture in 12 water skiers; 7 (58%) returned to preinjury sports, 5 (42%) were unable to return to sport, and 2 pursued delayed surgical repair [92]. A more recent study retrospectively reviewed 17 patients with complete proximal hamstring avulsions who underwent non-operative treatment; of those, 12 (70.5%) returned to sport, and in 10 strength at 45 and 90 degrees of flexion was found to be 62% and 66%, respectively, as compared to the contralateral leg [93]. Ferlic et al. retrospectively reviewed the records of 13 adolescents with ischial tuberosity avulsion fractures, of which 8 were managed non-operatively. All of the individuals with displacement <15 mm had excellent outcomes with conservative care. Among the four adolescents with displacement >15 mm who opted for conservative management, 50% reported excellent outcomes while 50% developed pseudoarthrosis and reported good outcomes, suggesting conservative care to be a reasonable treatment approach for minimally displaced (<15 mm) injuries [94]. A recent systematic review comparing conservative versus surgical treatment of pelvic apophyseal avulsion fractures among 596 adolescents across 14 studies (30% ischial tuberosity) found that there was no statistically significant difference in the success rate of surgery (88%) compared to conservative treatment (79%; $p = 0.09$), though return to sports was higher among the surgical group (93% vs. 80%; $p = 0.03$) at a mean follow-up of 12 months [95]. The majority of literature per-

taining to the treatment of hamstring avulsion injuries describes outcomes of surgical repair with no comparison to a conservative care group, limiting further conclusions. Additional, high-quality studies comparing operative and non-operative management of avulsion injuries are needed.

The benefit of incorporating modalities in the treatment of proximal hamstring injuries, particularly hamstring tendinosis, has also been suggested, including US, dry needling, soft tissue mobilization, and extracorporeal shock wave therapy (ESWT). However, evidence to support their use is inconsistent. While therapeutic US is often utilized following acute and chronic injury, there is no evidence to support beneficial effects on muscle or tendon healing [96, 97]. Similarly, limited evidence supports the use of trigger point dry needling, though one case report incorporating trigger point dry needling with eccentric exercises and lumbopelvic stabilization yielded good results [89]. Soft tissue mobilization combined with strengthening and stabilization exercises has been described in case reports and case series with athletes experiencing resolution of symptoms and return to activity [98–100]. However, to date, only low-level case reports have documented the benefit of soft tissue mobilization in conjunction with an eccentric exercise regimen [98, 100]. A well-studied modality is ESWT, which involves applying a device that generates and delivers shock waves to body tissues. Recently, applications to musculoskeletal disorders have become common, though the mechanism by which ESWT works is uncertain [101]. One RCT compared a progressive soft tissue mobilization and strengthening program with and without ESWT among 40 professional athletes with chronic PHT. They found that the ESWT group had a greater improvement in pain scores and Nirschl phase rating scale at 3 months, as well as a higher rate of return to sports [17]. Studies of ESWT have been conducted at other sites of tendinosis, including the Achilles tendon, rotator cuff, and common extensor tendon of the elbow, showing variable degrees of benefit [17, 101–104].

Interventional

Corticosteroids

Peritendinous corticosteroid injections have been used for the treatment of chronic PHT though there is limited evidence to suggest that steroid is beneficial, and there is an increasing body of literature demonstrating its risks. Two primary studies have investigated the effect of peritendinous corticosteroid injections in patients with PHT. In 2010, Nicholson et al. reported that there was a significant improvement in pain and level of athletic participation at a mean follow-up of 21 months following fluoroscopic-guided steroid injection. However, this was based on a retrospective case series of 18 athletes with 22 cases of MRI-confirmed PHT without control of other treatments during the study period [57]. Similarly, in a retrospective review of 65 patients receiving a US-guided steroid injection for presumed PHT (no diagnostic criteria defined), Zissen et al. found that 50% of patients reported moderate-to-complete resolution of symptoms for at least 1 month and 24% had symptom relief for more than 6 months [12]. While this study included a larger sample size and there was no procedure-associated adverse reaction, there was no control of additional treatments and no comparison group. Despite the benefits, the use of corticosteroid injections is controversial given the potential risks, including damage to the tenocytes, suppression of collagen synthesis, and risk for tendon rupture [57, 105–108]. The use of corticosteroid injection in the treatment of acute hamstring strain has not been well documented. In one retrospective review, 58 professional NFL players were treated with a landmark-guided corticosteroid injection for grades II–III hamstring strains. The average time to return to full practice was 7.6 (0–24) days and no complications were reported [109]. However, given the potential risks of corticosteroid injections and lack of high-quality evidence to support their use, the role of corticosteroid injections remains unclear and has fallen out of favor in clinical practice.

3.2.2. Percutaneous Needle Tenotomy or Fenestration

One retrospective review has analyzed the effectiveness of US-guided needle fenestration on pain in the tendons of the hip and pelvis, including PHT, which comprised 36.4%, or 8 of 22, patients. The range of time to follow-up was broad (1–70 months). When analyzing the entire study group, 82% had clinical improvement [110]. Since fenestration is often done when using platelet-rich plasma (PRP) or stem cells, discussed below, fenestration alone is a potential option in the treatment of PHT. No RCTs have been done to determine the effectiveness of fenestration alone in the treatment of hamstring tendinosis.

3.2.3. Regenerative Therapies: Platelet-Rich Plasma (PRP) and Stem Cells

Over the last decade, regenerative therapies for the treatment of muscle and tendon disorders have become more common. These include the use of PRP and stem cell injections. While no studies were identified that used stem cells, a number of studies have assessed the benefit of PRP for acute hamstring strains with mixed results. In 2014, Hamid et al. performed an RCT in which 28 patients with acute grade II hamstring strains received a progressive agility and trunk stabilization rehabilitation protocol with or without undergoing a PRP injection. The patients in the PRP group had a statistically significantly earlier return to play (26.7 ± 7.0 vs. 42.5 ± 20.6 days) as well as significantly lower pain scores [111]. It should be noted that there was no control arm with a sham injection in this study. In contrast, in 2015, Hamilton et al. performed a study in which 90 professional athletes with MRI-confirmed grade I–II hamstring strains were randomized to receive a standard rehabilitation program with PRP, platelet-poor plasma (PPP), or no injection. There was no significant difference in return to play between the PRP group and the rehabilitation-only group [112]. The median duration of return to play was 21 days (95% CI: 17.9–24.1) in the PRP group, 27 days (95% CI: 20.6–33.4) in the PPP group, and 25 days (95% CI: 21.5–28.5) in the no-injection group [112]. Similarly, Reurink et al. reported no significant difference in return to play (median 42 days in both groups) or reinjury rate (16% in the PRP group vs. 14% in the placebo group) among 80 athletes with MRI-confirmed hamstring strains (grade of strain specified, not specified) randomized to receive intramuscular PRP or sham (isotonic saline) injection [113]. A recent meta-analysis of three aforementioned RCTs showed no significant effect of PRP injections on the treatment of acute hamstring muscle-complex injuries when compared to control (HR, 1.03; 95% confidence interval, 0.87–1.22; $p = 0.73$) [73]. Lastly, out of ten NFL players with grade I or II acute hamstring strains, there was no significant difference in time to return to play between five players receiving PRP injection with a rehabilitation program and the five players receiving a rehabilitation program only (20 days in the PRP group and 17 days in the non-PRP group) [114]. The majority of studies identified did not demonstrate a clear benefit for PRP injections following acute hamstring muscle-complex injuries.

PRP has also been used in the treatment of chronic, often refractory, PHT. One retrospective case series of 12 individuals with MRI-confirmed, refractory, PHT found that individuals treated with landmark-guided PRP injection had a significant improvement in pain and Nirschl phase rating scale compared with individuals receiving physical therapy and NSAIDs with no injection [115]. In a slightly larger retrospective review of 18 consecutive patients with clinically diagnosed chronic PHT treated with US-guided PRP injection, 10 patients reported >80% improvement in pain at 6 months, with a mean improvement of 63% [116]. However, both of these studies were low-quality retrospective reviews with a number of limitations, including the small sample size, variable follow-up duration, and lack of standardized treatment. Most recently, Davenport et al. performed a prospective double-blind RCT comparing US-guided PRP injection to whole autologous blood injections in 15 patients with chronic PHT. Both groups demonstrated improvement in pain and function at 6 months without a significant difference between groups, suggesting PRP has no added benefit over whole blood [117]. Overall,

no conclusions can be made regarding the effectiveness or safety of PRP in the treatment of PHT. Large, prospective RCTs of image-guided PRP injections are needed.

Operative

Literature regarding surgical intervention for proximal hamstring tendon injury is largely focused on avulsion injuries. Specific indications cited for operative management include three-tendon avulsions or two-tendon avulsions that are retracted ≥2 cm [24]. Special consideration should be paid to two-tendon injuries where a third occult midsubstance or myotendinous junction rupture may also be present [24]. It has been advocated in the literature that avulsion injuries requiring surgery are important to diagnose early and are best managed within 4 weeks; delayed diagnosis can lead to a more difficult repair, potentially resulting in increased complications and inferior outcomes [118, 119]. However, good results have been reported for repair of chronic injuries [21, 120–122]. Patients with chronic proximal hamstring injuries can develop significant sciatic nerve compression from scar formation or myositis ossificans [21, 123]. Surgical repair with sciatic neurolysis and various techniques to limit scar recurrence have been reported for these cases [22, 120, 124].

The patient is positioned prone on the operating table with all bony prominences well padded. The table should be flexed to allow slight trunk flexion and the lower leg should also be elevated to allow slight knee flexion.

Incisions can either be transverse or longitudinal in nature. Transverse incisions are performed in the gluteal crease inferior to the ischial tuberosity. This offers improved access to avulsed tendons that insert transversely with the added benefit of improved cosmesis [120, 125]. However, for acute cases with significant retraction or chronic cases requiring significant mobilization, hamstring lengthening, or sciatic neurolysis, a longitudinal incision can be employed (Fig. 8.5).

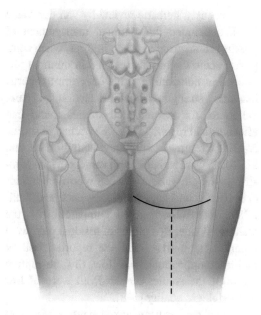

Fig. 8.5 Transverse and longitudinal incisions

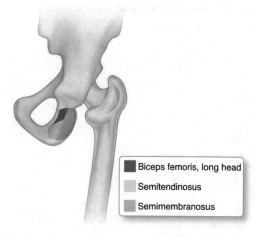

Fig. 8.6 Proximal hamstring insertion

Following incision, dissection is carried out through subcutaneous fat to the gluteal fascia. Attention must be turned to the posterior femoral cutaneous nerve and its branches as it runs deep to the fascia posteriorly crossing the long head of the biceps femoris in an oblique fashion. Once isolated and protected, the inferior border of the gluteus maximus is elevated superiorly by incising the gluteal fascia. The sciatic nerve can be identified distally and traced proximally; on average, it is found 1.2 cm lateral to the ischial tuberosity [19]. Next attention can be turned to avulsed tendon stumps. In chronic injuries, overlying scar tissue may need to be excised to accurately identify the tendon stumps. Once the tendon stumps have been isolated, they can be tagged with a high-strength suture. The tendons must be carefully mobilized in order to limit tension on the repair and minimize the amount of knee flexion needed to reapproximate the tendons to their origin. In patients with chronic injury or severe retraction, distal hamstring lengthening or Achilles allograft may be necessary.

Following hamstring tendon preparation, attention is turned to preparation of the ischial tuberosity. The anatomic insertional footprints for the hamstring tendons are on the lateral aspect of the ischial tuberosity (Fig. 8.6). The semitendinosus and biceps femoris share the more medial insertion with an oval footprint 2.7 cm in length by 1.8 cm in width, with the semimembranosus inserting more laterally. The semimembranosus insertion measures 3.1 cm in length by 1.1 cm in width and is crescent shaped [19]. Preparation of the insertion site involves periosteal elevation and curetting. Manual preparation of the site can be performed to allow a vascular bed for healing, though is not always necessary as suture anchors allow for bleeding into the repair site. Suture anchors are then placed in various number and configurations, depending on surgeon preference, to repair the tendons to bone. Fascia is subsequently repaired and the incision closed in layers.

Appropriate postoperative rehabilitation is crucial to the success of surgery. Patients are immediately fitted with a customized hip orthosis that restricts hip range of motion. The brace is locked at 90 degrees for 6 weeks while ambulating. They are non-weight bearing for 6 weeks with a scooter or crutches for mobility. Progressive passive and active range of motion protocols are strictly followed and are outlined in Table 8.3. After this initial postoperative rehabilitation, the general approach outlined earlier for non-operative management of hamstring injuries can be initiated.

Table 8.3 Postoperative rehabilitation protocol

Postoperative rehabilitation protocol

Week 0–1
  Gentle active extension to 45°
  Passive flexion
  Modalities as necessary to decrease swelling

Weeks 1–4
  Gentle active extension to 15°
  Passive flexion

Weeks 4–6
  Gentle active extension to 0°
  Passive flexion
  Quad sets with straight leg raise

Weeks 6–8
  Protected weight bearing with slow wean-off of crutches
  Discontinue brace
  Active and passive extension to 0°
  Begin zero resistance straight leg raise
  Patellar mobilization
  Quad-specific strengthening exercises

Weeks 8–12
  Being active flexion exercises
  Quad-specific strengthening exercises

Week 12
  Gradual hamstring strengthening exercises
  Stationary bike with both legs with gradual increased resistance
  Rowing/erg machine
  Aqua jogging/therapy
  Single knee bends

Week 16
  Return to run program
    Elliptical→Treadmill→Outdoor running
    Leg press to 90° with weights
    Leg curls with no hyperextension
    Sport-specific training with gradual return to agility exercises

Month 6
  Return to sports

Complications associated with proximal hamstring repair vary from neurologic injury and infection to repair failure and dissatisfaction with surgery [21, 122, 125]. Perioperative complications can include injury to local nerves: namely the sciatic nerve, the posterior femoral cutaneous nerve and its branches, and the inferior cluneal and perineal nerves potentially leading to chronic pain and loss of hip extension strength [118, 122, 126]. Other complications related to the proximity of surgical site to the perineal region include superficial and deep postoperative infections [21, 127].

A recent systematic review by van der Made et al. concluded that surgical management of proximal hamstring avulsion injuries, when comparing acute to chronic, resulted in minimal difference in outcome in terms of return to sports, hamstring strength, patient satisfaction, and pain. Outcomes for the included studies found that after surgical repair, 76–100% returned to sports, 55–100% returned to preinjury activity level, and 88–100% were satisfied with surgery. Mean hamstring strength varied between reporting studies (78–101%), and hamstring endurance and flexibility were fully restored compared with the unaffected side. Symptoms of residual pain were reported by 8–61%, and the reported risk of major complications was low (3% re-rupture rate). Of the studies included, all were of low methodologic quality [128].

Several studies have looked at return to play as an outcome measure following surgical intervention for proximal hamstring avulsion with good results. Birmingham et al. reported 21/23 (91%) athletes returned to sporting activity after repair [126]. Chalal et al. performed a retrospective review of 15 patients; of the 11 patients who participated in sports before surgery, 100% were able to return to sport, though 45% reported a decrease in their level of activity at a mean follow-up time of 36.9 months with strength measured at a mean of 78% of the contralateral leg [129]. In a series of 52 patients who underwent surgical repair for acute proximal hamstring avulsion, 23 (44%) reported that their injury occurred during sports activity. Of those individuals, 16 (69.5%) returned to the sport in which they were injured, while the other 6 were water skiers who preferred to avoid the sport for concern for reinjury, and 1 patient did not return as he had graduated [118]. Folsom et al. reported that 19/25 (76%) returned to sports following acute and chronic injury repairs when data were pooled [127]. In a study of ten professional and semiprofessional athletes, Konan and Haddad reported that 90% returned to sport with the tenth patient opting to not continue competing prior to surgery [130]. In a larger series, Lefevre et al. reported that of the 34 patients who participated in sports, 32 (94%) resumed activity; of these, 15 were athletes and 12 (80%) returned to sports at the same level [131]. More recently, Sandmann et al. performed proximal hamstring repairs on 15 patients and found 100% return to sport at mean follow-up of 56 months [132]. In a large case series, Subbu et al. reported a 108/112 (96.4%) return to sport rate; additionally, they found return to full sport was 9 weeks faster for early (<6 weeks) versus delayed repairs (6 weeks to 6 months) and 13 weeks faster for early versus late (>6 months) repairs [133]. Of note, none of the prior studies included a comparison group involving other treatment options.

Despite the reported success in return to sport from numerous individual case series, the data are less convincing in NFL athletes with proximal hamstring avulsions. A retrospective review of ten NFL athletes all managed surgically within 10 days found a return to play of 90%; however, only five of these athletes played in more than one game. This suggests that return to elite-level performance is less likely than return to sport in the recreational athlete [134].

There has been a lack of consensus in the orthopedic literature regarding indications and timing of surgical repair of proximal hamstring avulsions, though authors advocate that acute repair is superior to delayed repair. There have been numerous case series reporting good outcomes with repair of proximal hamstring avulsion injuries. Cohen et al. advocated that three-tendon injuries and two-tendon injuries with greater than 2 cm of retraction are absolute indications for surgery [24]. Relative indications include two-tendon injuries with suspicion for occult third myotendinous or midsubstance ruptures, injuries that have failed non-operative management, and those with sciatic nerve symptoms [24]. The authors recommend non-operative management for single-tendon injuries regardless of retraction and two-tendon injuries with less than 2 cm of retraction [24]. To our knowledge there are no studies with control groups comparing operatively and non-operatively treated proximal hamstring avulsions. A systematic review of surgical repair for these injuries found all studies analyzed to be of low methodologic quality and with minimal improvement in outcomes [128].

Of studies reviewed, there is very limited data related to functional outcomes in patients treated non-operatively [135].

In our experience the majority of patients, including high-level athletes, with proximal hamstring avulsion injuries can be treated initially without an operation. Conservative management with RICE—rest, ice, compression, and elevation—anti-inflammatories, and graduated stretching and strengthening regimens as outlined earlier may restore adequate function, thereby avoiding any risks associated with surgery.

Prognosis/Return to Play

Recovery time needed following acute hamstring injury has been shown to vary significantly among athletes. In a 2004 study of 60 professional male football players with clinically diagnosed hamstring strain, the median return to play time was 3 weeks, with a range of 4–56 days [25]. This study examined imaging findings associated with a prolonged recovery and found that tear size was proportional to recovery time. Specifically, increased longitudinal length of the tear on MRI and increased cross-sectional area on MRI and US were associated with a longer recovery period [25]. More recently, Cohen et al. created a detailed MRI classification system to analyze return to play in NFL athletes with acute hamstring strains. Thirty-eight injured players were analyzed using traditional MRI grade as well as this novel scoring system, described in Table 8.4 [136, 137]. The authors found that with increasing MRI grade and score, more games were missed. Specifically, they concluded that players with multiple muscles or tendons involved, >75% cross-sectional involvement, increased length of abnormal T2 signal in the sagittal plane, and complete tears with tendon end retraction had longer return to play compared to players with one muscle or tendon involved, <25% cross-sectional involvement, and no tendon retraction [137]. Other imaging features that have been associated with prolonged recovery include involvement of the biceps femoris tendon [25] and proximity to the ischial tuberosity [70,

Table 8.4 Novel MRI scoring system for return to play prediction

Points	Age, years	Muscles involved, N	Location	Insertion	Muscle injury, %	Retraction, cm	Long-axis T2 signal length, cm
0				No	0	None	0
1	≤ 25	1	Proximal		25	<2	1–5
2	26–31	2	Middle	Yes	50	≥2	6–10
3	≥ 32	3	Distal		≥75		>10

Table reproduced from original article by Cohen et al. [137]

138]. However, many have critiqued studies that use MRI to determine prognosis as they are often retrospective, unblinded, and involve univariate analysis without consideration of the clinical evaluation [139]. A recent review of 12 articles by Reurink et al. reported conflicting results within the current literature regarding the prognostic value of MRI findings for acute hamstring injuries. Ultimately, due to risk of bias within existing studies, they concluded there is currently no strong evidence that any MRI finding can help predict the return to play time after acute injury [139]. Of note, nearly all studies were focused on hamstring strains without mention of isolated proximal tendon disorders.

Clinical history and examination features may help predict recovery time. Determining the type of hamstring injury based on history and examination is important. Strain injuries involving the myotendinous junction typically require a shorter recovery period than injuries involving the proximal, free tendon [4, 5, 138, 140, 141]. Sprint-type myotendinous injuries took a mean of 16 weeks to return to preinjury activity level among a cohort of elite sprinters [4], while stretch-type proximal free tendon injuries took a mean of 50 weeks for return to preinjury activity level among a cohort of professional dancers who experienced acute pain while performing a split [4]. It is postulated that the increased recovery period for proximal tendon injuries is due to the decreased vascularity and increased remodeling time needed for tendons compared to muscles [140]. Of note, the recovery time of both groups in these studies was much longer than the previously cited averages among professional football players [2, 25, 142], emphasizing the significant variability among athletes and sports.

Physical examination findings on initial evaluation, including deficits in strength, decreased range of motion (ROM), and increased severity and duration of pain, have been associated with a prolonged recovery time. In fact, these findings were shown to be as good a predictor of recovery time as MRI following acute hamstring strain [63]. In this study, severity of injury by clinical examination was determined by measuring deficits with passive straight leg raise (i.e., measuring the angle of hip flexion at onset of pain on passive hip flexion with knee extended in supine), active knee extension (i.e., measuring knee flexion angle from vertical at the first sign of pain or resistance on active knee extension in supine), and strength (i.e., pain with strength testing at 15 and 90 degrees) compared to the asymptomatic side. The following prediction algorithm was used, with increasing pain and ROM restrictions on the above tests predicting an increased recovery duration: no pain and mildly decreased ROM with an estimated recovery of <7 days; mild pain and mildly decreased ROM with an estimated recovery of 7–14 days; moderate pain and moderately decreased ROM with an estimated recovery of 21–28 days; and moderate-severe pain and severely restricted ROM with an estimated recovery rate of >28 days. Incorporating information from short-term follow-up has been shown to further improve prognostication. A recent study by Jacobsen et al. found that while the findings on the initial examination by a therapist explained 50% of the variance in recovery time following acute hamstring injuries, the combination of findings at initial and 1-week follow-up examinations explained 93% of the variance. The evaluations in this study were extensive and will not be outlined in this chapter. Further, MRI offered no additional value regarding return to play time in this study [143]. Lastly, a recurrent hamstring injury has been shown to take up to twice as long to recovery as compared to the initial injury [65, 142]. The majority of research in this area has focused on hamstring strains or hamstring injury without specification of injury type. No studies have focused specifically on tendon injury or more chronic injuries. Return to sport following avulsion injury is detailed above in the surgical section as this literature has largely focused on surgical interventions.

Reinjury rates following proximal hamstring muscle-complex injuries are high, with reports as high as 30% [25]. However, predicting patients at high risk for reinjury has proven difficult. A recent retrospective review of 230 track and field athletes did find that recurrence rate was higher among proximal tendon injuries when compared to hamstring strains [141]. In contrast, multiple prospective investigations have not found that initial physical exam findings or severity of initial injury on MRI are associated with reinjury rates [9, 65, 144, 145]. The optimal criteria for return to play to minimize the risk of reinjury are currently unknown. While many studies cite full range of motion, full strength, and pain-free, full functional activities as requirements for return to play [9, 146], imaging abnormalities have been found to persist far beyond the period of clinical symptoms [25]. This prolonged period of healing may contribute to the high reinjury rate following acute proximal hamstring muscle-complex injuries [147].

Prevention

Given the high incidence of proximal hamstring injuries among athletes, as well as the high recurrence rates, methods to prevent future injury are of special interest. Most prevention strategies have focused on hamstring strains and have assessed modifiable risk factors, including inflexibility and weakness of the hamstrings and neighboring musculature.

Incorporation of eccentric hamstring exercises into training has been found to reduce the incidence of hamstring strains [142, 148, 149]. In one study, incorporation of eccentric hamstring strengthening in the training program for elite soccer players significantly reduced the incidence of hamstring strains (risk ratio, 0.43; 95% confidence interval, 0.19–0.98) [149]. In fact, a recent systematic review found that training programs that incorporated the Nordic hamstring eccentric exercise had a statistically significant reduction in hamstring injury risk ratio (IRR, 0.490; 95% confidence interval, 0.291–0.827; $p = 0.008$), with rates reduced up to 51% in the long term, compared to teams that did not incorporate any eccentric exercises for prevention [150]. In contrast, inclusion of a flexibility program has not been shown to reduce the incidence of hamstring strains [142, 149]. However, these conclusions are somewhat limited as few, high-quality studies have assessed stretching in the prevention of hamstring strains. Lastly, incorporation of neuromuscular control exercises and lumbopelvic stability have been suggested as another avenue for injury prevention, though studies on this topic are limited and further research is needed.

Conclusion

Most proximal hamstring injuries can be effectively treated with a non-operative approach using the rehabilitation protocol outlined. Non-operative management is effective and preferred for most PHT and myotendinous injuries. When initial non-operative management is incompletely effective, use of injections may facilitate recovery. While some advocate surgery for certain proximal hamstring tendon avulsions, especially in younger competitive athletes or if there is significant retraction, a thorough discussion about the risks and benefits of pursuing surgery early after the injury needs to take place, and a trial of non-operative management is very reasonable.

References

1. Verrall GM, Slavotinek JP, Barnes PG, Fon GT. Diagnostic and prognostic value of clinical findings in 83 athletes with posterior thigh injury: comparison of clinical findings with magnetic resonance imaging documentation of hamstring muscle strain. Am J Sports Med. 2003;31(6):969–73.
2. Feeley BT, Kennelly S, Barnes RP, Muller MS, Kelly BT, Rodeo SA, et al. Epidemiology of National Football League training camp injuries from 1998 to 2007. Am J Sports Med. 2008;36(8):1597–603.
3. Askling C, Lund H, Saartok T, Thorstensson A. Self-reported hamstring injuries in student-dancers. Scand J Med Sci Sports. 2002;12(4):230–5.
4. Askling CM, Tengvar M, Saartok T, Thorstensson A. Acute first-time hamstring strains during slow-speed stretching: clinical, magnetic resonance imaging, and recovery characteristics. Am J Sports Med. 2007;35(10):1716–24.
5. Askling CM, Tengvar M, Saartok T, Thorstensson A. Acute first-time hamstring strains during high-speed running: a longitudinal study including clinical and magnetic resonance imaging findings. Am J Sports Med. 2007;35(2):197–206.
6. Gidwani S, Bircher MD. Avulsion injuries of the hamstring origin - a series of 12 patients and management algorithm. Ann R Coll Surg Engl. 2007;89(4):394–9.
7. Chumanov ES, Schache AG, Heiderscheit BC, Thelen DG. Hamstrings are most susceptible to injury during the late swing phase of sprinting. Br J Sports Med. 2012;46(2):90.
8. Chumanov ES, Heiderscheit BC, Thelen DG. Hamstring musculotendon dynamics during stance and swing phases of high-speed running. Med Sci Sports Exerc. 2011;43(3):525–32.
9. Heiderscheit BC, Sherry MA, Silder A, Chumanov ES, Thelen DG. Hamstring strain injuries: recommendations for diagnosis, rehabilitation, and injury prevention. J Orthop Sports Phys Ther. 2010;40(2):67–81.
10. Sherry MA, Johnston TS, Heiderscheit BC. Rehabilitation of acute hamstring strain injuries. Clin Sports Med. 2015;34(2):263–84.
11. Fredericson M, Moore W, Guillet M, Beaulieu C. High hamstring tendinopathy in runners: meeting the challenges of diagnosis, treatment, and rehabilitation. Phys Sportsmed. 2005;33(5):32–43.
12. Zissen MH, Wallace G, Stevens KJ, Fredericson M, Beaulieu CF. High hamstring tendinopathy: MRI and ultrasound imaging and therapeutic efficacy of percutaneous corticosteroid injection. AJR Am J Roentgenol. 2010;195(4):993–8.
13. De Smet AA, Blankenbaker DG, Alsheik NH, Lindstrom MJ. MRI appearance of the proximal hamstring tendons in patients with and without symptomatic proximal hamstring tendinopathy. AJR Am J Roentgenol. 2012;198(2):418–22.
14. Thompson SM, Fung S, Wood DG. The prevalence of proximal hamstring pathology on MRI in the asymptomatic population. Knee Surg Sports Traumatol Arthrosc. 2017;25(1):108–11.
15. Fredberg U, Bolvig L. Significance of ultrasonographically detected asymptomatic tendinosis in the patellar and Achilles tendons of elite soccer players: a longitudinal study. Am J Sports Med. 2002;30(4):488–91.
16. Puranen J, Orava S. The hamstring syndrome. A new diagnosis of gluteal sciatic pain. Am J Sports Med. 1988;16(5):517–21.
17. Cacchio A, Rompe JD, Furia JP, Susi P, Santilli V, De Paulis F. Shockwave therapy for the treatment of chronic proximal hamstring tendinopathy in professional athletes. Am J Sports Med. 2011;39(1):146–53.
18. Lempainen L, Sarimo J, Mattila K, Vaittinen S, Orava S. Proximal hamstring tendinopathy: results of surgical management and histopathologic findings. Am J Sports Med. 2009;37(4):727–34.
19. Miller SL, Gill J, Webb GR. The proximal origin of the hamstrings and surrounding anatomy encountered during repair. A cadaveric study. J Bone Joint Surg Am. 2007;89(1):44–8.
20. Brucker PU, Imhoff AB. Functional assessment after acute and chronic complete ruptures of the proximal hamstring tendons. Knee Surg Sports Traumatol Arthrosc. 2005;13(5):411–8.
21. Wood DG, Packham I, Trikha SP, Linklater J. Avulsion of the proximal hamstring origin. J Bone Joint Surg Am. 2008;90(11):2365–74.
22. Chakravarthy J, Ramisetty N, Pimpalnerkar A, Mohtadi N. Surgical repair of complete proximal hamstring tendon ruptures in water skiers and bull riders: a report of four cases and review of the literature. Br J Sports Med. 2005;39(8):569–72.
23. Ali K, Leland JM. Hamstring strains and tears in the athlete. Clin Sports Med. 2012;31(2):263–72.
24. Cohen S, Bradley J. Acute proximal hamstring rupture. J Am Acad Orthop Surg. 2007;15(6):350–5.
25. Connell DA, Schneider-Kolsky ME, Hoving JL, Malara F, Buchbinder R, Koulouris G, et al. Longitudinal study comparing sonographic and MRI assessments of acute and healing hamstring injuries. AJR Am J Roentgenol. 2004;183(4):975–84.
26. McMaster PE. Tendon and muscle ruptures. Clinical and experimental studies on the causes and location of subcutaneous ruptures. J Bone Joint Surg. 1933;15:705.
27. Kannus P, Józsa L. Histopathological changes preceding spontaneous rupture of a tendon. A controlled study of 891 patients. J Bone Joint Surg Am. 1991;73(10):1507–25.
28. Gabbe BJ, Finch CF, Bennell KL, Wajswelner H. Risk factors for hamstring injuries in community level Australian football. Br J Sports Med. 2005;39(2):106–10.
29. Strocchi R, De Pasquale V, Guizzardi S, Govoni P, Facchini A, Raspanti M, et al. Human Achilles ten-

don: morphological and morphometric variations as a function of age. Foot Ankle. 1991;12(2):100–4.

30. Tuite DJ, Renström PA, O'Brien M. The aging tendon. Scand J Med Sci Sports. 1997;7(2):72–7.

31. Worrell TW. Factors associated with hamstring injuries. An approach to treatment and preventative measures. Sports Med. 1994;17(5):338–45.

32. Clark RA. Hamstring injuries: risk assessment and injury prevention. Ann Acad Med Singapore. 2008;37(4):341–6.

33. Croisier JL, Ganteaume S, Binet J, Genty M, Ferret JM. Strength imbalances and prevention of hamstring injury in professional soccer players: a prospective study. Am J Sports Med. 2008;36(8):1469–75.

34. Yeung SS, Suen AM, Yeung EW. A prospective cohort study of hamstring injuries in competitive sprinters: preseason muscle imbalance as a possible risk factor. Br J Sports Med. 2009;43(8):589–94.

35. van Dyk N, Bahr R, Burnett AF, Whiteley R, Bakken A, Mosler A, et al. A comprehensive strength testing protocol offers no clinical value in predicting risk of hamstring injury: a prospective cohort study of 413 professional football players. Br J Sports Med. 2017;51(23):1695–702.

36. Holmes GB, Lin J. Etiologic factors associated with symptomatic Achilles tendinopathy. Foot Ankle Int. 2006;27(11):952–9.

37. Malliaras P, Cook JL, Kent PM. Anthropometric risk factors for patellar tendon injury among volleyball players. Br J Sports Med. 2007;41(4):259–63; discussion 63

38. Fox AJ, Bedi A, Deng XH, Ying L, Harris PE, Warren RF, et al. Diabetes mellitus alters the mechanical properties of the native tendon in an experimental rat model. J Orthop Res. 2011;29(6):880–5.

39. Tsai WC, Liang FC, Cheng JW, Lin LP, Chang SC, Chen HH, et al. High glucose concentration upregulates the expression of matrix metalloproteinase-9 and -13 in tendon cells. BMC Musculoskelet Disord. 2013;14:255.

40. Gaida JE, Cook JL, Bass SL, Austen S, Kiss ZS. Are unilateral and bilateral patellar tendinopathy distinguished by differences in anthropometry, body composition, or muscle strength in elite female basketball players? Br J Sports Med. 2004;38(5):581–5.

41. Gaida JE, Alfredson L, Kiss ZS, Wilson AM, Alfredson H, Cook JL. Dyslipidemia in Achilles tendinopathy is characteristic of insulin resistance. Med Sci Sports Exerc. 2009;41(6):1194–7.

42. Magra M, Maffulli N. Genetic aspects of tendinopathy. J Sci Med Sport/Sports Med Australia. 2008;11(3):243–7.

43. Azevedo LB, Lambert MI, Vaughan CL, O'Connor CM, Schwellnus MP. Biomechanical variables associated with Achilles tendinopathy in runners. Br J Sports Med. 2009;43(4):288–92.

44. Creaby MW, Franettovich Smith MM. Retraining running gait to reduce tibial loads with clinician or accelerometry guided feedback. J Sci Med Sport/Sports Med Australia. 2016;19(4):288–92.

45. Kvist M. Achilles tendon injuries in athletes. Sports Med. 1994;18(3):173–201.

46. Nigg BM. The role of impact forces and foot pronation: a new paradigm. Clin J Sport Med. 1994;11:2–9.

47. Willems TM, De Clercq D, Delbaere K, Vanderstraeten G, De Cock A, Witvrouw E. A prospective study of gait related risk factors for exercise-related lower leg pain. Gait Posture. 2006;23(1):91–8.

48. Witvrouw E, Bellemans J, Lysens R, Danneels L, Cambier D. Intrinsic risk factors for the development of patellar tendinitis in an athletic population. A two-year prospective study. Am J Sports Med. 2001;29(2):190–5.

49. Mahieu NN, McNair P, Cools A, D'Haen C, Vandermeulen K, Witvrouw E. Effect of eccentric training on the plantar flexor muscle-tendon tissue properties. Med Sci Sports Exerc. 2008;40(1):117–23.

50. Riley G. The pathogenesis of tendinopathy. A molecular perspective. Rheumatology (Oxford). 2004;43(2):131–42.

51. Shiri R, Viikari-Juntura E, Varonen H, Heliövaara M. Prevalence and determinants of lateral and medial epicondylitis: a population study. Am J Epidemiol. 2006;164(11):1065–74.

52. Tsai WC, Hsu CC, Chen CP, Chang HN, Wong AM, Lin MS, et al. Ciprofloxacin up-regulates tendon cells to express matrix metalloproteinase-2 with degradation of type I collagen. J Orthop Res. 2011;29(1):67–73.

53. Tsai WC, Yang YM. Fluoroquinolone-associated tendinopathy. Chang Gung Med J. 2011;34(5):461–7.

54. Tsai WC, Hsu CC, Chou SW, Chung CY, Chen J, Pang JH. Effects of celecoxib on migration, proliferation and collagen expression of tendon cells. Connect Tissue Res. 2007;48(1):46–51.

55. Tsai WC, Hsu CC, Chang HN, Lin YC, Lin MS, Pang JH. Ibuprofen upregulates expressions of matrix metalloproteinase-1, −8, −9, and −13 without affecting expressions of types I and III collagen in tendon cells. J Orthop Res. 2010;28(4):487–91.

56. Hernández Rodríguez I, Allegue F. Achilles and suprapatellar tendinitis due to isotretinoin. J Rheumatol. 1995;22(10):2009–10.

57. Nicholson LT, DiSegna S, Newman JS, Miller SL. Fluoroscopically guided Peritendinous corticosteroid injection for proximal hamstring Tendinopathy: a retrospective review. Orthop J Sports Med. 2014;2(3):2325967114526135.

58. Chu SK, Rho ME. Hamstring injuries in the athlete: diagnosis, treatment, and return to play. Curr Sports Med Rep. 2016;15(3):184–90.

59. Koulouris G, Connell D. Evaluation of the hamstring muscle complex following acute injury. Skeletal Radiol. 2003;32(10):582–9.

60. Bencardino JT, Mellado JM. Hamstring injuries of the hip. Magn Reson Imaging Clin N Am. 2005;13(4):677–90, vi

61. Slavotinek JP, Verrall GM, Fon GT. Hamstring injury in athletes: using MR imaging measurements to compare extent of muscle injury with amount of time lost from competition. AJR Am J Roentgenol. 2002;179(6):1621–8.

62. Clanton TO, Coupe KJ. Hamstring strains in athletes: diagnosis and treatment. J Am Acad Orthop Surg. 1998;6(4):237–48.

63. Schneider-Kolsky ME, Hoving JL, Warren P, Connell DA. A comparison between clinical assessment and magnetic resonance imaging of acute hamstring injuries. Am J Sports Med. 2006;34(6):1008–15.

64. Koulouris G, Connell D. Hamstring muscle complex: an imaging review. Radiographics. 2005;25(3):571–86.

65. Koulouris G, Connell DA, Brukner P, Schneider-Kolsky M. Magnetic resonance imaging parameters for assessing risk of recurrent hamstring injuries in elite athletes. Am J Sports Med. 2007;35(9):1500–6.

66. Hickey JT, Timmins RG, Maniar N, Williams MD, Opar DA. Criteria for progressing rehabilitation and determining return-to-play clearance following hamstring strain injury: a systematic review. Sports Med. 2017;47(7):1375–387.

67. Mason DL, Dickens VA, Vail A. Rehabilitation for hamstring injuries. Cochrane Database Syst Rev. 2012;12:CD004575.

68. Malliaropoulos N, Papalexandris S, Papalada A, Papacostas E. The role of stretching in rehabilitation of hamstring injuries: 80 athletes follow-up. Med Sci Sports Exerc. 2004;36(5):756–9.

69. Sherry MA, Best TM. A comparison of 2 rehabilitation programs in the treatment of acute hamstring strains. J Orthop Sports Phys Ther. 2004;34(3):116–25.

70. Silder A, Sherry MA, Sanfilippo J, Tuite MJ, Hetzel SJ, Heiderscheit BC. Clinical and morphological changes following 2 rehabilitation programs for acute hamstring strain injuries: a randomized clinical trial. J Orthop Sports Phys Ther. 2013;43(5):284–99.

71. Askling CM, Tengvar M, Tarassova O, Thorstensson A. Acute hamstring injuries in Swedish elite sprinters and jumpers: a prospective randomised controlled clinical trial comparing two rehabilitation protocols. Br J Sports Med. 2014;48(7):532–9.

72. Askling CM, Tengvar M, Thorstensson A. Acute hamstring injuries in Swedish elite football: a prospective randomised controlled clinical trial comparing two rehabilitation protocols. Br J Sports Med. 2013;47(15):953–9.

73. Pas HI, Reurink G, Tol JL, Weir A, Winters M, Moen MH. Efficacy of rehabilitation (lengthening) exercises, platelet-rich plasma injections, and other conservative interventions in acute hamstring injuries: an updated systematic review and meta-analysis. Br J Sports Med. 2015;49(18):1197–205.

74. Kingma JJ, de Knikker R, Wittink HM, Takken T. Eccentric overload training in patients with chronic Achilles tendinopathy: a systematic review. Br J Sports Med. 2007;41(6):e3.

75. Langberg H, Kongsgaard M. Eccentric training in tendinopathy--more questions than answers. Scand J Med Sci Sports. 2008;18(5):541–2.

76. Murtaugh B, Ihm JM. Eccentric training for the treatment of tendinopathies. Curr Sports Med Rep. 2013;12(3):175–82.

77. Alfredson H, Pietilä T, Jonsson P, Lorentzon R. Heavy-load eccentric calf muscle training for the treatment of chronic Achilles tendinosis. Am J Sports Med. 1998;26(3):360–6.

78. Mafi N, Lorentzon R, Alfredson H. Superior short-term results with eccentric calf muscle training compared to concentric training in a randomized prospective multicenter study on patients with chronic Achilles tendinosis. Knee Surg Sports Traumatol Arthrosc. 2001;9(1):42–7.

79. Sussmilch-Leitch SP, Collins NJ, Bialocerkowski AE, Warden SJ, Crossley KM. Physical therapies for Achilles tendinopathy: systematic review and meta-analysis. J Foot Ankle Res. 2012;5(1):15.

80. Bahr R, Fossan B, Løken S, Engebretsen L. Surgical treatment compared with eccentric training for patellar tendinopathy (Jumper's knee). A randomized, controlled trial. J Bone Joint Surg Am. 2006;88(8):1689–98.

81. Jonsson P, Alfredson H. Superior results with eccentric compared to concentric quadriceps training in patients with jumper's knee: a prospective randomised study. Br J Sports Med. 2005;39(11):847–50.

82. Komi PV, Buskirk ER. Effect of eccentric and concentric muscle conditioning on tension and electrical activity of human muscle. Ergonomics. 1972;15(4):417–34.

83. Langberg H, Ellingsgaard H, Madsen T, Jansson J, Magnusson SP, Aagaard P, et al. Eccentric rehabilitation exercise increases peritendinous type I collagen synthesis in humans with Achilles tendinosis. Scand J Med Sci Sports. 2007;17(1):61–6.

84. Rees JD, Wolman RL, Wilson A. Eccentric exercises; why do they work, what are the problems and how can we improve them? Br J Sports Med. 2009;43(4):242–6.

85. Ohberg L, Alfredson H. Effects on neovascularisation behind the good results with eccentric training in chronic mid-portion Achilles tendinosis? Knee Surg Sports Traumatol Arthrosc. 2004;12(5):465–70.

86. Knobloch K, Kraemer R, Jagodzinski M, Zeichen J, Meller R, Vogt PM. Eccentric training decreases paratendon capillary blood flow and preserves paratendon oxygen saturation in chronic Achilles tendinopathy. J Orthop Sports Phys Ther. 2007;37(5):269–76.

87. Rees JD, Lichtwark GA, Wolman RL, Wilson AM. The mechanism for efficacy of eccentric loading in Achilles tendon injury; an in vivo study in humans. Rheumatology (Oxford). 2008;47(10):1493–7.

88. Beyer R, Kongsgaard M, Hougs Kjær B, Øhlenschlæger T, Kjær M, Magnusson SP. Heavy slow resistance versus eccentric training as treatment

for Achilles Tendinopathy: a randomized controlled trial. Am J Sports Med. 2015;43(7):1704–11.

89. Jayaseelan DJ, Moats N, Ricardo CR. Rehabilitation of proximal hamstring tendinopathy utilizing eccentric training, lumbopelvic stabilization, and trigger point dry needling: 2 case reports. J Orthop Sports Phys Ther. 2014;44(3):198–205.

90. Agre JC. Hamstring injuries. Proposed aetiological factors, prevention, and treatment. Sports Med. 1985;2(1):21–33.

91. Jarvinen TA, Jarvinen TL, Kaariainen M, Kalimo H, Jarvinen M. Muscle injuries: biology and treatment. Am J Sports Med. 2005;33(5):745–64.

92. Sallay PI, Friedman RL, Coogan PG, Garrett WE. Hamstring muscle injuries among water skiers. Functional outcome and prevention. Am J Sports Med. 1996;24(2):130–6.

93. Hofmann KJ, Paggi A, Connors D, Miller SL. Complete avulsion of the proximal hamstring insertion: functional outcomes after nonsurgical treatment. J Bone Joint Surg Am. 2014;96(12):1022–5.

94. Ferlic PW, Sadoghi P, Singer G, Kraus T, Eberl R. Treatment for ischial tuberosity avulsion fractures in adolescent athletes. Knee Surg Sports Traumatol Arthrosc. 2014;22(4):893–7.

95. Eberbach H, Hohloch L, Feucht MJ, Konstantinidis L, Sudkamp NP, Zwingmann J. Operative versus conservative treatment of apophyseal avulsion fractures of the pelvis in the adolescents: a systematical review with meta-analysis of clinical outcome and return to sports. BMC Musculoskelet Disord. 2017;18(1):162.

96. Markert CD, Merrick MA, Kirby TE, Devor ST. Nonthermal ultrasound and exercise in skeletal muscle regeneration. Arch Phys Med Rehabil. 2005;86(7):1304–10.

97. Rantanen J, Thorsson O, Wollmer P, Hurme T, Kalimo H. Effects of therapeutic ultrasound on the regeneration of skeletal myofibers after experimental muscle injury. Am J Sports Med. 1999;27(1):54–9.

98. McCormack JR. The management of bilateral high hamstring tendinopathy with ASTYM® treatment and eccentric exercise: a case report. J Man Manip Ther. 2012;20(3):142–6.

99. McCormack JR, Underwood FB, Slaven EJ, Cappaert TA. Eccentric exercise versus eccentric exercise and soft tissue treatment (Astym) in the Management of Insertional Achilles Tendinopathy. Sports Health. 2016;8(3):230–7.

100. White KE. High hamstring tendinopathy in 3 female long distance runners. J Chiropr Med. 2011;10(2):93–9.

101. Carulli C, Tonelli F, Innocenti M, Gambardella B, Muncibì F. Effectiveness of extracorporeal shockwave therapy in three major tendon diseases. J Orthop Traumatol. 2016;17(1):15–20.

102. Cacchio A, Paoloni M, Barile A, Don R, de Paulis F, Calvisi V, et al. Effectiveness of radial shockwave therapy for calcific tendinitis of the shoulder:

single-blind, randomized clinical study. Phys Ther. 2006;86(5):672–82.

103. Rasmussen S, Christensen M, Mathiesen I, Simonson O. Shockwave therapy for chronic Achilles tendinopathy: a double-blind, randomized clinical trial of efficacy. Acta Orthop. 2008;79(2):249–56.

104. Rompe JD, Furia J, Maffulli N. Eccentric loading versus eccentric loading plus shock-wave treatment for midportion Achilles tendinopathy: a randomized controlled trial. Am J Sports Med. 2009;37(3):463–70.

105. Paavola M, Kannus P, Jarvinen TA, Jarvinen TL, Jozsa L, Jarvinen M. Treatment of tendon disorders. Is there a role for corticosteroid injection? Foot Ankle Clin. 2002;7(3):501–13.

106. Scutt N, Rolf CG, Scutt A. Glucocorticoids inhibit tenocyte proliferation and tendon progenitor cell recruitment. J Orthop Res. 2006;24(2):173–82.

107. Wong MW, Tang YN, Fu SC, Lee KM, Chan KM. Triamcinolone suppresses human tenocyte cellular activity and collagen synthesis. Clin Orthop Relat Res. 2004;421:277–81.

108. Wong MW, Tang YY, Lee SK, Fu BS. Glucocorticoids suppress proteoglycan production by human tenocytes. Acta Orthop. 2005;76(6):927–31.

109. Shapses SA, Luckey MM, Levine JP, Timins JK, Mackenzie GM. Osteoporosis. Recommended guidelines and New Jersey legislation. New Jersey Med. 2000;97(11):53–7.

110. Jacobson JA, Rubin J, Yablon CM, Kim SM, Kalume-Brigido M, Parameswaran A. Ultrasound-guided fenestration of tendons about the hip and pelvis: clinical outcomes. J Ultrasound Med. 2015;34(11):2029–35.

111. Hamid MSA, Ali MRM, Yusof A, George J, Lee LPC. Platelet-rich plasma injections for the treatment of hamstring injuries: a randomized controlled trial. Am J Sports Med. 2014;42(10):2410–8.

112. Hamilton B, Tol JL, Almusa E, Boukarroum S, Eirale C, Farooq A, et al. Platelet-rich plasma does not enhance return to play in hamstring injuries: a randomised controlled trial. Br J Sports Med. 2015;49(14):943–50.

113. Reurink G, Goudswaard GJ, Oomen HG, Moen MH, Tol JL, Verhaar JA, et al. Reliability of the active and passive knee extension test in acute hamstring injuries. Am J Sports Med. 2013;41(8):1757–61.

114. Rettig AC, Meyer S, Bhadra AK. Platelet-rich plasma in addition to rehabilitation for acute hamstring injuries in NFL players: clinical effects and time to return to play. Orthop J Sports Med. 2013;1(1):2325967113494354.

115. Wetzel RJ, Patel RM, Terry MA. Platelet-rich plasma as an effective treatment for proximal hamstring injuries. Orthopedics. 2013;36(1):e64–70.

116. Fader RR, Mitchell JJ, Traub S, Nichols R, Roper M, Mei Dan O, et al. Platelet-rich plasma treatment improves outcomes for chronic proximal hamstring injuries in an athletic population. Muscles Ligaments Tendons J. 2014;4(4):461–6.

117. Davenport KL, Campos JS, Nguyen J, Saboeiro G, Adler RS, Moley PJ. Ultrasound-guided Intratendinous injections with platelet-rich plasma or autologous whole blood for treatment of proximal hamstring Tendinopathy: a double-blind randomized controlled trial. J Ultrasound Med. 2015;34(8):1455–63.

118. Cohen SB, Rangavajjula A, Vyas D, Bradley JP. Functional results and outcomes after repair of proximal hamstring avulsions. Am J Sports Med. 2012;40(9):2092–8.

119. Harris JD, Griesser MJ, Best TM, Ellis TJ. Treatment of proximal hamstring ruptures - a systematic review. Int J Sports Med. 2011;32(7):490–5.

120. Cross MJ, Vandersluis R, Wood D, Banff M. Surgical repair of chronic complete hamstring tendon rupture in the adult patient. Am J Sports Med. 1998;26(6):785–8.

121. Sallay PI, Ballard G, Hamersly S, Schrader M. Subjective and functional outcomes following surgical repair of complete ruptures of the proximal hamstring complex. Orthopedics. 2008;31(11):1092.

122. Sarimo J, Lempainen L, Mattila K, Orava S. Complete proximal hamstring avulsions: a series of 41 patients with operative treatment. Am J Sports Med. 2008;36(6):1110–5.

123. Jones BV, Ward MW. Myositis ossificans in the biceps femoris muscles causing sciatic nerve palsy. A case report. J Bone Joint Surg Br. 1980;62-B(4):506–7.

124. Haus BM, Arora D, Upton J, Micheli LJ. Nerve wrapping of the sciatic nerve with Acellular dermal matrix in chronic complete proximal hamstring ruptures and Ischial Apophyseal avulsion fractures. Orthop J Sports Med. 2016;4(3):2325967116638484.

125. Klingele KE, Sallay PI. Surgical repair of complete proximal hamstring tendon rupture. Am J Sports Med. 2002;30(5):742–7.

126. Birmingham P, Muller M, Wickiewicz T, Cavanaugh J, Rodeo S, Warren R. Functional outcome after repair of proximal hamstring avulsions. J Bone Joint Surg Am. 2011;93(19):1819–26.

127. Folsom GJ, Larson CM. Surgical treatment of acute versus chronic complete proximal hamstring ruptures: results of a new allograft technique for chronic reconstructions. Am J Sports Med. 2008;36(1):104–9.

128. van der Made AD, Reurink G, Gouttebarge V, Tol JL, Kerkhoffs GM. Outcome after surgical repair of proximal hamstring avulsions: a systematic review. Am J Sports Med. 2015;43(11):2841–51.

129. Chahal J, Bush-Joseph CA, Chow A, Zelazny A, Mather RC 3rd, Lin EC, et al. Clinical and magnetic resonance imaging outcomes after surgical repair of complete proximal hamstring ruptures: does the tendon heal? Am J Sports Med. 2012;40(10):2325–30.

130. Konan S, Haddad F. Successful return to high level sports following early surgical repair of complete tears of the proximal hamstring tendons. Int Orthop. 2010;34(1):119–23.

131. Lefevre N, Bohu Y, Naouri JF, Klouche S, Herman S. Returning to sports after surgical repair of acute proximal hamstring ruptures. Knee Surg Sports Traumatol Arthrosc. 2013;21(3):534–9.

132. Sandmann GH, Hahn D, Amereller M, Siebenlist S, Schwirtz A, Imhoff AB, et al. Mid-term functional outcome and return to sports after proximal hamstring tendon repair. Int J Sports Med. 2016;37(7):570–6.

133. Subbu R, Benjamin-Laing H, Haddad F. Timing of surgery for complete proximal hamstring avulsion injuries: successful clinical outcomes at 6 weeks, 6 months, and after 6 months of injury. Am J Sports Med. 2015;43(2):385–91.

134. Mansour AA 3rd, Genuario JW, Young JP, Murphy TP, Boublik M, Schlegel TF. National Football League athletes' return to play after surgical reattachment of complete proximal hamstring ruptures. Am J Orthop (Belle Mead NJ). 2013;42(6):E38–41.

135. Barry MJ, Palmer WE, Petruska AJ. A proximal hamstring injury--getting off a slippery slope. JAMA Intern Med. 2016;176(1):15–6.

136. Shelly MJ, Hodnett PA, MacMahon PJ, Moynagh MR, Kavanagh EC, Eustace SJ. MR imaging of muscle injury. Magn Reson Imaging Clin N Am. 2009;17(4):757–73. vii

137. Cohen SB, Towers JD, Zoga A, Irrgang JJ, Makda J, Deluca PF, et al. Hamstring injuries in professional football players: magnetic resonance imaging correlation with return to play. Sports Health. 2011;3(5):423–30.

138. Askling CM, Tengvar M, Saartok T, Thorstensson A. Proximal hamstring strains of stretching type in different sports: injury situations, clinical and magnetic resonance imaging characteristics, and return to sport. Am J Sports Med. 2008;36(9):1799–804.

139. Reurink G, Brilman EG, de Vos RJ, Maas M, Moen MH, Weir A, et al. Magnetic resonance imaging in acute hamstring injury: can we provide a return to play prognosis? Sports Med. 2015;45(1):133–46.

140. Askling C, Saartok T, Thorstensson A. Type of acute hamstring strain affects flexibility, strength, and time to return to pre-injury level. Br J Sports Med. 2006;40(1):40–4.

141. Pollock N, Patel A, Chakraverty J, Suokas A, James SL, Chakraverty R. Time to return to full training is delayed and recurrence rate is higher in intratendinous ('c') acute hamstring injury in elite track and field athletes: clinical application of the British athletics muscle injury classification. Br J Sports Med. 2016;50(5):305–10.

142. Brooks JH, Fuller CW, Kemp SP, Reddin DB. Incidence, risk, and prevention of hamstring muscle injuries in professional rugby union. Am J Sports Med. 2006;34(8):1297–306.

143. Jacobsen P, Witvrouw E, Muxart P, Tol JL, Whiteley R. A combination of initial and follow-up physiotherapist examination predicts physician-determined time to return to play after hamstring injury,

with no added value of MRI. Br J Sports Med. 2016;50(7):431–9.

144. Verrall GM, Slavotinek JP, Barnes PG, Fon GT, Esterman A. Assessment of physical examination and magnetic resonance imaging findings of hamstring injury as predictors for recurrent injury. J Orthop Sports Phys Ther. 2006;36(4):215–24.

145. Warren P, Gabbe BJ, Schneider-Kolsky M, Bennell KL. Clinical predictors of time to return to competition and of recurrence following hamstring strain in elite Australian footballers. Br J Sports Med. 2010;44(6):415–9.

146. Orchard J, Best TM, Verrall GM. Return to play following muscle strains. Clin J Sport Med. 2005;15(6):436–41.

147. Silder A, Heiderscheit BC, Thelen DG, Enright T, Tuite MJ. MR observations of long-term musculotendon remodeling following a hamstring strain injury. Skeletal Radiol. 2008;37(12):1101–9.

148. Askling C, Karlsson J, Thorstensson A. Hamstring injury occurrence in elite soccer players after preseason strength training with eccentric overload. Scand J Med Sci Sports. 2003;13(4):244–50.

149. Arnason A, Andersen TE, Holme I, Engebretsen L, Bahr R. Prevention of hamstring strains in elite soccer: an intervention study. Scand J Med Sci Sports. 2008;18(1):40–8.

150. Al Attar WS, Soomro N, Sinclair PJ, Pappas E, Sanders RH. Effect of injury prevention programs that include the Nordic hamstring exercise on hamstring injury rates in soccer players: a systematic review and meta-analysis. Sports Med. 2017;47(5):907–16.

151. Kilcoyne KG, Dickens JF, Keblish D, Rue JP, Chronister R. Outcome of grade I and II hamstring injuries in intercollegiate athletes: a novel rehabilitation protocol. Sports Health. 2011;3(6):528–33.

152. Mishra DK, Fridén J, Schmitz MC, Lieber RL. Anti-inflammatory medication after muscle injury. A treatment resulting in short-term improvement but subsequent loss of muscle function. J Bone Joint Surg Am. 1995;77(10):1510–9.

153. Rahusen FT, Weinhold PS, Almekinders LC. Nonsteroidal anti-inflammatory drugs and acetaminophen in the treatment of an acute muscle injury. Am J Sports Med. 2004;32(8):1856–9.

154. Järvinen MJ, Lehto MU. The effects of early mobilisation and immobilisation on the healing process following muscle injuries. Sports Med. 1993;15(2):78–89.

Lateral Gluteal Tendons

Gerard A. Malanga and Usker Naqvi

Abbreviations

GTPS   Greater trochanteric pain syndrome
ITB   Iliotibial band
MRI   Magnetic resonance imaging
NSAID Non-steroidal anti-inflammatory drug

Greater Trochanteric Pain Syndrome

Introduction

In 1848, Partridge initially proposed that lateral hip pain is due to greater trochanteric bursitis and described the removal of an enlarged bursa from underneath the gluteus maximus insertion [1]. However, modern radiologic and histologic studies have demonstrated that the trochanteric bursa is often not the primary source of pain or inflammation [2–4], leading to the more accurate term "greater trochanteric pain syndrome" (GTPS) [5]. GTPS is a clinical entity that includes disorders of the gluteal tendons, iliotibial band, and the bursae about the greater trochanter.

The incidence of GTPS has been estimated as 1.8 patients per 1000 per year [6]. The prevalence of GTPS in adults is estimated to be 17.6%, of which 11.7% of cases are bilateral and 5.9% unilateral [7]. Women are three times more likely to have GTPS than men [7]. In adults with low back pain, the prevalence of GTPS rises to 20–35% [7, 8]. Other factors associated with GTPS include iliotibial band tenderness and knee pain/osteoarthritis [7]. In addition, up to 17% of patients who undergo total hip arthroplasty eventually develop GTPS [9].

Among patients with GTPS, gluteal tendon pathology, particularly of the medius and minimus, appears to be the most common cause. Analysis of ultrasound images in patients with GTPS revealed that nearly 50% of patients had gluteal tendinosis, while 29% had iliotibial band thickening and 20% had trochanteric bursitis; notably, almost 80% of patients showed no signs of bursitis on ultrasound [4]. Analysis of MRI findings similarly revealed that over half of patients with GTPS had either tendinosis or tears of the gluteus medius or minimus tendons [3].

Anatomy

The gluteal muscle group, consisting of the gluteus maximus, medius, and minimus, is intimately involved in hip extension, abduction, and rotation. These muscles attach to the various facets of the greater trochanter of the femur

G. A. Malanga (✉)
New Jersey Regenerative Institute,
Cedar Knolls, NJ, USA

U. Naqvi
Las Vegas, Nevada, USA

© Springer Nature Switzerland AG 2021
K. Onishi et al. (eds.), *Tendinopathy*, https://doi.org/10.1007/978-3-030-65335-4_9

(see Fig. 9.1 and Table 9.1). Disorders of the gluteal tendons, therefore, frequently present with pain at the lateral hip. Tensor fascia lata

and the accompanying iliotibial band are implicated in snapping hip syndrome.

Gluteus Medius Tendinopathy

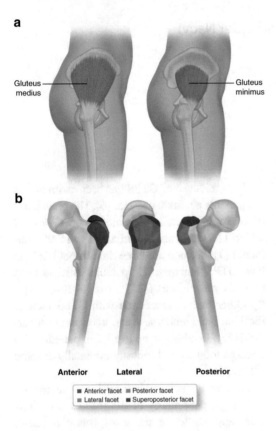

A 39-year-old avid runner presents with chief complaint of right lateral hip pain that had started after an increase in training volume. She recently began training for a marathon and has increased the frequency and duration of her runs. The pain initially only worsened with prolonged running but has now progressed to also hurting while walking. It occasionally radiates down the lateral thigh. She has difficulty sleeping on the right side due to tenderness localized to the right lateral hip. She also reports a history of chronic nonspecific low back pain. Her physical exam reveals full range of motion of the lumbar spine and hips. There is point tenderness about the right greater trochanter. Seated slump, straight leg raise, FABER, and Stinchfield's tests are negative. Resisted external derotation test is positive. What is the most likely diagnosis?

Fig. 9.1 Anatomy of the lateral hip. (**a**) Anatomy of the gluteus medius and minimus muscles. (**b**) Schematic drawing of the four facets of the greater trochanter: the anterior facet, lateral facet, posterior facet, and superoposterior facet, which represent the osseous attachment sites of the gluteus medius and gluteus minimus (AF) tendons and locations of the bursae

Clinical Presentation

Patients will typically complain of pain at the lateral hip, often worse with pressure or lying down on the affected side. The pain may radiate to the buttocks or down the lateral thigh. In severe tendinopathy, patients may complain of walking with a limp due to gluteal muscle weakness. The pain is worsened by prolonged standing, rising to a standing position, and sitting with the affected leg crossed [10, 11].

As discussed above, knee pain and low back pain are known to be associated with GTPS, so patients may complain about pain or longstanding problems in these areas. These complaints could represent referred pain from GTPS or, more likely, altered biomechanics from impaired gluteal muscles that affects low back and knee mechanics (see Table 9.2).

Physical Examination

Observation of gait and stance is useful in evaluating gluteal tendon pathology. The Trendelenburg gait pattern is indicative of gluteus medius or minimus weakness and is characterized by either

Table 9.1 Functions and attachments of lateral hip muscles

Muscle	Attachments	Function
Gluteus maximus	Ilium and dorsal sacrum to iliotibial band and gluteal tuberosity	Hip extension, external rotation, some abduction
Gluteus medius	Ilium to posterosuperior and lateral facets of the greater trochanter	Hip abduction, internal rotation
Gluteus minimus	Ilium to anterior facet of the greater trochanter	Hip abduction, internal rotation
Tensor fascia latae	Iliac crest and ASIS to iliotibial band	Hip abduction, flexion, internal rotation

Table 9.2 Differential diagnosis of GTPS

Greater trochanteric pain syndrome
  Gluteus medius tendon disorder
  Gluteus minimus tendon disorder
  Trochanteric bursitis
  Iliotibial band syndrome
  Referred pain from lower back or knee

a dropping pelvis to the unaffected side or a lateral trunk lean to the affected side [12]. This gives the patient a waddling appearance and occurs due to inability of the gluteal muscles to maintain pelvic stability. The Trendelenburg gait can be observed in 55% of patients [13]. Similarly, the Trendelenburg test (see Fig. 9.2) is performed

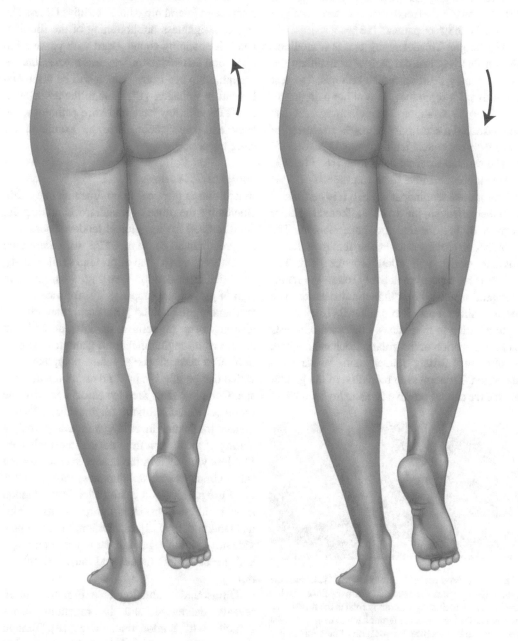

Fig. 9.2 Trendelenburg test. The test is performed by having the patient stand on the affected leg and raising the unaffected leg off the ground. The test is positive if the pelvis drops to the unsupported side

by having the patient stand on the affected leg and raise the unaffected foot off the ground. The test is positive if the pelvis drops on the unsupported side or if the trunk leans toward the supported side, indicating weakness of the gluteus medius or minimus. The Trendelenburg test has been shown to have a specificity as high as 94% for detecting gluteal tendon pathology [14, 15]. A positive Trendelenburg test can be observed in 68% of patients [13].

The fatigue Trendelenburg test is a modified version that requires the patient to maintain the Trendelenburg position for 30 seconds. The test is positive if it reproduces lateral hip pain during that time. The fatigue Trendelenburg test has demonstrated a sensitivity of 100% and specificity of 97% for gluteal tendinopathy [12, 16].

The resisted external derotation (see Fig. 9.3) test is a highly sensitive (88%) and specific (97%) test for gluteal tendinopathy [16]. It is performed with the patient supine and the affected leg in 90 degrees of hip flexion and knee flexion. The examiner externally rotates the femur as far as possible, which will often provoke pain. The patient is then asked to actively return the femur to neutral against the examiner's resistance. The test is positive if pain is reproduced [16].

In addition to these tests, other classical tests include palpation of the greater trochanter, which is often exquisitely tender, and resisted hip abduction. Tenderness to palpation of the greater trochanter can be positive in as many as 83% of

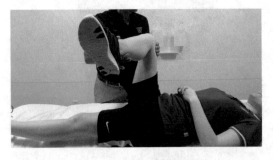

Fig. 9.3 Resisted external derotation test [12]. With the patient lying supine, the examiner passively flexes the hip and knee and maximally externally rotates the femur. The patient is asked to rotate the femur back to neutral against the examiner's resistance. Provocation of pain makes this a positive test

patients with gluteal tendinopathy [13]. Pain reproduced by resisted hip abduction is a sign that has shown specificity as high as 86%, while weakness with resisted hip abduction has demonstrated 80% sensitivity [14]. Weakness of the abductors can be seen in 64% of patients with gluteal tendon disorders [13].

The iliotibial band should also be examined as a source of lateral hip pain. A positive Ober's test suggests tightness or shortening of the iliotibial band. A snapping sound heard with passive hip abduction and adduction suggests coxa saltans or snapping hip syndrome, which will be discussed later in this chapter [17]. Due to the association of GTPS with low back and knee pathology, the back and knee should also be examined for completeness.

Diagnostic Workup

In addition to physical exam, imaging can aid in elucidating the cause of greater trochanteric pain. As discussed earlier, gluteal tendon disorder as the predominant cause of GTPS was determined by analysis of MRI and ultrasound studies [3, 4].

On MRI evaluation (see Fig. 9.4), an early sign of gluteal tendinopathy is soft tissue edema surrounding the tendon [18]. Focal disruption of tendon fibers suggests a partial tear and can appear as a longitudinal split. Complete disruption of tendon fibers suggests complete tear, which can be filled in by fluid or granulation tissue. Complete tears are also associated with the presence of avulsed bone fragment. The "bald" greater trochanter facet sign suggests complete tearing of the tendon from the greater trochanter. Fluid may be seen in the nearby submedius and subminimus bursae. Additionally, fatty atrophy, bony irregularity, and calcification at the tendon attachment are considered indirect signs of gluteal tendinopathy [18]. In addition, MRI can provide information regarding the articular cartilage and the other soft tissues and bursae about the hip.

Ultrasound evaluation (see Fig. 9.5) often reveals decreased and heterogenous echogenicity with tendon thickening [18]. Tendon thinning or anechoic defects within the tendon

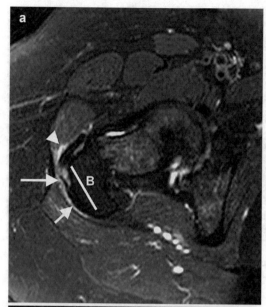

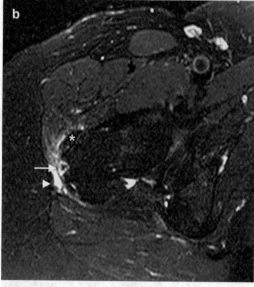

Fig. 9.4 MRI findings in gluteal tendinopathy. Axial T2 STIR. (**a**) Partial tear of the anterior third fibers of gluteus medius near the insertion on the lateral facet (line B). There is a focal tendon defect with fluid in the residual space. A low signal band of residual anterior third fibers is seen in this region (long arrow). The insertion of the middle and posterior third fibers on the lateral facet is intact (short arrow). (**b**) Partial tear of gluteus medius in a different patient with fluid surrounding the anterior fibers (arrow) separated from the remainder of the tendon. There is fluid in the submaximus bursa (arrowhead). Intrasubstance T2 hyperintensity (asterisk) and edema surrounding gluteus minimus suggest peritendinitis and low-grade tendinosis [18]

substance suggest partial or full thickness tears. Cortical irregularities may be seen at the attachment sites and the "bald" facet sign can be observed. Fluid distention may be observed in the bursae. Calcifications may be observed in the tendons; these can be aspirated under ultrasound guidance [18].

Treatments

Conservative

Physical therapy is often the starting point for treatment of gluteal tendinopathy. The goals should be to reduce pain, improve hip range of motion, and correct gait abnormalities to prevent falls and ensure safety. Activity modification and avoidance of painful positions may be necessary to allow for tendon healing. Stretching and soft tissue mobilization of the tensor fascia lata and iliotibial band can help to reduce pain and pressure over the greater trochanter [19]. One study comparing conservative treatments found that home exercise training had a success rate of 80% at 15-month follow-up, significantly better than corticosteroid injection [20]. While eccentric exercise has been shown to be beneficial for other tendinopathies, such as Achilles and patellar [21], no studies have evaluated its use in gluteal tendinopathy. In addition, there is little or no data on the value of manual treatments and therapeutic modalities in gluteal tendinopathy patients.

While non-steroidal anti-inflammatory drugs (NSAIDs) are often included in the general umbrella of conservative management, there has been little study specifically in GTPS patients. One study found statistically significant improvements in pain with oral etodolac 400 mg or topical diclofenac 3% [22]. Treatment with these medications demonstrated significant improvement in 2 weeks, with benefits that last through 6 weeks of follow-up [22]. No significant differences were found between groups; however, given the systemic effects of oral NSAID treatment, topical NSAID presents an attractive and equally effective alternative.

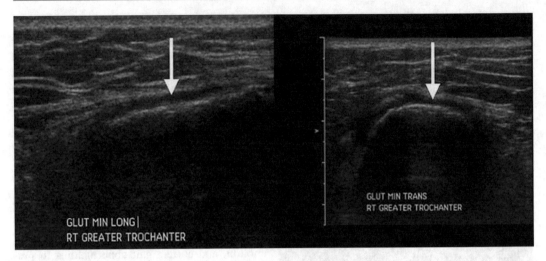

GLUT MIN TRANS
RT GREATER TROCHANTER

GLUT MIN LONG|
RT GREATER TROCHANTER

Fig. 9.5 Ultrasound findings in gluteal tendinopathy. Ultrasound longitudinal and transverse views. A "bald" greater trochanter appearance suggests absence of the gluteus minimus tendon signifying a complete tear (arrow) [18]

Interventional

Shockwave therapy (SWT) can be an effective treatment for GTPS. In a randomized controlled trial, radial SWT was found to have a success rate of 68% at 4 months follow-up; this improved to 74% after 15 months [20]. It was significantly superior to corticosteroid injection after 15 months; however, SWT did not show any significant improvement from baseline until 4 months after treatment [20], suggesting that it may provide a slower but more sustained treatment effect than corticosteroid injection.

Dry needling, in which a needle is directed into damaged tissue to induce mechanical trauma rather than to inject medication, has been compared against corticosteroid injection and was found to be non-inferior [23]. Both treatments resulted in significant improvement in pain over 6 weeks but were not significantly different from each other [23]. Another study compared ultrasound-guided tendon fenestration (see Fig. 9.6) with ultrasound-guided platelet-rich plasma (PRP) injection. Both treatments demonstrated significant improvements in pain compared to baseline but did not demonstrate significant differences compared to each other [24]. Taken together, the results of these studies reveal that dry needling can be as effective as either corticosteroid injection or PRP injection in the short term.

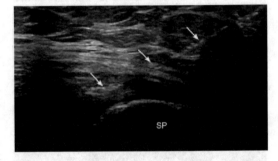

SP

Fig. 9.6 Needle fenestration of gluteus medius tendon. Gluteus medius fenestration. Ultrasound image long axis to the gluteus medius over the superoposterior (SP) facet of the greater trochanter shows 20-gauge needle and needle tip (*arrows*) within hypoechoic and thickened tendon segment (the left side of the image is superior) [45]

Corticosteroid injection is a common treatment for GTPS, stemming from the traditional belief that GTPS was due to an inflammatory bursitis. It has been shown to provide significant short-term benefit [20, 25]. However, in the long term, it has not shown superiority over other treatments for gluteal tendinopathy, including SWT [20], home exercises [20], physical therapy [26], oral analgesics [26], and dry needling [23]. No further benefit was demonstrated by the addition of fluoroscopic guidance compared to blind injections [27]. Ultrasound-guided corticosteroid injection has been studied and showed considerable short-term improvement but was not compared to blind or fluoroscopically guided injection head-to-head [25, 28]. These results for gluteal tendinopathy are in agreement with results for other tendons, such as Achilles and rotator cuff tendons, which show that corticosteroid injection can relieve pain in the short term but has no benefit for intermediate- or long-term relief [29]. In fact, performing no intervention at all provides better intermediate- and long-term benefits than corticosteroid injection [29].

The role of regenerative treatments for gluteal tendinopathy shows promise but remains to be elucidated. Injection of autologous tenocytes directly into the gluteal tendon under ultrasound guidance demonstrated significant improvement in pain through 24 months of follow-up in a case series of 12 female patients with gluteal tendinopathy who failed conventional conservative measures [30]. A multi-center, retrospective study found that PRP injection resulted in a 75% decrease in pain score, with 95% of patients reporting no pain disrupting daily activities at follow-up [31]. While this study was not limited to the gluteal tendons only, it was found that 81% of patients with gluteal tendinopathy who underwent PRP injection reported moderate improvement to complete resolution of symptoms [31]. One pilot study compared PRP to corticosteroid injection for GTPS and found no superiority of PRP; however, the injection was targeted to the trochanteric bursa and not the gluteal tendons, so these results should be interpreted cautiously with regard to treating gluteal tendinopathy [32]. Another study of intratendinous PRP injection under ultrasound guidance was found to provide statistically significant improvement compared to baseline but no difference compared to needle fenestration [24]. Current data supports the use of PRP, though its use exclusively in gluteal tendinopathy has not been studied in a randomized, controlled manner.

In an anatomical study of cadavers, researchers discovered that a branch of the femoral nerve innervates the periosteum of the greater trochanter. This may represent a potential target for intervention, such as nerve blocks or neurolysis, to reduce greater trochanteric pain. However, no studies have been performed in living humans to support any benefit from this treatment. In addition, this approach would only help to reduce the sensation of pain but would not address the underlying tendon disorder [9].

Operative

In refractory cases, surgical intervention may be performed. Operative gluteal tendon repair may be done endoscopically or as an open procedure. Studies have not compared the open approach to endoscopic [21], though the minimally invasive endoscopic surgery offers the benefits of a smaller incision, faster healing time, and less postoperative pain [21, 33]. Results for surgical repairs of the gluteal tendons are generally favorable for long-term improvement [21], with case series showing up to 95% of patients achieving resolution of pain through 12 months [34]. However, operative interventions have only been studied in case series and have not been compared to nonoperative treatments such as physical therapy, injections, or needle tenotomy. Still, patients who have failed other conservative measures may choose to consider surgical options.

Snapping Hip Syndrome

Introduction

Snapping hip syndrome, also known as coxa saltans, involves a catching or snapping sensation with movement at the hip. It may occur in up to 10% of the general population and is often seen in athletes such as dancers, weight lifters, runners, and soccer players [35, 36]. It is commonly divided into intraarticular and extraarticular types. Intraarticular causes of snapping hip syndrome include labral tears or loose bodies in the joint [37]. Extraarticular causes are further subdivided into internal and external types. Internal causes are typically attributed to disorders of the iliopsoas tendon, usually with snapping over the iliopectineal eminence, though snapping over a total hip arthroplasty, snapping at the lesser trochanter, and snapping of the iliofemoral ligament over the femoral head have also been described [37]. External causes are most common [38] and are typically attributed to the tensor fascia lata (TFL) and iliotibial band (ITB) or the anterior portion of the gluteus maximus tendon snapping over the greater trochanter [37] (Fig. 9.7) [38]. This chapter will focus on the external extraarticular type.

Case

A 17-year-old dancer presents with complaint of a snapping feeling over the outside of her right hip. It began about 3 months ago while dancing and has become progressively more frequent, now occurring in everyday activities like climbing stairs. Lately, she has also noticed some intermittent achiness occurring at the lateral right hip, especially at the end of dance practice. On physical exam, she has a positive Ober's test, and a snap could be felt and heard at the lateral hip while passively ranging the hip in flexion and extension. What is the most likely diagnosis?

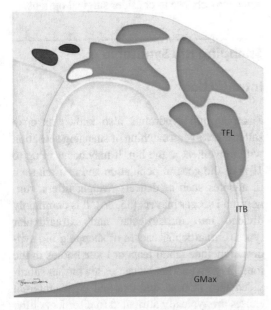

Fig. 9.7 Cross-sectional anatomy of the hip [38]. The anatomic relationship between gluteus maximus, tensor fascia lata, iliotibial band, and the greater trochanter is depicted here

Clinical Presentation

The hallmark feature of snapping hip syndrome is a palpable and/or audible snap that occurs with movement of the hip, often with flexion, extension, and rotation. Patients will often point to where they feel this occurring, which can help to differentiate external snapping hip (pointing to lateral hip) from internal or intraarticular (pointing to anterior and/or medial hip). In addition to the snap, patients may also feel a sensation of the hip dislocating, which is known as pseudosubluxation. There is often tenderness at the lateral hip [37]. Patients may complain of difficulty with running, stairclimbing, or carrying heavy loads due to snapping [36]. Some data suggest that total hip or total knee replacements may be risk factors for the development of external snapping hip, as portions of the ITB may be compromised intraoperatively [36].

Physical Exam

An important goal with physical exam in the snapping hip is to try to provoke the snapping. In external snapping hip syndrome, this can be provoked by internal/external rotation, flexion, extension, or a combination of these movements [36]. Patients often have already identified which movements provoke their snapping and can easily demonstrate this at the time of examination [38].

The Ober's test (Fig. 9.8) [12] can be used to evaluate for tightness of the TFL-ITB, which can predispose to snapping. It is performed by having the patient lie on an exam table on the unaffected side with both hip and knees flexed to 90 degrees. The examiner then passively abducts and extends the affected hip until it is in line with the body while maintaining the knee flexion at 90 degrees. The examiner then releases the affected leg, which should freely drop. If it remains abducted, this is a positive test, indicating tightness of the ITB. The modified Ober's test is performed similarly, except with the affected knee fully extended. Studies have demonstrated intrarater reliability to be similar for both tests at 0.90 for the Ober's test and 0.91 for the modified Ober's test [12].

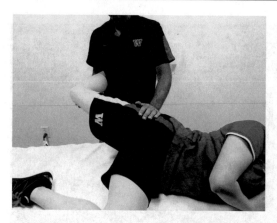

Fig. 9.8 Ober's test [12]. The patient is side-lying on the asymptomatic side with both knees and hips flexed to 90 degrees. The examiner places one hand on the affected hip and grasps the affected ankle with the other hand, abducting and extending the affected leg. Upon release, the affected leg will remain passively abducted if there is iliotibial band tightness

Diagnostic Workup

Plain radiographs are often the initial step because they can rule out other pathologies or allow for evaluation of hip morphology that may contribute to snapping, such as coxa vara, or small femoral neck angle [36]. Ultimately, however, there are no direct findings on plain radiographs to diagnose external snapping hip syndrome.

Ultrasound allows for evaluation of the involved tendons and identification of ITB or gluteus maximus tendon thickening, especially where they pass over the greater trochanter. Ultrasound examination is best performed with the patient in a side-lying position with the affected hip up. Dynamic ultrasound evaluation may allow for the snapping to be directly visualized by placing the probe directly over the greater trochanter and identifying the ITB and gluteus maximus tendons, where thickening and hypoechogenicity may be seen [39]. The hip should then be passively moved by the examiner and movement of the tendons observed [35]. Abrupt anterior movement of the ITB or gluteus maximus can be observed as the hip moves from extension to flexion [36] (Fig. 9.9) [38]. The

patient can often perform the movements that cause snapping while the examiner observes muscle activity on ultrasound [38]. Recording cine clips of this occurring can provide better confirmation than saving static images [38].

MRI may also be used to evaluate the hip and can show tendon or ITB thickening, as well as surrounding soft tissue edema [35]. However, these findings are largely nonspecific, and MRI lacks the ability to demonstrate dynamic movement.

Treatment

Conservative

External snapping hip syndrome can often be treated conservatively with stretching, hip abductor strengthening, activity modification, and NSAID's for pain [35]. There is often an imbalance between gluteus maximus activation and TFL activation, the correction of which becomes the focus of the physical therapy regimen [37]. Ultrasound-guided corticosteroid injection at the iliotibial band or at the trochanteric bursae can provide some relief of pain [35], though this is more useful to help the patient tolerate physical therapy more easily and does not address the mechanical cause of the snapping.

Surgical

There are various surgical options available for external snapping hip syndrome, with both open and endoscopic methods. The goal is to release the tendon or ITB, thus generating slack and eliminating snapping. Multiple techniques have been reported. However, the data supporting these are limited due to small sample sizes and lack of comparative studies between surgical approaches.

A popular open approach is the Z-plasty, which uses a Z-shaped cut and reattachment to loosen and lengthen the ITB. In a case series of nine patients who underwent this treatment, all but one achieved resolution of their symptoms [40]. In those with concurrent gluteus maximus tightness, making reapproximation of the ITB

Fig. 9.9 Ultrasound images of gluteus maximus movement [38]. (**a**) Transverse plane ultrasound images of the symptomatic left hip demonstrate normal position of the iliotibial band (arrows) over the greater trochanter (asterisks) at rest. The anterior margin of the gluteus maximus is posterior to the greater trochanter (arrowheads). (**b**) With the patient's stress maneuver, the anterior margin of the gluteus maximus (arrowheads) subluxed abruptly over the greater trochanter (asterisks); *A* anterior, *P* posterior

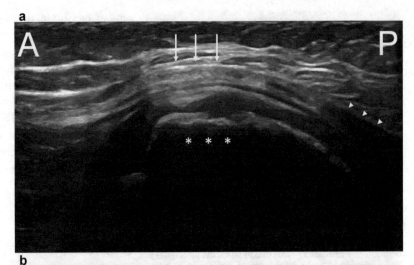

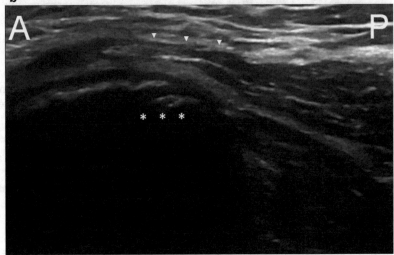

technically challenging, a modified Z-plasty technique calls for flexing and adducting the hip intraoperatively to allow for better approximation around the Z-shaped cut [41].

Endoscopic release of the ITB has been demonstrated to be effective in reducing pain, eliminating snapping, and promoting return to previous level of activity [42]. Ilizaliturri et al. [43] used a radiofrequency hook probe and a shaver under endoscopy to create a cross-shaped cut through the ITB, and then resected the resulting flaps to produce a diamond-shaped defect; after 2 years, they documented resolution of pain and snapping in all but one patient. Polesello et al. [44] described an endoscopic technique for releasing the gluteus maximus insertion on the femur,

resulting in the elimination of snapping; this technique, unlike others, allows for the ITB to remain intact.

Conclusion

Gluteal tendon disorders can largely be distilled down to two main syndromes: greater trochanteric pain syndrome and snapping hip syndrome. Gluteal tendinopathy, particularly of the gluteus medius and minimus tendons, is the leading cause of GTPS and lateral hip pain. Bursitis may occur as a secondary pathology. The fatigue Trendelenburg test and resisted external derotation test can often help make the diagnosis, though diagnosis is enhanced by MRI or ultrasound imaging showing degenerative changes of the gluteal tendons. Conservative treatment is typically successful and can include home exercises, physical therapy, SWT, dry needling, and PRP injection. Stem cell injection shows promise but will require more definitive study. Corticosteroid injection can provide short-term relief but is ultimately worse in the intermediate and long terms than no treatment at all. Surgical interventions can provide lasting relief in refractory cases.

External snapping hip syndrome is the subtype that involves the gluteal tendons and associated structures, particularly gluteus maximus, tensor fascia lata, and the iliotibial band. Tightness of one or more of these structures causes a mechanical snapping as they move abruptly over the greater trochanter, resulting in lateral hip pain. Patients commonly complain of a snapping sound or sensation and can readily identify movements that cause it. It is frequently reproducible on physical examination. Dynamic ultrasound evaluation can identify the structures involved and demonstrate the snapping movement in real time. Conservative treatments targeting the muscle tightness and imbalances that predispose to snapping are often effective; ultrasound-guided steroid injection can provide some pain relief. Refractory cases can be treated surgically, as both open and endoscopic techniques have proven effective.

References

1. Partridge M. Enlarged and thickened bursa, removed from underneath the fascial insertion of the gluteus maximus. Trans Path Soc London. 1848;1:153.
2. Silva F, Adams T, Feinstein J, Arroyo RA. Trochanteric bursitis: refuting the myth of inflammation. J Clin Rheumatol. 2008;14(2):82–6.
3. Kingzett-Taylor A, Tirman PF, Feller J, McGann W, Prieto V, Wischer T, et al. Tendinosis and tears of gluteus medius and minimus muscles as a cause of hip pain: MR imaging findings. AJR Am J Roentgenol. 1999;173(4):1123–6.
4. Long SS, Surrey DE, Nazarian LN. Sonography of greater trochanteric pain syndrome and the rarity of primary bursitis. AJR Am J Roentgenol. 2013;201(5):1083–6.
5. Leonard MH. Trochanteric syndrome: calcareous and noncalcareous tendonitis and bursitis about the trochanter major. J Am Med Assoc. 1958;168(2):175–7.
6. Lievense A, Bierma-Zeinstra S, Schouten B, Bohnen A, Verhaar J, Koes B. Prognosis of trochanteric pain in primary care. Br J Gen Pract. 2005;55(512):199–204.
7. Segal NA, Felson DT, Torner JC, Zhu Y, Curtis JR, Niu J, et al. Greater trochanteric pain syndrome: epidemiology and associated factors. Arch Phys Med Rehabil. 2007;88(8):988–92.
8. Tortolani PJ, Carbone JJ, Quartararo LG. Greater trochanteric pain syndrome in patients referred to orthopedic spine specialists. Spine J. 2002;2(4):251–4.
9. Genth B, Von During M, Von Engelhardt LV, Ludwig J, Teske W, Von Schulze-Pellengahr C. Analysis of the sensory innervations of the greater trochanter for improving the treatment of greater trochanteric pain syndrome. Clin Anat. 2012;25(8):1080–6.
10. Williams BS, Cohen SP. Greater trochanteric pain syndrome: a review of anatomy, diagnosis and treatment. Anesth Analg. 2009;108(5):1662–70.
11. Ebert JR, Retheesh T, Mutreja R, Janes GC. The clinical, functional and biomechanical presentation of patients with symptomatic hip abductor tendon tears. Int J Sports Phys Ther. 2016;11(5):725–37.
12. Malanga GA, Mautner K. Musculoskeletal physical examination: an evidence-based approach. Philadelphia: Elsevier Health Sciences; 2016.
13. Lindner D, Shohat N, Botser I, Agar G, Domb BG. Clinical presentation and imaging results of patients with symptomatic gluteus medius tears. J Hip Preserv Surg. 2015;2(3):310–5.
14. Woodley SJ, Nicholson HD, Livingstone V, Doyle TC, Meikle GR, Macintosh JE, et al. Lateral hip pain: findings from magnetic resonance imaging and clinical examination. J Orthop Sports Phys Therapy. 2008;38(6):313–28.
15. Cleland J, Koppenhaver S, Su J. Netter's orthopaedic clinical examination: an evidence-based approach. Philadelphia: Elsevier Health Sciences; 2015.
16. Lequesne M, Mathieu P, Vuillemin-Bodaghi V, Bard H, Djian P. Gluteal tendinopathy in refractory greater trochanter pain syndrome: diagnostic value of two clinical tests. Arthritis Care Res. 2008;59(2):241–6.
17. Redmond JM, Chen AW, Domb BG. Greater trochanteric pain syndrome. J Am Acad Orthop Surg. 2016;24(4):231–40.
18. Kong A, Van der Vliet A, Zadow S. MRI and US of gluteal tendinopathy in greater trochanteric pain syndrome. Eur Radiol. 2007;17(7):1772–83.
19. Wyss J. Therapeutic programs for musculoskeletal disorders. New York: Demos Medical Publishing; 2012.
20. Rompe JD, Segal NA, Cacchio A, Furia JP, Morral A, Maffulli N. Home training, local corticosteroid injection, or radial shock wave therapy for greater trochanter pain syndrome. Am J Sports Med. 2009;37(10):1981–90.

21. Reid D. The management of greater trochanteric pain syndrome: a systematic literature review. J Orthop. 2016;13(1):15–28.

22. Sarno D, Sein M, Singh J. (364) The effectiveness of topical diclofenac for greater trochanteric pain syndrome: a retrospective study. The Journal of Pain. 2015;16(4):S67.

23. Brennan KL, Allen BC, Maldonado YM. Dry needling versus cortisone injection in the treatment of greater trochanteric pain syndrome: a noninferiority randomized clinical trial. J Orthop Sports Phys Ther. 2017;47(4):232–9.

24. Jacobson JA, Yablon CM, Henning PT, Kazmers IS, Urquhart A, Hallstrom B, et al. Greater trochanteric pain syndrome: percutaneous tendon fenestration versus platelet-rich plasma injection for treatment of gluteal tendinosis. J Ultrasound Med. 2016;35(11):2413–20.

25. Labrosse JM, Cardinal E, Leduc BE, Duranceau J, Remillard J, Bureau NJ, et al. Effectiveness of ultrasound-guided corticosteroid injection for the treatment of gluteus medius tendinopathy. AJR Am J Roentgenol. 2010;194(1):202–6.

26. Brinks A, van Rijn RM, Willemsen SP, Bohnen AM, Verhaar JA, Koes BW, et al. Corticosteroid injections for greater trochanteric pain syndrome: a randomized controlled trial in primary care. Ann Fam Med. 2011;9(3):226–34.

27. Cohen SP, Strassels SA, Foster L, Marvel J, Williams K, Crooks M, et al. Comparison of fluoroscopically guided and blind corticosteroid injections for greater trochanteric pain syndrome: multicentre randomised controlled trial. BMJ. 2009;338:b1088.

28. Park KD, Lee WY, Lee J, Park MH, Ahn JK, Park Y. Factors associated with the outcome of ultrasound-guided trochanteric Bursa injection in greater trochanteric pain syndrome: a retrospective cohort study. Pain Physician. 2016;19(4):E547–57.

29. Coombes BK, Bisset L, Vicenzino B. Efficacy and safety of corticosteroid injections and other injections for management of tendinopathy: a systematic review of randomised controlled trials. Lancet. 2010;376(9754):1751–67.

30. Bucher TA, Ebert JR, Smith A, Breidahl W, Fallon M, Wang T, et al. Autologous tenocyte injection for the treatment of chronic recalcitrant gluteal tendinopathy: a prospective pilot study. Orthop J Sports Med. 2017;5(2):2325967116688866.

31. Mautner K, Colberg RE, Malanga G, Borg-Stein JP, Harmon KG, Dharamsi AS, et al. Outcomes after

ultrasound-guided platelet-rich plasma injections for chronic tendinopathy: a multicenter, retrospective review. PM R. 2013;5(3):169–75.

32. Ribeiro AG, Ricioli WJ, Silva AR, Polesello GC, Guimaraes RP. PRP in the treatment of trochanteric syndrome: a pilot study. Acta Ortop Bras. 2016;24(4):208–12.

33. Govaert LH, van Dijk CN, Zeegers AV, Albers GH. Endoscopic bursectomy and iliotibial tract release as a treatment for refractory greater trochanteric pain syndrome: a new endoscopic approach with early results. Arthrosc Tech. 2012;1(2):e161–e4.

34. Walsh MJ, Walton JR, Walsh NA. Surgical repair of the gluteal tendons. J Arthroplasty. 2011;26(8):1514–9.

35. Lee KS, Rosas HG, Phancao JP. Snapping hip: imaging and treatment. Semin Musculoskelet Radiol. 2013;17(3):286–94.

36. Lewis CL. Extra-articular snapping hip: a literature review. Sports Health. 2010;2(3):186–90.

37. Yen YM, Lewis CL, Kim YJ. Understanding and treating the snapping hip. Sports Med Arthrosc Rev. 2015;23(4):194–9.

38. Chang CY, Kreher J, Torriani M. Dynamic sonography of snapping hip due to gluteus maximus subluxation over greater trochanter. Skelet Radiol. 2016;45(3):409–12.

39. Bureau NJ. Sonographic evaluation of snapping hip syndrome. J Ultrasound Med. 2013;32(6):895–900.

40. Provencher MT, Hofmeister EP, Muldoon MP. The surgical treatment of external coxa saltans (the snapping hip) by Z-plasty of the iliotibial band. Am J Sports Med. 2004;32(2):470–6.

41. Nam KW, Yoo JJ, Koo KH, Yoon KS, Kim HJ. A modified Z-plasty technique for severe tightness of the gluteus maximus. Scand J Med Sci Sports. 2011;21(1):85–9.

42. Zini R, Munegato D, De Benedetto M, Carraro A, Bigoni M. Endoscopic iliotibial band release in snapping hip. Hip Int. 2013;23(2):225–32.

43. Ilizaliturri VM Jr, Martinez-Escalante FA, Chaidez PA, Camacho-Galindo J. Endoscopic iliotibial band release for external snapping hip syndrome. Arthroscopy. 2006;22(5):505–10.

44. Polesello GC, Queiroz MC, Domb BG, Ono NK, Honda EK. Surgical technique: endoscopic gluteus maximus tendon release for external snapping hip syndrome. Clin Orthop Relat Res. 2013;471(8):2471–6.

45. Malanga G, Mautner K. Atlas of ultrasound-guided musculoskeletal injections. 1st ed. New York: McGraw-Hill Education; 2014.

Quadriceps Tendon

10

Mark J. Sakr, Joseph M. Powers, Bryson P. Lesniak, David R. Espinoza, and Gregory V. Gasbarro

Abbreviations

AIIS	Anterior Inferior Iliac Spine
ASIS	Anterior Superior Iliac Spine
MRI	Magnetic Resonance Imaging
NSAID	Nonsteroidal Anti-inflammatory Drugs
PRP	Platelet Rich Plasma
RF	Rectus femoris
VI	Vastus intermedius
VL	Vastus lateralis
VM	Vastus medialis

Introduction

The quadriceps is comprised of four distinct muscles that stabilize the lower extremity through knee extension and proper patellar tracking within the inter-condylar fossa of the femur, also

M. J. Sakr (✉) · J. M. Powers
Northside Hospital Orthopedic Institute, Atlanta, GA, USA

B. P. Lesniak
Department of Orthopedic Surgery, University of Pittsburgh, Pittsburgh, PA, USA

D. R. Espinoza
The San Antonio Orthopedic Group (TSAOG), San Antonio, TX, USA

G. V. Gasbarro
Department of Orthopedic Surgery, Mercy Medical Center, Baltimore, MD, USA

known as the femoral groove. These actions are important for simple activities such as walking and standing upright. The quadriceps is critical to strenuous activities such as running, cutting, and traversing stairs or hills at an incline or decline. Injury to these muscles may result in increased stress on the proximal and distal tendons of the muscle group, thus predisposing to a wide array of tendon injury such as tendinitis, chronic tendinosis, partial tendon tear, or rupture. These types of injuries can range in prevalence from 2.5 to 14.4%, depending on the sport participated in by an athlete [1]. Recreational athletes and casual fitness seekers often are faced with issues stemming from repetitive motion of the quadriceps and strain on the tendon. Multiple intrinsic and extrinsic factors may play a role in predisposing someone to quadriceps tendinopathy and it is crucial to identify the correct diagnosis and degree of tendon pathology so that proper treatment modalities can be initiated and ultimately help prevent long-term sequelae of tendon injury.

Anatomy

The muscles that make up the quadriceps, from deep to superficial, include the vastus intermedius (VI), vastus medialis (VM), vastus lateralis (VL), and the rectus femoris (RF) (Fig. 10.1, Table 10.1). These muscles and their respective tendons must function in unison to allow for proper mechanics of the lower extremity.

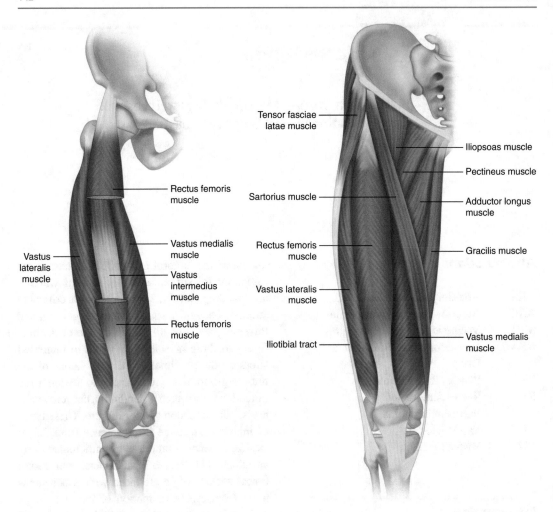

Fig. 10.1 Quadriceps anatomy

Table 10.1 Quadriceps anatomy

Muscle	Origin	Insertion	Arterial supply	Nerve innervation
Rectus femoris	Anterior inferior iliac spine & superior acetabulum	Superior patella and tibial tuberosity via the patellar tendon	Lateral circumflex femoral A.	Femoral N. (L2-L4)
Vastus medialis	Medial proximal femur	Superior medial patella and tibial tuberosity via patellar tendon	Lateral circumflex femoral A. and deep femoral A.	Femoral N. (L2-L4)
Vastus lateralis	Greater trochanter of the femur & gluteal tuberosity	Superior lateral patella and tibial tuberosity via patellar tendon	Transverse and lateral circumflex femoral A.	Femoral N. (L2-L4)
Vastus intermedius	Anterior and lateral femur	Superior patella and tibial tuberosity via patellar tendon	Lateral circumflex femoral A.	Femoral N. (L2-L4)

Proximally, the quadriceps musculature bind to their bony origins through fibrous tendons, which serve as anchors for muscle contraction and function. The vastus musculature arises from the femur, with the medialis primarily from the medial lip and lateralis from the lateral lip of the linea aspera. The intermedius has a more diverse origin, typically originating from the anterolateral aspect of the femur [54].

Detailed discussion of the rectus femoris is warranted given it is the most frequently implicated quadriceps muscle in injuries [64]. Multiple factors have been noted to play a role in RF injuries including its fusiform shape and extension across two joints [64]. Additionally, the RF may be subject to eccentric contraction and has a high percentage of type II fibers, both of which contribute to the RF relatively higher rate of injury [64]. A common mechanism of injury is kicking a ball due to the momentum-assisted transmission of force generated by the eccentrically loaded proximal muscles. This contraction pattern leaves the quadriceps vulnerable during various movements needed to kick a ball [6]. Predisposing factors for injury may include history of prior injury, poor conditioning, and fatigue [64]. Recent hamstring injury within the prior 8 weeks and any prior injury to the RF appears to be significant risk factors for RF injury as well [61].

The direct head of the rectus femoris originates from superior facet of the anterior inferior iliac spine (AIIS). The footprint on the AIIS has been described as broad based and "tear drop" shaped, situated just superior and anteromedial to the lateral most aspect of the acetabular rim. In normal morphology, a smooth concave wall of ilium is interposed between the acetabulum and AIIS, providing attachment site for the hip capsule, and the iliofemoral ligament on the lateral aspect [45]. The iliocapsularis muscle also arises from the AIIS along the inferior border, separated from the direct head of the RF by the AIIS ridge [45]. Cadaveric studies have revealed along the anterior medial region of the AIIS a "bare area"

with no tendinous attachment, important to note as this may be a safe zone for surgical decompression without involving the tendon [45].

The indirect head of the rectus femoris originates, slightly more inferiorly, from the superior acetabular ridge and hip joint capsule. A few centimeters beyond their origins, they fuse to form a conjoined tendon, with the direct head being the more superficial component. The superficial component of the conjoined tendon blends into the anterior fascia of the recuts musculature. The posterior component of the conjoined tendon, primarily from the indirect head, gives rise to an intrasubstance myotendinous junction spanning approximately two-thirds of the rectus musculature [55].

At the distal aspect of the quadriceps, multiple structures form the densely packed single anchor quadriceps tendon. The anatomy of the quadriceps tendon, although often simply described as a fusion of the tendinous contributions of the quadriceps musculature, is complex and variable. Historically, the quadriceps tendon was described as tri-laminar with superficial fibers from the RF, intermediate layer from VL and VM, and deep layer from the VI [20, 66]. More recent studies have suggested a more complex bilaminar, trilaminar, or tetralaminar structure with unequal contributions from the contributing tendons [67]. Grob et al. in 2016 described the quadriceps tendon as having "onion-like" layering and fibers arranged similarly to the husk of corn, further described as a trilaminar structure formed by six elements: lateral, deep medial, and superficial medial aponeuroses of VI, the VL, tensor VI, and rectus femoris [66]. Depending on the level at which the tendon is transected, there may be two, three, or four layers, further complicated by the fact that depending on the plane, the corresponding layers may be complete or incomplete. The VM contribution is interesting as it contributes to the quadriceps tendon with its medial insertion into all layers of the tendon. The tendon becomes increasingly thick until maximal thickness is reached at its insertion onto the patella [66]. Grob et al. note the variability of descriptions of the distal quadriceps tendon is likely due to the variability of fusion points of superficial and deep layers as well as the oblique orientation of the two-layered intermediate layer [66]. As the distal quadriceps tendon is frequently utilized as a graft, further research into the tendon is warranted to determine appropriateness of full versus partial thickness graft, exact harvest sites, and how tendon defects should be closed [66]. The quadriceps tendon is occasionally referred to as the suprapatellar tendon in the literature [67]. The superficial layer, originating from the RF, offers fibers that are continuous over the patella to contribute to the patellar tendon, occasionally referred to as the patellar ligament or infrapatellar tendon [67].

Adjacent to but distinct from the quadriceps musculature is the articularis genu, originating from the distal third of the femur and inserting on the proximal aspect of the supra-patellar bursa. The articularis genu acts as a tensor of the vastus intermedius during extension of the knee to retract the suprapatellar bursa proximally to prevent impingement of the synovial membrane within the patellofemoral joint space [2]. Recent research has confirmed the articularis genu does not contribute to the distal quadriceps tendon in any capacity [66].

Anterior Inferior Iliac Spine Apophysitis and Avulsion

A 12-year -old female presents with 2 months of progressive right anterior hip pain. There is no history of trauma or injury. She plays club soccer as a midfielder and is otherwise healthy. She initially noticed the pain while running and with kicking in practice. The pain is gradually worsening, limiting her ability to participate in sport. She denies feeling a "pop," and is able to ambulate with minimal discomfort. On physical exam, there is point tenderness over the AIIS with pain-

ful end range flexion of the hip and weakness with quadriceps testing.

Clinical Presentation

Pediatric and adolescent athletes are subject to chronic traction and repetitive microtrauma of the apophysis, leading to pain and inflammation termed apophysitis. The direct tendon of the rectus femoris originates from the apophyseal ossification center of the anterior inferior iliac spine. The indirect tendon, originating from the supra-acetabular ridge, is rarely involved in pediatric rectus injuries [44, 49, 52]. Unlike epiphyses, which are located at the ends of long bones and are responsible for longitudinal growth and circumferential remodeling, apophyses (also termed traction epiphyses) serve as the attachment site for tendons onto bone. Chronic loading of the apophyseal physes causes chondrocyte proliferation, hypertrophy, and inflammatory changes [42]. Additionally, explosive activities may result in the avulsion of the unfused apophysis due to strong contraction of the rectus femoris. These injuries are due to forceful contraction when transitioning from hip hyperextension and knee flexion to hip flexion with knee extension. The indirect head of the rectus femoris becomes more taut with increased hip flexion and is rarely involved in younger athletes [49]. Activities commonly associated with AIIS apophysitis and avulsion include kicking a ball, sprinting, and jumping [46, 48–51]. Historically, AIIS avulsions have been termed "sprinter's fractures" [45, 49]. The interval between appearance and closure of the apophysis serves as a window of vulnerability due to relative biomechanical weakness [44].

The median appearance AIIS apophysis for males is at 13.6 years of age and for females 14.0 years of age [43]. Table 10.2 describes the chronological age at appearance and closure of

Table 10.2 Age at appearance and closure of AIIS apophysis

Sex	First appearance	Median appearance	All appeared	First closure	Median closure	All closed
Male	11.1	13.6	15.3	13.9	16.3	17.5
Female	9.8	14.0	15.9	11.3	14.5	15.9

Adapted from Parvaresh et al. [43]

the AIIS apophysis. The general trend for pelvic apophyses is that of earlier appearance and closure for females than males, consistent with other areas of skeletal development. Importantly, younger patients are more likely to injury apophyses that appear earlier (i.e., AIIS) whereas older adolescents are more likely to injure later appearing ossifications centers (i.e., anterior superior iliac spine [ASIS]) [43, 44]. AIIS apophyseal avulsions are the second most common pelvic avulsion injury suffered by youth athletes, behind ischial tuberosity avulsions [51].

In AIIS apophysitis, symptoms will gradually worsen over time as the athlete continues to load the affected apophysis and microtrauma accumulates. On physical exam, there will be tenderness over the anterior hip along the AIIS but symptoms may be vague compared to the immediate disability seen in AIIS avulsion. The athlete may have minimal pain with walking, but as the quadriceps musculature is engaged with more vigorous activity such as sprinting, pain is reported. Hip range of motion is typically well maintained, although pain at end range flexion may be reported. If hip range of motion is asymmetrical, other etiologies should be considered. Strength will be reduced compared to the contralateral side.

In a more severe iteration of the above scenario, a true avulsion may occur at the apophysis. For AIIS avulsions, physical exam will reveal tenderness over the AIIS with variable presence of swelling and limited flexion of the hip. Strength will be more limited than with apophysitis given the added severity. Athletes should be queried regarding the presence of antecedent pain as avulsions may occur either on previously normal apophyses or in the setting of preexisting apophysitis [44].

Imaging

Radiographs

In cases where apophysitis is suggested by history and physical exam, radiographs may be considered unnecessary, as the findings are often nonspecific. If the diagnosis is in doubt, or if the patient has not responded to a typical treatment, radiographs may be obtained. In longer standing cases of apophysitis, radiographs may reveal irregularity or fragmentation of the apophyseal plate. Occasionally widening and sclerosis may be noted [52].

Radiographs will readily show avulsion injuries and are usually sufficient for diagnosis. The anteroposterior (AP) pelvis view allows for comparison of the affected and unaffected sides and normal apophyseal development. Of note, gonadal shields should not be used when performing radiography of the pediatric and adolescent pelvis [53]. In cases where AIIS injury has led to extra-articular impingement, AP pelvis with false-profile view may be utilized. The AP pelvis view may show low lying or prominent AIIS, associated with a "double cross-over sign" [45].

Ultrasound

Ultrasonography (US) may be employed in diagnosing and screening AIIS apophysitis and avulsions. The apophysis may appear as a "hetereogeneous vascularized psuedomass" in cases of apophysitis, due to underlying inflammation [52]. The AIIS ossification center will be displaced inferiorly in the case of avulsion. In younger athletes where the AIIS has yet to ossify and the apophysis cannot be visualized on radiographs, US may be of particular use. The cartilaginous AIIS may be visualized and compared to the unaffected side. Apophysitis and avulsions at multiple sites may exist simultaneously, and if screening with US, a thorough investigation of bilateral pelvic apophyses should be undertaken [44].

MRI

Magnetic resonance imaging (MRI) is not typically obtained for cases of uncomplicated apophysitis. If atypical in presentation, or in cases of treatment failure, MRI may be performed that will reveal enlargement and widening of the apophysis with conservation of the original shape of the AIIS apophysis. Increased signal intensity is expected on T2-weighted sequences about the apophysis, bone marrow, and adjacent soft tissue structures [52].

In cases of AIIS avulsion, those with ossified apophyses that have yet to fuse, MRI will reveal avulsion of the apophysis with associated marrow and soft tissue edema [49]. The size of the avulsed apophysis and measurement of gap should be noted [61]. In younger athletes, if the apophysis has yet to completely ossify, MRI may be considered the modality of choice to fully characterize these injuries. Fat suppressed T2-weighted and STIR sequences best image acute apophyseal injuries and will reveal edema. Osseous and musculotendinous involvement is also well characterized on these sequences [49]. In chronic injuries, T1-weighted sequences provide better anatomic detail and may reveal displaced osseous fragments [49]. Chronic apophyseal avulsion injuries may simulate aggressive bone lesions but the typical location in skeletally immature patients help to avoid misdiagnosis [61]. Recommended MRI protocol consists of "axial fat-suppressed T2-weighted or STIR series, coronal T1-weighted and fat-suppressed T2-weighted or STIR series, and a sagittal T2-weighted series" [49].

Treatment

AIIS apophysitis is treated conservatively and has an excellent prognosis. Often after a short period of rest, symptoms subside and the athlete may begin a gradual return to sport. Rehabilitative programs are commonly utilized, often under the direction of physical therapists. Pain control in the short term may be managed with topical application of ice and with use of nonsteroidal anti-inflammatory drugs (NSAIDs). Patients and parents should be counseled that the normal course of AIIS apophysitis is that of gradual improvement with time and complications are uncommon [52]. Traction hypertrophy is rarely seen in apophysitis, but can be associated with bony hypertrophy and development of prominence leading to restriction of hip motion and extra-articular impingement [45].

Acute AIIS avulsions are typically managed conservatively as well, unless avulsed beyond 2 cm. Initially, analgesia with NSAIDs, local application of ice, and rest are recommended. Crutches are initially used to assist in limiting weight bearing. Once able to walk with minimal discomfort crutches are discontinued and a progressive strengthening program may begin, often under the supervision of a physical therapist. Duration of time before return to play is variable, ranging from 3 weeks to 4 months. The variability is influenced by the patient's age, degree of displacement, and level of sport in which they participate. Additionally, compliance and commitment to rehabilitative protocols are important to maximize function and early return to sport [46].

The literature reveals little support for surgical treatment of AIIS apophysitis. However, a displaced AIIS avulsion can necessitate open surgical repair in certain populations such as high-level adolescent soccer players. Surgery may be indicated for AIIS avulsions beyond 2 cm or if severe rotational deformity is noted [45]. A Smith-Petersen anterior approach sparing the lateral femoral cutaneous nerve has been described [39]. The incision is carried distally from the ASIS toward the lateral border of the patella. The interval between the sartorius and tensor fascia lata is utilized to uncover the anterior surface of the rectus femoris. Careful identification of the indirect and direct heads of the rectus should be performed after clearing hematoma and debriding degenerative tissue. Techniques for fixation depend on the site of injury. Side-to-side repairs with nonabsorbable suture for mid-substance injuries can be performed [39]. Suture anchor fixation may be required for injuries at the enthesis, whereas avulsion-type injuries are typically repaired with cannulated screw fixation of the apophysis back down to the AIIS.

There have been case reports of bony exostoses developing after avulsion of the AIIS requiring arthroscopic debridement or open surgical resection [47]. This may be due to hematoma formation and subsequent exostoses formation within the tendon sheath itself, or from myositis ossificans within the rectus musculature. The development of hip impingement is a late complication and there may only be a remote history of injury as a youth [45].

Proximal Rectus Femoris Partial Tears, Avulsions, and Tendinopathy

A 32-year-old recreational athlete presents with acute onset of pain over the groin after kicking during a pick-up soccer game. He notes there was some mild aching pain over the area in the preceding 2 weeks. On physical exam, there is tenderness over the groin directly inferior to the AIIS. Pain is worsened with resisted knee extension. Passive range of motion is well maintained with mild discomfort at end range flexion.

Clinical Presentation

Proximal RF injuries are most commonly myotendinous or myoaponeurotic in nature, but occasionally proximal tendon tears and avulsions are encountered [44]. Proximal RF tendon avulsions account for approximately 1.5% of all hip lesions occurring during sport, and are more common in sports requiring sprinting and kicking [65, 68]. Accurate diagnosis is critical because long rehabilitation times may be required for proximal tendon tears [44, 61]. There is debate as to whether the direct or indirect head is more commonly implicated in proximal tendon tears and avulsions, partially due to the relative infrequency of these injuries [44, 64]. Regardless, either may be involved and conjoined tendon injuries may also be observed [44].

The direct head is under increased tension in early hip flexion. As hip flexion increases, the indirect head becomes more taut, and the direct head is placed under less tension [64]. Proximal RF injuries have been noted to occur during hip hyperextension and knee flexion or as a consequence of sudden eccentric contraction of the quadriceps [65]. Patients may describe a pop or tearing sensation at the time of injury. This may be accompanied by pain over the groin and anterior thigh with variable presence of ecchymosis and swelling depending on degree of injury [64].

The location of pain depends on which head of the RF is involved, with direct head injuries localized over the groin and indirect heard injuries presenting with more lateral or anterolateral pain [44, 64]. Given the lateral presentation of pain in indirect tendon injuries, misdiagnosis is common, especially in cases of chronic injury where initial trauma may be remote or the injury may be neglected [44].

On physical exam, ecchymosis may be present in acute cases and the patient will report tenderness at the origin of the tendons along the anterior hip accompanied by decreased function of the extensor tendon mechanism [64, 65]. In chronic cases, patients may report weakness with hip flexion and knee extension [65]. In cases of avulsions where significant muscle retraction has occurred, a palpable defect along the proximal RF may be appreciated. The retracted musculature may present as an anterior thigh mass, accentuated during quadriceps contraction [64].

Painful enthesopathic changes at the direct tendon due to overuse and repetitive trauma are uncommon. These patients may present with chronic hip pain and nonspecific clinic findings [44]. Patients with osteoarthritis of the femoroacetabular joint may develop paralabral and arthrosynovial cysts adjacent to or within the indirect tendon the RF leading to tendinopathy. These patients may report classic groin pain in addition to lateral or anterolateral hip pain. As with chronic indirect tendon tears and avulsions, the lateral nature of the symptoms may lead to initial misdiagnosis with the condition masquerading as gluteal tendinopathy [44]. Ultrasound can be utilized and will reveal hypoechoic thickening of the involved tendon, and occasionally intratendinous cysts [44].

Calcific tendinitis can affect the RF tendons, but is also rare. Apatite calcific densities may be identified on radiographs or advanced imaging, most commonly identified within the indirect head, just lateral to the tip of the acetabulum. The direct head is less commonly involved—calcification would be seen just inferior to the AIIS [44]. Calcific deposits in the direct head of the RF have been implicated in cases of internal snapping hip due to impingement with the overlying iliacus muscle [62]. Snapping due to calcific tendinitis of the direct head may be visualized dynamically under ultrasound [44]. Acute phase resorption of may present with acute onset of pain and limited motion of the hip. Visualizing tendinous calcifications under ultrasound, in addition to normal laboratory analysis, can help to differentiate acute resorption from more serious causes of hip pain such as septic arthritis [44].

Imaging

Radiographs

Radiographs are frequently the initial diagnostic study obtained in cases of proximal quadriceps tendon injury and are helpful in constructing a differential diagnosis. In adults, degenerative changes, femoroacetabular impingement, heterotopic ossification, and calcific tendinitis may be identified on plain radiographs [44]. Standard anteroposterior views are useful for visualizing the supra-acetabular rim, but the AIIS is not well delineated. The addition of false-profile or frog leg views allow for further characterization of the AIIS [44].

On plain radiographs, acute avulsions may reveal displaced osseous fragments, originating most commonly from the AIIS, and less commonly from the superior acetabular ridge [64]. Subsequent healing of these avulsed injuries may demonstrate sclerosis and osteolysis, not to be confused with infectious or malignant processes [64]. With time, heterotopic bone formation may be noted that can lead to impingement [45, 64].

Ultrasound

Evaluation of the proximal origins of the RF requires precise knowledge of underlying anatomy and thorough evaluation of both the affected and unaffected hip. The patient should be placed supine with the hip in neutral position. A high-frequency linear transducer is recommended for evaluation. After static scanning is performed, dynamic scanning may be considered to evaluate for snapping hip [44].

The direct tendon is best visualized in the axial plane scanning from ASIS to the AIIS. The probe may then be rotated 90 degrees in the sagittal plane to obtain long axis images of the direct tendon, which will appear as a hyperechoic fibrillary structure deep to the iliopsoas and sartorius musculature, originating from the AIIS. The indirect tendon is poorly visualized from this plane appearing as a hypoechoic structure along the lateral border of the direct tendon [44].

A lateral approach has recently been described to visualize the indirect tendon under ultrasound, but given the depth of the tendon, characterization may be difficult. Additionally, comparison views of the contralateral hip are recommended to evaluate for subtle changes consistent with tendinopathy or when chronic tearing is suspected. Sonographic evaluation of the indirect tendon via the lateral approach may be limited in the elderly due to fatty degeneration of the gluteal musculature [44]. The lateral approach to evaluate the indirect head is well described below by Moraux et al. [44]:

> Scanning the lateral hip in the axial plane, lateral to the anteroinferior iliac spine, localizing the indirect tendon underneath the gluteus muscles and overlying the supra-acetabular ridge and lateral iliofemoral ligament. When the tendon is identified, the transducer is positioned in an axial oblique plane with 30° obliquity on the lateral aspect of the hip. The indirect tendon appears as a convex thin echoic or hypoechoic structure underlying the gluteus minimus muscle, arising from the acetabular posterosuperior ridge and posterior capsule. In a case of insufficiently lateral transducer positioning, the tendon will appear hypoechoic because of its convexity and an anisotropy artifact. Then, the shor-axis view is obtained with a 90° transducer rotation; the tendon will appear as a thin and flat structure.

Alternatively, the indirect tendon may be visualized by scanning at the level of the conjoined tendon, just distal to the direct tendon, in the sagittal plane. The conjoined tendon will appear as a short echoic fusion of the direct and indirect tendons just inferior to the AIIS. Once identified, an ascending curvilinear sweeping motion along the course of the indirect tendon from distal aspect to origin on the supraacetabular ridge allows for visualization of the indirect tendon [44].

Limited literature exists describing acute proximal RF avulsion injuries under ultrasound.

Ultrasound should be considered to differentiate strains from partial tears or avulsions allowing for early accurate diagnosis, including field-side evaluation [44, 63]. Esser, et al., have described a case of proximal RF avulsion in a collegiate soccer player confirmed by ultrasound. Visualization of torn and retracted direct head of the RF was noted and dynamic scanning with active knee extension caused retraction of distal rectus femoris [63]. Chronic tears will appear thickened and hypoechoic with possible calcification noted [44].

In cases of tendinopathy, under ultrasound the affected tendon will appear hypoechoic and there will be increased tendon volume. Hyperemia may be noted within the tendon as well under power Doppler [19, 44]. In calcific tendinitis, calcification is well defined and hyperechoic in appearance. Large calcifications may present with posterior acoustic shadowing. Hyperemia under Doppler is variably present [44].

MRI

MRI is useful in confirming diagnosis of proximal RF tendon avulsion, grading tears and determining length of retraction [64]. Although tendon tears may be visible on axial images, oblique sagittal images parallel to the iliac wing are superior for delineating the exact nature of the tear and gap if present [61]. Proximal tendon injuries should be classified as partial or complete tears and if complete, margin quality and gap should be noted. Additionally, involvement of the direct, indirect or both heads should be specified [61]. Displaced osseous fragments are not well characterized on MRI [64]. For chronic injuries, MRI is also helpful for assessing tissue fibrosis as well as identifying pseudocyst formation that has been described [64].

Treatment

Most proximal RF tendon tears and avulsions are treated nonoperatively. High-level athletes, especially those whose sports involve repetitive kicking and sprinting, may be considered for earlier surgical intervention. Additionally, for patients who fail greater than 3 months of conservative

treatment and exhibit continued pain or weakness, surgery may be considered. Surgery is not indicated in patients with nondisplaced or minimally displaced avulsions and chronic tears in elderly patients [65]. There is no consensus on operative protocols [65].

Nonoperative

The largest case series of nonoperative management of proximal RF avulsions in athletes is Gamradt et al. series of 11 in the National Football League (NFL). These injuries, as previously noted, were found to be uncommon occurring approximately once per year in the NFL, and accounting for 1.5% of all hip injuries. Average return to play when excluding a single outlying athlete was 55.3 days, ranging from 21 to 84 days [68]. Gamradt et al. describe two cases with varying degrees of intervention to illustrate the lack of consensus on rehabilitation and differing impact on athletes. In one case, the athlete initially required a short period of protected weight bearing with crutches and use of NSAID, ice, and modalities. By week two, they progressed to active range of motion and isometrics, advancing to a resistance-training program by week four and a return to play with continued symptoms at week six. The athlete required a corticosteroid injection due to lingering symptoms the following season. To contrast, the other case presented was able to tolerate ambulation without difficulty and was able to resume light jogging at 9 days post injury. Full and unrestricted return to practice took place 2 weeks after injury and returned to games shortly thereafter with no long-term complications or limitations reported [68]. It would seem an individualized approach tailored to each patients' demands and degree of limitation is warranted with gradual progression back to sport as function normalizes.

Operative

Although there are no standardized protocols for proximal rectus femoris repair, Dean et al. describe one approach as follows. The patient is placed supine and the contralateral leg placed into full extension with sequential compression devices. The patient is draped, proximal to the

ASIS and distal to the knee. After identifying landmarks including the ASIS and greater trochanter, a 6-cm longitudinal incision just distal and lateral to the ASIS is made. This is extended distally using a Smith Petersen approach. Care should be taken to avoid the lateral femoral cutaneous nerve (LFCN) running medially to the ASIS deep to the inguinal ligament. Although the LFCN anatomy is variable, it most frequently crosses the interval between the tensor fascia lata and the sartorius 2–4 cm distal to the ASIS. The tensor fascia lata is retracted laterally, and in general, the sartorius and LFCN area retracted medially. The deep fascia is then identified and incised and the rectus femoris is identified. Once identified, the degree of retraction is assessed and the tendon and any adhesions are released from the surrounding tissues. Most often, the direct head is affected at the insertion on the AIIS. If both heads are affected, repair is performed on each separately. Devitalized tissue is removed from the tendon stump and a suture is passed through the direct head to assist with mobilization. The footprint on the AIIS is prepared by exposing the subchondral bone and a bleeding bed is created with a rasp to support healing. Suture anchors are placed over the footprint and the tendon is retracted to its origin. Of note, due to the small footprint on the AIIS, it may only be possible to place 1–2 anchors. The tendon is reattached in a double row fashion, initially placing an all suture anchor to establish the medial row. The suture from the anchor is passed deep to superficial through the tendon. Previously placed mobilization suture is then removed. Tension is applied while holding the sutures from the suture anchor to that tissue is well reduced against the bone. The sutures are tied over the tendon. A hole is drilled and the second anchor is then placed proximal to the first. Both strands are then passed through the second anchor and tissue tension should be assessed. Once satisfied, the anchor is placed into the bone socket and appropriate tension is obtained. If necessary, the hip can be flexed to decrease tension on the rectus tendon while being reattached. The tendon should cover both the anterior and inferior surfaces of the AIIS without excessive tension [65].

Postoperatively, to prevent active contraction of the rectus femoris, the patient is placed into a knee brace locked in extension for 6 weeks. The patient is restricted to nonweight bearing status during this period. Additionally, the patient is instructed to avoid active hip flexion. Postoperative arthrofibrosis is prevented with the use of a continuous passive motion machine from 0° to 90° for 6–8 hours per day. Formal physical therapy begins approximately 4 weeks postoperative with a focus on range of motion. Partial progressive weight bearing is started in week six and crutches are progressively weaned. The patient may discontinue crutches when able to walk without a limp and minimal pain. Eccentric strength training and running begin approximately 8 weeks after the procedure. Return to play is expected 4–6 months after surgery [65].

Proximal Quadriceps Myotendinous Injury

A 20-year-old male, collegiate soccer player presents post-match with acute onset of pain over the proximal right thigh after kicking the ball late in the second half. There was no antecedent pain and he is otherwise healthy. He is right leg dominant. He was able to continue playing with discomfort. In the training room post-match, he has a mildly antalgic gait. There is tenderness to palpation over the anterior third of the right thigh but no obvious defect or deformity. Manual muscle testing reveals relative weakness about the quadriceps.

Clinical Presentation

As previously discussed, the rectus femoris anatomy is complex with contributions from a direct and indirect tendinous origin proximally. There is intramuscular extension of the indirect tendon extending distally referred to as the central tendon or intramuscular tendon, and occasionally referenced as an intramuscular septum or central aponeurosis [26, 59, 69], This indirect myotendinous extension within the bipennate portion of the rectus is surrounded by the unipennate portion of the rectus, giving rise to unique "muscle-within-a-muscle" configuration [59]. Of note, a bipennate muscle has muscle fibers originating from two sides of a tendon (i.e., indirect head RF). A unipennate muscle has muscle fibers originating solely from one side of the tendon (i.e., direct head RF), and the tendon remains on one side of the muscle, blending superficially with the aponeurosis [59]. The indirect tendon of the RF is initially rounded in appearance and located within the medial aspect of the muscle. As it progresses distally, it flattens, rotates laterally and moves to the middle of the muscle belly. Distally, the deep tendon of the indirect tendon is flat and oriented more vertically, lying within the anterior muscle belly [26]. Given the long intermuscular myotendinous extension, the indirect head of the RF is subject to injury longitudinally. This can involve the myotendinous junction itself, or can result in an uncommon injury pattern called intramuscular degloving, where there is dissociation of the inner bipennate portion from the outer unipennate potion of the rectus femoris [59].

Rectus femoris myotendinous injuries occur most frequently in late adolescent and young adult males (average 18 years old, range 15–22) and are seen most commonly in soccer. The injury is typically sustained while kicking but has also been reported while sprinting. Myotendinous and intramuscular degloving injuries of the RF may occur on the dominant or nondominant leg [59]. Risk factors for RF injuries include short stature, preseason training, and recent injury to either the RF or hamstring musculature [61]. Additionally, environmental factors may contribute as RF injuries are seen more frequently in cold conditions [61].

Physical exam of patient who have sustained proximal RF myotendinous injuries is variable depending on the degree of injury. Less severe myotendinous injuries may present only with mild discomfort and slight weakness. More severe injuries, including intramuscular degloving injuries, can present with anterior thigh swelling due to intramuscular hematoma and retracted muscle fibers.

Imaging

Radiographs

There is limited literature available on utility of radiographs in evaluation of myotendinous RF injuries but they would be expected to be normal. Radiographs may be helpful in the evaluation of concomitant or alternate pathology such as AIIS avulsions.

Ultrasound

The literature on US evaluation of central tendon injuries is somewhat limited. Balius et al. identified 35 high-level Spanish soccer players with central tendon injuries evaluated under ultrasound. Only one patient suffered a grade III or degloving type injury. Grade I injuries revealed "ill-defined hyper or hypoechoic area without objective fibrillary discontinuity or inflammation of the fascia." Grade II injuries were notable for partial discontinuity of fibers [60]. For degloving injuries of the RF, correlating with MRI, one may expect to see a "bull's-eye" type pattern with discontinuity of the normal architecture: hyperechoic, rounded central bipennate fibers surrounded by anechoic fluid collection, finally surrounded around the periphery by the unipennate fibers (Fig. 10.2). Hyperemia may also be expected.

MRI

MRI may be utilized to fully characterize myotendinous and intramuscular degloving inju-

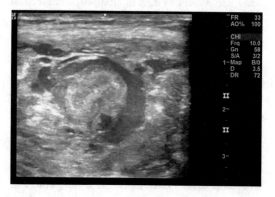

Fig. 10.2 Short axis ultrasound rectus femoris intramuscular degloving

ries of the RF. Kassarjian et al., recommended the following protocol in evaluation of myotendinous RF injuries:

> initial wide field of view images that include both hips and thigh and consists of: axial T1, axial STIR, and axial gradient echo sequences all of which extend from the anterior inferior iliac spine to the distal myotendinous junction of the rectus femoris. These images are not meant to be of high resolution but serve to accurately localize both acute and chronic injuries and allow evaluation of the contra-lateral hip and thigh both for comparison (e.g., of muscle bulk) and to assess for occult additional injuries. Subsequently, higher resolution images with a smaller field of view are obtained of the symptomatic rectus femoris. This includes T2 weighted sequences with fat suppression in the following planes: axial images in all cases, sagittal oblique images (paralleling the anterior inferior iliac spine) when proximal tendinous injuries are suspected, sagittal images when myotendinous injuries of the direct (superficial) component are suspected or when myofascial injuries are suspected, and coronal images when myotendinous injuries to the indirect (deep) component are suspected [61].

The tendon of the direct head is short and quickly fans to blend with the anterior fascia. This anatomy and quick transition make differentiation between grade I and II injuries difficult as well as differentiating between myotendinous versus myofascial injuries. High quality axial, sagittal and sagittal oblique images can facilitate in delineating the grade of these injuries. The tendon of the direct head may appear more hypointense than the fascia allowing for differentiation. Myotendinous injuries of the direct head will appear as edema along the intersection between the anterior fascia and muscle belly of the RF. Fluid and hematoma may track distally along the deep surface of the anterior fascia. This may be of importance if the collection is in close proximity to the sartorius crossing superficially. It is suggested that injuries in this area may carry a worse prognosis as the sartorius may compress and prevent clearance of breakdown products and prevent healing of the underlying injury [61].

The indirect head anatomy and long central extension is well described above. The complex anatomy and long course of the indirect head makes assessment with the classic three-point grading system traditionally used to classify injuries difficult. Grade I injuries may reveal edema extending into the musculature on both sides of the intact tendon. This resembles a feather due to the underlying bipennate architecture and is best visualized on coronal fat suppressed T2 images [26, 61].

Grade II injuries will reveal distortion of the muscle fibers and variable involvement of the tendon itself although the myotendinous junction will have fibers remaining [61]. Grade III injuries represent complete tears and there will be gapping of the myotendinous junction with variable degrees of retraction of the muscle and tendon themselves. Depending on the age of the injury the gap may be filled acutely with fluid, blood and debris or later with granulation tissue [61]. Kassarjian et al., noted the following poor prognostic factors that may be visualized on MRI: proximal injuries, the presence of perifascial fluid, changes visualized on T1-weighted images, and involvement of greater than 50% of cross-sectional area of the muscle [61]. The presence of perifascial fluid and lesions visible on T1-weighted images were associated with significantly longer recovery times [61]. Intramuscular degloving injuries on axial T2-weighted images will reveal separation of the outer unipennate from the inner bipennate myotendinous complex with associated intramuscular edema [59]. True myotendinous injuries of the indirect portion of the RF are relatively more common and appear as edema and fluid centered at the myotendinous junction [59]. On axial images this has been described as a "bull's-eye lesion" with edema surrounding the central tendon [61]. This injury is illustrated in Fig. 10.3. There is frequently evidence of edema in surrounding muscle groups as well. The average length of intramuscular RF degloving injuries is 9.9 cm, located 15.5 cm from the acetabular rim to the proximal most portion of the injury. On average, there is 1.2 cm of retraction [59]. The presence of atrophy and fatty infiltration may be observed in older injuries [6].

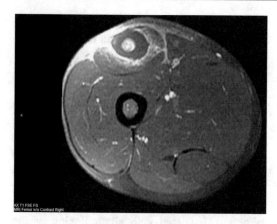

Fig. 10.3 Axial T1 MRI femur without contrast showing typical "bull's-eye lesion"

Treatment

Rehabilitative protocols are not standardized for proximal RF myotendinous injuries. Intramuscular tendon involvement often requires longer periods of rehabilitation compared to more peripheral injuries of the RF [26]. Return to play time for grade I and II central tendon RF injuries has been reported to average 27.7 and 46.3 days on average respectively [60]. Given the infrequency with which degloving RF injuries are encountered there is limited literature on return to play. It is more common for the myofibrils that attach to the central tendon to fail while the central tendon itself remains intact [26]. This results in increased stress on the intramuscular tendon and it has been hypothesized the indirect and indirect heads may begin to act independently of one another, resulting in shearing forces, possibly explaining longer rehabilitation times observed with higher grade injuries [26]. For intramuscular degloving injuries, the average return to play has been reported to range from 28–58 days, averaging 38.7 days [59].

In Balius et al. series athletes were treated with 2 weeks of absolute rest and local application of ice, compression and NSAIDs. Following this period, the athletes were gradually advanced over four stages of increasing intensity with the qualification that the athlete must be pain free

before progressing [60]. Kassarjian et al. recommended a short period of initial rest ranging from 1 to 5 days to allow for inflammation and pain to improve. Formal physical therapy is then initiated initially starting with careful mobilization and isometric contractions, advancing to isotonic contractions. Once able to complete these exercises without pain, eccentric exercises are initiated starting with manual resistance, progressing to more complex exercises with differing forms of resistance. Once pain free with eccentric resistance training, running may begin, gradually advancing back to sport specific drills [61]. Even once the athlete is able to return to play, some suggest limiting repetitive kicking and rapid deceleration running drills for 4 weeks due to potential for reinjury [61]. Of note, platelet rich plasma may accelerate scarring in myotendinous injuries but there is insufficient data to support routine use [61].

Distal Quadriceps Tendinopathy

A 42-year-old male presents with 3 month history of progressively worsening left anterior knee pain. He was recently instructed by his primary care physician to increase his physical activity. In order to do so, he has been jogging and playing pickup basketball that is a change from his previously sedentary lifestyle. He is a smoker and is overweight. The patient has tried a variety of over the counter treatments without improvement in symptoms. He localizes pain over the anterior knee along the quadriceps tendon but there is no palpable defect. He has slight weakness and discomfort with knee extension. He is able to bear weight and walk without discomfort, but when navigating stairs or jogging his pain returns.

Clinical Presentation

Distal quadriceps tendinopathy occurs less frequently than patellar tendinopathy, which is seen 4–5 times more frequently [70, 75]. Patients with quadriceps tendinopathy will complain of insidious onset of pain along the insertion of the quadriceps tendon at the insertion on the superior pole of the patella. Occasionally patients will provide history of recent increase in activities that may exacerbate such as jumping, running or kicking [70]. Running, especially hills, have been associated with quadriceps overuse injuries [4]. Quadriceps tendinopathy may also be observed in nonathletes, often associated with obesity [71]. Symptoms may range from mild pain after intense activity without functional impairment to pain during daily activity and inability to participate at any level of sport [75].

On physical exam, tenderness along the superior pole of the patella and the distal quadriceps tendon will be noted. In severe cases the patient's gait may be antalgic. Patients may note pain at end range flexion of the knee. Discomfort and potentially weakness with knee extension may be noted [70]. The presence of a palpable gap, swelling or effusion or other abnormalities should alert the clinician to presence of other potential etiologies. Weakness in context of comorbidities such as stroke or other ipsilateral limb injuries such as an occult fracture may complicate the diagnosis of quadriceps tendinopathy and additional, confirmatory imaging may be warranted [16].

Differential diagnosis for the patient with distal quadriceps tendinopathy includes patellofemoral pain syndrome, patellar tendinopathy, partial tears of the quadriceps or patellar tendons, and suprapatellar or infrapatellar bursitis [4]. Although rare, patellar stress fractures along the superior pole may masquerade as insertional quadriceps tendinopathy.

Imaging

Radiographs

Changes on radiographs would not be expected for most patients with uncomplicated quadriceps tendinopathy. Obtaining radiographs is helpful in constructing a differential diagnosis and evaluation of other causes of anterior knee pain. In long standing cases of quadriceps tendinopathy, radiographs may reveal calcific changes along the superior pole of the patella from osteophyte formation or occasionally intra-tendinous calcifications [70, 71].

Ultrasound

Normally the distal quadriceps tendon appears as multiple hyperechoic laminae with thin hypoechoic bands separating the layers. Due to the oblique insertion onto the patella, if the knee is in full extension the distal most insertion is not well visualized due to anisotropy. This is illustrated in Fig. 10.4. The insertion is better visualized with slight flexion of the knee [76]. Structural changes expected within the quadriceps tendon when investigated under ultrasound include thickening of the quadriceps tendon and hypoechoic areas. There may be variable presence of signal on power Doppler [74]. Additionally, in longer standing cases, calcifications may be noted [74]. Musculoskeletal ultrasound has grade 3 evidence for use in diagnosis of distal quadriceps tendinosis and other investigations often do not provide additional information [18, 58].

Visnes et al. prospectively followed a cohort of young elite athletes with serial exam and ultrasound. Those that were asymptomatic but noted to have hypoechoic changes or presence of neovascularization on ultrasound at baseline were more likely to develop symptoms over time. Ultimately, 16% of these initially asymptom-

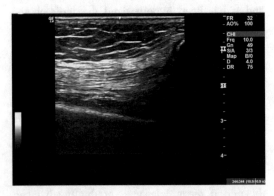

Fig. 10.4 Ultrasound – long-axis quadriceps tendon and insertion onto the superior pole of the patella. Note the anisotropy, seen as an anechoic streak, where the quadriceps tendon meets the patella. The insertion is better visualized with the knee in slight flexion

atic athletes with ultrasound changes went on to develop symptoms either of quadriceps or patellar tendinopathy [72]. Male athletes that developed symptoms were noted to have larger mean baseline quadriceps tendon thickness compared to athletes that remained asymptomatic [72]. For patients undergoing ultrasound of the knee for other reasons, if changes within the quadriceps tendon are noted, the provider should consider counseling the patient on potential development of symptoms as well as next steps in treatment.

MRI

The normal appearance of the quadriceps tendon is low signal fibers with intermediate signal fat interdigitating as seen in Fig. 10.5. The normal multilaminar structure should not be confused with partial tearing on MRI. Superficial fibers of the quadriceps tendon extend over the patella, as the prepatellar quadriceps continuation, blending with the patellar tendon as it inserts onto the tibial tubercle. Of note, the quadriceps fat pad lies deep to the quadriceps tendons insertion and anterior to the suprapatellar recess [56].

Tendinosis of the quadriceps tendon will appear as a thickened tendon with increased signal within the fibers [56]. This is well illustrated in Fig. 10.6. MRI is not typically required for diagnosis of quadriceps tendinopathy especially in cases where extension strength is maintained, and should be reserved for refractory cases or those with other abnormal features or where concomitant pathology is suspected [70].

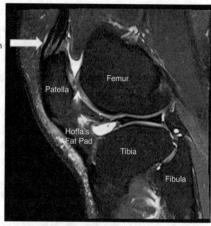

Fig. 10.6 MRI – moderate tendinopathic changes quadriceps tendon

Pappas et al. followed 24 asymptomatic collegiate basketball players with pre and post season knee MRI. A high prevalence of MRI documented changes consistent with quadriceps tendinopathy was noted in preseason scans, observed in 75% of the athletes. In post season scanning, 90% of knees were found to have changes on MRI consistent with quadriceps tendinopathy, but all of these athletes remained asymptomatic [73]. It is unclear, however, if changes observed on MRI may eventually develop symptoms consistent with quadriceps tendinopathy.

Treatment

Nonoperative treatment is the mainstay of treatment in quadriceps tendinopathy and is successful in the majority of cases [70]. Activity modification is often required initially in order to reduce symptoms. Physical therapy regimens should focus on flexibility, strength, and core stability of the quadriceps, hip, and core muscle groups. Flexibility of the hip flexors is of particular importance, as tight iliopsoas muscles may restrict hip extension and force the rectus femoris to become overloaded through increased hip flexion with activities such as kicking and jumping [5]. Eccentric strengthening programs for the extensor mechanism, as well as core, hip and pelvic muscles are focuses of physical therapy for quadriceps tendinopathy.

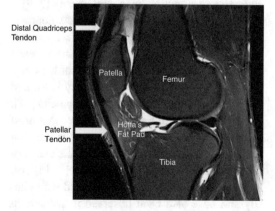

Fig. 10.5 MRI – normal quadriceps tendon

Some studies suggest that it is also important to focus on proprioceptive input with neuroplastic training regimens, ensuring short and long-term stability and proper biomechanics [25]. With most conservative measures of treating quadriceps tendinopathy, relief of pain is typically a measure of healing and can guide progression to initiate quadriceps, core, and hip strengthening. Proper strengthening and return to controlled movements effectively, begins the process of return to play after these injuries. The chronicity and severity of the condition can also dictate expected timing needed for rehabilitation and treatment prior to return to play. If the tendon injury is associated with a corresponding muscle strain, it is likely to have a more complicated recovery. The use of platelet rich plasma has been used anecdotally given success in other tendinopathies, such as patellar tendinopathy, but studies specifically investigating application of platelet rich plasma in the distal quadriceps tendon are lacking.

Distal Quadriceps Tendon Rupture

A 50-year-old male, with history significant for obesity, type II diabetes mellitus and hypertension presents after a slip and fall at his home while navigating wet steps on his front stoop. He is unable to bear weight and there is a palpable gap along his distal quadriceps tendon. He is unable to complete a straight leg raise.

Clinical Presentation

Quadriceps tendon ruptures are relatively uncommon, but devastating injuries, with an overall incidence is 1.37/100,000 per year [5]. Complete ruptures occur over four times more frequently in males than females [5]. These injuries primarily affect middle aged adults with a mean age of 50.5 in males and 51.7 in females [5]. Among all ruptures, the vast majority occur unilaterally but there are case series and case reports describing simultaneous, bilateral quadriceps tendon ruptures [12–14]. Once the tendon fails, the zone of injury may propagate resulting in disruption of

the retinacula and even nearby vascular structures leading to hematoma formation that may require surgical evacuation depending on severity and risk of damage to surrounding structures [15]. As quadriceps tendon ruptures typically affect middle-aged individuals, only a small number of cases reports describe this pathology in younger athletes [8].

The most common injury mechanism in quadriceps tendon ruptures is that of a suddenly contracted quadriceps muscle on a flexed knee with a planted foot, which leads to an eccentric contraction. This type of injury is most commonly seen in the nondominant leg, particularly with simple falls, falls downstairs, and sporting injuries with the lower extremity in this position [3]. The most common mechanism of injury is eccentric overload of the extensor mechanism as patients attempt to prevent falling with the foot planted and the knee partially flexed [8]. The rectus femoris is the only quadriceps muscle that traverses two joints and is at increased risk of tendon rupture. Additionally, there have been reports of quadriceps tendon tears due to direct blows sustained during contact sports [7].

Certain medications have also been implicated in predisposing individuals to quadriceps tendon injuries and rupture including anabolic steroids, statins, fluoroquinolones and prolonged use of local or systemic corticosteroids [7, 13]. Systemic diseases may lend an individual to quadriceps tendon injury including autoimmune disorders such as rheumatoid arthritis and systemic lupus erythematosus, diabetes, systemic endocrine dysfunction, gout, and obesity [7, 9].

Spontaneous ruptures, also termed nontraumatic ruptures, may occur in patients with underlying tendinopathy who present in the absence of trauma with tendon tears in areas of hypovascularity. This zone of hypovascularity is located 1–2 cm from the superior pole of the patella [11]. This is in contrast to traumatic ruptures that most frequently occur at the tendon osseous junction [24]. Case reports of bilateral spontaneous ruptures also exist although uncommon [9, 14, 16]. Bilateral injuries have been associated with obesity and have also been observed in patients in renal failure requiring hemodialysis [14, 16].

For quadriceps tendon rupture, physical exam will reveal pain localized over the superior pole of the patella in the distal thigh. The pain is often described as an immediate, intense tearing sensation at the time of rupture, while relief may be achieved by placing the extremity in knee extension [7, 8]. A diagnostic triad has been described that includes pain, inability to actively extend the knee and the presence of a suprapatellar gap [8]. If the physical exam is limited due to pain, consideration should be given to aspiration and injection with intra-articular anesthetic so the extensor mechanism can be more thoroughly assessed, although this may not be practical in all clinical settings [8]. The presence of a suprapatellar gap may be masked by the presence of a large hemarthrosis, and is a potential source of missed diagnosis [8]. The clinical picture can also be obscured if the medial and lateral patellar retinaculum remain intact. In this scenario, patients maintain some ability to extend the knee despite complete rupture of the tendon. Knee extension will be weaker compared to the contralateral side and an extensor lag may be present [8]. Similarly, the ability to bear weight on the extremity should not completely rule out quadriceps tendon rupture, as an intact retinaculum may allow for engagement of the extensor mechanism in the stance phase. Thorough and complete assessment of the hip and knee should also be completed. Associated pain and disability from quadriceps tendon rupture may distract the patient and clinician from associated injuries such as anterior cruciate ligament tears [10].

Imaging

Radiographs

Radiographs are commonly obtained as the initial diagnostic study for knee trauma including quadriceps tendon ruptures. Anteroposterior and lateral radiographs alone may reveal findings strongly suggestive of quadriceps tendon rupture including loss of quadriceps tendon shadow, suprapatellar mass, and suprapatellar calcific densities [17]. The loss of quadriceps tendon shadow has been noted to be present in 100% of cases [17]. Suprapatellar calcific densities may originate from avulsion of the patella or from calcification within the quadriceps tendon itself [17]. Additional findings may include joint effusion. A low-lying appearance of the patella termed patella baja is commonly noted (Fig. 10.7) [22, 57].

Ultrasound

Normal tendons are linear with fibrillary appearance and intermediate echogenicity. Rupture of the quadriceps tendon will reveal a loss of the normal echo texture and discontinuity of the fibers as well as hypoechoic to anechoic hematoma formation [8, 57]. Ultrasonography offers the advantage of contralateral comparison of the unaffected extremity. Dynamic evaluation during flexion and extension may also be undertaken to add additional diagnostic information and clarity to partial versus full thickness tears [57]. With contraction of the quadriceps or with distraction of the patella, the suprapatellar gap will be accentuated in full thickness tears [8].

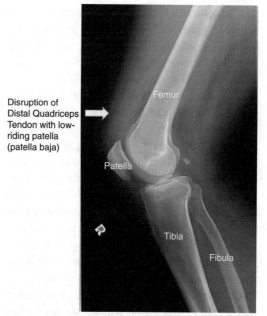

Disruption of Distal Quadriceps Tendon with low-riding patella (patella baja)

Femur

Patella

Tibia

Fibula

Fig. 10.7 Lateral knee radiograph demonstrating patella baja as seen quadriceps tendon rupture

Foley, et al., noted 100% sensitivity and specificity in diagnosis of quadriceps tendon high grade partial and complete tears under ultrasound retrospectively when compared with surgical correlation as the reference standard. For original nonretrospective ultrasounds, 96% of complete quadriceps tendon ruptures were correctly diagnosed [57]. Musculoskeletal ultrasound has grade 3 evidence for use in diagnosis of distal quadriceps tears and other investigations often do not provide additional information [18, 58].

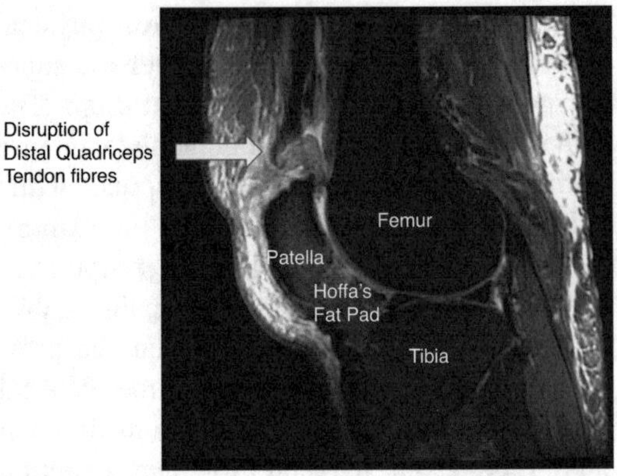

Fig. 10.8 MRI – T2 sagittal – full thickness quadriceps tendon tear

MRI

Magnetic resonance imaging (MRI) historically has been the modality of choice and has been reported to have 100% sensitivity, specificity, and positive predictive value in detecting quadriceps tendon rupture [21]. MRI permits analysis of the quadriceps tendon in the setting of extensive edema or hematoma and allows visualization of other pathology within the knee [22]. MRI consistently and accurately detects and localizes quadriceps tendon rupture and can be a valuable tool during preoperative planning [23]. Limitations include increased cost and decreased availability in the emergency setting. Indications for use are often reserved for cases in which the diagnosis may be equivocal on physical examination, radiographs or ultrasound. Concomitant intra-articular injuries are seen in 9.6% of cases, and if strong suspicion for injury beyond the quadriceps tendon tear itself, MRI should be obtained [57].

Ruptures more commonly occur at the tendon-osseous junction and partial tears are more frequent than complete ruptures [24]. MRI findings of complete rupture on sagittal images show fluid signal within a torn and retracted quadriceps tendon without direct fiber insertion into the superior pole of the patella [24]. Such findings can be appreciated as in Fig. 10.8. The patellar tendon may take on a wavy appearance in the setting of patella baja [24]. A large joint effusion, adjacent hematoma, and/or avulsed osseous fragments may also be appreciated as per Fig. 10.9a, b.

Complete ruptures of the quadriceps tendon will appear as fluid signal with a retracted tendon that migrates proximally. Fibers are not visualized inserting onto the patella as complete quadriceps tendon tears occur most frequently at the insertion. The patella itself will retract distally and, as a result of loss of tension, the patellar tendon will appear wavy in appearance (Fig. 10.8). Associated findings include hematoma, effusion and avulsion fragments. In cases of partial tears, the superficial most contribution from the rectus femoris is most frequently disrupted [56].

Treatment

Nonoperative

Low-grade distal quadriceps tendon tears may be treated nonoperatively [8, 57]. Treatment protocols are not standardized and vary by provider, but will typically consist of a period of immobilization in full extension followed by protected range-of-motion and gradual strengthening, usually under the guidance of a physiotherapist. Bracing may be discontinued once satisfactory strength and muscle control has been demonstrated, as well as ability to perform single leg raise without discomfort [8]. Although no studies have directly investigated aspiration of traumatic hemarthrosis in the setting of partial quadriceps tendon tears, consideration should be given to aspiration to improve pain and potentially accelerate recovery. This should be completed early in the treatment course before the hematoma has consolidated [8].

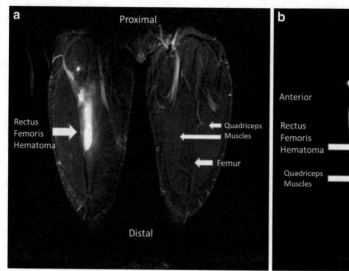
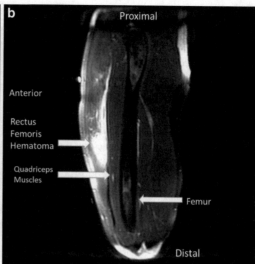

Fig. 10.9 (**a, b**) Rectus femoris hematoma.

Operative

Nonsurgical management of acute unilateral distal quadriceps tendon ruptures portend poor clinical results including long-term disability and weakness [27]. Consideration should be given to operative repair of high-grade partial thickness tears as well [57]. Delaying surgery of full thickness tears increases the difficulty of repair and may lead to less than satisfactory outcomes. Proximal tendon retraction away from the superior pole of the patella progresses rapidly over the first 72 hours after injury [7]. After 72 hours, difficulty with tendon-osseous apposition during repair may occur, however a 2008 case report highlighted successful delayed tendon repair at least 8 years after injury [28]. As such, early intervention is recommended, though delayed repair does not guarantee poor results [29, 30]. Many methods for surgical repair have been described, each of which has shown satisfactory results to achieve optimal functional outcome. The current literature, however, does not have randomized, controlled trials directly comparing the many surgical techniques [7].

For standard repairs, patients are placed supine on the operating room table with a bump under the ipsilateral greater trochanter. The use of a sidebar or sandbag can be employed to achieve intraoperative flexion at 30 degrees if desired. Alternatively, strategic use of sterile bumps can be employed. Nearly all techniques utilize a straight, midline longitudinal incision extending from proximal to the tear location to distal to the tibial tubercle. This permits adequate exposure of the underlying extensor mechanism. Full thickness medial and lateral soft tissue flaps are created to uncover the medial and lateral patellar retinaculum. Aspiration of the hematoma in the zone of injury and thorough debridement of fibrous and degenerative tissue are necessary to accurately identify healthy tissue planes and freshen the tendon edge for repair. Less common myotendinous or midsubstance ruptures can be treated with end-to-end primary repair with nonabsorbable sutures. More common tendon-osseous tendon tears may be repaired using a trans-osseous versus suture anchor techniques [30–33].

When performing the trans-osseous repair technique, an Allis or Lahey clamp can be used to tension the tendon distally after identifying and isolating its free edge. Two heavy, nonabsorbable sutures are placed in a locked, continuous fashion (Krakow) through the end of the tendon, leaving four suture limbs free at the distal stump. Next, attention is turned to preparing the patellar bone bed for healing. The superior pole is cleared of soft tissue and to a bleeding surface. The knee is flexed to 30 degrees and three 2-mm parallel drill holes through the patella are created in an anterograde fashion with care not to disrupt the articular surface. A suture passing device is then used to pass the free suture limbs from proximal-to-distal through the bone tunnels. Two limbs are passed through the central hole and a single limb is passed through the medial and lateral holes, respectively. The knee is then brought back into full extension and the suture limbs are tensioned as quadriceps excursion is analyzed. If sufficient tendon-osseous contact is achieved the sutures are tied over a bone bridge. The repair is reinforced with side-to-side repairs of retinacular defects. Suture irritation given the subcutaneous nature of the repair has been reported.

Alternative repair techniques with suture anchors for acute repairs or V-Y quadriceps turndown and/or soft tissue augmentation for chronic repairs have also been described in the literature [32, 34–37]. Suture anchors have been reported to provide multiple advantages over traditional methods [34, 35]. Potential advantages include reduced operative time, smaller surgical incisions, easy access to implantation site, better resistance of suture material, minimization of stress along the suture line with range of motion, higher strength of repair, and more consistent load-to-failure characteristics [32, 35, 38]. Bushnell et.al describe their use of two or three 5.0-mm suture anchors to secure the tendon with a modified Mason-Allen technique that limits soft tissue exposure [33]. Prior to skin closure, the knee is taken through a range of motion up to the "stress point" of the repair, defined by the position that excessive force is required for further flexion [34]. This "stress point" is used as a reference point for safe knee range of motion during early rehabilitation [34]. Richards, et.al describe a similar suture anchor technique but secure the tendon with a locking, continuous (Krakow) stitch supplemented with a side-to-side repair of the retinaculum [35]. Other methods of repair include the use of hamstrings autografts,

Dacron vascular grafts, polydioxanone (PDS) cord, carbon fiber, and synthetic prosthetic ligaments [34]. Two separate reports in 2008 describe novel techniques using free hamstrings autograft to treat chronically retracted and scarred quadriceps tendon ruptures not amenable to primary repair [36, 37].

Rehabilitation protocols after repair vary by surgeon and continue to be controversial in the literature. Goals of physical therapy include preventing quadriceps weakness and loss of knee motion. In general, most patients are placed in a removable knee immobilizer in full extension after surgery and are allowed to fully bear weight on the limb. Knee immobilizers or hinged knee braces allow the wound to be evaluated 48 hours later, whereas the traditional use of a cast makes wound inspection and management more cumbersome. Some authors have advocated for early range of motion though most surgeons still wait 4–6 weeks prior to permitting knee flexion with physical therapy over fear for the risk of rerupture [40, 41]. Disadvantages of cast immobilization include persistent pain, difficulty regaining motion, decreased patellar mobility, muscle weakness, loss of bone mass, poor cartilage nutrition, and patella baja [41]. Advocates of early motion starting 7 days after surgery cite improved tendon vascularity, earlier organization and remodeling of collagen fibers, and an increase in the number of collagen filaments and breaking strength of the tendon with controlled tension on the tendon [41]. Langenhan, et.al compared restrictive versus early range of motion rehabilitation protocols in 66 patients with a minimum 24 month follow-up [40]. No clinical difference was identified with the use of the IDKC subjective knee form, number of reruptures, or overall complication rate [40]. Patients in the restrictive protocol did return to work on average 10 days later than those in the early range of motion group, but this difference did not reach significance [40].

Several retrospective case series have studied the results of various methods of surgical repair techniques and rehabilitation protocols. Siwek, et.al evaluated outcomes on 36 ruptures and found good to excellent functional results in all patients treated within 72 hours, good results in three patients treated after a 2 weeks delay, and unsatisfactory results in three patients treated greater than 4 weeks after injury [29]. Another study reviewed 53 ruptures with varying surgical techniques and postoperative rehabilitation protocols [40]. No differences were identified among patients treated acutely, but operative delay led to poorer functional outcomes and decreased satisfaction scores [40]. Rasul, et.al immobilized 19 ruptures for 6 weeks after surgery [41]. Excellent results were noted in 17 patients who had early repair with good results in the two patients treated in a delayed fashion [41]. One study showed that 84% of working patients were able to return to their previous occupations [28]. However, more than 50% could no longer participate in their pre-injury recreational activities [28]. Among professional American football players, even with timely surgical repair, the rate of return to play in regular season games was 50% [8]. For those that did return to play, the average number of games after injury was 40.9 games [8].

Conclusion

The quadriceps is a unique complex of individual muscles and tendons that must work together in harmony to allow for a wide assortment of dynamic functions. However, given that the quadriceps is comprised of these separate components, its intrinsic complexity lends itself to potential for injury to yield improper function and subsequent damage with profound impact on mobility. Should injury occur, it is important to determine the mechanism of injury and true etiology of the derangement in order to proceed with the correct treatment plan for the patient. The wide array of dynamic function and injury mechanisms are what lead the multitude of treatment options when it comes to healing the quadriceps muscle group and their tendons.

References

1. Zwerver J, Bredeweg SW, van den Akker-Scheek I. Prevalence of Jumper's knee among nonelite athletes from different sports: a cross-sectional survey. Am J Sports Med. 2011;39(9):1984–8.
2. Woodley SJ, et al. Articularis genus: an anatomic and MRI study in cadavers. J Bone Joint Surg. 2012;94(1):59–67.
3. Ibounig T, Simons TA. Etiology, diagnosis and treatment of tendinous knee extensor mechanism injuries. Scand J Surg. 2016;105(2):67–72.
4. Fields KB. Running injuries – changing trends and demographics. Curr Sports Med Rep. 2011;10(5):299–303.
5. Clayton RAE, Court-Brown CM. The epidemiology of musculoskeletal tendinous and ligamentous injuries. Injury. 2008;39:1338–44.
6. Mendiguchia J, Alentorn-Geli E, Idoate F, Myer G. Rectus femoris muscle injuries in football: a clinically relevant review of mechanisms of injury, risk factors and preventive strategies. Br J Sports Med. 2013;47:359–66.
7. Boublik M, Schlegel T, Koonce R, Genuario J, Kinkartz J. Quadriceps tendon injuries in national football league players. Am J Sports Med. 2013;41(8):1841–6.
8. Ilan D, Tejwani N, Keschner M, Leibman M. Quadriceps tendon rupture. J Am Acad Orthop Surg. 2003;11(3):192–200.
9. Bhole R, Flynn J, Marbury T. Quadriceps tendon ruptures in uremia. Clin Orthop Relat Res. 1985;195:200–6.
10. McKinney B, Cherney S, Penna J. Intra-articular knee injuries in patients with knee extensor mechanism ruptures. Knee Surg Sports Traumatol Arthrosc. 2008;16:633–8.
11. Yepes H, Tang M, Morris S, Stanish W. Relationship between hypovascular zones and patterns of ruptures of the quadriceps tendon. J Bone Joint Surg. 2008;90:2135–41.
12. Neubauer T, Wagner M, Potschka T, Riedl M. Bilateral, simultaneous rupture of the quadriceps tendon: a diagnostic pitfall? Report of three cases and meta-analysis of the literature. Knee Surg Sports Traumatol Arthrosc. 2007;15(1):43–53.
13. David H, Green J, Grant A, Wilson C. Simultaneous bilateral quadriceps rupture: a complication of anabolic steroid abuse. J Bone Joint Surg. 1995;77(1):159–60.
14. Kim Y, Shafi M, Lee Y, Kim J, Kim W, Han C. Spontaneous and simultaneous rupture of both quadriceps tendons in a patient with chronic renal failure: a case studied by MRI both preoperatively and postoperatively. Knee Surg Sports Traumatol Arthrosc. 2006;14(1):55–9.
15. Kuri J II, DiFelice G. Acute compartment syndrome of the thigh following rupture of the quadriceps tendon: a case report. J Bone Joint Surg. 2006;88(2):418–20.

16. Kelly B, Rao N, St. Louis S, Kostes B, Smith R. Bilateral, simultaneous, spontaneous rupture of quadriceps tendons without trauma in an obese patient: a case report. Arch Phys Med Rehabil. 2001;82(3):415–8.

17. Kaneko K, DeMouy E, Brunet M, Benzian J. Radiographic diagnosis of quadriceps tendon rupture: analysis of diagnostic failure. J Emerg Med. 1994;12:225–9.

18. Henderson R, Walker B, Young K. The accuracy of diagnostic ultrasound imaging for musculoskeletal soft tissue pathology of the extremities: a comprehensive review of the literature. Chiropr Man Therap. 2015;23:31.

19. Giombini A, Dragoni S, Di Cesare A, Di Cesare M, Del Buono A, Maffulli N. Asymptomatic Achilles, patellar, and quadriceps tendinopathy: a longitudinal clinical and ultrasonographic study in elite fencers. Scand J Med Sci Sports. 2013;23:311–6.

20. Pfirrmann C, Jost B, Pirkl C, Aitzetmuller G, Lajtai G. Quadriceps tendinosis and patellar tendinosis in professional beach volleyball players: sonographic findings in correlation with clinical symptoms. Eur Radiol. 2008;18:1703–9.

21. Perfitt J, Petrie M, Blundell C, Davies M. Acute quadriceps tendon rupture: a pragmatic approach to diagnostic imaging. Eur J Orthop Surg Traumatol. 2014;24(7):1237–41.

22. Spector E, DiMarcangelo M, Jacoby J. The radiologic diagnosis of quadriceps tendon rupture. N J Med. 1995;92:590–2.

23. Kuivila T, Brems J. Diagnosis of acute rupture of the quadriceps tendon by magnetic resonance imaging: a case report. Clin Orthop Relat Res. 1991;262:236–41.

24. Yablon C, Pai D, Dong Q, Jacobson J. Magnetic resonance imaging of the extensor mechanism. Mag Reson Imaging Clin N Am. 2014;22(4):601–20.

25. Rio E, Kidgell D, Moseley G, Gaida J, Docking S, Purdam C, Cook J. Tendon neuroplastic training: changing the we think about tendon rehabilitation: a narrative review. Br J Sports Med. 2016;50:209–15.

26. Brukner P, Connell D. 'Serious thigh muscle strains': beware the intramuscular tendon which plays an important role in difficult hamstring and quadriceps muscle strains. Br J Sports Med. 2016;50:205–8.

27. Pocock C, Trikha S, Bell J. Delayed reconstruction of a quadriceps tendon. Clin Orthop Relat Res. 2008;466:221–4.

28. Konrath G, Chen D, Lock T, Goitz H, Watson J, Moed B, D'Ambrosio G. Outcomes following repair of quadriceps tendon ruptures. J Orthop Traumatol. 1998;12(4):273–9.

29. Siwek C, Rao J. Ruptures of the extensor mechanism of the knee joint. J Bone Joint Surg. 1981;63:932–7.

30. Meyer Z, Ricci W. Knee extensor mechanism repairs: standard suture repair and novel augmentation technique. J Orthop Traumatol. 2016;30:S30–1.

31. Maniscalco P, Bertone C, Rivera F, Bocchi L. A new method of repair for quadriceps tendon ruptures: a case report. Panminerva Med. 2000;42:223–5.

32. Kindya M, Konicek J, Rizzi A, Komatsu D, Paci J. Knotless suture anchor with suture tape quadriceps tendon repair is biomechanically superior to transosseous and traditional suture anchor–based repairs in a cadaveric model. Arthroscopy. 2017;33(1):190–8.

33. Bushnell B, Whitener G, Rubright J, Creighton R, Logel K, Wood M. The use of suture anchors to repair the ruptured quadriceps tendon. J Orthop Traumatol. 2007;21(6):407–13.

34. Richards D, Barber F. Repair of quadriceps tendon ruptures using suture anchors. Arthroscopy. 2002;18(5):556–9.

35. Rosa D, Lettera M, Iacono V, Cigala M, Maffulli N. Reconstruction of chronic tears of the quadriceps tendon with free hamstring autograft. Tech Knee Surg. 2008;7(1):27–30.

36. Franceschi F, Longo U, Ruzzino L, Rizzello G, Denaro V, Maffulli N. Chronic rupture of quadriceps tendon reconstruction with free semitendinosus tendon graft and suture anchors. Tech Knee Surg. 2008;7(1):31–3.

37. Kerin C, Hopgood P, Banks A. Delayed repair of quadriceps using the Mitek anchor system: a case report and review of the literature. Knee. 2006;13:161–3.

38. Rougraff B, Reeck C, Essenmacher J. Complete quadriceps tendon ruptures. Orthopedics. 1996;19:509–14.

39. West J, Keene J, Kaplan L. Early motion after quadriceps and patellar tendon repairs: outcomes with single-suture augmentation. Am J Sports Med. 2008;36(2):316–23.

40. Langenhan R, Baumann M, Ricart P, Hak D, Probst A, Badke A, Trobisch P. Postoperative functional rehabilitation after repair of quadriceps tendon ruptures: a comparison of two different protocols. Knee Surg Sports Traumatol Arthrosc. 2012;20(11):2275–8.

41. Rasul A, Fischer D. Primary repair of quadriceps tendon ruptures: results of treatment. Clin Orthop Relat Res. 1993;289:205–7.

42. Jaimes C, Jimenez M, Shabshin N, Laor T, Jaramillo D. Taking the stress out of evaluating stress injuries in children. Radiographics. 2012;32:537–55.

43. Parvaresh K, Upasani V, Bomar J, Pennock A. Secondary ossification center appearance and closure in the pelvis and proximal femur. J Pediatr Orthop. 2018;38(8):418–23.

44. Moraux A, Balbi V, Cockenpot E, Vandenbussche L, Miletic B, Letartre R, Khalil C. Sonographic overview of usual and unusual disorders of the rectus femoris tendon origin. J Ultrasound Med. 2018;37:1543–53.

45. Carton P, Filan D. Anterior inferior iliac spine (AIIS) and subspine impingement. Muscles Ligaments Tendons J. 2016;6(3):324–36.

46. Yildiz C, Yildiz Y, Ozdemir MT, Green D, Aydin T. Sequential avulsion of the anterior inferior iliac spine in an adolescent long jumper. Br J Sports Med. 2005;39:e31.

47. Novais E, Riederer M, Provance A. Anterior inferior iliac spine deformity as a cause for extra-articular hip impingement in young athletes after an avulsion fracture: a case report. Sports Health. 2017;10(3):272–6.

48. Rajasekhar C, Sampath Kumar K, Bhamra MS. Avulsion fractures of the anterior inferior iliac spine: the case for surgical intervention. Int Orthop. 2001;24:364–5.

49. Kjellin I, Stadnick M, Awh M. Orthopaedic magnetic resonance imaging challenge apophyseal avulsions at the pelvis. Sports Health. 2010;2(3):247–51.

50. Cardenas-Nylander C, Astarita E, Moya E, Bellotti V, Ciccolo F, Ribas FM. Internal fixation of the inferior iliac spine avulsion in adolescents: descriptions of two different surgical procedures. J Hip Preserv Surg. 2016;3(suppl 1):hnw030.019.

51. Rossi F, Dragoni S. Acute avulsion fractures of the pelvis in adolescent competitive athletes: prevalence, location and sports distribution of 203 cases collected. Skelet Radiol. 2001;30:127–31.

52. Arnaiz J, Piedra T, Marco de Lucas E, Maria Arnaiz A, Pelaz M, Gomez-Dermit V, Canga A. Imaging findings of lower limb apophysitis. Pediat Imaging. 2001;196:W316–25.

53. American Association of Physicists in Medicine Position statement on use of patient gonadal and fetal shielding, Policy number PP32-A, 2019.

54. Yoshida S, Ichimura K, Sakai T. Structural diversity of the vastus intermedius origin revealed by analysis of isolated muscle specimens. Clin Anat. 2017;30:98–105.

55. Gyftopoulos S, Sadka Rosenberg Z, Schweitzer M, Bordalo-Rodrigues M. Normal anatomy and strains of the deep musculotendinous junction of the proximal rectus femoris: MRI features. AJR. 2008;190:W182–6.

56. Yablon C, Pai D, Dong Q, Jacobson J. Magnetic resonance imaging of the extensor mechanism. Magn Reson Imaging Clin N Am. 2014;22:601–20.

57. Foley R, Fessell D, Yablon C, Nadig J, Brandon C, Jacobson J. Sonography of traumatic quadriceps tendon tears with surgical correlation. J Ultrasound Med. 2015;34:805–10.

58. Klauser A. Clinical indications for musculoskeletal ultrasound: a Delphi-based consensus paper of the European society of musculoskeletal radiology. Eur Radiol. 2012;22:1140–8.

59. Kassarjian A, Monica Rodrigo R, Maria SJ. Intramuscular degloving injuries to the rectus femoris: findings at MRI. AJR. 2014;202:W475–80.

60. Balius R, Maestro A, Pedret C, Estruch A, Mota J, Rodriguez L, Garcia P, Mauri E. Central aponeurosis tears of the rectus femoris: practical sonographic prognosis. Br J Sports Med. 2009;43:818–24.

61. Kassarjian A, Rodrigo RM, Santisteban JM. Current concepts in MRI of rectus femoris musculotendinous (myotendinous) and myofascial injuries in elite athletes. Eur J Radiol. 2012;81:3763–71.

62. Pierannunzii L, Tramontana F, Gallazzi M. Case report: calcific tendinitis of the rectus femoris: a rare case of snapping hip. Clin Orthop Relat Res. 2010;468(10):2814–8.

63. Esser S, Jantz D, Hurdle M, Taylor W. Proximal rectus femoris avulsion: ultrasonic diagnosis and nonoperative management. J Athl Train. 2015;50(7):778–80.

64. Ouellette H, Thomas B, Nelson E, Torriani M. MR imaging of rectus femoris origin injuries. Skelet Radiol. 2006;35:665–72.

65. Dean C, Arbeloa-Gutierrez L, Chahla J, Pascual-Garrido C. Proximal rectus femoris avulsion repair. Arthrosc Tech. 2016;5(3):545–9.

66. Grob K, Manestar M, Filgueira L, Ackland T, Gilbey H, Kuster M. New insight in the architecture of the quadriceps tendon. J Exp Orthop. 2016;3:32.

67. Waligora A, Johanson N, Hirsch B. Clinical anatomy of the quadriceps femoris and extensor apparatus of the knee. Clin Orthop Relat Res. 2009;467:3297–306.

68. Gamradt S, Brophy R, Barnes R, Warren R, Byrd T, Kelly B. Nonoperative treatment for proximal avulsion of the rectus femoris in professional American football. Am J Sports Med. 2009;37(7):1370–4.

69. Hasselman C, Best T, Hughes C, Martinez S, Garrett W. An explanation for various rectus femoris strain injuries using previously undescribed muscle architecture. Am J Sports Med. 1995;23(4):493–9.

70. Boden B. Knee and thigh overuse tendinopathy. In: Maffulli N, Renström P, Leadbetter WB, editors. Tendon injuries. London: Springer; 2005. p. 158–65.

71. King D, Yakubek G, Chughtai M, Khlopas A, Saluan P, Mont M, Genin J. Quadriceps tendinopathy: a review- part 1: epidemiology and diagnosis. Ann Transl Med. 2019;7(4):71.

72. Visnes H, Tegnander A, Bahr R. Ultrasound characteristics of the patellar and quadriceps tendons among young elite athletes. Scand J Med Sci Sports. 2015;25:205–15.

73. Pappas G, Vogelson M, Staroswiecki E, Gold G, Safran M. Magnetic resonance imaging of asymptomatic knees in collegiate basketball players: the effect of one season of play. Clin J Sport Med. 2016;26(6):483–9.

74. Pfirrmann C, Jost B, Pirkl C, Aitzetmüller G, Lajtai G. Quadriceps tendinosis and patellar tendinosis in professional beach bolleyball players: sonographic findings in correlation with clinical symptoms. Eur Radioldiol. 2008;18(8):1703–9.

75. King D, Yakubek G, Chughtai M, Khlopas A, Saluan P, Mont M, Genin J. Quadriceps tendinopathy: a review- part 2: classification, prognosis and treatment. Ann Transl Med. 2019;7(4):72.

76. Pasta G, Nanni G, Molini L, Bianchi S. Sonography of the quadriceps muscle: examination technique, normal anatomy, and traumatic lesions. J Ultrasound. 2010;13(2):76–84.

Patellar Tendon

11

11

Ronald Takemoto, Kevin Pelletier, Alex Miner, Abdullah Kandil, and Abdurrahman Kandil

Abbreviation

CD-US   Color Doppler ultrasound
GS-US   Gray scale ultrasound
HVIGI   High-volume image-guided injections
LIPUS   Low-intensity pulsed ultrasound
MRI   Magnetic resonance imaging
SLJ   Sinding-Larsen-Johansson
US   Ultrasound

Introduction

Patellar tendon disorders are a common source of anterior knee pain in both the recreational and serious athletes. Maurizio was the first to describe the association between jumping and patellar tendon pain in a study of volleyball players [1]. However, Blazina is credited for the term *jumper's knee* used to describe patellar tendon pain in athletes whose sport involves frequent jumping [2]. Sports that require the knee extensor mechanism to be used repetitively in explosive extension or eccentric flexion pose a risk of causing what is now referred to as *patellar tendinopathy*.

R. Takemoto (✉) · K. Pelletier · A. Miner · A. Kandil
Department of Physical Medicine and Rehabilitation, University of California Irvine, Orange, CA, USA
e-mail: ronald.takemoto@va.gov

A. Kandil
Department of Orthopedic Surgery, Stanford University, Redwood City, CA, USA

Volleyball, basketball, soccer, dancing, and Olympic-style weightlifting are all examples of sports that can cause patellar tendinopathy. Given the importance of the knee extensor mechanism in jumping, this condition can be quite disabling. In fact, 50% of athletes continue to endorse anterior knee pain 15 years after the initial diagnosis of patellar tendinopathy [3].

Anatomy

The patella is the largest sesamoid bone in the body and is connected at its inferior pole to the tibial tuberosity via the patellar tendon, or as some have labeled, the patellar ligament, since this attachment is from bone to bone. Proximally, the large quadriceps group of the vastus medialis, vastus lateralis, vastus intermedius, and rectus femoris attach to the superior aspect of the patella. As the quadriceps group has as its final attachment the tibial tuberosity, the term patellar tendon will be used for this chapter. The patellar tendon has a broad, flat origin at the distal aspect of the patella and then becomes thickened and narrow distally as it attaches to the tibial tuberosity (Fig. 11.1). Over 60% of the fibers of the patellar tendon are lateral to the apex of the distal pole of the patella [4]. Like the Achilles tendon, the patellar tendon lacks a true tendon sheath and is enveloped by paratenon, a two-layered membrane composed of epitenon and peritenon. Collagen fibrils are bundled into fascicles and are

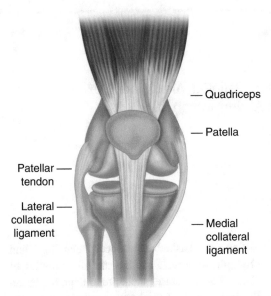

Fig. 11.1 Face-on view of R-knee

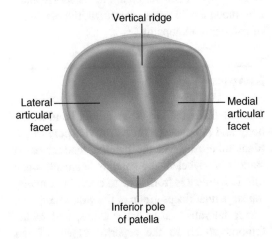

Fig. 11.2 Posterior surface of patella

mately 20–25% of the patella height [4] (see Fig. 11.2). One study of 22 dissected knees revealed that 16 of 22 knees were devoid of tendon attachment on the non-articulating posterior inferior pole, while 6 of the 22 knees did have a few fascicle attachments at that location [6]. The vascular supply to the patellar tendon is by anastomoses of the inferior lateral geniculate artery, inferior medial geniculate artery, and small vessels from Hoffa's fat pad [7]. The patellar tendon is innervated by the infrapatellar branch of the saphenous nerve and branches of the medial cutaneous femoral nerve, which form a plexus called the subsartorial plexus [4].

Extension of the knee is provided primarily by the large quadriceps muscle group. The power of this muscle group is enhanced by the addition of the patella, which increases the moment arm of the extensor mechanism. The moment arm is increased from 10% to 30% when the knee is flexed to 120 degrees and 30 degrees, respectively [8] (see Fig. 11.3). The patellar tendon is subjected to high tensile forces, especially with stair climbing and jumping. The tensile strength

surrounded by the endotenon. The fascicles are grouped together and surrounded by epitenon, which in turn is surrounded by peritenon [5].

Gross examination of the patella posteriorly reveals a large, smooth articular hyaline cartilage surface. This articulating surface is divided by a vertical ridge, which sits in the trochlear groove on the distal femur. The lateral articular facet is slightly larger than the medial articular facet. The inferior portion of the posterior patella (inferior pole) is non-articulating and represents approxi-

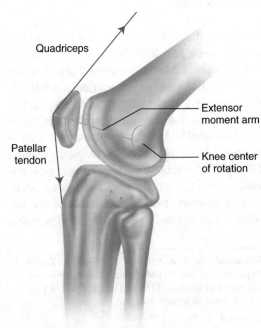

Fig. 11.3 Knee extensor moment arm at 50° of flexion

of the patellar tendon has been measured in studies to be 64 +/− 15 MPa in younger adults (29–50 years) and 53 +/− 10 MPa in older adults (64–93 years) [9]. The patellar tendon lengthens approximately 10% from full knee extension to 30 degrees of flexion. From 30 degrees to 110 degrees of flexion, there is no further change in patellar tendon length [10].

Patellar Tendinopathy Case

A 20-year-old collegiate basketball player presents with chronic infrapatellar pain that worsens when going up or down stairs and jumping. He recalls that the pain started when he was playing basketball as a senior in high school and says it has been slowly worsening ever since—though he denies any specific trauma to the knee. He states the pain used to occur only after practice but now is present during the first few minutes of practice as well. He is otherwise healthy, without any other medical problems. On examination, he is positive for the Royal London Hospital Test (see description under Section "Physical Examination"). He underwent physical therapy for 5 weeks without improvement. An injection of platelet-rich plasma was also not helpful. He presented to a university sports medicine specialty clinic, where he requested treatment that required minimal downtime. The patient opted for mechanical tendon scraping and was able to return to practice by next day with minimal pain; full activity was obtained by second week after the procedure.

Clinical Presentation

Blazina classified patellar tendinopathy into four stages, based primarily on the timing of patellar tendon pain [2]. The first stage is pain after activity; the second stage is pain at the beginning of activity that goes away after warming up but can return with fatigue; the third stage is constant pain at rest and with activity; and the fourth stage is complete patellar tendon rupture [2].

Skeletally mature individuals with patellar tendinopathy often present with anterior knee pain which must be distinguished from other conditions that can present similarly, such as patellofemoral pain syndrome and Hoffa's fat pad impingement [14]. Patients with patellar tendinopathy often describe the insidious onset of aching pain localized to the inferior pole of the patella, sometimes following a period of increased activity [14].

Skeletally immature individuals can also develop patellar tendinopathy, but there are pediatric-specific conditions that can present similarly which must be ruled out, such as Sinding-Larsen-Johansson (SLJ) syndrome [13]. The typical patient with SLJ syndrome is a physically active adolescent who has recently undergone a rapid growth spurt [17]. The pathophysiology of SLJ syndrome involves a repetitive traction force on the patellar growth plate by the patellar tendon that results in strain of this growth plate before completion of secondary ossification. This results in avulsion of the distal patellar ossicles, manifesting as anterior knee pain. This could potentially be mistaken for patellar tendinopathy. With a similar pathophysiology as SLJ syndrome but involving a repetitive traction force on the tibial tubercle apophysis by the patellar tendon, Osgood-Schlatter disease similarly causes strain on the apophyseal joint and results in avulsion of the tibial tubercle [17]. While this condition also causes knee pain, the location of the pain would be more toward the distal aspect of the patellar tendon, which would be atypical in cases of patellar tendinopathy.

Both intrinsic and extrinsic causes have been implicated in patellar tendinopathy. Intrinsic causes include tight quadriceps and hamstrings, weak VMO muscle, increased Q-angle, abnormalities of the distal pole of the patella, rotational deformities (increased femoral anteversion, excess tibial torsion), genu varum/valgus, patella alta, leg length difference, male sex, reduced ankle dorsiflexion, foot abnormalities, obesity, inflammatory disease, and fluoroquinolone usage [11]. Extrinsic causes include overtraining with increases in frequency and intensity, errors in specific sport technique, playing surfaces that are harder, and footwear.

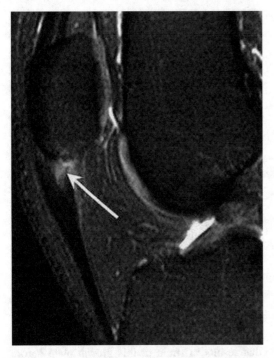

Fig. 11.4 T2 MRI of the knee demonstrating signal change (*arrow*) in the posterior aspect of the proximal patellar tendon [49]

The primary location of patellar tendinopathy is at the tendon-bone interface at the inferior pole. Traditional theory of the cause of patellar tendinopathy was secondary to overuse [13]. Recently, patellar tendon impingement at the distal patella has been proposed. These conclusions were primarily based on the location of tendon abnormalities by MRI scans at the dorsal aspect of the proximal insertion of the patellar tendon [45] (see Fig. 11.4). From these findings, it has been theorized that patellar tendinopathy may be an adaptive process secondary to impingement and compressive forces [14]. Further studies will need to clarify this issue.

Several authors have studied excised tissues of the patellar tendon at the inferior pole of the patella in athletes with patellar tendinopathy. The tendon is often enlarged in this area with loss of demarcation of the collagen bundles and an increase in mucoid degeneration, intra-tendinous calcifications, and fibrinoid necrosis [15]. In chronic cases, inflammatory cells are typically sparse. Recently, neovascularization has been demonstrated in chronic patellar tendinopathy [16]. These results tend to suggest that most patients suffering from patellar tendinopathy appear to have a tendinosis pathologically.

Complete patellar tendon rupture is an uncommon occurrence but one that is important to recognize. Patients presenting with a ruptured patellar tendon are typically going to be athletes who are less than 40 years old. The mechanism of injury involves explosive contraction of the quadriceps resisted by a flexed knee. The patient may also recall hearing a "pop" at the time of injury, followed by severe anterior knee pain. Finally, take note of medical conditions and medications that have been associated with weakening tendons, such as hyperparathyroidism, quinones, and steroids [12].

Physical Examination

On examination, the clinician should first perform a thorough visual inspection of the spine and lower extremities, assessing for muscular atrophy or disproportion of the quadriceps; genu varum, valgum, or recurvatum; positioning of the patella at rest; swelling, erythema; scars; pes cavus or planus and leg length discrepancy, as well as any side-to-side asymmetry in the above findings [18].

The clinician should then palpate both knees, starting on the unaffected side. This should include palpation of the entire length of the patellar tendon from proximal to distal with the knee resting in full extension. Take note of discrete areas of palpable thickening along the patellar tendon, which if present is more likely to occur toward the proximal end of the tendon [17]. However, a more likely finding in cases of patellar tendinopathy is tenderness to palpation of the patellar tendon—typically at or near the inferior pole of the patella [20]. Next, the clinician should perform the Royal London Hospital Test, which is considered positive if there is tenderness to palpation of the patellar tendon when the knee is resting in full extension (patellar tendon relaxed) but no longer tender to palpation of the same spot when the knee is placed in 90 degrees of flexion (patellar tendon more taut) [21]. This test is more specific than only testing for tenderness to palpation of the patellar tendon when the knee is resting in full extension [21].

Infrapatellar fat pad syndrome is a condition believed to result in pain secondary to Hoffa's fat pad irritation, and it may be mistaken for patellar tendinopathy given its proximity to the patellar tendon. One way to distinguish between the two is by performing the *Hoffa test*. The clinician holds the patient's knee in 30–60 degrees of flexion with one hand, while applying firm pressure with the thumb of the opposite hand just medial or lateral to the patellar tendon. The knee is then brought to full extension while maintaining pressure on the fat pad with the thumb. Increased pain in the fat pad with this maneuver is considered a positive test [20].

Finally, in cases of complete patellar tendon rupture, the patient will likely be unable to ambulate as knee extension is no longer associated with quadriceps contraction, given the disruption of the extensor mechanism. The patient will likely experience rapid swelling of the affected knee, as the result of hemarthrosis.

Diagnostic Imaging

Plain Radiography (X-Ray)

As a soft-tissue structure, the patellar tendon is poorly if at all visualized on X-ray imaging. However, X-rays can sometimes prove quite helpful while working up patellar tendinopathy and even patellar tendon rupture. For example, one may see a deposit of radiolucent material just distal to the most inferior aspect of the patella likely representing hydroxyapatite, which in a symptomatic patient can represent calcific patellar tendinosis. Furthermore, the position of the patella can also provide indication of whether there is a complete patellar tendon rupture. A so-called "high-riding" patella is radiographic support for the diagnosis of the patellar tendon rupture. Moreover, the clinician may be able to appreciate a piece of avulsed patellar bone from the inferior pole of the patella, as patellar avul-

sion fractures are often found in cases of patellar tendon rupture [12].

Ultrasonography (US)

The benefits of US are contingent upon the skill of the clinician. When used properly, US can elucidate dynamic, real-time images that can be obtained relatively quickly, inexpensively, and without exposure to radiation. A skilled ultrasonographer can use this technology to help determine the presence of patellar tendinopathy. A normal patellar tendon under gray scale ultrasound (GS-US) would have a near uniform width, tendon fibers arranged in parallel, and a relatively homogeneous intra-tendinous echogenicity [19].

To investigate the patellar tendon for pathology, the knee is first examined in partial flexion as this lengthens the tendon fibers, making it easier to comment on their general appearance [19]. A US image of a patient with patellar tendinopathy may demonstrate localized widening of the tendon, an irregular arrangement of tendon fibers, and an area of intra-tendinous hypoechogenicity indicative of collagen disruption [19]. However, it is important to note that areas of hyperechogenicity within the patellar tendon can also be indicative of patellar tendinopathy, likely representing intra-tendinous calcifications [47] (see Fig. 11.5).

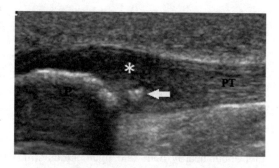

Fig. 11.5 Gray-scale ultrasound long-axis of patellar tendon (pt) showing a thickened proximal patellar tendon with an area of hypoechogenicity (*asterisk*) representing collagen disruption and an area of hyperechogenicity (*arrow*) representing an intratendinous calcification [50]. Proximal is left side of screen. Patella (P)

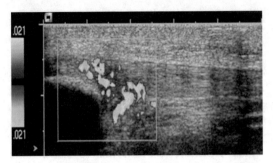

Fig. 11.6 Color Doppler ultrasound revealing neovascularization [51]

When the color Doppler function is utilized (CD-US) to examine a patellar tendon with tendinopathy, the resultant image may reveal the presence of blood flow not found in a healthy patellar tendon—this is referred to as *neovascularization* [19] (see Fig. 11.6). Neovascularization is best visualized with the knee in full extension as this lessens the mechanical constriction of the small intra-tendinous blood vessels by surrounding soft tissue structures [19].

Compared to MRI, US performed by an experienced examiner has proven equally specific, yet more sensitive in the detection of clinically diagnosed patellar tendinopathy [19]. Additionally, GS-US and CD-US were shown not to significantly differ in terms of sensitivity and specificity, although a positive CD-US may be more likely to determine if a patient is symptomatic [22].

Magnetic Resonance Imaging (MRI)

MRI is also useful in the evaluation of anterior knee pain. Along with US, it can be used to detect patellar tendon pathology, as abnormal appearing areas on both imaging modalities have been corroborated with histological evidence of tendon pathology [22]. MRI can also capture information about nearby bone and ligamentous structures that may be of interest. Although MRI is less operator-dependent than US, it has a lower specificity for patellar tendinopathy and is more expensive [19].

Similar to US, MRI can detect the patellar tendon widening commonly seen in patellar tendinopathy [14]. Pathological tendons have also been shown to have an increased signal intensity on both T1- and T2-weighted images [19]. In such cases, the signal abnormality is commonly found on the posterior aspect of the proximal patellar tendon [46] (see Fig. 11.4).

MRI can also be useful in identifying injuries to structures near the patellar tendon that may be confounding the clinical picture. For instance, it could reveal hemorrhage, inflammation, and fibrosis in the infrapatellar fat pad [17].

While imaging remains a useful tool in the diagnosis of patellar tendinopathy, it alone cannot be used to make the diagnosis of patellar tendinopathy. MRI and US testing can provide an image of the patellar tendon that appears normal when the clinical evidence strongly supports a diagnosis of patellar tendinopathy and vice versa [22].

Treatment

Conservative

In the treatment of patellar tendinopathy, exercise therapy is the cornerstone of an evidence-based approach [23]. The most extensively studied exercise regimens focus on progressive weight load bearing starting with isometric exercises and progressing to eccentric exercises [24]. Programs utilizing eccentric contractions with decline squats have been successful in alleviating symptoms and returning athletes to sport [24]. Performing a squat on a 25 degree decline board maximizes the eccentric load through the patellar tendon by limiting passive and active calf tension (see Fig. 11.7). A typical decline squat program consists of 3 sets of 15 repetitions twice daily of single-leg eccentric squats with an upright torso on a decline board [25]. While many studies have focused specifically on the decline squat, a comprehensive rehabilitation program ideally focuses on multiple types of exercises with gradual progressive loading protocols, moving from isomet-

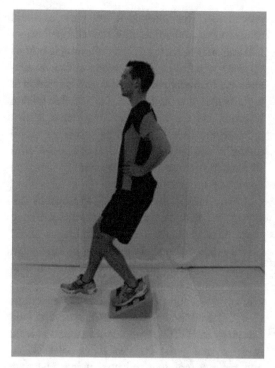

Fig. 11.7 Single-leg decline squat performed with an upright torso to 90 degrees of knee flexion or maximum angle allowed by pain [52]

ric loading, then to isotonic loading, and then to energy storage loading exercises. These comprehensive protocols are more practical approaches compared to programs emphasizing only one exercise [25].

These comprehensive progressive exercise programs emphasize progressive load tolerance of the tendon, musculoskeletal unit, and kinetic chain while addressing biomechanical risk factors [24]. Dose-dependent pain is a key feature of patellar tendinopathy rehabilitation [26]. As a result, a reasonable training regimen is likely to produce short-term symptom aggravation. Pain provocation up to 24 hours after energy-storage activities is acceptable during rehabilitation [26]. An appropriate rehabilitation approach will recognize deficits at the hip, knee, ankle, and foot regions. Additionally, addressing associated features of patellar tendinopathy including quadriceps and hamstring flexibility along with weight-bearing ankle dorsiflexion range of motion may also provide benefit [25].

Eccentric loading programs may also have very good outcomes with partial patellar ruptures of less than 10 mm. However, partial ruptures >20 mm are unlikely to respond to exercise therapy alone and should be operated on promptly if not responding to therapy. Complete patellar tendon rupture requires surgical consultation and should be repaired within 1 month of injury [27].

Extracorporeal shockwave therapy (pulsed ultrasound) is another noninvasive approach that has also received recent attention. There have been some positive results noted in existing studies utilizing extracorporeal shockwave protocols; however, studies do not support objective benefits with treatment against placebo. Significant variability exists between reported dosing and treatment regimens, but the best results (though still not statistically significant against placebo) utilize intermediate dose and fewer sessions [28].

Low-intensity pulsed ultrasound (LIPUS) has also been applied to patellar tendinopathy and though with unclear clinical benefits to date. LIPUS involves an application of ultrasound wave that has spatial-averaged temporal intensity equal to or lower than 100 mW/cm^2. Various protocols have been studied. For patellar tendon, one such protocol utilized 2 ms bursts of 1.0 MHz sine waves repeating at 100 Hz produced by a modified ultrasound therapy device. However, this study did not show any benefit against placebo in a randomized double-blinded trial [29].

Non-surgical Interventional Treatment

When patellar tendinopathy does not respond to the above conservative options, several minimally invasive approaches can be considered. Multiple injection techniques exist for treatment of patellar tendinopathy including platelet-rich plasma (PRP) injections, steroid injections, and polidocanol injections. A recent study on PRP as a treatment for patellar tendinopathy demonstrated that ultrasound-guided PRP injection with dry needling and exercises accelerates the recovery from patellar tendinopathy, but the benefit dissipates over time [30]. The

International Olympic Committee consensus paper on the role of PRP in tendon injuries states that there is a lack of well-designed studies to support the use of PRP in clinical settings [31]. It is important to note that PRP formulation varies, with possibility of varying benefits depending on both the formulation and the pathology type treated. Currently, PRP injection is believed to work by recruiting tenocytes/collagen-producing cells to the injured site through its paracrine mechanism, resulting in ultimate collagen synthesis [24]. Recent literature has generally not supported the use of corticosteroid injections as beneficial in the treatment of patellar tendinopathy [32]. Most treatment modalities utilized in treatment of patellar tendinopathy act in some way to induce an inflammatory response to promote a level of healing beyond the damage induced by therapy, and thus logically, the use of corticosteroids to counteract all inflammation is counterproductive [32].

Other recent approaches target the neovascularization process, which is thought to play a role in the pathophysiology of patellar tendinopathy and has been gaining popularity in recent years. The foundation of these approaches is the utilization of Doppler ultrasound to identify areas of high blood flow indicating neovascularization. In one such approach, polidocanol, an irritant that damages the cell lining of blood vessels causing them to fibrose and occlude, is injected outside the tendon at the entrance of the transversal vessels as they enter the injured part of the tendon from the dorsal side [33]. One study compared ultrasound and color Doppler ultrasound-guided polidocanol injections (with 6–8 weeks of follow-up and repeat injection up to three times for residual symptoms) vs ultrasound and color Doppler-guided arthroscopic debridement up to 12 months posttreatment [33]. This study found that patients had a lower visual analogue score and were more satisfied with arthroscopic shaving than sclerosing injections [33]. However, another study found patients to have similar continued lasting benefits after receiving either treatment at 3–5 years of follow-up [34]. When comparing these treatment approaches, it is important to realize that arthroscopic debridement is a surgical

procedure. This means it requires standard arthroscopic evaluation with standard anteromedial and anterolateral surgical arthroscopic portals for entry of a full-radius blade shaver used to separate the Hoffa fat pad from the patellar tendon at high blood flow regions of the patellar tendon insertion. While studies to date have shown arthroscopic debridement to be superior to sclerosing injections, this comparison is between a surgical procedure (though minimally invasive) and a non-surgical one.

Newer novel "less invasive" approaches targeting the neovascularization process utilizing ultrasound guidance for non-surgical methods have been developed. Two such approaches that have been described for the treatment of chronic tendinopathy (symptoms more than 3 months) are high-volume image-guided injections (HVIGI) and percutaneous mechanical needle scraping. In HVIGI, Doppler ultrasound is used to detect and grade areas of neovascularization, and patients are then injected using 21-gauge needle with a combination of local anesthetic and steroid followed by 30 mL of normal saline to separate the Hoffa fat pad from the posterior tendon surface [35]. Alternatively, ultrasound-guided percutaneous mechanical needle scraping utilizes ultrasound for guidance of mechanical separation of the Hoffa fat pad from the posterior tendon surface utilizing an 18-gauge 2-inch needle [36] (see Fig. 11.8). Recent literature on

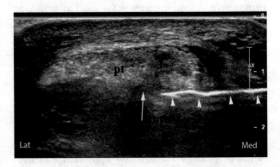

Fig. 11.8 Short-axis image of the left patellar tendon (pt) with medial to the right of the screen. An 18-gauge needle (*short arrowheads*) is guided to the interface (*long arrow*) between the posterior aspect of the tendon and Hoffa fat pad (hf). The needle is then used to mechanically separate the two layers, effectively disrupting the bridging neovessels and associated neonerves [36]

HVIGI in Achilles and patellar tendinopathy concludes that there is still insufficient evidence for HGIVI therapy for chronic tendinopathy that has failed conservative treatment [37]. HVIGI and ultrasound-guided percutaneous mechanical needle scraping have been described in case series and case reports, and authors of these papers have suggested that ultrasound-guided percutaneous needle scraping is a better tolerated procedure [36]. Thus far, case studies have presented promising results with these novel procedures, but a randomized study comparing high-volume image-guided injections or percutaneous ultrasound-guided needle scraping with arthroscopic-guided debridement techniques has not yet been performed [36].

Surgical Treatment

While most cases of patellar tendinopathy can be managed non-surgically, some recalcitrant cases may benefit from surgical management. Surgery is indicated in patients with persistent symptoms and functional impairment that have failed at least 6 months of conservative management [38]. If patients continue to have pain interfering with physical activity after a course of physical therapy, injections, and other non-operative interventions, then surgery can be considered. About 10% of patients treated for patellar tendinosis undergo surgery [38]. Goals of surgery include removal of tendinopathic tissue, stimulation of biologic healing through debridement, and re-establishing vascularity to the diseased tendon.

There is strong evidence to support surgical treatment for cases of chronic patellar tendinosis in patients with severe baseline symptoms who have failed conservative management [39]. One study demonstrated that the overall success rate of surgical management for symptomatic relief was greater than 80% [40]. Most studies to date have been retrospective in nature however [40]. Multiple surgical options exist for the treatment of patellar tendinosis including the following [39]:

1. Open longitudinal tenotomy with excision of pathology +/− resection of the inferior pole of the patella
2. Open, multiple, longitudinal tenotomie
3. Arthroscopic debridement and/or patellar tenotomy
4. Arthroscopic vs. open drilling or resection of the inferior pole of the patella

Open surgical excision of diseased tissue and drilling of the inferior pole involve making a longitudinal incision centered on the patellar tendon, followed by exposing the paratenon and reflecting it longitudinally. The tendon is then longitudinally incised and diseased tissue is excised and debrided. Finally, the inferior pole of the patella may be drilled to promote bleeding and dispersion of healing factors to the tendon [24]. Another open procedure involves the excision of necrotic tendon, followed by multiple longitudinal tenotomies placed in the tendon. There was subjective improvement in all athletes and an 87.5% return to previous level of sport at a mean of 8.1 months (range 3–12 months) [41].

Patients requiring surgery for insertional patellar tendinosis may also be treated arthroscopically. A diagnostic arthroscopy is first performed to rule out chondral and meniscal pathology. The inferior pole of the patella is then resected, which exposes the diseased tissue in the proximal patellar tendon, which is then excised [42].

There is no clear superiority of open vs. arthroscopic management of insertional patellar tendinosis [15]. Surgical outcome studies in the literature have demonstrated variability. One study did a systematic review that showed that the mean rate of success for surgical treatment of patellar tendinosis was 87% for open treatment and 91% for arthroscopy [43]. The mean return to sport time was 3.9 months for arthroscopy and 8.3 months for open treatment. However, another study showed the success rate of returning to sporting activity was only 54% in the open treatment group and 46% in the arthroscopic group [40].

Recovery following surgery, even with a good to excellent result, can take up to 6–12 months.

Rehabilitation consists of early weight-bearing and full range of motion as tolerated. After 2 weeks, patient may progress to eccentric squat exercises and quadriceps strengthening. Return to sport is guided by completion of at least 3 months of rehabilitation and return of pain-free strength and range of motion [44].

Patellar tendon ruptures are rare, with an incidence of approximately 0.6% [45]. Patellar tendon ruptures tend to occur when a violent contraction of the quadriceps is resisted by the flexed knee, i.e., during landing after a jump. The estimated force to disrupt a normal patellar tendon has been reported to be as high as 17.5 times body weight [46]. Given that such a force is needed to rupture a healthy tendon, it seems likely that ruptures occur in areas of preexisting disease at the tendon-bone interface. Immediate surgical repair is the standard of care with an isolated patellar tendon rupture. Outcome after repair is related to the length of time between injury and surgical repair. The many different types of surgical repair are beyond the scope of this chapter and may include end-to-end suturing, transosseous reinsertion, or re-attachment via suture anchors [47]. In the past, the knee was locked in extension for up to 6 weeks, but recent treatment protocols allow for earlier and more aggressive rehabilitation [48].

Surgical intervention is a reasonable option in patients with chronic refractory patellar tendinosis who have failed 6 months of conservative therapy. Choice of open versus arthroscopic approach should be based on surgeon preference due to similar clinical outcomes. With the chronic nature of patellar tendinopathy, and the fact that in some studies only half of active athletes make it back to pre-injury levels, further research and studies are needed for more effective treatment options.

References

1. Maurizio E. La tendinite rotulea del giocatore di pallavolo. Arch So Tosco Umbra Chir. 1963;24:443–5.
2. Blazina MF, Kerlan RK, Jobe F, Carter VS, Carlson GJ. Jumper's knee. Orthop Clin North Am. 1973;4:665–78.
3. Kettunen JA, Kvist M, Alanen E, Kuhala U. Long term prognosis in jumper's knee in male athletes. A prospective follow-up study. Am J Sports Med. 2002;30:689–92.
4. Fox AJS, Wanivenhaus F, Rodeo SA. The basic science of the patella: structure, composition and function. J Knee Surg. 2012;25(2):127–41.
5. Tan SC, Chan O. Achilles and patellar tendinopathy: current understanding of pathophysiology and management. Disabil Rehabil. 2008;30(20–22):1608–15.
6. Basso O, Johnson DP, Amis AA. The anatomy of the patellar tendon. Knee Surg Sports Traumatol Arthrosc. 2001;9:2–5.
7. Pang J, Shen S, Pan WR, Jones IR, Rozen WM, Taylor GI. The arterial supply of the patellar tendon: anatomical study with clinical implications for knee surgery. Clin Anat. 2009;22(3):371–6.
8. Kaufer H. Patellar biomechanics. Clin Orthop Relat Res. 1979;(144):51–4.
9. Johnson GA, Tramaglini DM, Levine RE, Ohno K, Choi NY, Woo SL. Tensile and viscoelastic properties of human patellar tendon. J Orthop Res. 1994;12(6):796–803.
10. DeFrate LE, Nha KW, Papannagari R, Moses JM, Gill T, Li G. The biomechanical function of the patellar tendon during in-vivo weight-bearing function. J Biomech. 2007;40(8):1716–22.
11. Reinking MF. Current concepts in the treatment of patellar tendinopathy. Int J Sports Phy Ther. 2016;11(6):854–66.
12. Saragaglia D, Pison A, Rubens-Duval B. Acute and old ruptures of the extensor apparatus of the knee in adults (excluding knee replacement). Orthop Traumatol Surg Res. 2013;99(1 Suppl):S67.
13. Zaid A, Duri A, Aichroth PM. Patellar tendonitis: clinical and literature review. Knee. 1996;3(1–2):95–8.
14. Johnson DP, Wakeley CJ, Watt I. Magnetic resonance imaging of patellar tendonitis. J Bone Joint Surg Br. 1996;78(3):452–7.
15. Rosso F, Bonasia DE, Cottino U, Dettoni F, Bruzzone M, Rossi R. Patellar tendon: from tendinopathy to rupture. Asia-Pacific J Sports Med Arthrosc Rehabil Technol. 2015;2(4):99–107.
16. Alfredson H, Ohberg L. Neovascularization in chronic painful patellar tendinosis-promising results after sclerosing neovessels outside the tendon challenge the need for surgery. Knee Surg Sports Traumatol Arthrosc. 2005;13(2):74–80.
17. Hiemstra LA, Kerslake S, Irving C. Anterior knee pain in the athlete. Clin Sports Med. 2014;33:437–59.
18. Rossi R, Dettoni F, Bruzzone M, Cottino U, D'Elicio D, Bonasia DE. Clinical examination of the knee: know your tools for diagnosis of knee injuries. Sports Med Arthrosc Rehabil Ther Technol. 2011;3:25–36.
19. Torres SJ, Zgonis MH, Bernstein J. Patellar tendinopathy. Univ Pa Orthop J. 2012;22:12–20.
20. Lester JD, Watson JN, Hutchinson MR. Physical examination of the patellofemoral joint. Clin Sports Med. 2014;33:403–12.

21. Maffulli N, Oliva F, Loppini M, Aicale R, Spezia F, King JB. The Royal London Hospital Test for the clinical diagnosis of patellar tendinopathy. Muscles Ligaments Tendons J. 2017;7(2):315–22.

22. Warden SJ, Kiss ZS, Malara FA, Ooi AB, Cook JL, Crossley KM. Comparative accuracy of magnetic resonance imaging and ultrasonography in confirming clinically diagnosed patellar tendinopathy. Am J Sports Med. 2007;35:427–36.

23. Sharma P, Maffuli N. Tendon injury and tendinopathy: healing and repair. J Bone Joint Surg Am. 2005;87(1):187–202.

24. Rodriguez-Merchan EC. The treatment of patellar tendinopathy. J Orthop Traumatol. 2013;14(2):77–81.

25. Malliaras P, Cook J, Purdam C, Rio E. Patellar tendinopathy: clinical diagnosis, load management, and advice for challenging case presentations. J Orthop Sports Phys Ther. 2015;45(11):887–98.

26. Kountouris A, Cook J. Rehabilitation of Achilles and patellar tendinopathies. Best Pract Res Clin Rheumatol. 2007;21:295–316.

27. Ramseier LE, Werner CM, Heinzelmann M. Quadriceps and patellar tendon rupture. Injury. 2006;37(6):516–9.

28. Wang CJ, Ko JY, Chan YS, Weng LH, Hsu SL. Extracorporeal shockwave for chronic patellar tendinopathy. Am J Sports Med. 2007;35:972–8.

29. Warden SJ, Metcalf BR, Kiss ZS, Cook JL, Purdam CR, Bennell KL, et al. Low-intensity pulsed ultrasound for chronic patellar tendinopathy: a randomized, double-blind, placebo-controlled trial. Rheumatology (Oxford). 2008;47(4):467–71.

30. Dragoo JL, Wasterlain AS, Braun HJ, Nead KT. Platelet-rich plasma as a treatment for patellar tendinopathy, a double-blind, randomized controlled trial. Am J Sports Med. 2014;42(3):610–8.

31. Engebretsen L, Steffen K, Alsousou J, Anitua E, Bachl N, et al. IOC consensus paper on the use of platelet-rich plasma in sports medicine. Br J Sports Med. 2010;44:1072–81.

32. Everhart JS, Cole D, Sojka JH, Higgins JD, Magnussen RA, et al. Treatment options for patellar tendinopathy: a systematic review. Arthroscopy. 2017;33(4):861–72.

33. Willberg L, Sunding K, Forssblad M, Fahlstrom M, Alfredson H. Sclerosing polidocanol injections or arthroscopic shaving to treat patellar tendinopathy/jumper's knee? A randomized controlled study. Br J Sports Med. 2011;45(5):411–5.

34. Sunding K, Willberg L, Werner S, Alfredson H, Forssblad M, Fahlström M. Sclerosing injections and ultrasound-guided arthroscopic shaving for patellar tendinopathy: good clinical results and decreased tendon thickness after surgery—a medium-term follow-up study. Knee Surg Sports Traumatol Arthrosc. 2015;23(8):2259–68.

35. Morton S, Chan O, King J, Perry D, Crisp T, Maffulli N, Morrissey D. High volume image-guided injections for patellar tendinopathy: a combined retrospective and prospective case series. Muscles Ligaments Tendons J. 2014;4(2):214–9.

36. Hall MM, Sathish R. Ultrasound-guided scraping for chronic patellar tendinopathy: a case presentation. PM R. 2016;8(6):593–6.

37. Barker-Davies RM, Nicol A, McCurfir I, Watson J, et al. Study protocol: a double blind randomized control trial of high volume image guided injections in Achilles and patellar tendinopathy in a young active population. BMC Musculoskelet Disord. 2017;18:204–16.

38. Ogon P, Maier D, Jaeger A, Suedkamp NP. Arthroscopic patellar release for the treatment of chronic patellar tendinopathy. Arthroscopy. 2006;22(4):462:e1–5.

39. Coleman BD, Khan KM, Maffulli N, Cook JL, Wark JD. Studies of surgical outcome after patellar tendinopathy: clinical significance of methodological deficiencies and guidelines for future studies. Victorian Institute of Sport Tendon Study Group. Scand J Med Sci Sports. 2000;10(1):2–11.

40. Coleman BD, Khan KM, Kiss ZS, Bartlett J, Young DA, Wark JD. Open and arthroscopic patellar tenotomy for chronic patellar tendinopathy. A retrospective outcome study. Victorian Institute of Sport Tendon Study Group. Am J Sports Med. 2000;28(2):183–90.

41. Shelbourne KD, Henne TD, Gray T. Recalcitrant patellar tendinosis in elite athletes: surgical treatment in conjunction with aggressive postoperative rehabilitation. Am J Sports Med. 2006; 34(7):1141–6.

42. Alaseirlis DA, Konstantinidis GA, Malliaropoulos N, Nakou LS, Korompilias A, Maffulli N. Arthroscopic treatment of chronic patellar tendinopathy in high level athletes. Muscles Ligaments Tendons J. 2012;2(4):267–72.

43. Brockmeyer M, Diehl N, Schmitt C, Kohn DM, Lorbach O. Results of surgical treatment of chronic patellar tendinosis (Jumper's knee): a systematic review of the literature. Arthroscopy. 2015;31(12):2424–9.

44. Ferretti A, Conteduca F, Camerucci E, Morelli F. Patellar tendinosis: a follow-up study of surgical treatment. J Bone Joint Surg Am. 2001;84(12):2179–85.

45. Clayton RAE, Court-Brown CM. The epidemiology of musculoskeletal tendinous and ligamentous injuries. Injury. 2008;39(12):1338–44.

46. Zernicke RF, Garhammer J, Jobe FW. Human patellar-tendon rupture. J Bone Joint Surg Am. 1977;59(2):179–83.

47. Roudet A, Boudissa M, Chaussard C, Rubens-Duval B, Saragaglia D. Acute traumatic patellar tendon rupture: early and late results of surgical treatment of 38 cases. Orthop Traumatol Surg Res. 2015;101(3):307–11.

48. Marder RA, Timmerman LA. Primary repair of patellar tendon rupture without augmentation. Am J Sports Med. 1999;27(3):304–7.

49. Crema MD, Murakami A. Chapter 25, Imaging of volleyball injuries. In: Imaging in sports-specific musculoskeletal injuries, vol. 674: Springer; 2016.

50. Bianchi S, Martinoli C. Chapter 14, Knee. In: Ultrasound of the musculoskeletal system, vol. 681: Springer; 2007.

51. Alfredson H, Willberg L, Ohberg L, Forsgren S. Chapter 27, Ultrasound and Doppler-guided arthroscopic shaving for the treatment of patellar tendinopathy/jump-er's knee: biological background and description of method. In: Anterior knee pain and patellar instability. 2nd ed. London: Springer; 2011. p. 368.

52. Rudavsky A, Cook J. Physiotherapy management of patellar tendinopathy (jumper's knee). J Physiother. 2014;60(3):122–9.

Distal Hamstring, Pes Anserine, and Popliteal Tendons

12

Christopher Urbanek, Christopher McCrum,
Bryson P. Lesniak, and Jeanne M. Doperak

Abbreviations

MRI	Magnetic resonance imaging
NSAID	Non-steroidal anti-inflammatory drug
OA	Osteoarthritis
PATB	Pes anserinus tendinobursitis
US	Ultrasound

Introduction

Hamstring pathology involving the biceps femoris, semitendinosis, or semitendinosis are some of the most common injuries in sports. Acute injuries are common with sprinting, jumping, or high energy ballistic activities [1–3]. While the vast majority of tears occur at the proximal hamstrings, rare instances of distal tears have been reported in the literature [4, 5]. Overuse injury to the distal hamstring resulting in tendon inflam-mation is equally rare but should not be over-looked by the medical provider [6]. Another entity encountered in this region of the body is pes anserine tendinobursitis (PATB).

Anatomy

The distal hamstrings and their attachments have some unique properties that lay the groundwork for increased risk of injury. Starting laterally, the biceps femoris inserts into the iliotibial band, posterolateral capsule, lateral tibial condyle, and the head of the fibula [2]. This broad attachment is speculated to be one possible contributor to its predisposition to injury [7]. Medially, the semi-membranosus continues its course from the ischial tuberosity medial and deep to the semiten-dinosus before separating into five distal inser-tions. The anterior, direct, and inferior arms anchor semimembranosus to the medial tibial condyle. The capsular arm inserts on the poste-rior oblique ligament. The oblique popliteal liga-ment attaches to both the posterior joint capsule and the arcuate ligament [8]. The extensive distal insertion of semimembranosus makes it a marked contributor of stability to the knee [1]. Semiten-dinosus tendon joins with that of gracilis and sar-torius to form the most posterior and distal aspects of the pes anserinus [4, 9]. As these three tendons attach to the medial tibia, they form a shape said to resemble a goose's foot, hence its

C. Urbanek (✉)
Department of Family Medicine, East Carolina
University, Greenville, NC, USA
e-mail: urbanekc17@ecu.edu

C. McCrum
Department of Orthopedic Surgery, University of
Texas Southwestern, Dallas, TX, USA
e-mail: mccrumcl@upmc.edu

B. P. Lesniak · J. M. Doperak
Department of Orthopedic Surgery, University of
Pittsburgh, Pittsburgh, PA, USA
e-mail: lesniakbp@upmc.edu; doperakjm@upmc.edu

© Springer Nature Switzerland AG 2021
K. Onishi et al. (eds.), *Tendinopathy*, https://doi.org/10.1007/978-3-030-65335-4_12

literal Latin moniker. Deep to the pes anserinus lies the pes anserine bursa, a common site of irritation [10] (Fig. 12.1).

Distal hamstring pathology is varied, but, in general, injury commonly occurs at the myotendinous junction during an eccentric load. This is biomechanically more likely given the course over the hip and knee joint instead of only a solitary joint [1, 2]. Gait analysis with sprinters demonstrates risk of injury is highest with the hamstrings contracting eccentrically just before heel strike in a maximally lengthened position

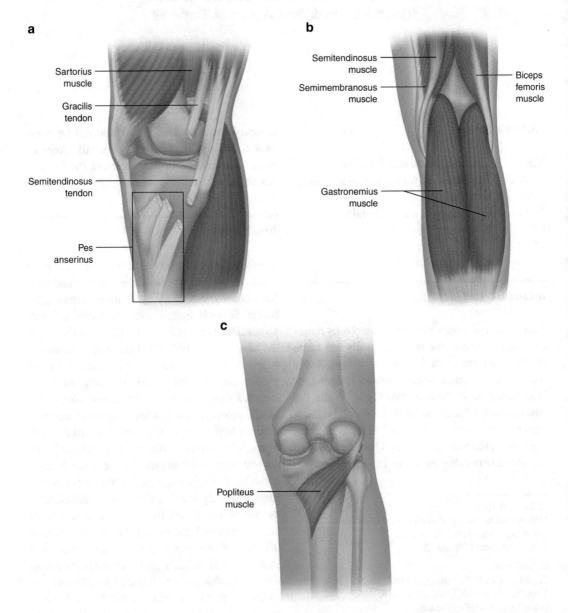

Fig. 12.1 Anatomy: (**a**) Medial knee depicting sartorius, gracilis, and semitendinosus tendons and their convergence on the tibia at the pes anserinus. (**b**) Posterior knee with relative positions of hamstring and gastrocnemius tendons and muscle. (**c**) Posterior knee depicting course of popliteus tendon and muscle

[3]. The one exception to this is the short head of the biceps femoris which, due to its origin just medial to the linea aspera, intermuscular septum, and lateral supracondylar line, only crosses the knee [1, 2, 6]. Innervation is also unique for the short head of the biceps femoris. All of the hamstring muscles are innervated by the tibial division of the sciatic nerve, except for the short head of the biceps femoris which is innervated by the peroneal branch. Dual innervation and potential resultant discordant muscular activation may be a reason as to why biceps femoris has the greatest rate of tears of the three hamstring muscles [6]. Muscle weakness is thought to predispose to injury in several ways. A classic teaching is that side-to-side hamstring strength discrepancy of >10 to 15% or a quadriceps-to-hamstring strength ratio of <0.6 places the athlete at greater risk [3]. However, meta-analysis looking at comparative strength testing at higher arc speeds demonstrates no greater risk [11]. Similarly, flexibility is controversial with some studies suggesting pre-season flexibility as a predictor of in-season injuries and other studies showing no correlation between passive or active range of motion and rate of injuries This remains an area of debate and need for ongoing research [3, 11]. The one risk factor almost unanimously agreed on is prior injury. Reinjury risk is not inconsequential at 12–31% [3]. Much like factors contributing to initial injury, the causes for reinjuries vary but include familiar mechanisms such as fatigue, strength imbalance, scar tissue formation, impaired flexibility, and incomplete rehabilitation among many others [12]. Finally, osteoarthritis has a strong association with pes anserine bursitis. In one study looking at symptomatic patients with knee osteoarthritis (OA), pes anserine bursitis was found as high as 20% when confirmed with musculoskeletal ultrasonography. Other studies without radiographic confirmation have found a correlation as high as 46% [13]. While there is some overlap between the posterior hamstring tendons and the pes anserinus via the semitendinosus, the pes anserinus will be discussed in greater detail later in this chapter.

Another tendinous injury to this region of human body includes pes anserine region tendinopathy. The pes anserinus refers to the anteromedial tibial attachment of the sartorius, gracilis, and semitendinosus tendons as they converge in roughly triangular arrangement reminiscent of a goose's foot. It is from this conjoined tendon's configuration that the complex derives its name [9, 10]. From proximal to distal the tendons insert linearly into the tibia: sartorius, gracilis, then semitendinosus [9, 10]. At this position, these muscles act first as flexors of the knee, but also as dynamic stabilizers controlling against valgus and external rotation stress [14]. Careful dissection studies have revealed that the tendon of sartorius integrates into the superficial fascial layer of the medial knee, whereas the tendons of gracilis and semitendinosus attach to the deep fascia [9, 10]. Accessory bands of the pes anserine tendons are not uncommon, particularly as found at the gracilis and semitendinosus tendons [10]. These can be bifid or trifid tendons that, while having little implication in the study of tendinopathy and bursopathy, may be considerations as the gracilis and semitendinosus can be harvested for utilization in anterior cruciate ligament (ACL) reconstruction [10]. Deep to the pes anserinus is the pes anserine bursa. Again, in studies utilizing careful dissection and injection of blue ink gelatin, the medial border is consistently at the insertion of the pes anserinus tendons with a roughly irregular circular shape spanning superior and posterior [10]. This superoposterior course has clinic significance as it takes the bursa close to the inferior fibers of the infrapatellar nerve, a structure that should be well avoided during injection of the bursa [10].

Irritation of the pes anserine tendons and/or the underlying bursa is typically referred to as pes anserinus tendinobursitis (PATB) or pes anserinus tendinobursitis syndrome [14]. This name exemplifies some of the knowledge gaps in the exact pathogenesis. It is unclear whether the pain syndrome is a tendinosis, a bursitis, or both [14, 15]. Better understanding of the etiology could be useful in understanding pathogenesis; however, studies to elucidate the risk factors for PATB are limited. It is suggested that PATB is more common in overweight females with concomitant knee osteoarthritis [14]. Mechanically, a wider pelvis and increased Q-angle would antagonize the pes anserine tendons potentially resulting in PATB. Some studies suggest that diabetes mellitus can be a predisposing factor [14]. One case–control study attempted to define the risk factors for PATB. Their findings confirmed that valgus deformity at the knee, with or without collateral instability, was a clear risk factor for PATB [15]. As the study used sex and age as matched variables, they were unable to determine how PATB was affected by those factors, but their data supports a distribution of PATB favoring older females [15]. They did not find a correlation between PATB and diabetes mellitus [15]. In these areas, more research is certainly needed. One area with clear association is concomitant knee osteoarthritis. Several recent studies have utilized diagnostic musculoskeletal ultrasound (US) to confirm the clinical diagnosis of PATB in patients with known OA [13, 16]. In one study, PATB prevalence was higher in symptomatic patients with knee OA than in symptomatic adults without OA at 20% versus 2.5% [13, 17]. Also noted was increasing bursal size associated with osteoarthritis grade [13]. Specific ultrasonographic changes will be discussed later in this section.

A third potential site of tendon injuries in this area is popliteal tendon injuries. The popliteus is a muscle located on the posterolateral aspect of the knee. The muscle originates within a depression on the anterior aspect of the lateral femoral condyle, posterior and distal to the lateral collateral ligament (LCL), and wraps around the lateral knee, beneath the LCL, to insert into the posteromedial aspect of the tibia. The arcuate ligament arises from the popliteus tendon, which can attach to the lateral meniscus or meniscofemoral ligaments. The muscle is innervated via a branch of the tibial nerve, which inserts on the deep surface of the popliteus muscle belly. Vascular supply is provided via a branch of the popliteal artery [18].

The popliteus mainly functions to unlock the knee, in order to allow for knee flexion. Contraction of the muscle when the knee is loaded leads to internal rotation of the tibia relative to the femur, and it is the only structure that has the mechanical

advantage to produce internal rotation of the tibia on the femur during gait. In addition, as a result of fibrous connections to the lateral meniscus or meniscofemoral ligament, it may also serve to control meniscal movement throughout knee range of motion [19–21].

Finally, the last group of tendons in this region is that of calf musculature. The posterior knee is the locale for the origin of the triceps surae musculature. The gastrocnemius, soleus, and plantaris muscles originate proximally, and provide power for plantarflexion at the ankle, while the gastrocnemius and plantaris are biarticular muscles that cross the knee, thus also contribute to knee flexion (Table 12.1).

The gastrocnemius muscle has two heads proximally, with the origin of the medial head on the medial condyle of the femur and the lateral head on the lateral femoral condyle, both proximal to the articular surface of the posterior condyles. This muscle is innervated via a branch from the tibial nerve, and it receives its vascular supply from tributaries of the sural artery. The plantaris muscle also crosses the knee and ankle joints. It originates on the lateral supracondylar ridge of the femur, just proximal to the origin of the lateral head of the gastrocnemius. Plantaris is innervated by tibial nerve, and the sural arteries provide arterial supply. Finally, the solus originates on the posterior fibula and medial border of the tibia, and it is innervated by the tibial nerve as well, although vascular supply is provided by a combination of the popliteal artery, posterior tibial artery, and peroneal artery. All three tendons insert on the posterior calcaneus, and they are found in the superficial posterior compartment of the leg [18].

Distal Hamstring Tendinopathy

A 22-year-old collegiate baseball player with no previous medical history presents with chief complaint of sudden onset posteromedial right knee pain. He was sprinting to the home base when he felt a sudden onset pain with a sense of "pop" two days ago. On examination, there is a focal swelling at the posterior medial tibial con-

Table 12.1 Anatomy of posterior knee

Muscle	Origin	Insertion	Innervation	Vascular supply
Semi-membranosis	Upper outer quadrant of ischial tuberosity	Posterior aspect of the medial condyle of the tibia	Tibial nerve	Branches from internal iliac, popliteal and profundal femoris artery
Semi-tendinosis	Upper inner quadrant of the Ischial tuberosity	Upper part of the medial surface of tibia	Tibial nerve	Branches from internal iliac, popliteal and profundal femoris artery
Bicep femoris	Upper inner Ischial tuberosity	Styloid process of fibula	Tibial nerve	Branches from internal iliac, popliteal and profundal femoris artery
Sartorius	Inferior portion of anterior inferior iliac spine	Medial tibia	Femoral nerve	Femoral artery
Gracilis	Lower half of pubis, pubic ramus and ischial ramus	Medial tibia	Obturator nerve	Obturator artery
Gastronemius	Medial head: medial condyle of femur Lateral head: lateral femoral condyle	Posterior calcaneus	Tibial nerve	Sural artery
Soleus	Posterior fibula and medial tibia	Posterior calcaneus	Tibial nerve	Popliteal, posterior tibial and peroneal artery
Plantaris	Lateral supercondylar ridge of femur	Posterior calcaneus	Tibial nerve	Sural artery
Popliteus	Lateral femoral condyle	Posterior medial tibia	Tibial nerve	Popliteal artery

dyle area and he notes some difficulty in flexing the knee due to a tenderness. On passive extension of the knee joint, he notes radiation of pain from the area of the tibial condyle to medial posterior mid-thigh. He denies a recent use of fluoroquinolones or a history of anabolic steroid use.

Clinical Presentation

Most athletes will complain of a sudden sharp pain in the posterior distal thigh with acute distal hamstring injuries. This can be associated with a sense of, or even audible, popping and is very similar to proximal and myotendinous junction hamstring injuries discussed in the previous chapter, with the exception of slightly distally located site of pain. This usually occurs during running, jumping, or kicking. There is usually an energetic, rapid stretch into hip flexion and knee extension or an eccentric load in that maximally stretched position [1–3]. Typically, they are limited in any further participation in their activity. Falling is not uncommon. Chronic or acute on chronic injuries can present with decreased motion, cramping, or a coarse, stiff gait in which they attempt to avoid concurrent hip flexion and knee extension [3].

Rupture of the distal hamstrings are particularly rare and usually associated with damage to the cruciate ligaments [5]. There is one case report of a professional football player with complete tearing of both the semimembranosus tendon and biceps femoris without involvement of the cruciate ligaments [5]. As this athlete denied use of fluoroquinolones and anabolic steroids which could increase the risk of tendon rupture, it further supports eccentric loading as the responsible mechanism [5].

In young endurance athletes and older individuals who present with insidious pain in the posterior medial knee, overuse semimembranosus tendinopathy needs to be considered in the differential diagnosis for medial knee pain [6].

Physical Examination

Initial assessment can start as early as watching the athlete walk as noted above. They will often favor the affected extremity with a rigid, stiff gait [3]. The entirety of the posterior thigh should be exposed to evaluate for ecchymosis. In minor acute injuries or in cases of overuse tendinopathy, there may be no ecchymosis, whereas avulsion or myotendinous injuries can have significant ecchymosis [3]. Palpation should start at the proximal origin and continue to the distal insertions evaluating for both pain and defect. It can be helpful to palpate for defect with the muscle relaxed and again under tension; even still, detecting defects can be difficult due to the deep nature of the muscles [1]. Comparing range of motion of the bilateral lower extremities at the hips and knees can be useful in defining injury and determining severity. Increased popliteal angle, assessed by flexing the hip to 90 and then passively extending the knee, associated with posterior thigh pain can indicate hamstring pathology [3]. Strength testing should also be compared bilaterally. An eccentric load can be recreated by positioning the patient in the prone position with the knee flexed to 90°. The patient actively flexes the knee while the examiner extends the knee to 30°. Positive findings while recreating the provocative mechanism may guide diagnosis [3]. There are three special tests that have demonstrated moderate to high validity in the diagnosis of hamstring tendinopathy and strain: the bent-knee stretch test, the modified bent-knee stretch test, and the Puranen-Orava test [3]. With the bent-knee stretch test, the patient is supine with the tested hip and knee in maximal flexion. The knee is then slowly passively extended. In the modified version, the patient is again supine with maximal hip and knee flexion. This time, however, the knee is rapidly passively extended. The Puranen–Orava test consists of the patient standing with the hip flexed at 90°. The knee is brought into active extension and maintained on a support. While the examinations are developed for proximal hamstring injuries originally, posterior thigh/distal thigh/knee pain may indicate distal hamstring tendinopathy [3].

Diagnostic Workup

X-Ray

Diagnosis of hamstring tendinopathy/tear can often be accomplished through history and physical examination; however, diagnostic imaging plays an important role in defining the extent of injury, evaluating associated structures for pathology, and prognosticating return to play. The initial study of choice has traditionally been X-ray. While plain film radiographs do not visualize pathologic tendon or muscle directly, they can be useful in evaluating for avulsion fractures. While these can occur at the insertions of all three distal hamstring tendons, semitendinosus avulsions are believed to be most common [7].

Musculoskeletal Ultrasound

With increasing access to portable or even pocketable units and improving resolution, musculoskeletal ultrasound (US) is becoming a more widely used imaging modality in the assessment of athletic injury. It offers the advantage of being able to evaluate muscular, tendinous, ligamentous, and osseous structures in a dynamic examination with immediate bilateral comparison if needed. Furthermore, it has no exposure to radiation and a lower cost than magnetic resonance imaging (MRI). Though there has not been direct comparison for distal hamstring tendon injuries, several studies have compared the accuracy of diagnostic ultrasound to MRI for proximal hamstring tendinopathy, generally resulting in comparable diagnostic accuracy [7]. US tended to have higher sensitivity during the acute phase and this phenomenon was attributed to the high sensitivity of US for fluid collections. Depth of injury generally affects ultrasonographic assessment though distal hamstring tendons are generally well visualized regardless of body habitus [7]. Doppler US can indicate inflammation, neovascularization, or healing; processes that may be associated with tendinopathy. No study has attempted return to play analysis for distal hamstring tendinopathy/tear.

Magnetic Resonance Imaging

MRI is the most widely used imaging modality in the assessment of hamstring injury. It is capable of evaluating deep tissues and bony edema regardless of habitus that may be associated with tendinopathy/tear [8]. Low-grade strains have a classic appearance of edema or hemorrhage at the myotendinous junction, around the intramuscular tendon, or surrounding the myofascial junction; this is best visualized on fat-suppressed T2-weighted sequences [8]. All fibers will be intact to qualify as a grade 1 strain. In the grade 2 injury pattern, muscle fiber disruption is apparent within T1 sequences [8]. Typically, the injury becomes occupied by hematoma [8]. While rare, a grade 3 strain is represented by complete disruption of the tendon or myotendinous junction [8]. Equally rare, distal avulsion injuries are best assessed with MRI and concomitant injuries such as anterior cruciate ligament (ACL) and posterior crucate ligament (PCL) injuries, osseous avulsions, posterolateral corner injuries, and joint effusion can be further evaluated [8]. Cohen et al. have developed a scoring system correlating extent of injury on MRI to time to return to play; however, their focus is on proximal hamstring pathology [22]. Based on 38 National Football League (NFL) athletes with acute hamstring strains, their novel MRI scoring system takes into consideration age, number of muscles involved, location, insertional involvement, percent cross-sectional injury, cm retraction, and cm long-axis T2 signal length [22]. Return to play was then organized into two main groups based on their score [22]. Rapid return to play, the first group, if score < 10 and would likely return in less than 1 week [22]. Prolonged recovery, the second group, if score > 15 and would return in greater than 2–3 weeks [22]. Scores between 10 and 15 fell in between [22]. An MRI-based grading system for distal hamstring tendon injury has not been published.

Treatment

Conservative

Management of distal hamstring tendon injury is dependent on an accurate diagnosis based on the above information. The type, timing, and extent of injury can dictate the appropriate treatment plan. For the vast majority of injuries, conservative management is sufficient in returning to play. While many studies demonstrate a reinjury rate as high as 31%, many of these do not differentiate between proximal, intramuscular, and distal injuries. There is no published data evaluating reinjury rate specific to the distal hamstring tendons. Still, a complete rehabilitation program is essential in the management of distal hamstring pathol-

ogy [3]. For minor injuries, activity modification, relative rest, non-steroidal anti-inflammatory drugs (NSAIDs), ice, or compression can treat or palliate symptoms. While NSAIDs may be commonly used to treat the pain associated with tendon injury, their role is not clearly defined. In vitro studies demonstrate an inhibitory effect by both ibuprofen and celecoxib on tendon cell migration and proliferation [23, 24]. Conversely, a rat study evaluating NSAIDs and tendon healing following Achilles tendon transection revealed an increase in maximum stress in the rats treated with parecoxib between days 6–14 [25]. Those treated with parecoxib for the first five days had decreased maximum stress and force-at-failure [25]. These findings may support a delayed initiation of NSAID therapy of at least six days post injury. Traditionally used therapeutic modalities like electrical stimulation and therapeutic ultrasound can be used as well. A randomized controlled trial with professional athletes looking at proximal hamstring tendinopathy demonstrated that shockwave therapy was a superior modality compared to treatment with NSAIDs, physiotherapy, and hamstring muscle group exercise program [26]. This could likely be extrapolated to distal hamstring tendinopathy as well. Considering that risks for reinjury include muscle strength discrepancy and flexibility limitation, physical therapy should be directed as correcting these deficiencies [3]. An eccentric strengthening program, while the mainstay of tendinopathy rehabilitation, will also address the core mechanical dysfunction associated with hamstring injuries. General conditioning, a seemingly obvious treatment, should not be overlooked as there is a correlation between fatigue and reinjury [12]. More severe injuries will take a longer time to heal and a slower progression initially. Crutches may be necessary to off-load the limb initially and prevent the particularly painful combination of hip flexion and knee extension. A compression wrap applied distal to proximal with elastic bandage (Ace™) can help reduce swelling. Rehab should progress slowly, first focusing on desensitization, then range of motion, eventually strength, and finally a sport-specific progression prior to return to play.

Interventional

More invasive options have been utilized for proximal hamstring tendon or intramuscular injuries, but none looking specifically at the distal hamstring tendon. A study out of the NFL has looked at intramuscular injection of corticosteroid as an early intervention that could prevent significant disability [27]. It is proposed that by disrupting the inflammatory response, those professional athletes studied were able to return to play sooner without any observed complications [27]. Theoretical risks include injection, post injection pain flare, fat atrophy, hypopigmentation, and with any peritendinous injection, risk of tendon rupture [27]. This treatment could be considered for distal hamstring tendon, particularly if involving a myotendinous junction component; however, there are no published studies evaluating this.

Hypertonic dextrose therapy or prolotherapy has gained popularity in the management of tendinopathies. There have been no dedicated studies looking at prolotherapy for the distal hamstring tendons. However, a recent well performed systematic review evaluated the effectiveness and safety of prolotherapy for lower limb tendinopathies/fasciopathies, specifically Achilles tendon, plantar fascia, and Osgood–Schlatter disease [28]. It is speculated that prolotherapy is effective by reversing the neovascularization of tendinosis and inducing wound healing to eliminate damaged tissues and form new collagen [28]. Of the eight studies in their review, no adverse effects were reported [28]. In the Achilles tendinopathy group, there was moderate evidence of improved pain with associated patient satisfaction [28]. Ultrasound assessment correlated with their subjective improvement [28]. Likewise, in the plantar fasciitis group 80% of the patients had good to excellent outcomes in pain reduction [28]. In the sole Osgood–Schlatter study, prolotherapy was superior to lidocaine injection with 67% of the prolotherapy group returning to asymptomatic sport participation at 3 months compared to only 23% of the lidocaine group [28]. Applying these findings to the distal hamstring tendons, prolotherapy too would be an option to promote tendon healing without significant adverse effects. More research specific to management of distal hamstring pathology with dextrose prolotherapy is needed.

This author is unaware of published data specifically for platelet-rich plasma (PRP) in distal hamstring injury. However, a meta-analysis of 16 randomized controlled trials by Miller et al. in 2017 concluded that injection of PRP is more efficacious than control injections in patients with symptomatic tendinopathy [29]. While this meta-analysis did assess PRP composition for neutrophil content (comparing leukocyte count to whole blood), their findings did not report efficacy difference between neutrophil-rich or neutrophil-poor preparations [29]. Studies on PRP are promising, but as of yet there are no level 1 studies with long-term follow-up for the distal hamstrings. Further research is certainly needed.

Operative

Surgical intervention for distal hamstring injuries is a rare event and has been reserved for tendon ruptures. In one study looking at 25 distal semitendinosus tendon ruptures in elite-level athletes, all of them received conservative management; 42% ultimately required surgery [30]. Furthermore, operative management essentially cut recovery time in half [30]. Another case study and literature review described a semimembranosus tendon rupture and biceps femoris avulsion fracture of the conjoint attachment of the LCL [5]. While semimembranosus ruptures are commonly associated with injuries to the cruciate ligaments, in this case there was no intra-articular damage following an isolated hyperextension injury [5]. In this somewhat unique case, surgical repair is directed at solely at the hamstring tendons without having to consider cruciate reconstruction [5]. Initially the lateral aspect is approached by identifying and protecting the peroneal nerve [5]. Popliteus insertion and LCL origin are exposed and evaluated for integrity [5]. Primary repair of the biceps femoris is performed using suture anchors within the fracture donor site of the fibula [5]. Posteromedially, the semimembranosus is identified along with its distal, fanned insertion [5]. The two ends are approximated and primary repair performed via high-tensile sutures [5]. Immobilization is maintained with the knee in 90° of flexion for 2 weeks before unlocking [5]. Passive full extension should be achieved by 4 weeks [5]. Strengthening can begin by 8 weeks [5]. Once full range of motion (ROM) is painless and strength is symmetric, the athlete can initiate a sport-specific rehab program [5].

Pes Anserinus Tendinopathy

A 62-year-old female who enjoys hiking with a known history of left moderate tricompartmental osteoarthrosis presents with 2-month history of increased pain at left medial knee. On further history, her pain is in the area slightly distal to the joint line and pain increases with palpation as well as resisted knee flexion.

Clinical Presentation

The typical PATB patient will often present with anteromedial or posteromedial knee pain which is worse with ascending or descending stairs [14, 17]. There may be a preceding blunt trauma to the area or a history of repetitive stress as is common with distance runners [17]. They may report swelling in the area of the pes anserinus insertion, but this is not always present [14]. Diagnostic criteria for PATB was first described in 1985 by Larson and Baum consisting of: anteromedial knee pain worse with going up, pain and stiffness in the morning lasting up to 1 hour, difficulty with arising from a chair or car, night pain, and difficulty bending the knee along with tenderness over the area of the pes anserine bursa [14]. This constitution of symptoms remains accurate in the description of PATB.

Physical Examination

Similar to the clinic presentation, the examiner will note tenderness over the pes anserinus, with or without accompanying edema from the underlying bursa. There may be pain with both active and passive motion of the knee as the tendons rub against the inflamed bursa. Strength testing with flexion and adduction may be

impaired secondary to effort in the setting of pain. Ligamentous and neurological testing of the knee is unrevealing.

Diagnostics

Laboratory
While not necessary for diagnosis, aspiration of bursal fluid typically reveals an aseptic aspirate without inflammatory cells or with mononuclear cells and no crystals [14].

X-Ray
Plain film radiographs may demonstrate arthritic changes, typically of the medial compartment, but without overt indication of tendinopathy or bursitis [14]. Often the first imaging modality, for perhaps no logical reasons other than the fact that X-ray was the initial orthopedic imaging historically, is typically unrevealing for the diagnosis of PATB except to demonstrate the presence or absence of underlying knee OA.

Musculoskeletal Ultrasound
Utilization of ultrasound is becoming a more popular imaging modality due to its lower cost, more immediate application with ability to compare bilaterally, and lack of ionizing radiation. In normal ultrasound evaluation of the pes anserinus, the tendons demonstrate a uniform fibrillar echotexture without thickening (Fig. 12.2a, b). The underlying bursa is not distended and typically not visualized. Ultrasound findings of PATB consist of loss of fibrillar echotexture and thickening of the pes anserine tendons [16, 31]. Bursal fluid appears anechoic below the tendons [31]. However, these changes are not consistently present in patients with clinically diagnosed PATB. In a study looking at patients with symptomatic knee OA with radiographic findings and clinical symptoms of PATB, only 7.7% of patients demonstrate sonographic changes consistent with PATB [31]. A similar study in patients with clinical and radiographic knee OA and a clinical diagnosis of PATB, 25.1% of the patients with both knee OA and PATB had findings of bursopathy [16]. Sample size and presence of

Fig. 12.2 Ultrasound images: (**a**) Sagittal oblique view of normal pes anserinus tendons superficial to distal fibers of MCL (arrow). Tendons of sartorius (open arrow), gracilis (arrowheads), and semitendinosus (open arrowheads) may appear anisotropic due to their curvature around the medial proximal tibia. (**b**) Transverse view of normal pes anserinus tendons (arrows, primarily sartorius) seen in long axis inserting on medial proximal tibia

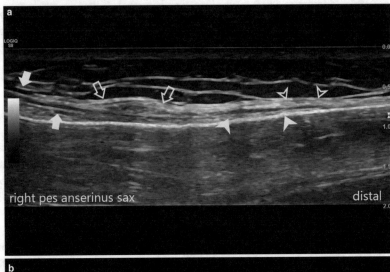

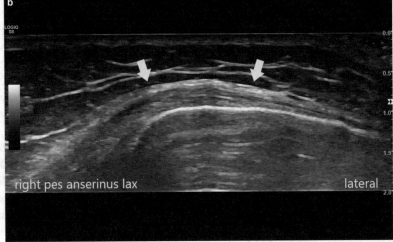

PATB symptoms may result in differing outcomes compared to the study that found a prevalence of PATB of 20% in knee OA patients without PATB symptoms [13].

Magnetic Resonance Imaging

Magnetic resonance imaging (MRI) can be utilized as an additional means of evaluating PATB. Beyond this, it is a useful tool in differentiating other causes of pain and swelling from PATB. MRI has the ability to evaluate deeper knee structures and can be complimentary to ultrasound. In acute PATB, high-intensity signal deep to or interdigitating between the pes anser-

ine tendons best seen in T2 sequences is a classic finding [32]. This of course occurs in the absence of any communication between the cystic structure and the joint, and when there is no damage to the medial meniscus or medial collateral ligament (MCL) [32, 33]. The bursa often demonstrates a heterogeneous signal intensity accompanied by synovial thickening [33]. Fluid signal intensity can help differentiate from other cystic structures such as pigmented villonodular synovitis (PVNS) which will have low intensity due to hemosiderin content or synovial hemangiomas [33].

Treatment

Conservative

Treatment for PATB is wholly conservative. Early treatment can begin with activity modification, relative rest, ice, and NSAIDs. While the etiologic contributors are not entirely understood, suspected risk factors should be mitigated wherever possible. Weight loss should be encouraged if body mass index (BMI) is greater than 25. Emphasis should be placed on blood sugar control with diabetic patients. Those with osteoarthritis should engage in tolerated exercises. Medial unloader braces may be utilized for medial compartment arthropathy.

Interventional

Beyond initial conservative measures, injectable corticosteroid can provide notable relief. In one study comparing bursal injection of corticosteroid to naproxen, the steroid group reported 70% significant improvement and 30% resolution at 1 month compared to 58% and 5% respectively in the naproxen group [14]. Another study was able to demonstrate both a reduction in pain and an improvement in ultrasonographic findings following corticosteroid injection [31].

Given the superficial location of the pes anserine bursa, the injection is relatively straight forward. However, accuracy of landmark guided injection is surprisingly poor relative to an ultrasound guided approach. In a study comparing the two techniques as performed by an experienced physiatrist, accuracy with ultrasound was between 92 and 100% compared to "blind" at 17–50% [34]. With this degree of accuracy disparity, it is recommended to utilize ultrasound guided injection regardless of the injectate so long as the appropriate equipment and training is available.

Similar to the previously discussed management of distal hamstring tendinopathy, there are no published studies on utilization of prolotherapy specific to the pes anserinus. Again, many studies looking at the efficacy and safety of prolotherapy on other tendons can be utilized in consideration for clinical application. There is, however, one published study on the use of intrabursal diclofenac injection. One group received nine 1 mL injections of diclofenac three times per week (mesotherapy dosing), the other group received 50 mg PO diclofenac daily for 3 weeks [35]. Both groups had a decrease in pain, but only the mesotherapy group had ultrasonographic improvement [35].

Platelet rich plasma may also be an effective injectate in the treatment of PATB. A military study looking at the utility of PRP for chronic PATB found that 84.8% of their subjects had complete or near-complete pain relief by 6 months [36]. No adverse reactions were reported [36]. While ongoing studies and standardized protocols are needed for PRP, this appears to be a promising option.

Operative Management

While there may be consideration of arthroscopic debridement or bursectomy, there are no published studies demonstrating surgical benefit for acute or chronic PATB.

Popliteus Tendon Tendinopathy

A 21-year-old male soccer player presents with a 3-month history of posterolateral knee pain that started during a match suddenly. He describes the event where he was going for a 50/50 ball when his knee hyperextended and externally rotated when going for a 50/50 ball. He was noted to have gait abnormality immediately, and developed posterolateral knee region swelling. On examination in the clinic, he complains of palpation tenderness at lateral knee although he has no laxity with varus stress of the knee. There was no PCL laxity and dial test was negative.

Clinical Presentations

Injury to the popliteus tendon occurs along a spectrum, ranging from simple tendinitis through complete rupture of the tendon. Chronic overuse can lead to tendinitis. Trauma can also lead to a rupture of the popliteus tendon, generally through a forced hyperextension or external rotation mechanism [37, 38], although injuries to this tendon are most often seen in conjunction to injury to the remainder of the posterolateral knee structures [39], with less than 10% of popliteal ruptures occurring in isolation [7, 39].

Popliteal tendon rupture can present with a clinically benign history, with no evidence of trauma, or following an acute trauma, such as a forced hyperextension or forced external rotation of the knee. Generally, patients present with symptoms similar to those of a lateral meniscal injury. Patients often note persistent laterally based knee pain with effusion. Pain is often more pronounced with stairs and squats [37].

Patients with snapping popliteal tendon generally present with a spontaneous onset of snapping over the posterolateral aspect of the knee. Snapping popliteus tendon syndrome generally presents in a young, active patient population, most often found in runners. This can either occur insidiously or following a twisting injury to the knee, or even knee to knee collisions, such as those occur in ice hockey [40].

Physical Examination

Examination of patients with tendinitis of the popliteus or snapping popliteus tendon often has no effusion or ligament instability. With either of these injuries, there can be lateral tenderness along the popliteal tendon. Snapping popliteal tendon can be noted through palpation between the lateral epicondyle and lateral joint line, most commonly while varus load is applied to the knee (such as in figure-of-4 position) and bringing the knee into extension. The pop generally occurs around 20–30° flexion [40].

Partial tearing or complete avulsion of the popliteal tendon may be found in conjunction with a hemarthrosis, as only a thin synovial membrane separates the tendon from the joint [38, 41]. When evaluating knee stability of these patients, there is no increased laxity to anterior or posterior drawer or Lachman testing, no pivot shift instability, and no increased laxity on dial testing, as these tests would only be positive in the context of a more profound ligamentous injury to the knee. Patients may be tender to palpation over the lateral joint line, and this may extend to the lateral femoral condyle, along the path of the tendon [38]. Passive external rotation of the tibia on the femur may produce pain. Garrick and Webb describe an active functional test (Garrick's Test) in which the hip and knee of a supine patient is flexed to 90°, the leg is internally rotated, and the patient is instructed to oppose the external rotation force of the physician [42]. Pain or inability to maintain this position would suggest popliteus injury.

Diagnostic Workup

X-Ray

Standard radiographs, including anteroposterior (AP) and lateral views of the knee, should be the first step in evaluating this injury with imaging. In addition to providing information on the presence or absence of degenerative changes, radiographs may also show an avulsed fragment of the lateral condyle with complete avulsion of the popliteus [41, 43].

Ultrasound

Ultrasonography can also be used for assessment of the popliteal tendon. Placing the ultrasound probe along the lateral-proximal to medial-distal axis at the level of the popliteus tendon provides a view of the tendon, which can be followed to evaluate for differences in thickness or an absence of continuity of the tendon [44]. Ultrasound provides a 33%, 100%, 100%, 33%, and 50% sensitivity, specificity, negative predictive value, positive predictive value, and accuracy, respectively, with regard to popliteal tendon injuries [45]. Furthermore, dynamic examination can help diagnose snapping of the popliteal tendon over the lateral femoral condyle [46].

Magnetic Resonance Imaging

While MRI can often be negative in the case of snapping popliteus tendon syndrome [40], MRI scan is helpful in providing a definitive diagnosis of injury to the popliteus. Some authors suggest that a coronal oblique plane is best utilized to achieve optimal visualization of the popliteus tendon [47]. The appearance of this tendon varies based on the degree of damage to this structure. Complete tears of the popliteus tendon can be noted by an interruption of the course of the tendon from its origin to insertion, which appears on the scan as a retracted mass of tendon that is surrounded by fluid. Partial injury to the tendon may appear as irregular contour of the tendon, with high-signal intensity edema around the tendon [47]. Additionally, since only fat should be found behind the popliteus tendon, fluid in this area suggests a capsular injury with fluid in the popliteal bursa [48]. The majority of injuries to the popliteal occur in the muscular or musculotendinous area of the popliteus, so edema or disorganized muscle fibers in this area with high signal intensity changes are suggestive of injury [38].

Treatments

Conservative

Tendinopathy of the popliteal tendon is most commonly treated with simple conservative management. Non-steroidal anti-inflammatory medications can be used for pain control, and activity modification should take place to avoid exacerbating activities, specifically running and plyometric sports. A therapy course can be utilized, with focus on eccentric strengthening of the quadriceps, as well as focus on stretching the hamstrings and posterior structures of the knee, in order to help reduce the strain on the popliteus [49]. Snapping popliteus tendon syndrome can most often be successfully treated with similar methods, by simply resting patients and avoiding aggravating activities [40].

Interventional

Injection of a strained popliteus has been advocated in select, refractory cases. Generally, this procedure is done under ultrasound, which results in a high degree of accuracy of the injection. Injection of steroid has been shown to provide reliable pain relief in otherwise refractory cases [44, 50].

Conservative treatment of isolated popliteal tendon ruptures can often provide good outcomes

without reconstruction [41, 51], even in the context of professional athletes [52]. Following a short period of immobilization, patients should undergo a therapy program with focus on minimizing strain on the popliteus as described above.

Operative

Snapping popliteus and tendinitis of the popliteus lack surgical indication, and surgery is rarely indicated for isolated injury of the popliteus tendon, especially outside of the context of injury to the posterolateral corner of the knee. However, in the context of an acute, complete rupture of the popliteus, some suggest operative management with arthroscopy and primary repair of the avulsed popliteus [37, 41].

If a patient has been taken to the operating room for arthroscopy, popliteus rupture can be noted during routine arthroscopy, where the lateral gutter and popliteal hiatus should be closely evaluated. This structure can be noted in the popliteal hiatus in the posterolateral aspect of the lateral compartment of the knee [52]. However, given less than 50% of the tendon length can be noted arthroscopically, and the femoral insertion and musculoskeletal junction cannot be evaluated arthroscopically, arthroscopic evaluation alone is not sufficient to rule out injury to this structure [53]. Probing the popliteus tendon arthroscopically may increase the sensitivity of arthroscopy, as this technique may demonstrate laxity of the popliteus tendon [41].

Once the tendon injury has been confirmed, an incision may be made laterally over the lateral condyle of the femur. The iliotibial (IT) band is sharply split to expose the lateral condyle, and the avulsed popliteus tendon is identified, often retracted medially toward the insertion. There may be an avulsed bony fragment attached to the tendon. If there is an avulsed bony fragment, this may be reduced and fixed with a screw [41]. Alternatively, suture anchors can be utilized to reduce and fix the tendon to the anatomic insertion site on the lateral femoral condyle, especially if there is insufficient bone to allow for screw fixation [39].

In the context of snapping popliteus tendon syndrome, surgical exploration reveals the popliteal tendon to appear grossly normal or thickened. Confirmation of diagnosis can be done by visualizing the tendon snap over the lateral femoral condyle when the knee is brought into extension. Treatment can consist of either releasing the popliteus tendon from its origin on the lateral femoral condyle and tenodesing the tendon to the proximal aspect of the fibular collateral ligament via non-absorbable suture, or simply resecting the popliteus tendon [54].

Proximal Triceps Surae Tendon Tendinopathy

A 31-year-old jiu jitsu practitioner experienced severe sharp posterior knee pain in his support leg when posting for a kick 3 months ago and he presents today as the posterior knee pain had not improved. He reports it felt "like he got shot in the back of the calf." He noted some swelling over posterior knee and calf area then. Despite pain, he continued to compete/practice. He presents with limp and difficulty with resisted plantar flexion and pain in posterior knee with stretching of triceps surae muscles.

Clinical Presentation

The most common condition affecting these structures proximally is "tennis leg", first described in 1883 as "Lawn Tennis Leg" [55], which is a condition described by rupture of either the medial head of the gastrocnemius or rupture of the plantaris, although the lateral head can be injured as well [56]. When examining the etiology of proximal calf strains and tears, the gastrocnemius is injured in about 49% of cases (with the medial head composing 95% of these injuries compared with only 5% lateral head injuries), while the soleus was involved in 46.2% of cases and the plantaris in only 5% of cases. Furthermore, multiple muscles are injured in >60% of cases [57].

Although the most common presentation of "tennis leg" is an acute tearing sensation in the proximal posterior calf, generally during jumping or sprinting, about 20% of patients may experience prodromal calf soreness before injury. Athletes who train more frequently or with high-tempo activities are more susceptible to injury, as fatigue or overtraining may play a role in this condition [56]. Master athletes, and moreover "weekend warriors," are more likely to sustain injury to the proximal calf muscles than their younger or less active counterparts, specifically those athletes between 30 and 50 years old [58].

While the above muscular injuries are by far the most common injuries to the proximal gastrocnemius, few case reports exist demonstrating calcification with and without tendinopathy [59, 60]. Tendon calcification may be as high as 31.9% in patients with calcium pyrophosphate deposition disease (CPPD) [61]. With similarly low reported cases in literature, isolated tendon tear or avulsion injuries can occur with similar mechanisms as described above [62, 63]. There is a relative paucity of data on proximal gastrocnemius tendon injuries.

Physical Examination

Physical examination should include a full examination of the knee and neurovascular structures of the leg. Knee examination should reveal stability of the knee in all planes, without joint line pain or mechanical symptoms. Mild injury to the proximal triceps surae generally present with pain posteriorly on the calf, up to the insertion of the effected muscle. The clinician should note whether pain is localized medially or laterally proximally (associated with proximal gastrocnemius injury), deep and distal (associated with soleus injury), or between the heads of the gastrocnemius (may be associated with injury to the plantaris). Mechanism of injury may also vary between the muscle injured, with gastrocnemius and plantaris injury most often occurring with an eccentric calf contraction with the ankle flexed and the knee extended, and the soleus most commonly is injured due to repetitive dorsiflexion with the knee bent [56].

Patients with injury to the proximal calf may walk with a plantarflexed ankle or bent knee, in order to minimize strain across the injured muscle [64]. More severe injury, such as complete rupture of a head of the gastrocnemius, may present with a palpable defect in the muscle. Furthermore, severe injury may present with an impressive amount of ecchymosis and swelling. Strength testing can be performed by both manual evaluation of ankle plantarflexion and knee extension, as well as asking the patient to perform single leg heel raises [56].

Importantly, care should be taken if a patient appears to have pain out of proportion to their mechanism on injury on examination, especially in the context of calf swelling. Rarely, rupture of the medial head of the gastrocnemius can be accompanied by injury to the supplying arterial structures and can lead to a compartment syndrome. Suspicion for this condition should be high, if in addition to severe pain, patients have pain with passive range of motion of the ankles and toes. This condition necessitates immediate diagnosis, which can be confirmed via compartment pressure measuring, indicated by difference in compartment pressure of <20 mmHg compared to the diastolic blood pressure. This condition is treated by emergent fasciotomy of the effected compartment(s), while delayed treatment or missed diagnosis can lead to complete functional loss of the affected compartments, including insensate nerves and necrosis of the musculature [65–67]. Additionally, venous thromboembolism can present with similar symptoms of calf swelling and pain, and should be considered when evaluating patients with these symptoms [56].

Diagnostic Imaging

X-Ray
Since standard plain radiographs are likely to be negative in the context of injury to the proximal calf, this modality of imaging may not be routinely obtained for evaluation of these injuries.

Ultrasound
Ultrasonography, however, has been shown to have excellent sensitivity and specificity with regard to confirming the diagnosis of injury to the proximal calf, with sensitivity and specificity similar to that of MRI [14]. With injury, ultrasound may reveal diffuse hypoechoic changes to the injured muscle, disruption of normal fiber patterns, and localized hypoechoic changes surrounding the injury [56]. Ultrasound evaluation can provide additional utility, as one can examine for the presence of deep vein thrombosis. However, the reliability of ultrasound is operator dependent.

Magnetic Resonance Imaging
MRI scan can also evaluate proximal calf injuries, and may be able to reveal lesions missed by ultrasound and provide a more accurate assessment of the extent of injury. High signal intensity fluid will be noted around the injured structures in both partial and complete injuries, and can extend into the superficial posterior compartment, signifying the presence of a hematoma (Fig. 12.3). Furthermore, complete injury may show dissociation at the musculotendinous junction of the muscle or an avulsion from the proximal origin of the injured muscle [68].

Unfortunately, MRI and ultrasound are not useful in predicting return to play or assessing the risk for re-injury. Although athletes may be held from competition until physical exam and imaging normalizes, some athletes are able to return to competition and training without any issues, despite persistent abnormal imaging [69].

Treatments

Conservative
The vast majority of injuries to the proximal calf resolve with simple conservative management. Acute injuries are immediately managed with rest, ice, elevation, and compression, which encourage minimal hematoma formation and help promote early healing [56]. Furthermore, compression sleeves may help alleviate symptoms and help minimize swelling, and may even speed return to running, especially if initiated early in treatment [70].

More severe injuries can be managed early with a walking boot with heel lifts, in order to reduce the strain at the injury site. However,

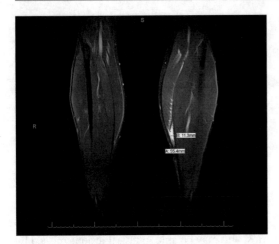

Fig. 12.3 MRI of a medial gastrocnemius tear

when patients can walk with no limp, these devices should be discontinued, in order to prevent stiffness during and following recovery [56].

Therapy begins with gentle stretching after recovery from the initial injury, generally at about 2 weeks. The cornerstone of physical therapy for any calf injury is eccentric strengthening of the calf as healing allows. A course of therapy will also work on achieving improved hamstring flexibility, as tightness can pre-dispose to recurrent injury [71].

Return to sports can range between weeks and 3 to 4 months, depending on the severity of injury. Return is based on regaining calf strength, as measured by single leg raises, as well as ability to run pain free without a limp [56].

Operative

Surgery for injury to the medial head of the gastrocnemius is rarely indicated. The majority of injuries heal uneventfully. Furthermore, several reports have suggested that chronic injuries that do not respond to conservative management may be successfully treated with surgery [71, 72]. In order to do so, an incision is made longitudinally over the posterior calf, and the sural nerve is identified and protected. The scarred tendon of the medial head of the gastrocnemius is identified and elevated. A Z-lengthening of the tendon can be performed if extra length is needed to reach the insertion on the posterior medial condyle, and can be attached with suture anchors. Postoperatively,

the foot is splinted in plantarflexion, and heel lifts are then placed and progressively removed at 2 weeks postoperatively, at which point they are then gradually advanced to eccentric strengthening and return to sport [71].

References

1. Clanton T, Coupe K. Hamstring strains in athletes: diagnosis and treatment. J Am Acad Orthop Surg. 1998;6:237–48.
2. Ali K, Leland J. Hamstring strains and tears in the athlete. Clin Sports Med. 2012;31(2):263–72.
3. Ahmad C, Redler L, Ciccotti M, Maffulli N, Longo U, Bradley J. Evaluation and management of hamstring injuries. Am J Sports Med. 2013;41(12):2933–47.
4. Lempaninen L, Sarimo J, Mattila K, Heikkila J, Orava S. Distal tears of the hamstring muscles: review of the literature and our results of surgical treatment. Br J Sports Med. 2007;41:80–3.
5. Aldebeyan S, Boily M, Martineau P. Complete tear of the distal hamstring tendons in a professional football player: a case report and review of the literature. Skeletal Radiol. 2016;45:427–30.
6. Bylund W, DeWeber K. Semimembranosus tendinopathy one cause of chronic posteriormedial knee pain. Sports Health. 2010;2(5):380–4.
7. Koulouris G, Connell D. Hamstring muscle complex: an imaging review. Radiographics. 2005;25:571–86.
8. Rubin D. Imaging diagnosis and prognostication of hamstring injuries. AJR. 2012;199:525–33.
9. LaPrade R, Engebretsen A, Ly T, Johansen S, Wentorf F, Engebretsen L. The anatomy of the medial part of the knee. J Bone Joint Surg Am. 2007;89:2000–10.
10. Lee J, Kim K, Jeong Y, Lee N, Han S, Lee C, Kim K, Han S. Pes anserinus and anserine bursa: anatomical study. Anat Cell Biol. 2014;47:127–31.
11. Freckleton G, Pizzari T. Risk factors for hamstring muscle strain injury in sport: a systematic review and meta-analysis. Br J Sports Med. 2013;47:351–8.
12. Croisier J. Factors associated with recurrent hamstring injuries. Sports Med. 2004;34(10):681–95.
13. Uysal F, Akbal A, Gokmen F, Adam G, Resorlu M. Prevalence of pes anserine bursitis in symptomatic osteoarthritis patients: an ultrasonographic prospective study. Clin Rhematol. 2015;34:529–33.
14. Helfenstein M, Kuromoto J. Anserine syndrome. Rev Bras Reumatol. 2010;50(3):313–27.
15. Alvarez-Nemegyei J. Risk factors for pes anserinus tendinitis/bursitis syndrome: a case control study. J Clin Rheumatol. 2007;13(2):63–5.
16. Toktas H, Dundar U, Adar S, Solak O, Ulasli A. Ultrasonographic assessment of pes anserinus tendon and pes anserinus tendinitis bursitis syndrome in patients with knee osteoarthritis. Mod Rheumatol. 2015;25(1):128–33.

17. Rennie W, Saifuddin A. Pes anserine bursitis: incidence in symptomatic knees and clinical presentation. Skeletal Radiol. 2005;34(7):395–8.
18. Scott WN. Insall & Scott surgery of the knee. Philadelphia: Elsevier; 2018.
19. Basmajian J, Lovejoy J. Functions of the popliteus muscle in man. A multifactorial electromyographic study. J Bone Joint Surg Am. 1971;53(3):557–62.
20. Jones C, Keene G, Christie A. The popliteus as a retractor of the lateral meniscus of the knee. Arthroscopy. 1995;11(3):270–4.
21. Mann R, Hagy J. The popliteus muscle. J Bone Joint Surg Am. 1977;59(7):924–7.
22. Cohen S, Towers J, Zoga A, Irrgang J, Makda J. Hamstring injuries in professional football players: magnetic resonance imaging correlation with return to play. Sports Health. 2011;3(5):423–30.
23. Tsai WC, Hsu CC, Chen CP, Chen MJ, Lin MS, Pang JH. Ibuprofen inhibition of tendon cell migration and down-regulation of paxillin expression. J Orthop Res. 2006;24:551–8.
24. Tsai WC, Hsu CC, Chou SW, Chung CY, Chen J, Pang JH. Effects of celecoxib on migration, proliferation and collagen expression of tendon cells. Connect Tissue Res. 2007;48:46–51.
25. Virchenko O, Skoglund B, Aspenberg P. Parecoxib impairs early tendon repair but improves later remodeling. Am J Sports Med. 2004;32:1743–7.
26. Cacchio A, Rompe JD, Furia JP, Susi P, Santilli V, De Paulis F. Shockwave therapy for the treatment of chronic proximal hamstring tendinopathy in professional athletes. Am J Sports Med. 2011;39(1):146–53.
27. Levine W, Bergeld J, Tessendorf W, Moorman C. Intramuscular corticosteroid injection for hamstring injuries. A 13-year experience in the National Football League. Am J Sports Med. 2000;20(3):297–300.
28. Sanderson L, Bryan A. Effectiveness and safety of prolotherapy injections for management of lower limb tendinopathy and fasciopathy: a systematic review. J Foot Ankle Res. 2015;8:57.
29. Miller LE, et al. Efficacy of platelet-rich plasma injections for symptomatic tendinopathy: systemic review and meta-analysis of randomized injection-controlled trials. BMJ Open Sport Exerc Med. 2017;3(1)
30. Cooper D, Conway J. Distal semitendinosus ruptures in elite-level athletes; low success rates of nonoperative treatment. Am J Sports Med. 2010;38(6):1174–8.
31. Yoon H, Kim S, Suh Y, Seo Y, Kim H. Correlation between ultrasonographic findings and the response to corticosteroid injection in pes anserinus tendinobursitis syndrome in knee osteoarthritis patients. J Korean Med Sci. 2005;20(1):109–12.
32. Forbes J, Helms C, Janzen D. Acute pes anserine bursitis: MR imaging. Radiology. 1995;194(2):525–7.
33. McCarthy C, McNally E. The MRI appearance of cystic lesions around the knee. Skeletal Radiol. 2004;33(4):187–209.
34. Finnoff J, Nutz D, Henning P, Hollman J, Smith J. Accuracy of ultrasound-guided versus unguided pes anserinus bursa injections. PM&R. 2010;2(8):732–9.
35. Saggini R, Di Stefano A, Dodaj I, Scarcello L, Bellomo R. Pes anserine bursitis in symptomatic osteoarthritis patients: a mesotherapy treatment study. J Altern Complement Med. 2015;21(8):480–4.
36. Rowicki K, Płomiński J, Bachta A. Evaluation of the effectiveness of platelet rich plasma in treatment of chronic pes anserinus pain syndrome. Ortop Traumatol Rehabil. 2014;16(3):307–3018.
37. Davalos E, Barank D, Varma R. Two cases of chronic knee pain caused by unusual injuries to the popliteus tendon. Joints. 2016;4(1):62–4.
38. Guha A, Gorgees K, Walker D. Popliteus tendon rupture: a case report and review of the literature. Br J Sports Med. 2003;37(4):358–60.
39. Recondo J, Salvador E, Villanúa J, Barrera M, Gervás C, Alústiza J. Lateral stabilizing structures of the knee: functional anatomy and injuries assessed with MR imaging. Radiographics. 2000;20:S91–S102.
40. Cooper D. Snapping popliteus tendon syndrome. A cause of mechanical knee popping in athletes. Am J Sports Med. 1999;27(5):671–4.
41. Naver L, Aalberg J. Avulsion of the popliteus tendon. A rare cause of chondral fracture and hemarthrosis. Am J Sports Med. 1985;13(6):423–4.
42. Garrick JG, Webb DR. Sports injuries: diagnosis and management. Philadelphia: WB Saunders; 1990:251–256.
43. Nakhostine M, Perko M, Cross M. Isolated avulsion of the popliteus tendon. J Bone Joint Surg Br. 1995;77(2):242–4.
44. Chang K-V, Hsiao M-Y, Hung C-Y, Özçakar L. An uncommon cause of posterior knee pain: diagnosis and injection for popliteus strain using ultrasonography. Pain Med. 2016;17(4):795–6.
45. Sekiya J, Swaringen J, Wojtys E, Jacobson J. Diagnostic ultrasound evaluation of posterolateral corner knee injuries. Arthroscopy. 2010;26(4):494–9.
46. Shukla D, Levy B, Kuzma S, Stuart M. Snapping popliteus tendon within an osteochondritis dissecans lesion: an unusual case of lateral knee pain. Am J Orthop (Belle Mead NJ). 2014;43(9):E210–3.
47. Yu JS, Salonen DC, Hodler J, Haghighi P, Trudell D, Resnick D. Posterolateral aspect of the knee: improved MR imaging with a coronal oblique technique. Radiology. 1996;198(1):199–204.
48. Deutsch A, Mink J. Magnetic resonance imaging of musculoskeletal injuries. Radiol Clin North Am. 1989;27(5):983–1002.
49. Petsche T, Selesnick F. Popliteus tendinitis: tips for diagnosis and management. Phys Sportsmed. 2002;30(8):27–31.
50. Smith J, Finnoff J, Santaella-Sante B, Henning T, Levy B, Lai J. Sonographically guided popliteus tendon sheath injection: techniques and accuracy. J Ultrasound Med. 2010;29(5):775–82.
51. Gruel J. Isolated avulsion of the popliteus tendon. Arthroscopy. 1990;6(2):94–5.
52. Burstein D, Fischer D. Isolated rupture of the popliteus tendon in a professional athlete. Arthroscopy. 1990;6(3):238–41.

53. Ferrari D. Arthroscopic evaluation of the popliteus: clues to posterolateral laxity. Arthroscopy. 2005;21(6):721–6.

54. Westrich G, Hannafin J, Potter H. Isolated rupture and repair of the popliteus tendon. Arthroscopy. 1995;11(5):628–32.

55. Fineberg M, Duquin T, Axelrod J. Arthroscopic visualization of the popliteus tendon. Arthroscopy. 2008;24(2):174–7.

56. Powell R. Lawn tennis leg. Lancet. 1883;122(3123):44.

57. Fields K, Rigby M. Muscular calf injuries in runners. Curr Sports Med Rep. 2016;15(5):320–4.

58. Koulouris G, Ting A, Jhamb A, Connell D, Kavanagh E. Magnetic resonance imaging findings of injuries to the calf muscle complex. Skeletal Radiol. 2007;36(10):921–7.

59. Pereira ER, Brown RR, Resnick D. Prevalence and patterns of tendon calcification in patients with chondrocalcinosis of the knee: radiologic study of 156 patients. Clin Imaging. 1998;22:371–5.

60. Iguchi Y, Ihara N, Hijioka A, Uchida S, Nakamura T, Kikuta A, Nakashima T. Calcific tendonitis of the gastrocnemius. J Bone Joint Surg. 2002;84-B:431–2.

61. Yang BY, Sartoris DJ, Resnick D, Clopton P. Calcium pyrophosphate dihydrate crystal deposition disease: frequency of tendon calcification about the knee. J Rheumatol. 1996;23:883–8.

62. Watura C, Harries W. Isolated tear of the tendon to the medial head of gastrocnemius presenting as a painless lump in the calf. BMJ Case Rep. 2009;2009. bcr01.2009.1468

63. Watura C, Ward A, Harries W. Isolated partial tear and avulsion of the medial head of gastrocnemius tendon presenting as posterior medial knee pain. BMJ Case Rep. 2010;2010. bcr.2009.2278

64. Campbell J. Posterior calf injury. Foot Ankle Clin. 2009;14(4):761–71.

65. Delgado G, Chung C, Lektrakul N, Azocar P, Botte M, Coria D, Bosch E, Resnick D. Tennis leg: clinical US study of 141 patients and anatomic investigation of four cadavers with MR imaging and US. Radiology. 2002;224(1):112–9.

66. Pai V, Pai V. Acute compartment syndrome after rupture of the medial head of gastrocnemius in a child. J Foot Ankle Surg. 2007;46(4):288–90.

67. Russell G, Pearsall A, Caylor M, Nimityongskul P. Acute compartment syndrome after rupture of the medial head of the gastrocnemius muscle. South Med J. 2000;93(2):247–9.

68. Tao L, Jun H, Muliang D, Deye S, Jiangdong N. Acute compartment syndrome after gastrocnemius rupture (tennis leg) in a nonathlete without trauma. J Foot Ankle Surg. 2016;55(2):303–5.

69. Megliola A, Eutropi F, Scorzelli A, Gambacorta D, De Marchi A, De Filippo M, Faletti C, Ferrari F. Ultrasound and magnetic resonance imaging in sports-related muscle injuries. Radiol Med. 2006;111(6):836–45.

70. Slavotinek J. Muscle injury: the role of imaging in prognostic assignment and monitoring of muscle repair. Semin Musculoskelet Radiol. 2010;14(2):194–200.

71. Kwak H-S, Lee K-B, Han Y-M. Ruptures of the medial head of the gastrocnemius ("tennis leg"): clinical outcome and compression effect. Clin Imaging. 2006;30(1):48–53.

72. Jennings A, Peterson R. Delayed reconstruction of medial head of gastrocnemius rupture: a surgical option. Foot Ankle Int. 2013;34(6):904–7.

Peroneal Tendons

13

Mary E. Caldwell, Marc Gruner, Miguel Pelton,
Daniel Dean, Francis Xavier McGuigan,
and Arthur Jason De Luigi

Abbreviations

IPR	Inferior peroneal reticulum
MRI	Magnetic resonance imaging
NSAID	Nonsteroidal anti-inflammatory drug
PB	Peroneal brevis
PL	Peroneal longus
POPS	Painful os peroneum syndrome
PRP	Platelet-rich plasma
SPR	Superior peroneal retinaculum
US	Ultrasound

M. E. Caldwell (✉)
Department of Physical Medicine and Rehabilitation,
Virginia Commonwealth University,
Richmond, VA, USA

M. Gruner
Department of Rehabilitation Medicine, Georgetown
University, Washington, DC, USA
e-mail: marc.gruner@medstar.org

M. Pelton
Tidewater Orthopedics, Suffolk, VA, USA

D. Dean · F. X. McGuigan
Department of Orthopedic Surgery, MedStar Health,
Washington, DC, USA
e-mail: francis.mcguigan@medstar.org

A. J. De Luigi
Department of Physical Medicine and Rehabilitation,
Mayo Clinic, Scottsdale, AZ, USA

Introduction

The peroneal tendons are important dynamic lateral stabilizers of the ankle and hindfoot that when damaged are a source of significant pain and dysfunction which impair activity and quality of life. Certain anatomic factors can predispose an individual to peroneal tendon pathology. They include but are not limited to a cavus-shaped hindfoot, a shallow fibular retinacular groove, and certain hyperlaxity ligamentous disorders [1]. Peroneal tendon injuries are often overlooked causes of lateral ankle pain and ankle instability [2]. Given that the peroneal tendons are important stabilizers and movers of the ankle, they are a common location for tendinopathy in the lower extremity due to the repetitive mechanical stresses they endure [3, 4].

Peroneal tendon pathology, as discussed in this chapter, will not only include a discussion on tendinopathy, but also peroneal tendon interstitial tears, tendon rupture, tendon subluxation and dislocation, and painful os peroneum syndrome [1, 4].

A brief review of tendinopathy is included here with regard to acute tendinopathy, chronic tendinopathy, and tenosynovitis [1, 5]. Acute tendinopathy may be followed by chronic tendinopathy in an abnormal healing response where the tendon does not heal and pain persists [6, 7]. For instance, after tendon injury, there is an acute inflammatory response followed by a persistent chronic inflammatory response, collagen matrix deposition, and tendon remodeling. This results in a persistently painful and weak tendon (see Chaps. 1 and 2 for more details) [2, 8–10]. In order to define between acute and chronic tendon pathologies, these authors agree with expert consensus and recommend doing so based on the duration of clinical symptoms. Acute can be considered in someone with symptoms of less than 6 weeks of duration, while chronic should be considered in someone with persistent symptoms of more than 6 weeks of duration [11].

We further do not recommend defining acute as "tendinitis" [12]. Tendinitis was a "pathologic" term based around the thought that only acute tendinopathy involved an inflammatory state, which is not correct [13]. Multiple studies have now demonstrated that inflammation can be present in chronic tendinopathic tendons as well [9, 14]. Interestingly, the types of inflammatory cells in a chronic tendinopathy may differ from those in acute tendinopathy [9].

Tenosynovitis, which can be seen with tendinopathy, is an inflammatory process affecting the sheath of a tendon and can present as both fluid around the tendon or within the tendon itself. The cause of tenosynovitis is broad but can include idiopathic, infectious, autoimmune, systemic disorders, overuse, and chronic degeneration [15].

A thorough knowledge of how the various peroneal conditions (tendinopathy, partial tears, tendon rupture, tendon subluxation and dislocation, and painful os peroneum syndrome) present can help the practicing physician, not only to correctly diagnose the condition, but also to direct treatment to all the underlying contributors to the pathology. This chapter will cover lateral ankle anatomy, physical examination, imaging studies, and common case presentations of peroneal pathological conditions with their pertinent nonoperative and operative treatment options.

Anatomy

Regarding the peroneal tendons, common areas of pathology and their cause rely on understanding this anatomy and the mechanisms of action of the muscles. The peroneus longus (PL) and peroneus brevis (PB) muscles lie in the lateral compartment of the leg. The PB originates from the distal two-thirds of the lateral fibula and travels directly posterior to the lateral malleolus within the retromalleolar groove, which is a fibrocartilaginous ridge located at the posterolateral fibula, covered by the superior and inferior peroneal retinaculum (SPR and IPR). It then inserts onto the tuberosity at the fifth metatarsal base [7]. The PL originates from the upper two-thirds of the proximal lateral fibula and travels over retromalleolar groove deep to SPR and IPR. It then travels within the cuboid notch of the cuboid and inferior to peroneal tubercle of calcaneus before inserting on both the medial cuneiform and the base of the first metatarsal [7, 8].

At the level of distal fibula, peroneal tendons are stabilized by several soft tissue structures. First, the SPR extends about four centimeters (cm) proximal to the lateral malleolus to the level of the tip of fibula. It attaches anteriorly to the malleolus and posteriorly to the lateral wall of the calcaneus and Achilles tendon. The SPR serves to counteract peroneal tendon subluxation with dorsiflexion and eversion movements of the foot. Second, the calcaneofibular ligament stabilizes peroneal tendon translation medially at this level. Third, the retromalleolar groove accentuates the concavity of distal fibula and plays an important role in preventing subluxation of the tendons. Lastly, at approximately two to three cm distal to the lateral malleolus, the tendons pass underneath in the common sheath of the IPR. The IPR anteriorly connects with the extensor retinaculum of the foot and posteriorly attached to calcaneus. The IPR helps to direct and concentrate the pull of both tendons [8–10].

The PB everts, abducts, and plantarflexes the foot and also depresses the first ray [16]. The PB is also the primary abductor of the forefoot [16]. Both muscles are innervated by the superficial peroneal nerve. Both tendons receive their blood supply through branches of the posterior peroneal artery.

An os peroneum is a round fibrocartilaginous (osseous in 20% of cases) structure that may be present within the PL tendon at the level of calcaneocuboid articulation in up to 40% of the popu-

Fig. 13.1 Anatomy of
peroneal tendons

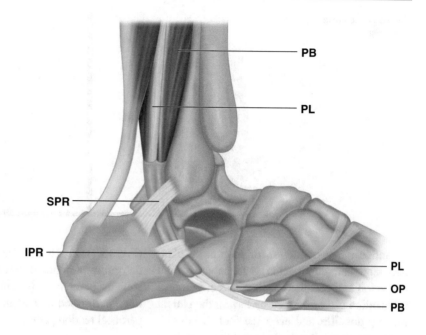

lation [17]. It acts as a sesamoid and fulcrum to
increase the mechanical advantage of the peroneus longus. The implications of aberrant func-
tioning of this will be discussed later.

Anatomic variations of the peroneal muscle exist and are an important source of the PB
and PL pathologies as they can overcrowd the
retromalleolar groove and cause laxity of the
SPR. First, the PB muscle belly can be low lying
and extend below the superior margin of the SPR
[18]. Second, the peroneus quartus is an anomalous muscle which can contribute to stenosis as
well. It is present in about 6–22% of subjects
[19]. Its origin lies at the distal aspect of the PB
right before it travels through the SPR. The peroneus quartus then travels with PL and PB before
inserting onto the peroneal tubercle.

For normal anatomy, refer to Fig. 13.1 for
reference.

Clinical Examination

Examination of both lower extremities is vital
to making a diagnosis and uncovering all contributing factors in any case of suspected pero-

neal pathology. Exam begins with inspection,
palpation, passive and active range of motion,
strength testing, and provocative tests. Close
inspection of the ankle and course of the peroneal tendons will often reveal swelling, though
this may be subtle in chronic cases. Inspection
must include standing assessment for ankle
varus and arch structure, while also looking for
lateral ankle swelling. Standing inspection is
included because patients with hindfoot varus
and cavovarus deformities place increased forces
on the lateral tendons which can lead to tendon
overuse [20]. Palpation both at rest and with
active firing of the tendons should be included.
Sobel et al. described that pain with eversion and
dorsiflexion and manual pressure against the retromalleolar groove is a positive test for PB tendinopathy [21]. The clinician should also check
for tendon enlargement and tenderness along the
path of the entire tendon(s) [16]. The location of
pain with palpation can often indicate the type of
pathology present. For example, pain and swelling at the calcaneocuboid junction may raise
suspicion for an os peroneum syndrome versus
pain more proximally might indicate a standard
tendinopathy.

Fig. 13.2 Coleman block test

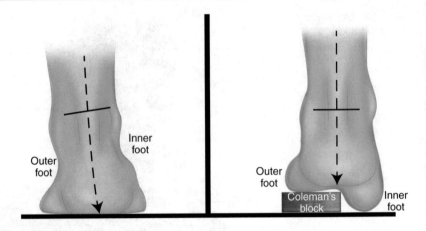

Active range of motion of the ankle (plantarflexion and dorsiflexion) and subtalar joint (inversion and eversion) are measured. Peroneal subluxation can be elicited by having the patient actively dorsiflex and evert the foot. It is helpful to have the patient do this repetitively, making a circling motion with the foot. A painful click indicates peroneal subluxation; alternatively, repetitive dorsiflexion and plantarflexion may also provoke subluxation [16]. These maneuvers should be performed with the practitioner palpating posterior to the lateral ankle lightly to appreciate subluxation but not to reduce subluxation.

Sensory testing of the sural, superficial peroneal, deep peroneal, and plantar nerves is routinely performed. Strength testing of the peroneal tendons should be obtained by resisted eversion and resisted plantarflexion of the great toe. Strength testing is critical for diagnosing peroneal tendon pathology. Often pain or weakness with resisted eversion is present [16]. First ray plantarflexion can elicit pain in PL pathology, especially if the pain is localized to the cuboid notch [21, 22]. Single stance heel raise with pain on the plantar lateral foot may indicate PL pathology [21].

Special tests that assess for lateral ankle and subtalar joint stability should be included, such as the varus inversion stress test [21] and anterior drawer. A Coleman block test can be used to assess the flexibility of any varus deformity

(Fig. 13.2) [11, 18, 21]. The degree of fixed varus deformity portends different orthotic options as well as potential adjuvant surgical procedures to be performed in tandem with the treatment of peroneal tendon pathology.

Imaging Studies

Radiographs

In all suspected peroneal tendon pathologies, weight bearing foot and ankle radiographs remain the mainstay for imaging modalities. They can quickly detect anatomical contributions to the pain, including an os peroneum, hypertrophic peroneal tubercle, subtalar degeneration, or a lateral talus osteochondral defect [23, 24]. On the oblique foot view, an avulsion or calcification at the base of the fifth metatarsal may be seen indicative of a peroneus brevis tear. A fleck avulsion off the lateral aspect of distal fibula may also be seen which is indicative of traumatic disruption of the SPR. An os peroneum may also be seen in the lateral ankle or oblique foot views [23]. It may appear fragmented or degenerative reinforcing a physical examination that suggests os peroneum syndrome. Assessment of the hindfoot alignment may be augmented with a Harris heel view, which allows visualization of the peroneal tubercle and retromalleolar groove [23, 24].

Comparison views of the contralateral foot may be beneficial to assess for any generalized finding bilaterally versus unilateral discrepancies in the symptomatic limb [23].

Ultrasound

If the clinician has ultrasound available, it is very reasonable to assess the tendons with ultrasound [25, 26]. Examination under US begins with the patient lying supine with the knee flexed at 30 degrees, and the foot resting on a pillow [25]. Start with the axial (short axis) view from superior to distal at the supramalleolar region scanning slowly down over the tunnel to the inframalleolar region [25]. It is important to note that at the supramalleolar region, the tendons can be examined together, while at the inferior malleolar region, the tendons should be examined separately to avoid anisotropy. After obtaining short axis images, longitudinal images are taken. It is important to scan from above the malleolus all the way down to the insertional site of the PB on the base of the 5th metatarsal and the PL on the base of the 1st metatarsal looking for a fibrillar pattern to the tendons [27]. Both ankles should be imaged to compare any differences between the pathologic and normal side. Following static imaging, dynamic imaging is taken. For dynamic assessment, the transducer is placed over the lateral malleolus while the patient goes through resisted dorsiflexion and eversion motion [28] [25].

Chronic tendinopathy is suggested by thickening of tendons and a change from homogenous tendon structure to heterogeneous tendon structure (loss of normal fibrillar echotexture). As discussed above, tendinopathy can also be associated with tenosynovitis. Tenosynovitis on ultrasound would demonstrate increased fluid content in the tendon sheath, thickening of the sheath with or without increased vascularity, and peritendinous subcutaneous edema [29]. The edema would display as hypoechoic ring around the tendon in the transverse view [30]. Color Doppler is important for assessing the tendon and surrounding sheath for neovascularization, as this may be associated with causing pain, though neovascularization can also be seen in asymptomatic patients [31]. It is also important to note if there are echogenic structures within the sheath, which would suggest more of an acute exudative tenosynovitis and should prompt the clinician to consider the etiology [15, 30].

Having advanced tendinopathy is believed to be a risk factor for various peroneal tendon tears. The diagnosis of peroneal tendon tear under ultrasound has shown to be 100% sensitive and 90% specific [32]. Diagnostic ultrasound may demonstrate an anechoic line in the short axis view of PB or PL consistent with a split tear in the tendon [33]. A peroneus brevis tear is demonstrated on ultrasound image Fig. 13.3d with its MRI correlate for comparison (Fig. 13.3a–c).

With real-time imaging capability, US is the imaging modality of choice for an evaluation of peroneal tendon subluxation and is often seen with an SPR tear [33]. SPR tears are graded based on a classification scheme developed by Eckert and Davis and modified by Oden. A grade I injury is most common and is an elevation of the retinaculum from the fibula with subluxation of the tendons between the bone and periosteum, a grade II injury is elevation of the fibrocartilaginous ridge from the fibula, a grade III injury is defined by a small cortical avulsion, and a grade IV injury is a tear of the SPR from its calcaneal attachment [34, 35]. If there is no SPR injury, the tendons can still have intrasheath instability that can be seen on dynamic US. There are two types: an intertendinous intrasheath switch of the tendons or the PL can sublux through a PB longitudinal split tear [33].

Given accessibility and low cost combined with above advantages, our authors believe US should be the first line diagnostic tool when evaluating injuries at the lateral ankle.

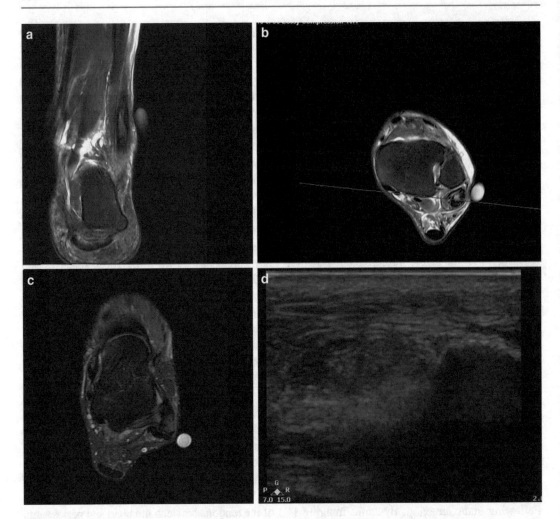

Fig. 13.3 (**a–d**) Displayed by MRI, both coronal (**a**) and axial (**b, c**), classic "boomerang" sign of the peroneus longus going in between the split tear of the peroneus brevis. US correlate is included (**d**). (Images courtesy of Dr. Jessalyn Adam (Sports Medicine, Mercy Orthopaedic Specialty Hospital) and Dr. Peter Haar (Musculoskeletal Radiology at Virginia Commonwealth University))

Magnetic Resonance Imaging (MRI)

MRI can be used to help diagnose tendinopathy, tendon tears, and tenosynovitis; though it can be difficult to delineate these with an MRI [36]. Most peroneal tendon subluxations or dislocations are transient and are rarely seen on MRI, and ultrasound (US) is superior for detecting such dynamic pathologies [37]. In conjunction with an evaluation of the peroneal tendons, the supporting structures such as the calcaneofibular ligaments, the posterior talofibular ligaments, and the ankle syndesmotic ligaments are also

assessed. Anatomical variants or ganglion cysts can also be visualized well on MRI [38].

Normal tendons exhibit low signal intensity in all image protocols due to the low water content. The peroneus brevis is flat or has mildly crescentic appearance at the retromalleolar groove, whereas peroneus longus has a more ellipsoid cross section. Pathology is indicated by the presence and degree of increased signal intensity. MRI can be helpful to help diagnose longitudinal split tears, partial thickness tears, full thickness tears, and complete tears of the peroneal tendons, especially if surgical treatment is being considered in recalcitrant cases to conservative therapy [39]. MRI has shown to have fair diagnostic ability (83% sensitivity and 75% specificity) for detection of a PB tear in correlation with intra-operative findings [39]. All of these structures should appear as thin bands of low signal intensity. Partial thickness tears of either the peroneus brevis or longus can show as thinned or thickened tendons with irregular intermediate signal or hyperintense signal. A complete tendon tear will not only show increased signal intensity in a portion of the tendon, but also a separation of the tendon into two or more sections. The most common tear seen on MRI is a longitudinal split tear of the PB and the PL fills the gap between two components of the PB. This is well visualized on both axial and coronal cuts [40].

Pathological Conditions and Treatment Options

Case 1: Peroneal Tendinopathy

A 31-year-old male triathlete presents with 3 months history of pain at the lateral ankle. Pain is most exacerbated by long runs. His past medical history is significant for multiple ankle sprains since he was a soccer player back in college. Physical exam is notable for tenderness in the tendon to palpation at the inferior posterior margin of lateral malleolus. Radiograph is normal. Ultrasound demonstrates peroneal brevis and longus tendon thickening, heterogeneous changes to the tendon's echogenicity, and power Doppler revealed neovascularity of the tendons at the distal fibula. There is no tendon sheath swelling and no subluxation noted on a dynamic ultrasound. The patient responds well to formal physical therapy and conservative management including anti-inflammatories, modified running schedule, and ankle strengthening with eccentric exercises.

Clinical Presentation and Treatment

The patient with suspected tendinopathy will often complain of gradual onset of lateral ankle pain, possibly associated with swelling and tenderness behind the lateral malleolus or along the course of the tendon [41]. The pain typically is reported to occur after activity but it may be present at rest [2, 41]. Often, peroneal tendinopathy may be associated with a history of ankle sprain(s), calcaneal or ankle fracture [31, 42, 43]. Defining acute vs chronic pathology, again, is typically defined by symptom duration as discussed already in this chapter. Chronic tendinopathy changes occur most commonly at hypo-vascular areas in the lateral ankle which are located at the turn around the distal fibula and the level of the cuboid tunnel, correlating to physical exam [44–46]. Other risk factors for tendinopathy include an anatomic variant or a ganglia from the ankle joint [25, 41, 47].

Nonoperative Treatment

Conservative measures include pain control with anti-inflammatories or acetaminophen, protection, relative rest, ice, and compression [2]. With regard to relative rest of the injured tendon, this will require the patient to decrease repetitive loading on the tendon. The duration depends on the patient's activity level [2, 4, 48]. There is not a clear recommendation for the duration of rest [2]. Braces are helpful to offload the tendon. Consider the use of an ankle brace or lateral heel wedge orthosis. Alternatively, using a rocker-bottom boot, a short leg weight bearing cast, or controlled ankle motion (CAM) boot for 3–4 weeks is plausible in patients with significant pain [22, 41]. Orthotics in particular have little evidence to support their efficacy with correcting foot alignment to offload the lateral ankle but they may help by modifying the vector strength on the lateral osseous insertion [16, 49, 50].

Physical therapy should include stretching, strengthening, and the use of a biomechanical ankle platform system (BAPS) board [41]. Eccentric training has shown to be quite possibly the most effective treatment for chronic tendinopathy [51]. The studies have shown that progressive use of the tendon over a certain period of time (20–30 exercise sessions) leads to activation of senescent tendon-specific stem cells, resulting in healing of the tendon injury [50, 52].

Anti-inflammatory treatment such as nonsteroidal anti-inflammatory drugs (NSAIDs) and corticosteroids can reduce inflammation and provide short-term pain relief in both acute and chronic tendinopathy. However, they may have a negative impact on structural healing and do not appear to change long-term outcomes [2, 9, 52–55].

It may be reasonable to also consider extracorporeal shock wave therapy (ESWT), ablation with a sclerosing agent, or transcutaneous glyceryl trinitrate patches, though none of these have directly been studied in peroneal tendinopathy [56]. ESWT may stimulate cell activity, increase blood flow, and increase collagen synthesis. The type of shock wave generator, wave type, intensity, frequency, and number of shocks can vary [50]. Sclerosing agents could be used to block areas of neovascularization which is believed to be part of the chronic pain experienced by patients [57]. Lastly, nitrate patches may result in better mechanical structure of the tendon during the healing process as free radicals can stimulate fibroblast proliferation [5].

If inflammation of the tendon sheath and synovium (tenosynovitis) is present, a corticosteroid injection could be helpful [58]. Otherwise, in tendinopathy without synovitis, no significant clinical benefits have been observed and there is a lack of strong evidence for local steroid injections for tendon disorders [59]. Studies have shown short-term pain improvement, but recurrence of pain is common [50, 54]. The general consensus is that intra-tendinous injections of corticosteroids should be avoided due to the increased risk of tendon rupture [59–61].

Regarding *orthobiologics,* the use of platelet-rich plasma (PRP) in chronic peroneal tendinopathy has been investigated in cohort studies. In patients with chronic peroneal tendinopathy who fail conservative treatment and undergo PRP injections, there was improved functional outcomes and pain scores [62, 63]. Further, the measurement of tendon thickness/hyperemia after PRP was reduced on US [62]. Such studies suggest that PRP may be an option in patients that fail other conservative treatments; however, trials that are randomized, controlled, and double-blinded are warranted. Stem cells can be considered for use in tendon pathologies; however, to our knowledge, there is little evidence to support their use with regard to peroneal pathologies [50].

Operative Treatment

In most instances, peroneal tendinopathy and tenosynovitis respond well to conservative management [43, 64]. However, if symptoms persist despite 3 months of nonoperative treatment, surgery can be considered.

Open tenosynovectomy with debridement is the most common surgical approach for chronic tendinopathy and/or tenosynovitis, though there is not a large prospective study on clinical outcomes comparing open versus endoscopic repair [18, 43]. Of note, failure to address cavovarus hindfoot alignment, associated peroneal tears, anatomical variants, or lateral ankle instability may result in incomplete pain relief [43].

Simple open repair is performed in the lateral decubitus or often the modified lateral decubitus position. All bony prominences are well padded including at the fibular head and lateral malleolus of the nonoperative leg. A bean bag or peg board can be used to hold the patient in the position. An axillary roll is inserted to protect the brachial plexus during the procedure. A thigh tourniquet is applied and inflated. A curvilinear incision is made following the contour of the tendons just posterior to the fibula depending on the levels and amount of associated pathology. The sheath should be incised in a longitudinal fashion and the tendons should be inspected for degeneration, flattening, and fraying. Degenerate tendon, including areas of erythema, synovitis, and granulation tissue should be debrided [43]. At this point any anatomical variants or biomechanical abnormalities should also be addressed [43]. If there is a tendon split tear associated with tendinopathy, then the tear should be repaired (see tendon tear surgery discussion to follow). The tendon sheath may or may not be re-approximated [43].

Tendoscopy or arthroscopic management can be performed for simple tenosynovectomy [65]. It is also performed in the lateral decubitus position. For comparison of technique to open repair, the procedure is reviewed here. Two tendoscopy portals are employed during the procedure. They are located proximal and distal to the lateral malleolus. The distal portal is located 1.5 to 2 cm distal to the tip of the fibula. The proximal portal, located 2–3 cm proximal to the tip of the fibula, is made under direct visualization. To establish the portholes, a blunt dissection technique is utilized to decrease the risk of injury to the sural nerve. A 2.7 mm small joint arthroscopy is used for the evaluation [18, 65].

After surgery (from a tenosynovectomy) postoperatively, the patient is placed in a back slab, cast or boot (depending on surgeon preference), made non weight bearing for 2 weeks, followed by weight bearing in a cast for 4 more weeks. Strengthening and range of motion can start once cast is removed [18].

Case 2: Peroneal Subluxation and Dislocation

A 21-year-old Olympic skier fell 1 week ago and presented to the clinic with right lateral ankle pain associated with recurrent painful lateral ankle region popping/snapping. He reports the popping is notable when skiing down-hill and making turns to the left. When out of skiing boots, he notes active dorsiflexion and eversion results in increased pain, but only ankle circumduction would result in occasional pop. On exam he is tender to palpation at the retromalleolar groove and reports pain with resisted eversion. Anterior drawer, talar tilt test, and squeeze tests were negative. An x-ray was unremarkable. A dynamic ultrasound demonstrated an elevated superior peroneal retinaculum with bony avulsion. Patient was placed in a boot for 6 weeks and underwent physical therapy. Patient's symptoms did not improve with conservative care and the patient underwent a peroneal groove-deepening procedure with repair of the superior peroneal retinaculum. He was able to return to skiing after a year.

Clinical Presentation and Treatment

Acute dislocation of the peroneal tendons out of the retromalleolar groove could occur when a patient reports a forceful passive dorsiflexion/inversion mechanism of injury (Fig. 13.4a, b) [16, 66]. This is common in multiple populations but was first reported in skiers falling over their skis [16]. This is commonly seen in an athlete that cuts laterally or with a history of eversion/

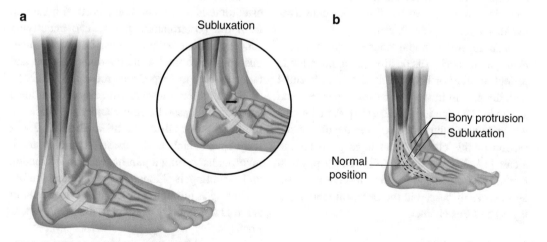

Fig. 13.4 (**a, b**) Vector forces moved peroneal retinaculum from normal position and can result in subluxation without SPR tear and with SPR tear

dorsiflexion mechanism of ankle injury where there is likely disruption of the SPR that holds the tendons in the retromalleolar groove [16, 41, 66]. Sometimes, patients can have intrasheath subluxation without SPR disruption [67]. The tendon or tendons may reduce on their own or stay dislocated. An injury to superficial peroneal retinaculum makes patients prone to future tendon dislocation and relocation. In both acute and chronic injuries, patients also report snapping or clicking with movements such as dorsiflexion, eversion, or simply, circumduction [66, 68]. Patients sometimes note weakness in eversion due to biomechanical changes along with worsening pain if overlooked.

Nonoperative Treatment

Things to consider for treatment options include if the injury is acute vs chronic and if the patient is an athlete vs not [11]. Expert consensus from the 2018 Ankle and Foot Associates (AFAS) of the European Society of Sports traumatology, Knee surgery and Arthroscopy (ESSKA) concluded that for acute dislocation in a nonathletic patient, conservative therapy is reasonable to trial. If pain and symptoms persist after 3 months, consider surgery. If there is an acute or chronic dislocation in an *athlete*, surgical management is recommended [11]. This is recommended due to recurrent peroneal instability recurring up to 50% of the time after conservative management [18, 69, 70].

With regard to initial conservative management in an acute dislocation in a nonathletic patient, casting or booting should be performed with the patient in the plantarflexed position and a 2 cm heel wedge for 6 weeks [11]. Patients with a type 3 Oden injury, discussed in the ultrasound section of this chapter, tend to respond best to a cast [34, 35]. Casting is followed by physical therapy and other options for conservative management as discussed in the peroneal tendinopathy case of this chapter.

Operative Treatment

Peroneal subluxation with SPR tears can be addressed in four different manners: direct superficial retinaculum repair, tissue transfer to reinforce the SPR, bone block procedures, and groove deepening procedures.

Experts report that the SPR should always be repaired in all types of peroneal instability if an open repair is performed, while during an endoscopic procedure, it is a reasonable option [11]. Remember, for any repair, the tendons are also assessed for tendinopathy, tears, and tenosynovitis, and this should also be treated accordingly. In SPR repair, the fibrocartilaginous ridge is sacrificed and the SPR is reattached to the retromalleolar groove [18]. The tensioning used to relocate must be closely assessed to prevent stenosis from the repair and complications postoperatively [11].

In athletes with peroneal instability and SPR tear, the retromalleolar groove should be deepened. This can be done either endoscopically or by open repair. Endoscopically is favored due to the possibility of earlier rehabilitation and sooner return to play [11]. Groove deepening procedures are commonly used in conjunction with superficial peroneal retinacular reconstruction in athletes with a shallow retromalleolar groove or deficiency of the fibrocartilaginous ridge. Further, rates of return to sport have been shown to be higher in athletes who underwent both groove deepening and SPR repair [71]. In this procedure, the tendons are dislocated and an osteotome is used to elevate a cortical bone flap from the posterolateral fibula. The underlying cancellous bone is burred down before the osseous flap is returned to its previous position and tamped down to deepen the groove [18, 72, 73].

If the athlete presents with chronic peroneal subluxation, tissue transfer could also be used to reinforce the repair of the SPR. The Ellis Jones technique, which is the most commonly used, involves harvesting a part of the Achilles tendon and rerouting it through a bony tunnel before anchoring it through a drill hole in the fibula to serve as a secondary restraint of the peroneal tendons [74].

In non-athletes undergoing surgery for peroneal instability with SPR tear, the tendons should be reduced into the groove. Groove deepening can also be considered but there is an expert consensus on this matter [11].

Bone block procedures are another option for chronic peroneal subluxation, but rarely used any longer secondary to complication related to hardware irritation and nonunion. This involves making a sagittal plane osteotomy at the tip of the distal fibula. The lateral fragment is translated posteriorly and fixed into place. The translated fibula serves as a lateral buttress to peroneal tendon subluxation. This procedure is mentioned for historical perspective [75].

Patients with intrasheath subluxation without SPR tears do well with groove deepening alone, though studies are lacking [18, 67].

Case 3: Peroneal Tendon Tears (Isolated and Combined)

A 42-year-old female trail runner with a history of left lateral ankle pain for 3 years presents with worsening of pain in left lateral ankle since a recent ankle sprain 2 months ago. Patient has performed office-based physical therapy in the past for her ankles, which helps with pain reduction some, and does maintain her home exercise program. After long runs, she will have subtle lateral ankle swelling that takes a few days to resolve even before her recent ankle sprain but denies any other symptoms. On physical exam, pain is focal to just posterior to lateral malleolus and pain reproducible with varus inversion stress at that location. She also has subtle cavovarus on exam and radiograph. Running gait demonstrates excessive subtalar and ankle varus moment pattern. Diagnostic ultrasound demonstrates anechoic line in the short axis view of peroneus brevis tendon at the level of the distal fibula consistent with a split tear in the tendon. Patient started in new course of physical therapy for 8–12 weeks and was fit for custom orthotics. Patient had 40% relief in symptoms after 3 months, therefore surgical referral was placed and the patient underwent tendoscopy with repair.

She was able to resume running within 12 weeks and reported free of pain and swelling.

Clinical Presentation and Treatment

Patients with partial tendon tears may report anywhere from "mild" to "severe" pain posterior and inferior to the lateral malleolus or at the proximal fibula [41]. There may also be pain reported at the plantar aspect of the foot [41]. Patients may report a history similar to those with chronic tendinopathy stating they have persistent swelling and tenderness [76] [20]. Tendon tears are most commonly associated and often reported with a recent history of an ankle sprain or trauma, but can also be secondary to poor biomechanics and chronic overuse [77, 78]. Risk factors for tendon tears include subluxation of the tendons, history of multiple ankle sprains, corticosteroid use, quinolone use, anatomical variation such as peroneal tubercle hypertrophy, or cavovarus [41, 73, 79]. PL tears often occur at the level of the inferior retinaculum to the cuboid notch, while PB tears often occur at the distal tip of the fibula [80–82]. Prevalence of PB tears in the general population is not well known, but it is possibly anywhere from 11% to 38% [45]. Isolated PL tears are less common than isolated PB tears and it is also more likely to have tears in both tendons rather than just the PL [77].

Rupture of the tendon(s) can occur but is uncommon compared to partial tears and tendinopathy incidence. A rupture, like a partial tear, can be both acutely trauma related or could be secondary to chronic degeneration of the tendon [45]. Some patients may have no pain or symptoms but demonstrate foot deformity, while others may have mild to severe pain [11].

Nonoperative Treatment

With regard to partial tendon tears (split tears), similar to tendinopathy care, surgical therapy is considered after 3 months of conservative care without improvement in symptoms. Conservative care is universally recommended first, but there is limited and varied outcome on the success of conservative care [11]. For ruptured tendons, if the patient is asymptomatic and inactive, conservative care is appropriate [11]. Approach to conservative care is reviewed in the tendinopathy "Nonoperative Treatment" section of this chapter and again includes anti-inflammatory medications, physical therapy, and activity modification, while considering bracing, casting, orthotics, and orthobiologics [43].

Operative Treatment

Surgical options for partial tears include (1) primary debridement and tubularization, (2) autograft or allograft, and (3) tenodesis. Ruptured tendons in the symptomatic and highly active patient should be addressed by tenodesis or grafting. Tendon transfer could also be considered in complete ruptures [11, 84]. As stated before, failure to also address cavovarus hindfoot alignment, associated peroneal tears, anatomical variants, or lateral ankle instability may result in incomplete pain relief [43].

Surgical outcomes for tendon tears vary but overall seem beneficial to the patient (level IV and V evidence) [11, 20, 81, 83, 85–87].

Repair of peroneal tendon tears has been categorized by multiple authors to help determine which type of surgery to perform [20, 83, 88]. Sobel et al. recommended dividing the type of tear into four different grading systems (based on partial vs full thickness split tears) in order to determine the type of repair [88]. Krause and Brodsky recommended the type of repair be based on the 50% rule: If less than 50% of the tendon is involved, then excise and perform a tubularization of the tendon, while if greater than 50% of the cross-sectional area is involved, then perform a tenodesis [83]. Redfern and Myerson suggested that intraoperative findings should dictate the type of repair [20].

Expert consensus from the 2018 Ankle and Foot Associates (AFAS) of the European Society of Sports traumatology, Knee surgery and Arthroscopy (ESSKA) agreed that initial repair, no matter what degree of partial tear or percentage of the tendon involved, the surgeon should aim to preserve the tendon (s) with *primary debridement and tubularization* [11]. This process involves excision of the unhealthy tissue

and re-approximation of the healthy tendon fibers with running 2-0 to 4-0 sutures. The repair is tested in dorsiflexion and plantarflexion to make sure impingement or stenosis does not occur. The wounds are washed and closed in a layered fashion and the patient is placed in a splint in relative eversion at the subtalar joint.

If tendon tears are deemed irreparable with tubularization, then grafting or tenodesis of the peroneal tendons may be performed. The ESSKA-AFAS recommends single stage grafting over tenodesis [11, 89].

Although technically difficult, *autograft* preserves the independent action of each tendon and preserves their normal excursion and therefore maximizes function return [11]. *Autograft* is recommended over allograft, typically hamstring or foot extensor tendon [11, 18, 90]. If using an allograft, peroneal or semitendinosus allograft is used to reconstruct peroneal tendon tears with large defects [91].

For grafting the peroneal sheath is identified and opened surgically. The fibro osseous tunnel is inspected and a tenosynovectomy and tenolysis are routinely performed. The ruptured ends of the tendon or areas of tendinopathy are debrided until healthy appearing tendon is encountered. The defect length is measured and an appropriately sized graft is chosen. If the peroneus brevis is completely avulsed off of the fifth metatarsal then a suture anchor device or interference screw technique may be used to secure the graft to the base of the fifth metatarsal [18]. Alternatively, if a cuff of normal peroneus brevis is present distally a Pulvertaft weave used to secure the graft to the native tendon with braided non-absorbable sutures [92]. Closure and immobilization are accomplished as previously stated for tendon repairs.

Tenodesis involves the same operating room set up as a tendon debridement. Once the tendon is deemed irreparable the frayed ends are cleaned to a stable edge and then sewn to the intact tendon proximal and distal to the rupture site with 2-0 or 3-0 nonabsorbable sutures. The tendon is then taken through dorsiflexion and plantarflexion, eversion and inversion to observe for any stenosis occurring as a result of the increased tendon bulk. The wound is then washed and closed in a layered fashion and the ankle is immobilized as described above for repair.

The typical postoperative rehabilitation for these procedures includes non-weight bearing for 2 weeks in a back slab or boot until the first wound check, followed by 6 weeks of protected weight bearing in a boot [18]. The patient would begin physical therapy about three to 4 weeks post op, and transition to regular shoe wear as tolerated at 8 weeks postop with anticipated return to full activity at about 6 months.

Case 4: Painful Os Peroneum Syndrome (POPS)

A 17-year-old elite male soccer player presents to clinic with chronic right ankle pain for 1 year. He states the pain is at the lateral ankle, and points just distal and anterior to lateral malleolus. He says he has had many ankle inversion sprains in the past and despite wearing an ankle brace for the last 6 months, he has recurrent swelling and pain in this location. He has had prior physical therapy and did not have much improvement in his pain or swelling. On exam, pain is reproducible at the level of the calcaneocuboid articulation with palpation, varus inversion stress test, single stance heel rise, and resisted plantarflexion of the first ray. Oblique radiograph of the foot, as well as other views, demonstrates os peroneum. MRI was ordered and demonstrates edema within the os peroneum and a peroneus longus split tear at the level of the cuboid tunnel. Patient was placed in cast for 8 weeks without improvement and subsequently underwent surgery with excision of the os peroneum and repair of peroneus longus tendon.

Clinical Presentation and Treatment

Given the os peroneum is located at the calcaneocuboid articulation in the PL tendon, pain is often reported in the plantar lateral foot [21]. The presentation can be either acute or chronic. If there is an acute presentation, the patient frequently reports a history of trauma or of an inversion/supination sprain [22]. Patients may

complain of worse pain with plantarflexion and heel raising during walking [93]. POPS may be secondary to (1) an acute fracture or diastasis of a multipartite os peroneum after supination/inversion injury because the os compresses against the cuboid with strong contraction of the PL muscle, (2) chronic fracture with callus and resulting stenosing tenosynovitis, (3) partial tear or rupture of the tendon proximal or distal to the os peroneum, or (4) the PL tendon being entrapped between a hypertrophied peroneal tubercle and the Os [21, 93]. Therefore, if an os peroneum is present on imaging, tendinopathy, tears, and ruptures must always be considered [93].

Nonoperative Treatment

POPS should be managed in a similar fashion to other peroneus longus tendon tears as discussed above. Nonoperative management should initially be attempted, prior to surgical options, if there isn't a complete rupture of the PL or if there is an asymptomatic fracture. Symptomatic nondisplaced fractures without PL function disruption can specifically be managed conservatively by non-weight bearing for 2 weeks, followed by partial weight bearing for 2 weeks. Symptomatic PL rupture with an intact os peroneum or symptomatic displaced fractures with loss of PL function should be managed surgically [11].

Operative Treatment

Traditional surgical management involves os peroneum excision and subsequent end-to-end repair of the tendon or tenodesis [11]. Because of the plantar lateral position of the ossific fragment, end-to-end repair of the tendon is difficult, results in a shortened tendon, and increases the risk of sural nerve damage [94]. Results from a retrospective study with a small sample size demonstrate that os peroneum excision with associated peroneus longus tendon debridement and tenodesis to an intact peroneus brevis tendon leads to significant clinical improvement [94]. As described above, however, tenodesis to the peroneus brevis tendon proximally significantly alters the excursion and line of pull of both tendons. It is our practice to excise the os perineum and transplant it into the lateral calcaneus along its normal pathway with the use of an interference screw. This technique preserves the independent function of the peroneus longus tendon and its line of pull.

Conclusion

Pathology of the peroneal tendons is an underdiagnosed cause of lateral ankle pain. Tendinopathy of the peroneal tendons can be acute or chronic. Partial tears are very common and should be considered in someone with lateral ankle pain. Other common pathologies include peroneal tendon subluxation and os perineum syndrome, which should be included in the differential diagnosis. Physical exam and the use of US or MRI verify the pathology suspected based on the patient's history and symptoms. Nonoperative management such as immobilization, bracing, NSAIDs, orthotics, and physical therapy is traditionally attempted first for the management of peroneal tendon pathology. For patients who fail nonoperative management, there are several surgical options available including tendon debridement, tenosynovectomy, tendon tubularization, grafting, and tenodesis depending on the pathology type. Associated conditions including peroneal tendon subluxation, os perineum syndrome, cavovarus deformity, and lateral ankle instability should be addressed at the time of surgical management. With appropriate management following expert consensus, as current evidence is predominately levels IV and V, patients with peroneal pathology can have good outcomes [11].

References

1. Ozbag D, Gumusalan Y, Uzel M, Cetinus E. Morphometrical features of the human malleolar groove. Foot Ankle Int. 2008;29(1):77–81.
2. Simpson MR, Howard TM. Tendinopathies of the foot and ankle. Am Fam Physician. 2009;80(10):1107–14.
3. McKeon POHJ, Bramble D, et al. The foot core system: a new paradigm for understanding intrinsic foot muscle function. Br J Sports Med. 2015;49:290.
4. Murrell GA. Understanding tendinopathies. Br J Sports Med. 2002;36(6):392–3.
5. Murrell GA. Using nitric oxide to treat tendinopathy. Br J Sports Med. 2007;41(4):227–31.
6. Puddu G, Ippolito E, Postacchini F. A classification of Achilles tendon disease. Am J Sports Med. 1976;4(4):145–50.
7. Wilson JJ, Best TM. Common overuse tendon problems: a review and recommendations for treatment. Am Fam Physician. 2005;72(5):811–8.
8. Khan KM, Cook JL, Bonar F, Harcourt P, Astrom M. Histopathology of common tendinopathies. Update and implications for clinical management. Sports Med. 1999;27(6):393–408.
9. Jomaa G, Kwan CK, Fu SC, Ling SK, Chan KM, Yung PS, et al. A systematic review of inflammatory cells and markers in human tendinopathy. BMC Musculoskelet Disord. 2020;21(1):78.
10. Andarawis-Puri N, Flatow EL, Soslowsky LJ. Tendon basic science: development, repair, regeneration, and healing. J Orthop Res. 2015;33(6):780–4.
11. van Dijk PA, Miller D, Calder J, DiGiovanni CW, Kennedy JG, Kerkhoffs GM, et al. The ESSKA-AFAS international consensus statement on peroneal tendon pathologies. Knee Surg Sports Traumatol Arthrosc Off J ESSKA. 2018;26(10):3096–107.
12. Maffulli N, Khan KM, Puddu G. Overuse tendon conditions: time to change a confusing terminology. Arthroscopy J Arthrosc Relat Surg Off Publ Arthrosc Assoc North Am Int Arthrosc Assoc. 1998;14(8):840–3.
13. Rees JD, Wilson AM, Wolman RL. Current concepts in the management of tendon disorders. Rheumatology. 2006;45(5):508–21.
14. Tang C, Chen Y, Huang J, Zhao K, Chen X, Yin Z, et al. The roles of inflammatory mediators and immunocytes in tendinopathy. J Orthop Transl. 2018;14:23–33.
15. Adams JE, Habbu R. Tendinopathies of the hand and wrist. J Am Acad Orthop Surg. 2015;23(12):741–50.
16. Roster B, Michelier P, Giza E. Peroneal tendon disorders. Clin Sports Med. 2015;34(4):625–41.
17. Oh SJ, Kim YH, Kim SK, Kim MW. Painful os peroneum syndrome presenting as lateral plantar foot pain. Ann Rehabil Med. 2012;36(1):163–6.
18. Davda K, Malhotra K, O'Donnell P, Singh D, Cullen N. Peroneal tendon disorders. EFORT Open Rev. 2017;2(6):281–92.
19. Zammit J, Singh D. The peroneus quartus muscle. Anatomy and clinical relevance. J Bone Joint Surg. 2003;85(8):1134–7.
20. Redfern D, Myerson M. The management of concomitant tears of the peroneus longus and brevis tendons. Foot Ankle Int. 2004;25(10):695–707.
21. Sobel M, Pavlov H, Geppert MJ, Thompson FM, DiCarlo EF, Davis WH. Painful os peroneum syndrome: a spectrum of conditions responsible for plantar lateral foot pain. Foot Ankle Int. 1994;15(3):112–24.
22. Philbin TM, Landis GS, Smith B. Peroneal tendon injuries. J Am Acad Orthop Surg. 2009;17(5):306–17.
23. Bashir WA, Lewis S, Cullen N, Connell DA. Os peroneum friction syndrome complicated by sesamoid fatigue fracture: a new radiological diagnosis? Case report and literature review. Skelet Radiol. 2009;38(2):181–6.

24. Hyer CF, Dawson JM, Philbin TM, Berlet GC, Lee TH. The peroneal tubercle: description, classification, and relevance to peroneus longus tendon pathology. Foot Ankle Int. 2005;26(11):947–50.

25. Bianchi S, Delmi M, Molini L. Ultrasound of peroneal tendons. Semin Musculoskelet Radiol. 2010;14(3):292–306.

26. Jacobson JA. Musculoskeletal ultrasound: focused impact on MRI. AJR Am J Roentgenol. 2009;193(3):619–27.

27. BF DI, Fraga CJ, Cohen BE, Shereff MJ. Associated injuries found in chronic lateral ankle instability. Foot Ankle Int. 2000;21(10):809–15.

28. Wu CH, Shyu SG, Ozcakar L, Wang TG. Dynamic ultrasound imaging for peroneal tendon subluxation. Am J Phys Med Rehabil. 2015;94(6):e57–8.

29. Shewmaker DM, Guderjahn O, Kummer T. Identification of peroneal tenosynovitis by point-of-care ultrasonography. J Emerg Med. 2016;50(2):e79–81.

30. Chew K, Stevens KJ, Wang TG, Fredericson M, Lew HL. Introduction to diagnostic musculoskeletal ultrasound: part 2: examination of the lower limb. Am J Phys Med Rehabil. 2008;87(3):238–48.

31. Chang A, Miller TT. Imaging of tendons. Sports Health. 2009;1(4):293–300.

32. Grant TH, Kelikian AS, Jereb SE, McCarthy RJ. Ultrasound diagnosis of peroneal tendon tears. A surgical correlation. J Bone Joint Surg Am. 2005;87(8):1788–94.

33. Draghi F, Bortolotto C, Draghi AG, Gitto S. Intrasheath instability of the peroneal tendons: dynamic ultrasound imaging. J Ultrasound Med. 2018;37(12):2753–8.

34. Eckert WR, Davis EA Jr. Acute rupture of the peroneal retinaculum. J Bone Joint Surg Am. 1976;58(5):670–2.

35. Oden RR. Tendon injuries about the ankle resulting from skiing. Clin Orthop Relat Res. 1987;216:63–9.

36. Kijowski R, De Smet A, Mukharjee R. Magnetic resonance imaging findings in patients with peroneal tendinopathy and peroneal tenosynovitis. Skelet Radiol. 2007;36(2):105–14.

37. Wang XT, Rosenberg ZS, Mechlin MB, Schweitzer ME. Normal variants and diseases of the peroneal tendons and superior peroneal retinaculum: MR imaging features. Radiographics Rev Publ Radiol Soc N Am. 2005;25(3):587–602.

38. Major NM, Helms CA, Fritz RC, Speer KP. The MR imaging appearance of longitudinal split tears of the peroneus brevis tendon. Foot Ankle Int. 2000;21(6):514–9.

39. Lamm BM, Myers DT, Dombek M, Mendicino RW, Catanzariti AR, Saltrick K. Magnetic resonance imaging and surgical correlation of peroneus brevis tears. J Foot Ankle Surg Off Publ Am Coll Foot Ankle Surg. 2004;43(1):30–6.

40. Taljanovic MS, Alcala JN, Gimber LH, Rieke JD, Chilvers MM, Latt LD. High-resolution US and MR imaging of peroneal tendon injuries. Radiographics Rev Publ Radiol Soc N Am. 2015;35(1):179–99.

41. Heckman DS, Gluck GS, Parekh SG. Tendon disorders of the foot and ankle, part 1: peroneal tendon disorders. Am J Sports Med. 2009;37(3):614–25.

42. Gray JM, Alpar EK. Peroneal tenosynovitis following ankle sprains. Injury. 2001;32(6):487–9.

43. Heckman DS, Reddy S, Pedowitz D, Wapner KL, Parekh SG. Operative treatment for peroneal tendon disorders. J Bone Joint Surg Am. 2008;90(2):404–18.

44. Baumhauer JF, Nawoczenski DA, DiGiovanni BF, Flemister AS. Ankle pain and peroneal tendon pathology. Clin Sports Med. 2004;23(1):21–34.

45. van Dijk PA, Lubberts B, Verheul C, DiGiovanni CW, Kerkhoffs GM. Rehabilitation after surgical treatment of peroneal tendon tears and ruptures. Knee Surg Sports Traumatol Arthrosc Off J ESSKA. 2016;24(4):1165–74.

46. Petersen W, Bobka T, Stein V, Tillmann B. Blood supply of the peroneal tendons: injection and immunohistochemical studies of cadaver tendons. Acta Orthop Scand. 2000;71(2):168–74.

47. Geller J, Lin S, Cordas D, Vieira P. Relationship of a low-lying muscle belly to tears of the peroneus brevis tendon. Am J Orthop. 2003;32(11):541–4.

48. Gorter K, de Poel S, de Melker R, Kuyvenhoven M. Variation in diagnosis and management of common foot problems by GPs. Fam Pract. 2001;18(6):569–73.

49. Hennessy MS, Molloy AP, Sturdee SW. Noninsertional Achilles tendinopathy. Foot Ankle Clin. 2007;12(4):617–41. vi-vii

50. Kaux JF, Forthomme B, Goff CL, Crielaard JM, Croisier JL. Current opinions on tendinopathy. J Sports Sci Med. 2011;10(2):238–53.

51. Alfredson H, Pietila T, Jonsson P, Lorentzon R. Heavy-load eccentric calf muscle training for the treatment of chronic Achilles tendinosis. Am J Sports Med. 1998;26(3):360–6.

52. Khan KM, Scott A. Mechanotherapy: how physical therapists' prescription of exercise promotes tissue repair. Br J Sports Med. 2009;43(4):247–52.

53. Magra M, Maffulli N. Nonsteroidal antiinflammatory drugs in tendinopathy: friend or foe. Clin J Sport Med Off J Can Acad Sport Med. 2006;16(1):1–3.

54. Andres BM, Murrell GA. Treatment of tendinopathy: what works, what does not, and what is on the horizon. Clin Orthop Relat Res. 2008;466(7):1539–54.

55. Chisari E, Rehak L, Khan WS, Maffulli N. Tendon healing in presence of chronic low-level inflammation: a systematic review. Br Med Bull. 2019;132(1):97–116.

56. Mead MP, Gumucio JP, Awan TM, Mendias CL, Sugg KB. Pathogenesis and Management of Tendinopathies in sports medicine. Transl Sports Med. 2018;1(1):5–13.

57. Knobloch K. The role of tendon microcirculation in Achilles and patellar tendinopathy. J Orthop Surg Res. 2008;3:18.

58. Barile A, La Marra A, Arrigoni F, Mariani S, Zugaro L, Splendiani A, et al. Anaesthetics, steroids and platelet-rich plasma (PRP) in ultrasound-guided mus-

culoskeletal procedures. Br J Radiol. 2016;89(1065): 20150355.

59. Paavola M, Kannus P, Jarvinen TA, Jarvinen TL, Jozsa L, Jarvinen M. Treatment of tendon disorders. Is there a role for corticosteroid injection? Foot Ankle Clin. 2002;7(3):501–13.

60. Borland S, Jung S, Hugh IA. Complete rupture of the peroneus longus tendon secondary to injection. Foot. 2009;19(4):229–31.

61. Tose J. Complete rupture of the peroneus longus tendon secondary to injection. Foot. 2010;20(2–3):99.

62. Dallaudiere B, Pesquer L, Meyer P, Silvestre A, Perozziello A, Peuchant A, et al. Intratendinous injection of platelet-rich plasma under US guidance to treat tendinopathy: a long-term pilot study. J Vasc Interv Radiol JVIR. 2014;25(5):717–23.

63. Unlu MC, Kivrak A, Kayaalp ME, Birsel O, Akgun I. Peritendinous injection of platelet-rich plasma to treat tendinopathy: a retrospective review. Acta Orthop Traumatol Turc. 2017;51(6):482–7.

64. Lui TH. Endoscopic synovectomy of peroneal tendon sheath. Arthrosc Tech. 2017;6(3):e887–e92.

65. van Dijk CN, Kort N. Tendoscopy of the peroneal tendons. Arthroscopy J Arthrosc Relat Surg Off Publ Arthrosc Assoc N Am Int Arthrosc Assoc. 1998;14(5):471–8.

66. Brukner P, Khan K. Brukner and Khan's clinical sports medicine. 4th ed. North Ryde: McGraw-Hill Education; 2012.

67. Guelfi M, Vega J, Malagelada F, Baduell A, Dalmau-Pastor M. Tendoscopic treatment of peroneal Intrasheath subluxation: a new subgroup with superior peroneal retinaculum injury. Foot Ankle Int. 2018;39(5):542–50.

68. Raikin SM. Intrasheath subluxation of the peroneal tendons. Surgical technique. J Bone Joint Surg Am. 2009;91(Suppl 2 Pt 1):146–55.

69. McLennan JG. Treatment of acute and chronic luxations of the peroneal tendons. Am J Sports Med. 1980;8(6):432–6.

70. Ferran NA, Oliva F, Maffulli N. Recurrent subluxation of the peroneal tendons. Sports Med. 2006;36(10):839–46.

71. van Dijk PA, Gianakos AL, Kerkhoffs GM, Kennedy JG. Return to sports and clinical outcomes in patients treated for peroneal tendon dislocation: a systematic review. Knee Surg Sports Traumatol Arthrosc Off J ESSKA. 2016;24(4):1155–64.

72. Saragas NP, Ferrao PN, Mayet Z, Eshraghi H. Peroneal tendon dislocation/subluxation – case series and review of the literature. Foot Ankle Surg Off J Eur Soc Foot Ankle Surg. 2016;22(2):125–30.

73. Vega J, Batista JP, Golano P, Dalmau A, Viladot R. Tendoscopic groove deepening for chronic subluxation of the peroneal tendons. Foot Ankle Int. 2013;34(6):832–40.

74. Thomas JL, Sheridan L, Graviet S. A modification of the Ellis Jones procedure for chronic peroneal subluxation. J Foot Surg. 1992;31(5):454–8.

75. Deng E, Shi W, Jiao C, Xie X, Jiang D, Chen L, et al. Reattachment of the superior peroneal retinaculum versus the bone block procedure for the treatment of recurrent peroneal tendon dislocation: two safe and effective techniques. Knee Surg Sports Traumatol Arthrosc Off J ESSKA. 2019;27(9):2877–83.

76. Giza E, Mak W, Wong SE, Roper G, Campanelli V, Hunter JC. A clinical and radiological study of peroneal tendon pathology. Foot Ankle Spec. 2013;6(6):417–21.

77. Dombek MF, Lamm BM, Saltrick K, Mendicino RW, Catanzariti AR. Peroneal tendon tears: a retrospective review. J Foot Ankle Surg Off Publ Am Coll Foot Ankle Surg. 2003;42(5):250–8.

78. Else B, Emel TJ, Kern T, Cavanagh LE, Allen TW. Peroneus longus rupture at its origin managed with platelet rich plasma. J Am Osteopath Assoc. 2015;115(10):622–4.

79. Deben SE, Pomeroy GC. Subtle cavus foot: diagnosis and management. J Am Acad Orthop Surg. 2014;22(8):512–20.

80. Slater HK. Acute peroneal tendon tears. Foot Ankle Clin. 2007;12(4):659–74, vii.

81. Sammarco GJ. Peroneus longus tendon tears: acute and chronic. Foot Ankle Int. 1995;16(5):245–53.

82. Rademaker J, Rosenberg ZS, Delfaut EM, Cheung YY, Schweitzer ME. Tear of the peroneus longus tendon: MR imaging features in nine patients. Radiology. 2000;214(3):700–4.

83. Krause JO, Brodsky JW. Peroneus brevis tendon tears: pathophysiology, surgical reconstruction, and clinical results. Foot Ankle Int. 1998;19(5):271–9.

84. Seybold JD, Campbell JT, Jeng CL, Short KW, Myerson MS. Outcome of lateral transfer of the FHL or FDL for concomitant peroneal tendon tears. Foot Ankle Int. 2016;37(6):576–81.

85. Demetracopoulos CA, Vineyard JC, Kiesau CD, Nunley JA 2nd. Long-term results of debridement and primary repair of peroneal tendon tears. Foot Ankle Int. 2014;35(3):252–7.

86. Squires N, Myerson MS, Gamba C. Surgical treatment of peroneal tendon tears. Foot Ankle Clin. 2007;12(4):675–95, vii.

87. Bahad SR, Kane JM. Peroneal tendon pathology: treatment and reconstruction of peroneal tears and instability. Orthop Clin North Am. 2020;51(1):121–30.

88. Sobel M, Geppert MJ, Olson EJ, Bohne WH, Arnoczky SP. The dynamics of peroneus brevis tendon splits: a proposed mechanism, technique of diagnosis, and classification of injury. Foot Ankle. 1992;13(7):413–22.

89. Pellegrini MJ, Glisson RR, Matsumoto T, Schiff A, Laver L, Easley ME, et al. Effectiveness of allograft reconstruction vs tenodesis for irreparable peroneus brevis tears: a cadaveric model. Foot Ankle Int. 2016;37(8):803–8.

90. Nishikawa DRC, Duarte FA, Saito GH, de Cesar Netto C, Monteiro AC, Prado MP, et al. Reconstruction of the

peroneus brevis tendon tears with semitendinosus tendon autograft. Case Rep Orthop. 2019;2019:5014687.

91. Mook WR, Parekh SG, Nunley JA. Allograft reconstruction of peroneal tendons: operative technique and clinical outcomes. Foot Ankle Int. 2013;34(9):1212–20.

92. Marsland D, Stephen JM, Calder T, Amis AA, Calder JDF. Strength of interference screw fixation to cuboid vs pulvertaft weave to peroneus brevis for tibialis posterior tendon transfer for foot drop. Foot Ankle Int. 2018;39(7):858–64.

93. Chagas-Neto FA, de Souza BN, Nogueira-Barbosa MH. Painful Os Peroneum syndrome: underdiagnosed condition in the lateral midfoot pain. Case Rep Radiol. 2016;2016:8739362.

94. Stockton KG, Brodsky JW. Peroneus longus tears associated with pathology of the os peroneum. Foot Ankle Int. 2014;35(4):346–52.

Anterior/Dorsal Ankle Tendons

14

Kenneth Mautner, Katherine Nanos
and Ashley McCann

Abbreviations

EDL   extensor digitorum longus
EHL   extensor halluces longus
MRI   magnetic resonance imaging
NSAID nonsteroidal anti-inflammatory drug
TA   tibialis anterior
US   ultrasound

Overview

The following will be discussed throughout this chapter, in order:

- Tibialis anterior
- Extensor digitorum longus
- Extensor hallucis longus
- Peroneus tertius

K. Mautner
Department of Orthopedic Surgery, Emory University, Atlanta, GA, USA
e-mail: kmautne@emory.edu

K. Nanos (✉)
Strive Physiotherapy and Sports Medicine, Toronto, ON, Canada

A. McCann
Department of Family Medicine, Morehouse School of Medicine, Atlanta, GA, USA

Tibialis Anterior (TA)

Introduction/Anatomy

The tibialis anterior (TA) muscle originates on Gerdy's tubercle on the proximal lateral tibia, along the proximal 2/3 of the lateral surface of the tibia, and the anterior surface of the interosseous membrane [1, 2]. Its tendon is the largest and most medial tendon of the anterior ankle [3] (Figs. 14.1 and 14.2). Its insertion sites can vary [4]; however, most often the tendon inserts on the medial plantar surface of the medial cuneiform (dominant slip) and distally on the plantar surface of the base of the first metatarsal (thin slip) [1, 2, 4, 5]. The TA tendon is secured to the anterior aspect of the ankle and foot by the both superior and inferior extensor retinaculum along with the other foot extensor tendons [5]. The proximal TA tendon is surrounded by a synovial sheath, while the distal few centimeters of the tendon are enveloped by a paratenon [4].

The TA is responsible for 80% of ankle dorsiflexion [4], and is the main foot inverter while in dorsiflexion (along with tibialis posterior). It also aids in suspending the foot arch, participates in foot adduction (with extensor hallucis longus) [2], and supination of the rearfoot [5]. It is part of the anterior compartment of the leg and receives its blood supply from the anterior tibial artery proximally, and branches of the medial tarsal artery distally [5]. It is innervated by the deep

Fig. 14.1 Tendons of
the ankle dorsum, lateral
view

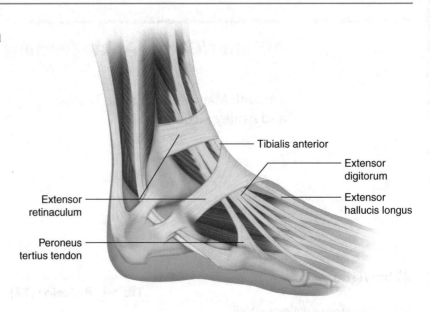

Tibialis anterior

Extensor
digitorum

Extensor
hallucis longus

Extensor
retinaculum

Peroneus
tertius tendon

peroneal nerve which receives contributions from L4 and L5 nerve roots [2].

Lesions of the tibialis anterior (TA) tendon have been infrequently reported in the literature to date, though the pathology does occur. Like other conditions of the ankle extensor compartment, TA tendinopathy is a commonly missed diagnosis at clinical presentation, due to a low index of clinical suspicion and potentially subtle findings on physical examination [4]. Distal tendinopathy is more commonly described, often affecting the band inserting onto the medial cuneiform [5]. It is possible that the distal tendon is more vulnerable to degeneration due to its naturally poor blood supply, which in turn, limits its reparative abilities [6]. Tendon pathology at the level of the ankle deep to the superior extensor retinaculum also exists. It is typically reported as an overuse injury in runners and race walkers in the setting of an increase in training distance, particularly with up and downhill components [6, 7], or in football kickers and soccer players who repeatedly and forcefully dorsiflex a plantarflexed foot against resistance, placing eccentric force on the TA and its tendon [7]. Other proposed etiologies for TA tendon pathology include tight-fitting or high-heeled footwear and elevated body mass index due to the increased load this places on the medial longitudinal arch [4]. The relationship between TA tendinopathy

and midfoot arthropathy has been suggested in the literature, but is unclear [5, 6].

Rupture of the TA is also relatively uncommon, and to date, has predominantly been reported in case reports and small case series [8]. When it occurs, it can be spontaneous or secondary to trauma, and tends to rupture between the extensor retinaculum and insertion [3, 5]. Spontaneous rupture is most commonly seen in older patients [3]. Rupture can be brought on by movements that induce sudden plantarflexion and eversion in a dorsiflexed foot [9, 10], subjecting an already degenerated tendon to notable eccentric loading [10, 11]. Patients with preexisting conditions such as inflammatory arthropathies, gout, diabetes, infections, hypothyroidism, ischemia, lupus, or patients receiving chronic steroids (oral or intratendinous injections) are more at risk for spontaneous rupture secondary to tendon degeneration [10, 11]. Younger patients tend to rupture their tendons in more acute/traumatic settings [3].

Tibialis Anterior Tendinopathy

A 29-year-old ultra-marathon runner presents with a 2-day history of anteromedial ankle pain that had started after completing a predominantly down-hill 50 kilometer trail run. On exam-

Fig. 14.2 Tendons of
the ankle dorsum, dorsal
view

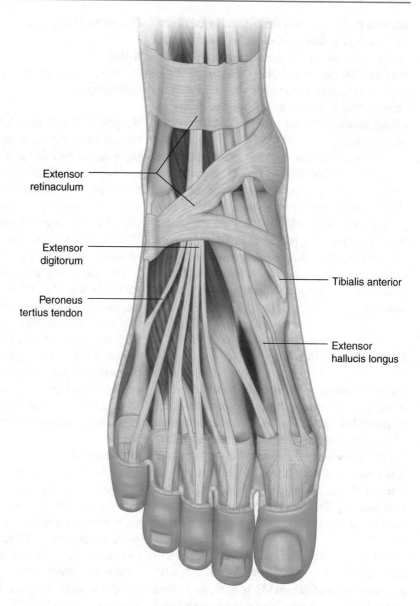

Extensor
retinaculum

Extensor
digitorum

Peroneus
tertius tendon

Tibialis anterior

Extensor
hallucis longus

*ination, her pain became worse with active
dorsiflexion of the ankle, and a subtle "puffiness"
over the anteromedial ankle was noted.*

Clinical Presentation

TA tendinopathy affecting the distal tendon is
most commonly seen in overweight females,

ages 50–70 years [5] and presents with a burning
sensation along the medial midfoot [4–6]. Pain
can be exacerbated at night, secondary to the
increased tension placed on the tendon while
relaxing in the supine position or laying prone
with the feet passively plantarflexed [4–6].
Dorsomedial foot swelling can be appreciated in
some [6], as well as relative plantarflexion of the
first metatarsal during active foot dorsiflexion

[4]. Due to its infrequent description in the literature, the natural history of distal TA tendinopathy is not well known. As previously noted, more proximal TA tendon pathology also exists at the level of the ankle, deep to the superior extensor retinaculum, typically as an overuse injury in young, athletes who do a lot of down- or uphill running [4, 6].

A patient with TA tendon rupture may note weakness with dorsiflexion [3, 11], and in some cases may present with a steppage or foot-slapping gait, gait incoordination and/or a propensity to toe-drag [8, 10, 11]. Pain associated with this injury is typically mild [10, 11]. Foot drop can sometimes be misdiagnosed as L4-L5 radiculopathy or peroneal nerve palsy [11]. Stress fracture is an important differential diagnosis to consider.

Physical Examination

On examination, a patient with distal TA tendinopathy may demonstrate dorsomedial foot swelling [6], as well as relative plantarflexion of the first metatarsal during active dorsiflexion [4]. They may also have point tenderness at the tendon's distal insertion [6], pain with resisted dorsiflexion [6], and difficulty with heel walking. There is a high incidence of concurrent Achilles tendon contracture/tightness as well.

In the case of tendon rupture, the patient will no longer have a palpable or visible tendon, even during active dorsiflexion [3]. Instead, the tendon stump may form a lump that can be appreciated on the anteromedial aspect of the distal leg [3, 10]. The patient may demonstrate weakness with active dorsiflexion, though this action may be preserved to some degree due to the role that the other extensor tendons play in assisting dorsiflexion [3, 11]. Because of this compensation, TA tendon rupture can sometimes go unnoticed for extended periods of time [8]. However, in other cases, patients with TA tendon rupture may present with a high-steppage or foot-slapping gait, gait incoordination and/or a propensity to toe-drag [8, 10, 11].

Diagnostic Workup

X-Ray
X-ray has a minimal role in helping diagnose TA tendinopathy.

Magnetic Resonance Imaging
Magnetic resonance imaging (MRI) is a key imaging modality used in the accurate diagnosis of TA tendinopathy [4]. High signal intensity (linear vs diffuse), split tears, tendon thickening, peritendinous edema and synovitis, as well as soft tissue edema overlying the affected tendon can be appreciated [11, 12]. In some instances, associated pathologies such as midfoot arthropathy can also be seen [6, 12]. Occasionally, bony edema can be observed along the medial aspect of the foot on the plantar surface [6]. Per the literature, a majority of abnormalities tend to occur in the zone approximately 3 cm away from the tendon insertion [6]. In the case of tendon rupture, MRI is the imaging modality of choice for diagnosis and can also be helpful for planning surgical repair and potential graft selection [10, 11]. Discontinuity and tendon retraction of the proximal tendon segment can be seen [11].

Ultrasound
Ultrasound (US) can also be helpful in identifying and characterizing TA tendon pathology. When using US, it is important for the sonographer to examine both insertional bands to ensure complete evaluation. Ultrasound of distal TA tendinopathy will reveal a thickened, hypoechoic tendon [3]. Neovascularity may also be noted using the color Doppler function. In complete ruptures, US can be helpful in confirming that the palpable mass is in fact tendon, as a subcutaneous lump viewed underneath the skin can easily be misdiagnosed as a tumor or cyst to the naked eye [3]. In these cases, an effusion can also be appreciated within the tendon sheath [3].

Treatment

Conservative
Initial conservative treatment for distal TA tendinopathy includes relative rest, custom orthotics

that provide support to the medial longitudinal arch and reduce load on the tendon, short-term use of nonsteroidal anti-inflammatory drugs (NSAIDs), rehabilitation, and night splints [6, 7, 12]. Other factors to consider addressing include correction of training errors, Achilles tendon stretching, optimization of equipment (e.g., footwear), and overall health (e.g., smoking, weight reduction) [7]. From a physical therapy perspective, as with other tendinopathies, eccentric strengthening helps promote the formation of new collagen [7]. In cases of tenosynovitis, immobilizing the ankle in a walking boot for a short period of time can be helpful in calming acute inflammation as well [7]. Due to its infrequent occurrence, no strict guidelines for TA tendon rupture management have been established [10].

In the case of an elderly patient with a rupture who is a poor surgical candidate or does not have a high baseline level of activity, conservative treatment may be preferred [8, 10], including physical therapy or an ankle-foot orthosis [8]. However, advanced age is not a contraindication for surgical treatment in the appropriate (active) candidate [8]. Patients with TA tendon rupture who undergo conservative treatment should be counseled regarding the potential functional outcomes, including persistent gait abnormalities [8]. Patients with partial tears also tend to do well with conservative treatment [10]. A study by Dooley et al. recommended conservative treatment for patients with a delay of diagnosis of more than 3 months, as outcomes may be suboptimal and the surgery more complicated [10].

Interventional

Peritendinous injections with corticosteroids can be effective in modulating pain related to TA tendinopathy or tenosynovitis [5]. As with any corticosteroid injection used to treat tendon-related pain, careful attention should be paid toward avoiding intratendinous injection, as the literature has shown that corticosteroids have deleterious effects and may put the patient at risk for tendon rupture. The use of ultrasound can improve accuracy of guiding the needle into the tendon sheath or the peritendinous tissue [5].

Currently, there is a paucity of literature addressing the role of orthobiologics or other minimally invasive procedures including tenotomy in the treatment of conditions involving the TA tendon.

Operative

Recalcitrant TA tendinopathy unresponsive to conservative measures may require surgical intervention. In these cases, tendinopathic tissue can be debrided. Different approaches to repair exist. One study by Grundy et al. suggested that the presence of more than 50% of normal tendon post-debridement, longitudinal split tears may be repaired, whereas when less than 50% of normal tendon remains, the tendon may be augmented with an extensor hallucis longus (EHL) tendon transfer [12]. Alternatively, some believe that an EHL transfer should be performed in any case beyond mild tendinopathy [12]. In addition, concomitant Achilles tendon contractures should always be diagnosed and an Achilles lengthening or gastrocnemius release offered at time of surgery.

Surgical repair of TA tendon ruptures can offer better functional outcomes as it aims to normalize gait patterns by restoring the actions of the TA. Additionally, it works to prevent potential sequelae of TA tendon rupture, such as the development of claw toe deformity from flexor/extensor imbalance [8, 9].

Direct/primary tendon repair is uncommon but ideal when the tendon ends can be approximated or when the tendon can reach its insertion [8, 10]. If neither can be achieved, then interpositional tendon grafts can be used [10]. Common autologous graft sources include the plantaris, EHL, peroneus longus, and Achilles tendons. A study by Sammarco et al. (2009) recommended that tendon repair be performed in all cases, regardless of age, when the patient is symptomatic with an unsteady or slapping gait or weakness and fatigability due to lack of dorsiflexion strength. Additionally, primary repairs tend to be performed when the pathology is diagnosed within 3 months of injury [8]. Surgical patients should be counseled regarding possible continuing dorsiflexion weakness compared with the contralateral foot. According to a systematic review performed by Christman-Skieller et al. in 2015, there is a need for further studies regarding the treatment of TA tendon ruptures. Larger, randomized studies with validated scoring systems for pre- and postoperative function would offer more insight into the best treatments for these injuries [8].

Extensor Digitorum Longus (EDL)

Introduction/Anatomy

The extensor digitorum longus (EDL) originates on the lateral condyle of the tibia, the head and proximal three quarters of the anterior aspect of the fibula and the proximal portion of the interosseous membrane [2]. After passing deep to the inferior extensor retinaculum, its four tendon slips insert on the dorsal aspect of the middle and distal phalanges on their respective digits, II–V [2, 4] (Figs. 14.1 and 14.2). EDL is responsible for extension of toes II–V and participates in dorsiflexion of the ankle [2, 4]. It is also part of the anterior compartment of the leg, receiving its blood supply from the anterior tibial artery and nerve supply from the deep peroneal nerve, which has contributions from L4 and L5 nerve roots [2].

Extensor Digitorum Longus Tendinopathy

A 35-year-old ultramarathon runner presents with pain over the dorsal aspect of his ankle. He is amidst training for a century race that is coming up in 4 weeks. On examination, you notice excessive pronation of his affected ankle, as well a relative weakness and pain with extension of his toes.

Clinical Presentation

EDL tendinopathy is uncommon but can be a result of overuse, and per the literature, it accounts

for 14% of injuries sustained by ultramarathon runners [13]. The entity known as "ultramarathoner's ankle" [4, 13, 14] is inflammation at the anterior ankle, attributable to excessive pronation, tight-fitting shoes, muscle imbalance, eccentric overload, and the shuffling gait that can be characteristic of an ultramarathon runner [13, 14] which requires relatively more movement about the ankle as compared to a typical running gait [13]. There is an additional case report in the literature by Kobayashi et al. that identified talar head impingement and exostosis as a possible cause for EDL tendinopathy [14]. Accounts of EDL rupture in the literature are extremely rare.

Physical Examination

Patients with EDL tendinopathy may present with tenderness and swelling along the course of the tendon at the dorsal aspect of the ankle [14]. They can exhibit crepitus or triggering at the inferior extensor retinaculum [14] and toe extension may be weak and/or painful. As with TA tendinopathy, Achilles tendon contracture/tightness may also be present.

Diagnostic Workup

Similar to the TA tendon, both MRI and ultrasound can be helpful diagnostic tools and findings will be similar in the tendinopathic EDL tendon. Fluid can be seen distending the tendon sheath in the case of tenosynovitis [4]. Ultrasound can be used dynamically to assess for tendon partial versus complete tearing/laceration and identifying tendon edges in the case of complete tears [4]. Fusiform tendon thickening, increased intrasubstance signal intensity, and partial or complete tendon fiber tearing can be seen on MRI [4].

Treatment

Conservative/Interventional
Conservative treatment for EDL tendinopathy is effective in most cases and can include NSAIDs,

taping, immobilization in acute tendinitis (not tendinopathy), orthotics, and peritendinous corticosteroid injections [14]. As in the case of the TA tendon, there is a paucity of literature addressing the role of biologics or other minimally invasive procedures including tenotomy in the treatment of conditions involving the EDL. However, based on the theories of their mechanisms of action and the current clinical indications for their use, their role in the treatment of EDL tendinopathy can be considered. They would not be suitable for use in the cases of more acute inflammatory conditions or complete tearing of the EDL tendon.

Operative

Although rarely mentioned in the literature, surgical treatment of a lacerated or ruptured EDL tendon is indicated to preserve gait, improve extension, and prevent toe clawing. Talus spurs can be removed in the same setting. Surgery for EDL tendinopathy or tenosynovitis is only indicated in recalcitrant cases in athletes who are severely impaired [14]. Tenosynovectomy can be considered, and in these cases, surgeons are careful to maintain the integrity of the extensor retinaculum in order to prevent postoperative "bowstringing" of the tendons in the anterior ankle [14]. Careful attention should also be paid in order to avoid injury to the superficial peroneal nerve [14]. The role of Achilles lengthening or gastrocnemius release is unclear and requires further study.

Extensor Hallucis Longus (EHL)

Introduction/Anatomy

The extensor hallucis longus (EHL) muscle originates from the middle 2/3 of the anterior potion of the fibula and adjacent interosseous membrane and descends vertically between the tibialis anterior (TA) and extensor digitorum longus (EDL) muscles to become tendinous at the distal third of the tibia. The EHL tendon obliquely courses deep to the superior and inferior extensor retinacula before inserting medially onto the dorsal surface

of the distal phalangeal base of the hallux [15] (Figs. 14.1 and 14.2). The tendon inserts as an expansion of a thin, triangular, aponeurotic sheath that covers the dorsal surface of the distal phalangeal base. There is considerable anatomic variation of the EHL tendon and its insertion, including one to three muscle bellies and tendons and a shared muscle slip with the EDL tendon [16]. The EHL is supplied by the anterior tibial artery and is innervated by the deep peroneal nerve [17]. The principle function of the EHL is to extend the hallux, although the EHL tendon also contributes to overall foot dorsiflexion and inversion.

Injuries to the extensor compartment of the ankle are often overlooked yet require prompt diagnosis and treatment to preserve function and produce a desirable outcome [9]. Any structure within the ankle extensor compartment is subject to injury, with the most frequent injuries involving the tendons, most commonly the TA tendon followed by the EHL and EDL tendons. Injury to the ankle extensor compartment is relatively uncommon, in part because the straight course of the extensor tendons compared with that of other tendons in the ankle protects them from biomechanical stress [18].

Injuries to the EHL tendon include tenosynovitis, more chronic tendinopathy, and tendon tear or a rupture. Given the superficial location of the EHL tendon it is especially vulnerable to penetrating trauma and laceration during industrial accidents [19]. It is reported in one study that 88% of EHL tendon disruption is due to lacerations [20]. Closed tendon ruptures, which are caused by active tendon contraction against resistance, are unusual and typically are associated with a predisposing cause such as mechanical overuse, inflammatory arthritis, infection, diabetes mellitus, crystal deposition disease, or midfoot arthropathy [19, 20]. Mechanical impingement by bone spurs or tight-fitting, high-laced boots can also be a predisposing factor. Sports-related injuries incurred during activities such as ultramarathon running [21] and tae kwon do [22] and iatrogenic injury after arthroscopic thermal ablation have also been described [23].

Extensor Hallucis Longus Tendinopathy

A 34-year-old male runner presents with complaints of worsening pain along the dorsal aspect of the left great toe for 2 months. The patient reported a pain level of 2–3/10 without movement. Pain worsened with active and passive flexion and extension of the great toe to a level of 7–8/10.

Clinical Presentation

EHL tendinopathy can occur as a result of acute injury and overuse injury. Overexerting the tendons, such as excessive running, especially running uphill or downhill as the tendon has to work hard to control the foot or running on icy surfaces can also put added stress on the tendon. Degenerative changes in the tendon due to aging or other factors such as excessive pes planus can also be a source of injury. Tight calf muscles, which pose greater resistance to the action of extensor tendons or pes planus, as well as Ill-fitting shoes, especially shoes that irritate the top of the foot can be detrimental to the EHL tendon.

Physical Examination

Examination for EHL pathology starts with inspection for local swelling, redness, or skin laceration. Bare foot gait analysis typically shows drooping of the great toe with loss of extension in mid-stance.

Palpation of the tendon with and without resistance is paramount in detecting tenderness, weakness, and tendon gap formation in case of rupture or laceration. Deep peroneal nerve irritation or loss of sensation may accompany an EHL injury at the level of the midfoot.

Diagnostic Workup

With US and MRI imaging, fluid is seen distending the tendon sheath with tenosynovitis of either mechanical or inflammatory origin. Any amount of fluid within the extensor tendon sheath is indicative of disease. Both modalities are useful for assessing intrasubstance tearing, usually present in more chronic injury. If there is complete rupture with tendon retraction, US may be advantageous over MRI to locate torn tendon edges [24].

MRI findings include fusiform tendon thickening, increased intrasubstance signal intensity, and frank fiber discontinuity, reflecting tendinosis, partial tear, and complete tear, respectively [24].

Ultrasonography is a noninvasive, operator-dependent imaging modality useful for diagnosis of injuries to the ankle extensor compartment [25]. It is important that a skilled sonographer evaluates bilateral EHL tendons to ensure a complete and accurate assessment of the injured tendon. The superficial location of the EHL allows easy depiction on US [24]. Ultrasound of a distal EHL tendinopathy will reveal loss of normal fibular structure with increased spacing of the hyperechoic fibrillar lines and generally reduced echogenicity often associated with thickening of the tendon. Power Doppler may show tendon neovascularization and sometimes calcification may be presents. A tear may be seen as a hypoechoic area that interrupts the ligament fibers, extending across the ligament in a full thickness complete tear. Dynamic imaging during muscle contraction or passive movement is often helpful [26].

Treatment

Both nonsurgical and surgical treatments of EHL tendon tears have been advocated. Lacerations of the EHL tendon distal to the extensor expansion compartment may not cause significant loss of function or tendon retraction and thus may be treated conservatively. Conversely, more proximal lacerations create significant tendon retraction and function loss and require surgical intervention, particularly in young patients [27].

The literature is inconsistent regarding surgical repair of the EHL, with some authors advocating allowing spontaneous healing. Complications of nonsurgical treatment may result in plantar flexion deformity of the hallux joint (hammer toe), while surgical complications include painful scar, tendon adhesions, limitation of motion, and rerupture [28].

Conservative/Interventional

The location of the EHL tendon pathology is critical to the potential success of non-operative management. In cases where laceration occurs distal to the extensor expansion of the EHL, hallux dorsiflexion function is preserved and nonoperative treatment should be the first line [27].

The initial treatment involves rest and pain relief. For nontraumatic tendinopathy, avoiding stressful activities, cold therapy, and anti-inflammatory drugs help to control pain and swelling. The actual treatment depends upon the cause of the problem. Calf muscle stretching helps to reduce the stiffness of calf muscles and reduce stress on the extensor tendons. Eccentric strengthening of the extensor muscles also improves their resistance to overuse injury. Using padding in the forefoot area helps to relieve pressure and orthotics can be used to help support the foot and rest overworked tendons. Arch supports can be used to correct faulty biomechanics especially when the foot over-pronates causing stress to the extensor tendons.

For tendinosis, as the main problem is failed healing, there are certain new treatments which promote healing by increasing growth factor activity in the area (platelets have growth factors that may facilitate healing for chronic tendinopathy). These include needling the affected tendon to promote bleeding and thus platelet activity, or by injecting a person's own blood or platelets (derived from the blood) in the area. It should be remembered that tendon injuries are slow to heal, therefore it is important that a proper healing period be provided, usually weeks to months [13].

Operative

In cases of EHL laceration proximal to the extensor expansion, surgical intervention should be considered to address the loss of joint extension. There has been a trend toward primary surgical repair of acute tendon injuries or surgical reconstruction if tendon retraction prevents tension-free tendon opposition; however, few studies have used patient-rated objective outcome mea-

sures to quantify function after repair [19]. The most cited complication of EHL tendon repair is painful scar formation, which can occur in as many as 38% of patients [29].

Chronic multifocal closed rupture of the EHL tendon is a very rare disease. Although primary suture could be performed, tendon graft is used when primary suture is not possible. Many structures that could be used as donor graft exist in the foot such as the plantaris, peroneus tertius, extensor digitorum longus (EDL) slip, extensor digitorum brevis (EDB), and extensor hallucis brevis (EHB) [30]. Two details must be considered when performing autologous graft repair. The first is the length of the graft tendon. Among those tendons that are used as free graft, shorter grafts can be obtained from the EDL, EDB, and EHB. The plantaris and peroneus tertius tendons are used when a longer graft length is needed. The second thing is that the diameter of the graft tendon should be similar to that of the damaged tendon to prevent adhesion due to fibrotic projections that would develop at both ends of the tendon due to unequal anastomosis. For large gaps, the semitendinosus tendon has been shown to provide a sufficient length and diameter similar to the EHL tendon for repair [31].

Peroneus Tertius

Introduction/Anatomy

The peroneus tertius (PT) muscle arises from the lower 1/3 of the anterior surface of the fibula, from the lower part of the interosseous membrane, and from an intermuscular septum between it and the peroneus brevis muscle. The tendon, after passing under the superior extensor retinaculum and inferior extensor retinaculum of the foot in the same canal as the extensor digitorum longus, is inserted into the dorsal surface of the base of the metatarsal bone of the fifth digit (Figs. 14.1 and 14.2). The peroneus tertius tendon or fibularis tendon is innervated by the deep peroneal nerve (L5, S1), unlike other peroneal muscles which are innervated by the superficial peroneal nerve, since the peroneus tertius is a member of the anterior compartment. The anterior tibial artery is the blood supply for the peroneus tertius. There is no primary action but secondarily the peroneus tertius assists with weak dorsiflexion of the ankle joint and to evert and extend the foot [32]. The prevalence of the PT muscle ranges from 49% to 94% in anatomic studies by Ramirez and Rourke, and congenital absence of the muscle has not been associated with an increased risk of ankle ligamentous injury [33–35]. This may explain why the PT tendon is often used as an autograft for other vital tendon injuries.

Injury to the peroneus tertius tendon is rare, with no previously reported cases in the literature. Therefore, there is little information pertaining to the clinical significance, diagnostic maneuvers, and therapeutic options for patients presenting with PT injury or rupture. It is important to understand this rare anatomic variant and the potential for associated pathology when considering the management of patients who present with injury involving the peroneus tertius tendon [32].

Peroneus Tertius Tendinopathy

A 21-year-old avid runner presents with 2 months of vague lateral right foot pain. States that the pain is more of a tightness and worse with ambulation. She denies fall or other injury. Of note, the patient increased her running mileage by 30% over the last 3 months and incorporated long distance running on uneven surfaces. There is mild local swelling along the medial aspect of the fifth metatarsal.

Clinical Presentation

A strain or injury can be caused to the peroneus tertius tendon due to overuse. This can be seen in those involved with long distance running on uneven surfaces. Prolonged standing at one place without any movement such as those people who work as greeters or security guards can also injure or strain the peroneus tertius muscle and lead to tendon pain as well.

Some of the activities that can cause peroneus tertius injury are sudden forceful twisting motion of the ankle, prolonged immobilization of the leg such as during a fracture, wearing tight bands around the leg, or even wearing high heels.

Physical Examination

Examination for peroneal tertius pathology starts with inspection for local swelling, redness or skin laceration.

Palpation of the tendon with and without resistance is paramount in detecting tenderness, weakness, and tendon gap formation in case of rupture or laceration.

Diagnostic Workup

There is little information pertaining to the diagnostic physical exam maneuvers or imaging for patients presenting with peroneus tertius injury or rupture. MRI findings can include elevated signal around the common peroneal tendon sheath, consistent with tenosynovitis of the peroneus tertius or even evidence of rupture if the tendon variant is identified. Ultrasound can also be used to look for typical findings expected with tendinopathy.

Treatment

Conservative/Interventional
Any sort of damage or injury to the peroneus tertius tendon will result in ankle and heel pain and problems with ambulation. Treatment for peroneus tertius tendon injury acutely is normally conservative with use of analgesics, hot and cold packs, gentle stretching exercises and limited or non-weight bearing on the affected foot for a few days. Usually, it takes a couple of weeks for the peroneus tertius tendinitis to resolve although the natural history has not been well studied given the rarity of the diagnosis.

Operative

Our literature search yielded no reports for operative treatment of PT. Surgery is only indicated for PT harvest as an autograft.

References

1. Wheeless CR. Wheeless' textbook of orthopaedics. Wheeless Online. Duke Orthopedics, 27 Sept. 2016. Web. 07 Jan. 2017.
2. Thompson JC. Netter's concise orthopedic anatomy. 2nd ed. Philadelphia: Elsevier; 2010.
3. Bianchi S, Martinoli C. Ultrasound of the musculoskeletal system. Berlin: Springer; 2007.
4. Ng JM, Rosenberg ZS, Bencardino JT, et al. US and MRI imaging of the extensor compartment of the ankle. Radiographics. 2013;33:2047–64.
5. Varghese A, Bianchi S. Ultrasound of tibialis anterior muscle and tendon: anatomy, technique of examination, normal and pathologic appearance. J Ultrasound. 2014;17:113–23.
6. Beischer AD, et al. Distal tendinosis of the tibialis anterior tendon. Foot Ankle Int. 2009;30(11):1053–9.
7. Simpson MR, Howard TM. Tendinopathies of the foot and ankle. Am Fam Physician. 2009;80(10):1107–14.
8. Christman-Skieller C, Merz MK, Tansey JP. A systematic review of tiialis anterior tendon rupture treatments and outcomes. Am J Orthop. 2015;44(4):E94–9.
9. Markarian GG, Kelikian AS, Brage M, Trainor T, Dias L. Anterior tibialis tendon ruptures: an outcome analysis of operative vs nonoperative treatment. Foot Ankle Int. 1998;19(12):792–802.
10. Sammarco VJ, Sammarco GJ, Henning C, Chaim S. Surgical repair of actute and chronic tibialis anterior tendon ruptures. J Bone Joint Surg. 2009;91(2):325–32.
11. Nabil JK, El-Khoury GY, Saltzman CL, Brandser EA. Rupture of the anterior tibial tendon: diagnosis by MR imaging. Am J Roentgenol. 1996;167(2):351–4.
12. Grundy JRB, O'Sullivan RM, Beischer AD. Operative management of distal tibialis anterior tendinopathy. Foot Ankle Int. 2010;31(3):212–9.
13. Moore D. Extensor Digitorum Longus (L5). Orthobullets. University of Washington; 2017. Web. 07 Jan. 2017.Bishop.
14. Kobayashi H, Sakurai M, Kobayashi T. Extensor digitorum longus tenosynovitis caused by talar head impingement in an ultramarathon runner: a case report. J Orthop Surg. 2007;15(2):245–7.
15. Sarrafian SK, Kelikian AS. Anatomy of the foot and ankle: descriptive, topographic, functional. 3rd ed. Philadelphia: Lippincott Williams & Wilkins; 2011. p. 120–62, 223–291

16. Tezer M, Cicekcibasi AE. A variation of the extensor hallucis longus muscle (accessory extensor digiti secundus muscle). Anat Sci Int. 2012;87(2):111–4.
17. Moore D. Extensor Hallucis Longus (L5). Orthobullets. Medical Illlustrations; 1997. Web. 10 Mar 2017.
18. Scheller AD, Kasser JR, Quigley TB. Tendon injuries about the ankle. Orthop Clin North Am. 1980;11(4):801–11.
19. Al-Qattan MM. Surgical treatment and results in 17 cases of open lacerations of the extensor hallucis longus tendon. J Plast Reconstr Aesthet Surg. 2007;60(4):360–7.
20. Scaduto AA, Cracchiolo A 3rd. Lacerations and ruptures of the flexor or extensor hallucis longus tendons. Foot Ankle Clin. 2000;5(3):725–36.
21. Kobayashi H, Sakurai M, Kobayashi T. Extensor digitorum longus tenosynovitis caused by talar head impingement in an ultramarathon runner: a case report. J Orthop Surg (Hong Kong). 2007;15(2):245–7.
22. Lee KT, Choi YS, Lee YK, Lee JP, Young KW, Park SY. Extensor hallucis longus tendon injury in taekwondo athletes. Phys Ther Sport. 2009;10(3):101–4.
23. Tuncer S, Aksu N, Isiklar U. Delayed rupture of the extensor hallucis longus and extensor digitorum communis tendons after breaching the anterior capsule with a radiofrequency probe during ankle arthroscopy: a case report. J Foot Ankle Surg. 2010;49(5):490. e1–3.
24. Ng JM, Rosenberg ZS, Jenny T. Bencardino, Restrepo-Velez Z, Ciavarra GA, Adler RS. US and MR imaging of the extensor compartment of the ankle. RadioGraphics. 2013. Web. 10 Mar 2017.
25. Fessell DP, Vanderschueren GM, Jacobson JA, et al. US of the ankle: technique, anatomy, and diagnosis of pathologic conditions. Radiographics. 1998;18(2):325–40.
26. Morvan G, Busson J, Wybier M, Mathieu P. Ultrasound of the ankle. Eur J Ultrasound. 2001;14:73–82.
27. Kass JC, Palumbo F, Mehl S, Camarinos N. Extensor hallucis longus tendon injury: an in-depth analysis and treatment protocol. J Foot Ankle Surg. 1997;36(1):24–7.
28. Jahss MH. Disorders of the hallux and the first ray. In: Jahss MH, editor. Disorders of the foot and ankle, vol. II. Philadelphia: W.B. Sauners Company; 1991. p. 943–1174.
29. Floyd DW, Heckman JD, Rockwood CA Jr. Tendon lacerations in the foot. Foot Ankle. 1983:8–14.
30. McGlamry ED. McGlamry's comprehensive textbook of foot and ankle surgery. Philadelphia: Wolters Kluwer/Lippincott Williams & Wilkins Health; 2012.
31. Park HG, Lee BK, Sim JA. Autogenous graft repair using semitendinous tendon for a chronic multifocal rupture of the extensor hallucis longus tendon: a case report. Foot Ankle Int. 2003;24:506–8.

32. Derrick E, et al. Peroneus tertius tendon tear: a rare cause of lateral ankle pain. Ed. Alexander Muacevic and John R Adler. Cureus. 2016;8(4):e577. *PMC*. Web. 12 March 2017.

33. Rourke K, Dafydd H, Parkin IG. Fibularis tertius: revisiting the anatomy. Clin Anat. 2007;20:946–9.

34. Witvrouw E, Borre KV, Willems TM, Huysmans J, Broos E, De Clercq D. The significance of peroneus tertius muscle in ankle injuries: a prospective study. Am J Sports Med. 2006;34:1159–63.

35. Ramirez D, Gajardo C, Caballero P, Zavando D, Cantín M, Suazo G. Clinical evaluation of fibularis tertius muscle prevalence. Int J Morphol. 2010;28:759–64.

Medial Ankle/Plantar Foot Tendons

15

Rohit Navlani and Stephanie A. Giammittorio

Abbreviations

CT	Computed tomography
FDL	Flexor digitorum longus
FHL	Flexor hallucis longus
MRI	Magnetic resonance imaging
NSAID	Non-steroidal anti-inflammatory drug
PRP	Platelet rich plasma
PTT	Posterior tibialis tendon
PTTD	Posterior tibial tendon dysfunction
TAL	Tendon Achilles lengthening
US	Ultrasound

Tibialis Posterior

Introduction/Anatomy

The tibialis posterior muscle originates from the posterior aspect of the interosseous membrane and the medial posterior borders of the tibia and fibula (Fig. 15.1). It then travels down to wrap around the posteromedial aspect of the ankle (Fig. 15.2). It passes below the plantar calcaneonavicular ligament

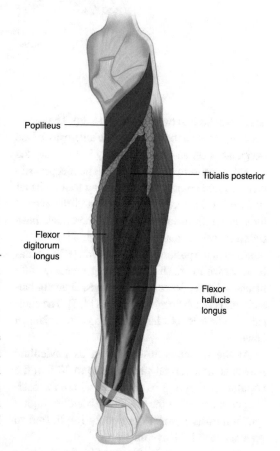

Fig. 15.1 Proximal anatomy of medial ankle muscle/tendon constructs

R. Navlani (✉)
Department of Anesthesiology and Perioperative Medicine, University of Pittsburgh, Pittsburgh, PA, USA
e-mail: navlanir@upmc.edu

S. A. Giammittorio
Riverside Medical Group Orthopedics and Sports Medicine, Williamsburg, VA, USA

Fig. 15.2 Distal
anatomy of the medial
ankle tendons

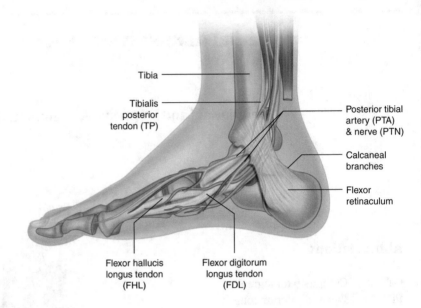

Tibia

Tibialis
posterior
tendon (TP)

Posterior tibial
artery (PTA)
& nerve (PTN)

Calcaneal
branches

Flexor
retinaculum

Flexor hallucis
longus tendon
(FHL)

Flexor digitorum
longus tendon
(FDL)

and then splits into two slips (Fig. 15.3a). The super-ficial slip goes on to insert onto the tuberosity of the navicular bone, and it occasionally inserts onto the medial cuneiform (Fig. 15.3b). The deeper slip divides again before finally attaching to the plantar surfaces of the second cuneiform and the second through fourth metatarsals [1–3]. There have been cadaveric studies that have shown variations on the insertion of the posterior tibialis tendon (PTT). It has been shown to attach to the spring ligament, fifth metatarsal base, flexor hallucis brevis, abductor hal-lucis, and even the peroneus longus [4, 5]. The clini-cal significance of these variations is unknown however.

At the navicular insertion, an os naviculare may exist as a normal variant in up to 28% of the population. A type 2 os navicular where the ossi-cle is connected to the navicular bone through a synchondrosis is most commonly implicated to predispose to PTT dysfunction.

The arterial supply for the tibialis posterior arises from the muscular branches of the sural, peroneal, and posterior tibial arteries. The blood supply is poorest when the tendon is passing behind the medial malleolus, making it prone to rupture [6]. The innervation is derived from the tibial nerve [L4, L5] [1–3].

The tibialis posterior primarily functions to invert the foot. It also plays a role in adduction of the foot and plantarflexion at the ankle [1, 2]. In addition, tendon of posterior tibialis muscle serves as the primary dynamic stabilizer of the medial longitudinal arch of the foot, the calcaneonavicu-lar ligament, or the spring ligament, serves as the primary static stabilizer [1–7]. During the normal toe-off stage of gait, the posterior tibialis muscle helps to support the medial longitudinal arch by locking the transverse tarsal joint (or talocalcaneo-navicular joint in this case) and in turn locking the hindfoot and midfoot in place. Conversely, during heel strike to the foot flat stage of gait, the tendon allows for unlocking of these joints, which allows for a smooth transition from a dorsiflexed phase to the neutral flat foot phase [7, 8].

Posterior Tibialis Tendinopathy

A 23-year-old post-collegiate female distance runner presents with chief complaint of 2-month history of pain localized the right medial ankle with running since beginning to run on trails. On physical exam the patient had tenderness to pal-pation posterior to the medial malleolus. She had flattening of the medial longitudinal arch on the right compared to the left with increased hindfoot

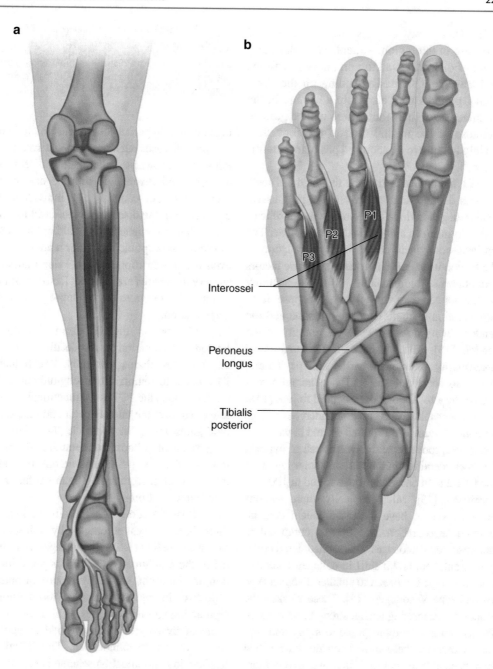

Fig. 15.3 (**a**, **b**): PTT anatomy and distal insertion of the tibialis posterior tendon

valgus. She had an antalgic gait with medial ankle pain while toeing off. She was unable to walk on her toes or do single leg toe raise due to pain. She has medial ankle pain and weakness with resisted ankle inversion and plantarflexion.

Clinical Presentation

The presentation is typically insidious. Patients typically complain of pain along the medial side of the foot and ankle, along the path of the

PTT. There may or may not be associated swelling in the region. Patients typically complain of difficulty walking on uneven surfaces, and traversing steps. Depending on the chronicity, patients may also note a change in the architecture of their foot. There will be gradual collapse of the medial arch of the foot, ultimately leading to an acquired pes planus deformity [6, 8–12].

PTT tendinopathy may be the result of acute injuries or more commonly chronic progressive tendon degeneration. The etiology is multifactorial with intrinsic and extrinsic components. The intrinsic component comes from degradation of the tendon itself, which is due to extrinsic factors like abnormal biomechanics [10]. The anatomy of the tendon is believed to predispose it to degeneration as there is no mesotendon and the tendon sheath does not span the entirety of the tendon [13]. The presence of the anatomical abnormality mentioned earlier, os naviculare, may also accelerate the PTT degeneration process or be a focal point of structural failure [14].

Biomechanically, the tendon undergoes a large amount of strain as it is pulled around in the retromalleolar groove repetitively. An area of hypoxia has been identified in the retromalleolar region of the PTT and in one study it was found in 100% of specimens [15]. Microscopically, these tendons are observed to have increased mucin content, myxoid degeneration, and fibrosis compared to non-diseased tendons, as well as disordered collagen orientation, and a shift in collagen composition from type I collagen to smaller diameter type III and type V collagen [15]. These weaken the tendon by decreasing tensile strength. As a result, the tendon is now more prone to injury and rupture. However, there have been no studies that have been able to confirm if this area is truly more commonly affected in PTT tendinopathy or tendon rupture.

Although physiologic PTT degeneration is expected with aging or overuse, many risk factors such as obesity, iatrogenic exposure to steroids, along with a variety of systemic diseases also play a role (Table 15.1) [8]. Examples of systemic illnesses include common diseases such as

Table 15.1 Risk factors for the development of PTTD [16]

Risk factors
Hypertension, obesity, diabetes mellitus, corticosteroid therapy, lupus, gout, rheumatoid arthritis, accessory navicular bone

diabetes and hypertension, but also include more complex diseases such as seronegative arthropathies [17]. Systemic inflammatory disease such as lupus and rheumatoid arthritis are typically seen in younger patients [17]. Individuals with connective tissue diseases are believed to exhibit slower tendon regeneration, making this population more susceptible to further tendon injury or even a possible rupture [13]. Prior trauma and surgery to the area are also risk factors that might result in a progression of subsequent tendon degeneration.

Dysfunction of the PTT from long standing tendon degeneration is a leading cause of acquired pes planus deformity. Recall that the PTT helps to maintain the longitudinal arch of the foot. Once the PTT is dysfunctional, it can no longer support the talonavicular and calcaneocuboid joints during the gait cycle [7–9]. This leads to subsequent collapse of the arch and development of acquired pes planus deformity. Patients may also suffer from spring ligament failure and sinus tarsi syndrome [10].

PTT dysfunction was initially divided into three basic stages or classes by Johnson and Strom in 1989 [11]. The three stages were based off of the condition of the tibialis posterior tendon, the hindfoot, subjective reports of pain and objective findings such as the "too-many-toes" sign and single-heel-rise test [11]. Based on the stage of dysfunction, conservative or operative treatment was recommended. The initial PTT dysfunction classification scheme is summarized in Table 15.2 [11, 12, 18].

The initial grading system did have its shortcomings, however. It only addressed one cause of the acquired flat foot deformity, the posterior tibialis tendon [19]. It did not take into account the importance of the naviculocuneiform joint, tarsometatarsal joints, the spring ligament complex, or the deltoid ligament which all play a key

Table 15.2 PTTD classification by stages. This table describes the original three stages described by Johnson and Strom [11, 12, 18]

	Stage I	Stage II	Stage III
Tendon pathology	Tenosynovitis or degeneration of the tendon	Elongation and degeneration of the tendon	Elongation and degeneration of the tendon
Subjective findings	Pain at medial ankle	Pain at medial and lateral ankle	Pain at medial and lateral ankle
Deformity	No deformity	Flexible pes planus deformity	Fixed pes planus deformity
Objective findings	Mild weakness, but patient will be able to complete single heel rise	Significant weakness, extreme difficulty or inability to perform single heel rise Positive "too many toes sign"	Inability to perform a single leg heel rise Positive "too many toes sign" Crepitus with tibiotalar motion

role in maintaining the arch of the foot [20, 21]. The plantar calcaneonavicular ligament, which is also referred to as the spring ligament complex, comprises three individual ligaments spanning from the calcaneus to the navicular on the underside of the foot. This ligamentous complex helps to maintain the medial longitudinal arch of the foot and provides support to the head of the talus. If the complex becomes damaged or torn, the medial arch becomes compromised with downward displacement of the talus that can result in a flatfoot deformity [20]. As discussed previously, the posterior tibial tendon along with the spring ligament complex helps to provide the structural integrity of the medial arch. If the medial arch of the foot is compromised, leading to instability of the midfoot, specifically the medial column by causing sag of the naviculocuneiform or tarsometatarsal joints. If this medial column instability is not addressed it can lead to poor outcomes and persistent deformities in patients [19, 22].

Multiple authors have made attempts to modify the existing system in efforts to correct the limitations [11, 12, 18, 22]. Though there have been multiple other grading systems developed, the validity has not been studied and usefulness has yet to be determined. All of the aforementioned should be considered when determining what surgical interventions may be required to obtain a successful outcome.

Table 15.3 Differential diagnosis of the acquired flat foot [23]

Rupture of the spring ligament complex
Degenerative arthritis of the ankle joint
Arthritis of the talonavicular joint
Posttraumatic tarsometatarsal joint arthritis
Inflammatory arthritis of the hindfoot
Charcot foot secondary to underlying neuropathy
FHL or FDL tendinopathy

As with any clinical problem, having a broad differential diagnosis is very important. When evaluating a patient with possible posterior tibial tendinopathy it is also important to consider bony, ligamentous, joint-related pathologies. Please refer to Table 15.3 for further details [23].

Physical Examination

Clinical findings can vary based on severity of the PTT tendinopathy. Some of the key exam findings are highlighted here.

The exam should begin with inspection of the patient. There may be subtle gait changes secondary to alterations in ankle and forefoot kinematics, such as increased dorsiflexion and abduction of the forefoot or increased plantarflexion and eversion of the hindfoot [24]. The patient may have a limited ability to walk secondary to impaired balance or severe pain [8–10, 12]. Ideally the examiner should be evaluating the patient from posterior to anterior to fully access any abnormal angulations. Inspection of the foot and ankle may reveal pes planus, or abnormal angulation at the hindfoot or forefoot as mentioned above. There may even be protrusion of the talar head secondary to subluxation [11]. There may also be notable swelling along the posterior tibialis tendon.

The "too-many-toes" sign was described by Johnson and Strom. When viewing the patient's foot from a posterior direction, the patient will have more toes visible on the lateral aspect of the affected foot due to forefoot abduction (Fig. 15.4) [11].

Next, the PTT should be palpated from its origins to the insertion to elicit any tenderness and evaluate for any associated swelling. Palpation of the tendon may also demonstrate irregularities within the tendon such as thickening or synovitis. It may be absent if there was a rupture of the tendon. Pes planus deformities can be broadly characterized into being flexible or fixed. A flexible deformity is where the foot maintains a normal arch at rest, but once there is contact with the ground the angulation deformities are noted. In contrast, the rigid foot deformities are present whether the patient is bearing weight or not. Thus, noted deformities in angulation should be

examined to determine if they are flexible or fixed, as this plays a major role in determining treatment options [11, 12, 18].

The range of motion of the ankle and the intrinsic joints of the foot should be examined. The tibialis posterior muscle strength should also be tested by having the patient plantarflex and invert against resistance. This may elicit pain and/or weakness [12, 18].

A double-leg toe raise can be performed to help differentiate between a flexible and rigid flatfoot. As the patient goes from bilateral flat foot stance to standing on their toes, the hindfoot should go into varus angulation. In PTT tendon, the patient's heel on the affected foot will be stuck in hindfoot valgus during this maneuver [8–12]. Typically, patients with stage I dysfunction, as characterized by the Johnson and Strom classification, will be able to perform this maneuver, while later stages will not [11, 12].

The single heel rise test is another special test often used in the diagnosis of PTT tendinopathy [8, 12]. The patient is asked to lift the unaffected leg off the ground and attempt to perform a single leg toe raise on the affected limb. Patients with PTT tendinopathy will have extreme difficulty performing this task in earlier stages and complete inability in later stages [11, 12].

Hintermann described a third special test that can be used to diagnose PTT tendinopathy. During his study, he noted that patients with PTT tendinopathy had absence of the signs mentioned above 20–35% of the time [25]. He went on to describe the first metatarsal raise sign. The patient is asked to stand on both feet. The examiner then grabs the tibia of the affected lower extremity being tested and externally rotates it. If PTT tendinopathy is present, the head of the first metatarsal will be elevated. In his study, it had 100% sensitivity [25].

Imaging

Although the diagnosis of PTT tendinopathy can be made with a careful history and physical examination, imaging studies help the clinician

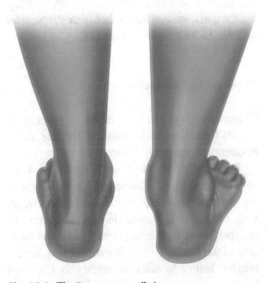

Fig. 15.4 The "too many toes" sign

in confirming the diagnosis, ruling out other pathologies and in planning both interventional and operative procedures.

X-Ray

Radiographs can be obtained to help evaluate for abnormal alignment and other bony changes [26]. Typically, anteroposterior and lateral weight-bearing images of the foot as well as the ankle mortise view are obtained. The specific radiographic terminologies used in this section are illustrated in Fig. 15.5 below. Radiographs in the early stages of disease may be normal. In the AP view, an increase in the talo-first metatarsal angle can be seen, known as the Meary angle [26]. There may also be increased talonavicular uncoverage seen on the AP images. This refers to the amount of talar head that is not in contact with the navicular due to forefoot abduction [26]. The lateral images may also show an increase in the Meary angle.

The Meary angle is the angle created between two lines, one drawn from the center of longitudinal axes of the talus and the other from the first metatarsal. The talocalcaneal angle is the angle formed by the intersection of the lines down the centers of the talus and calcaneus bones. The first metatarsal angle is measured from the ground and the line bisecting the first metatarsal. Finally, the calcaneal pitch can be measured using the ground and the calcaneal inclination axis. The normal

Meary angle is 0 degree. An angle >4 degrees indicates pes planus. The degree of angulation correlates to the severity of the deformity. Angles less than 15 degrees are mild, 15–30 degrees are considered moderate, and greater than 30 degrees are severe [27]. The normal calcaneal inclination axis is 17–32 degrees. The normal medial cuneiform-floor height is between 15 and 25 mm [26–29].

There may be decreased calcaneal pitch and medial cuneiform-floor height, indicating that there is collapse of the arch [26, 28]. In the ankle mortise view, talar tilt may be seen. This is typically seen in stage IV disease, as described by the modified Johnson classification, and is attributed to deltoid ligament insufficiency [26, 28]. Insufficiency of the deltoid ligament can lead to instability of the medial ankle and subsequent lateral tilt of the talus and hindfoot valgus deformity [28]. The collapse of the longitudinal arch can also be seen. There is a decrease in the calcaneal inclination axis, Meary angle, and the medial cuneiform-floor height [26–29].

These radiographic findings were studied by Younger in 2005. The above radiographic findings were found to be significantly different when comparing patients with PTT tendinopathy versus normal controls. These findings were found to be statistically significant [29]. Along with the above findings, there may also be non-specific findings of soft tissue swelling, or fine changes in the architecture of the tendon itself.

Tenography is an older imaging technique that involves injecting the synovial sheath with contrast material. Using fluoroscopy, the dye can be visualized and any irregularities in the tendon itself can be identified. Tenography has largely been replaced by ultrasound and MR imaging, modalities that are capable of yielding cross-sectional images of all of the ankle tendons and their surrounding structures [30].

Computed Tomography

Computed tomography (CT) has also been used in the diagnosis of PTT tendinopathy [31]. It appears to have more of a role in diagnosis of tendon ruptures. It is not commonly used as MRI and ultrasound provide superior imaging and less radiation exposure than CT scans [28].

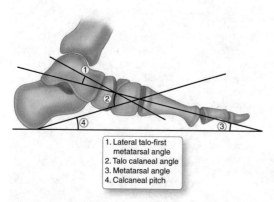

1. Lateral talo-first metatarsal angle
2. Talo calcaneal angle
3. Metatarsal angle
4. Calcaneal pitch

Fig. 15.5 A lateral weight-bearing image of the foot depicting the various angles: Meary angle, talo-calcaneal angle, metatarsal angle, and calcaneal pitch

Magnetic Resonance Imaging

Magnetic resonance imaging (MRI) is currently considered a useful imaging method for evaluation of PTT tendinopathy due to its soft tissue resolution, and multiplanar imaging ability. It also has a wider field of view than ultrasound allowing visualization beyond what can otherwise be reasonably covered [28, 32, 33]. It can identify any misalignment, bony changes, and even bony edema. MRI has a sensitivity of 95%, specificity of 100%, and accuracy of 96% in diagnosing PTT tendinopathy [33]. MRI can also assess the surrounding tendons and ligaments, and is especially useful if surgery is planned as part of the treatment course [12, 18, 34, 35]. Conti et al. described a classification system based on MRI appearance of the PTT which was found to be a better guide to outcomes when compared to intraoperative surgical findings [32]. Some of the major drawbacks of MRI are the high cost and lack of accessibility to the general population. These barriers can lead to delay of care, as compared to ultrasound where the diagnosis can be made in the office, potentially on the first visit. The scans are typically longer than radiographs and CT images and hence require more cooperation from the patient. Table 15.4 shows MRI classification of PTT tendinopathy as described by Conti et al. along with associated clinical findings [32].

Ultrasound

Ultrasound (US) has been described to be a valuable tool and has an increasing role in the evaluation of PTT tendinopathy [28, 36]. Arnoldner et al. compared 18 MHz high-resolution ultrasound to 3 T MRI and concluded that US was actually slightly more accurate than 3 T MRI when diagnosing PTT tendinopathy [37]. The probe is placed just behind the medial malleolus, to view the tibialis posterior in short axis. Once identified, the posterior tibialis tendon is followed from the myotendinous junction down to the insertion point in both short and long axis. The posterior tibialis tendon normally has homogenous, echogenic, longitudinal fibers, with minimal or no fluid adjacent to the tendon [28, 36, 37]. The normal diameter of the PTT ranges from 4 to 6 mm. With tendinosis, it can become thickened. The tendon will also appear heterogenous and become hypoechoic [36]. In cases of tenosynovitis, fluid may be seen around the tendon. Another classic sign of tenosynovitis on US would be the presence of a "target sign" on the transverse view although trace fluid around PTT may be normal [36]. Doppler signal is not normally found in the synovial lining and can be diagnostic of tenosynovitis [10].

Ultrasound does have some clear advantages when compared to the other modalities. It is noninvasive, low cost, and radiation-free. It is also

Table 15.4 MRI classification of tibialis posterior tendon degeneration from Conti et al. [32]

MRI classification of tibialis posterior tendon degeneration					
Stage	Type IA	Type IB	Type II	Type III	Type IIIB
MRI findings	Few longitudinal splits No intrasubstance degeneration	Increased number of longitudinal splits Increased tendon width	Tendon narrowed Long longitudinal splits Intramural tendon degeneration	Diffuse tendon swelling Uniform degeneration A few intact strands of tendon	Complete rupture of tendon Replacement by scar tissue
Clinical findings	Short duration, minimal tenderness, swelling, no heel valgus	Same as IA, but duration of symptoms is extended to 6–12 months	Increased valgus deformity	Decreased inversion strength Marked heel valgus Duration >2 years	All signs and symptoms of prior stages

possible to confirm the clinical suspicion on the first visit and allows for a precisely targeted intervention all in a single visit, effectively eliminating the need for subsequent visits. One of the major drawbacks is that it is operator dependent and requires someone who is highly skilled in obtaining and interpreting the images. It has even been recommended as a tool for routine screening for early PTT tendinopathy by some authors [38].

Other imaging modalities that have also been used to study PTT tendinopathy include nuclear imaging. Three-phase bone scanning, or scintigraphy, and single-photon emission CT scanning have been used specifically. These imaging modalities do not seem to add any information that would change management at this time [39].

Treatment

Conservative

Non-operative management is typically reserved for early-stage disease such as patients with stage I PTT tendinopathy and certain patients with stage II and greater PTT tendinopathy that are not surgical candidates [40, 41]. Treatment typically includes a combination of protection, relative rest, immobilization, icing, stretching, and strengthening exercises, and the use of additional modalities and medications [8, 11, 12, 18, 40, 41]. As PTT tendinopathy can be due to underlying diseases, such as diabetes, hypertension, and even inflammatory diseases such as rheumatoid arthritis and lupus, the underlying medical conditions should also be appropriately treated with pharmacotherapies as indicated [18].

First line therapy includes relative rest with immobilization. This involves cessation of activities that may be exacerbating the condition and placing the affected lower extremity in a walking cast, controlled ankle motion [CAM] boot, brace or an ankle foot orthosis [AFO]. As mentioned above, patients with adult acquired pes planus show several kinematic abnormalities secondary to hindfoot and forefoot dysfunction [24]. This leads to increased energy cost of walking as well

as pain. Orthotic treatment aims to reduce these abnormalities, with the goal to improve symptoms and allow for restoration of natural function.

There have been many studies validating the success of foot orthoses and braces, with success rates from 67% to 89% [41–44]. The main types of orthotics utilized in these studies included the University of California- Berkeley Lab orthotic, CAM boots, and low-profile articulating AFO (LAFO) or other AFOs. These types of devices have shown great utility in treating patients with PTT tendinopathy and helping them avoid surgery even after 8 years of follow-up [41–44]. The average age of patients evaluated in the Nelson study was 57.1 with an average BMI of 34.1 [41]. Chao et al. demonstrated that flexible pes planus deformities can be managed using the UCBL device along with good to excellent results in 67% of the patient population [44]. The UCBL has been reported to provide the same level of correction to the hindfoot and ankle deformities as calcaneal osteotomy [45].

The more progressive pes planus deformities can be managed by CAM boots and LAFOs with great success, as demonstrated by Nielsen and others [41, 42, 46]. The LAFO can minimize the progression of PTT tendinopathy by reducing the flatfoot deformity without completely restricting the motion of the ankle [42]. These devices also help to maintain the heel in neutral position and reduce the tension on the posterior tibialis tendon [8, 42]. Although these orthotics have shown great benefit in treating PTT tendinopathy alone, the addition of physiotherapy and rehabilitation has also been shown to help [43, 47–49].

Physical therapy plays a key role in the treatment of PTT tendinopathy [8, 11, 12, 18, 40–44, 47–49]. The emphasis is placed on tibialis posterior strengthening and recruitment. The symptoms can be quite painful in the acute stages. Patients will typically start with range of motion, stretching, and isometric exercises such as resisted foot inversion ensuring there is no movement at the ankle. The patient can then be progressed to concentric exercises such as inversion and eversion using a TheraBand. The later stages of rehabilitation will focus on further strengthening with eccentric exercises and improving balance/proprioception [48]. The basic principle of eccentric exercise is to increase the resting length of the tendon by progressively loading it with increased resistance. The theory is that it will lead to less strain and increase the strength of the tendon preventing it from further reinjury. This is thought to occur via an increase in collagen cross-linking which impacts tendon remodeling [50].

Clinical response in patients completing an eccentric training program has been well documented in the literature. Kulig et al. performed a randomized control trial comparing the use of orthotics alone, or in combination with eccentric/concentric exercises. There was an improvement in all groups, but the most marked improvement was in the group using orthotics plus eccentric exercise. Reduction in pain and increase in functionality has been shown after completion of 3-month regimens [48]. The decrease in symptoms was maintained at 6 -month follow-up following completion of the regimen. These improvements in function and pain were assessed using various methods including the foot function index, visual analogue scale, and single heel raise [48]. Despite these clinical improvements, no significant changes were seen in tendon morphology when studied under ultrasonography [48].

Analgesia has routinely been achieved with over the counter medications. Some consideration should be given to the use of acetaminophen over nonsteroidal anti-inflammatory drugs (NSAIDs) outside of the acute phase of injury. Ibuprofen, a NSAID, has been shown to inhibit collagen repair [51]. There has been no evidence published showing that NSAIDs are superior to acetaminophen in achieving pain relief in PTTD. They can be used in the treatment for symptom relief, but it should be noted that they have not been shown to improve long-term outcomes [51, 52].

Interventional

Some authors have used corticosteroid injections in addition to the above treatment modalities in the management of PTT tendinopathy to help with management of severe pain symptoms [41]. However, there has been a risk of tendon rupture associated with these injections and thus they have not been commonly utilized in conservative management [18, 31, 32]. Of note, the reported cases of tendon rupture were without ultrasound guidance. Without image-guidance, injection of the posterior tibial tendon has been limited because the tibialis posterior tendon is a weight-bearing structure, and the potential risk of tendon rupture with injection of cortisone into the tendon itself.

Other more novel approaches to treating tendinopathy are now on the horizon, such as autologous growth factor injections/platelet rich plasma (PRP). Currently there is no literature on the efficacy of PRP in treatment of PTT tendinopathy [53]. PRP is still in its early development phases and further high quality randomized controlled trials need to be conducted before it can be recommended for the treatment of PTT tendinopathy. Physicians may use this modality of treatment in patients that have not had success with other treatment modalities.

Operative

If conservative management fails for greater than 6 months, or there is progression in the deformity or worsening of symptoms, then surgical consultation can be considered [46]. The operative management is dictated by the stage of the deformity and location of symptoms. Some risk factors identified for requiring surgery are prior orthotic use, prior corticosteroid injections, higher body mass index, and longer disease course [54].

Stage I Dysfunction

If conservative management fails, then surgical treatment with tenosynovectomy, tendon debridement, and decompression can be attempted [34, 55–57]. Teasdall and Johnson reported an 84% success rate with surgical synovectomy and debridement in cases of persistent stage I PTT dysfunction [55]. Their study evaluated 19 patients with an average age of 56. The average length of follow-up was 30 months. A successful outcome was considered if the patient had complete resolution of pain symptoms, subjective improvement in physical function, and ability to perform a single limb heel rise test [55]. This was done via the traditional open approach with a curvilinear incision along the medial ankle over the course of the posterior tibial tendon. However, there have been documented drawbacks using this approach such as wound infection, pain, scar contracture, and longer hospital stay [56].

Many advances have been made since the addition of tendoscopy, which can be described as "endoscopy of the tendon sheath" [58]. Chow et al. had shown great success in using this approach in treatment of stage I PTT dysfunction [56]. The advantages of this procedure are cosmetic (only two 4 mm scars), less postoperative pain, and lower complication rate than with traditional open procedures. There is also no need for immobilization for wound protection. No complications were found associated with the tendoscopy procedure and it reduced postoperative pain and hospital stay [56]. Tendoscopy has only been shown to be useful in stage I and stage II posterior tibial tendon dysfunction in the literature [56, 59].

Stage II Dysfunction

Multiple surgical approaches have been described to address stage II PTT dysfunction depending on the deformities present. These include a combination of flexor digitorum longus (FDL) tendon transfer, calcaneal osteotomy, tendon Achilles lengthening (TAL)/gastrocnemius recession, forefoot correction osteotomy, and spring ligament repair [12, 18, 34, 57, 60]. Myerson et al. found that patients with stage II PTT dysfunction who were treated with a combination of calcaneal osteotomy and FDL tendon transfer had a success rate of as high as 97%. His initial publication included 32 patients, with a mean age of 58 years who on an average had 2.5 years of symptoms before surgical correction [12, 60]. Those findings have been confirmed by multiple other studies with equally as high rates of success [61, 62].

The FDL tendon is typically the tendon used during transfer surgeries [23, 34, 60–66] which is discussed in further detail in the FDL segment of this chapter. Other tendons have been used for

transfer including the flexor hallucis longus (FHL) tendon, peroneus brevis tendon, and a split tibialis anterior graft technique [64, 65, 67]. Sammarco et al. successfully transferred the FHL tendon in addition to a medial calcaneal osteotomy with good results, but not superior to those with FDL tendon transfers. The study included 19 patients, with the mean age being 58. The average body mass index (BMI) was 32.6 kg/m² in the sample population [64]. The same results were found with peroneus brevis tendon transfers [67]. The technique using a split graft of the tibialis anterior is known as the Cobb reconstruction and has been shown to have good outcomes in over 90% of patients at 5-year follow-up in a study containing 32 patients [65].

Stage III and IV Dysfunction

These two stages are both treated with triple arthrodesis techniques in combination with TAL. In the case of stage IV PTT dysfunction, the addition of a deltoid ligament reconstruction may be required [66]. Tibiotalocalcaneal arthrodesis has also been attempted with success in severe stage IV tendinopathy [34, 68]. However, even after surgical intervention, up to 50% of patients may still have symptoms [69].

A summary of the commonly used approaches and their indications is listed in Tables 15.5 and 15.6 [12, 34, 55–57, 61, 62, 64, 65, 67, 70].

Tendon Transfer

The basic tendon transfer principles were outlined by Bluman and Dowd in 2011 [71]. They outlined five basic properties that the ideal tendon transfer must possess. Those properties are strength, excursion, similar direction, and attachment, ideally being in phase with the tendon that is being replaced, and that it serves a single function [71]. The relative strengths and excursions of the tendons of the foot and ankle were studied in detail by Silver et al. in 1985; Table 15.7 summarizes their findings [72]. The relative strength was calculated by taking the cross-sectional area of the individual muscle over the total cross-

Table 15.5 Surgical treatment options for PTTD, with their indications and short descriptions [12, 34, 55–57, 61, 62, 64, 65, 67, 70]

Intervention	Description	Indication
Tenosynovectomy	Removal of inflammatory tissue with the goal of decreasing pain If a tear is located, it should also be repaired	Stage I resistant to conservative management
Osteotomy	Surgical removal of a piece of the calcaneal bone in efforts to correct any hindfoot valgus present	Stage II with hindfoot deformity
Tendon transfer	Transfer of the FDL tendon onto the navicular adjacent to the tibilais posterior insertion If there is damage to the spring or deltoid ligaments it should be repaired	Stage II with a flexible pes planus deformity
Lateral column lengthening	The calcaneus is lengthened using a bone allograft with the goal of producing increased forefoot adduction	Stage II disease with >40% talonavicular Uncoverage
Arthrodesis	Surgical fusion of adjacent bones to immobilize joints. Multiple have been used in the treatment of PTTD (isolated subtalar arthrodesis, triple arthrodesis)	Stage II–IV disease
TAL or gastrocnemius recession	Release of the involved muscle leading to the ankle plantarflexion contracture	Stage II disease with plantarflexion contracture

Table 15.6 Summary of the diagnosis and treatment of posterior tibialis tendon tendinopathy

Stage	Clinical findings	Imaging	Treatment
I	Tenderness along posterior tibial tendon, normal anatomy	Normal	Conservative treatment: Immobilization, orthosis, NSAIDS If conservative management fails consider tenosynovectomy
II	Supple hindfoot valgus, flexible/fixed forefoot varus	Hindfoot valgus Increased Meary angle Loss of calcaneal pitch and medial cuneiform floor height Talonavicular uncoverage	Orthosis Surgery consult Consider calcaneal osteotomy, TAL or gastrocnemius recession Flexor digitorum longus transfer Lateral column lengthening
III	Rigid hindfoot valgus, forefoot abduction, pain in sinus tarsi	Loss of subtalar joint space, hindfoot valgus	Surgery consult Consider triple arthrodesis ± lateral column lengthening Custom bracing if not surgical candidate
IV	Supple/rigid ankle valgus	Hindfoot and ankle valgus	Surgery consult Consider triple arthrodesis ± deltoid reconstruction

sectional area of the muscles in the limb. A muscle with a relative strength of 4 has twice of strength of one with a relative strength of 2.

There are many reasons why the FDL is preferred over other tendons in the treatment of PTT dysfunction. The FDL tendon normally runs adjacent to the PTT. This allows for the tendon sheath and neurovascular structures to stay intact during the transfer [73]. As they have a similar course down the extremity into the foot and ankle, the tension of the pulley can be maintained. Since they are adjacent, the same incision that is used to expose the PTT can be used to harvest the tendon of the FDL [74]. The tibialis posterior and the FDL are in phase during the gait cycle, allowing for an "in phase" tendon transfer, leading to improved functional outcomes [73, 74]. In phase muscles are considered synergistic and allow for restoration of normal function much easier than out of phase muscles would. The function of the FDL is also preserved after tendon transfer due to the connections it has

Table 15.7 Comparison of relative strength of tendon properties of the medial foot. The information for the above table was obtained from Silver et al. [72]

Tendon	Relative strength	Excursion (cm)
PTT	6.4	4.1
FDL	1.8	4.8
FHL	3.6	4.8

between the FHL and the quadratus plantae attachments at the distal aspect of the FDL tendon [73–75].

The FDL tendon does have disadvantages, with some authors noting it to be the weakest of the potential donor tendons [72, 74]. One study noted that the FDL tendon transfer failed after an average time of 14.7 months, and patients required subsequent triple arthrodesis procedures [32]. Newer research has been emerging studying the FDL and FHL tendons in closer detail. One recent anatomy study found that the FHL may be the better donor for tendon transfer to restore lost function, but harvesting the FDL seems to be more suitable to prevent long-term functional damage to surrounding neurovascular structures [76]. However, most clinicians continue to prefer the FDL transfer over others due to several reasons mentioned above, mainly the preservation of function and the neurovascular bundle.

Flexor Hallucis Longus

Introduction/Anatomy

The FHL muscle originates from the posterior aspect of the lower fibula and interosseous membrane, lateral to the flexor digitorum longus (FDL) muscle (Fig. 15.6). It courses distally underneath the flexor retinaculum and within the tendon sheath, to attach at the posterior talus and calcaneus. The tendon sheath and bony surfaces of the talus and calcaneus form the tarsal tunnel under which the tendon passes [3, 77]. This fibro-osseous tunnel is a key location for pathology and will be discussed later in the chapter. The tendon then continues down the ankle into the foot, between the medial and lat-

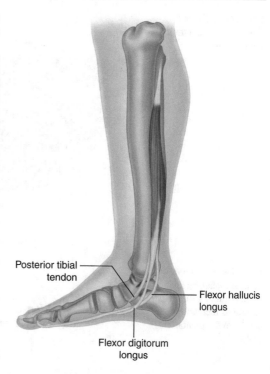

Fig. 15.6 FHL anatomy and the origin and insertion of the flexor hallucis longus

eral tubercles of the talus, along the groove within the sustentaculum tali. Another key area along the path to the tendon's insertion onto the base of the distal phalanx of the hallux is when it courses dorsally over the flexor digitorum longus. There is a complex interconnection that occurs between the two muscle tendons referred to as the "master knot of Henry." There is typically a fibrous slip that connects the FDL and FHL tendons together (Fig. 15.7). The tendon sheaths of the two usually communicate, which facilitates the transfer of inflammation between the adjacent tendons [14]. The knot of Henry is typically located over the navicular and medial cuneiforms [14]. The tendon then continues down the distal aspect of the foot, passing deep to the inter-sesamoid ligament and plantar plate (Fig. 15.8), before finally inserting onto the distal phalanx of the hallux [7].

The blood supply to the FHL arises from the peroneal branch of the posterior tibial and medial plantar arteries. The primary innervation to the

Fig. 15.7 FHL and
FDL tendons and their
intersection

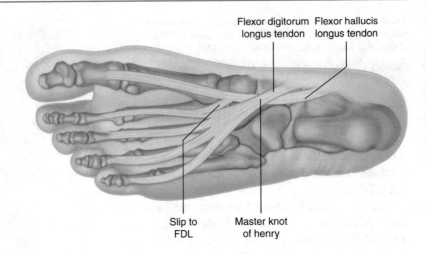

Flexor digitorum Flexor hallucis
longus tendon   longus tendon

Slip to   Master knot
FDL   of henry

Fig. 15.8 Great toe
metatarsophalangeal
joint, depicting the FHL
tendon as it courses
caudal to the plantar
plate

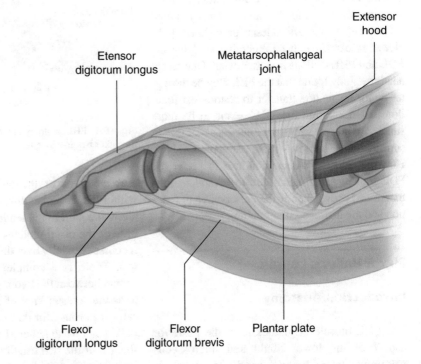

Etensor
digitorum longus

Metatarsophalangeal
joint

Extensor
hood

Flexor
digitorum longus

Flexor
digitorum brevis

Plantar plate

muscle arises from the tibial nerve and from the sciatic nerve roots S1 and S2. The primary functions of the FHL are plantarflexion of the first metatarsophalangeal (MTP) and interphalangeal joint of the hallux [1, 3, 77]. It is the antagonist of the extensor hallucis longus muscle.

There have been many cadaveric studies performed and not many anatomic variants have been identified in the FHL [78]. There have been case reports of missing FHL muscle and tendon in patients [35]. Instead in that patient, the tendon originated from the flexor digitorum longus. Surprisingly

the patient was able to maintain normal function prior to injury. There has also been a report of an accessory FHL muscle belly and accessory tendon slip causing tarsal tunnel syndrome. In this case the accessory muscle belly was causing impingement of the tibial nerve within the tarsal tunnel [40]. There are some variations in anatomy that occur at the knot of Henry mentioned earlier. These variations do not seem to play a role in the pathogenesis of tendinopathy, but do have some importance when considering tendon transfer in the treatment of posterior tibialis tendon tendinopathy [79].

The main function of the FHL is plantarflexion of the hallux, or great toe, at the interphalangeal and metatarsophalangeal joints [3]. It also aids in plantarflexion and supination at the ankle and subtalar joints. It also serves as the primary resistant to passive dorsiflexion at the first MTP joint [49].

Flexor Hallucis Longus Tendinopathy

A 23-year-old ballet dancer complains of progressive posteromedial left ankle and plantar foot pain since starting en pointe 3 months ago. On physical exam, patient had tenderness to palpation at the posteromedial ankle and plantar first MTP joint. She had decreased range of motion at the first MTP. The pain was reproduced with passive extension of the first toe and resisted first interphalangeal flexion.

Clinical Presentation

As with the other forms of tenosynovitis described in this chapter, the etiology is often secondary to overuse, rather than any specific trauma [47]. It has often been described as "dancer's tendonitis" as it is often seen in classic ballet or "en pointe" dancers [80]. This excess plantarflexion places increased strain on the FHL tendon, leading to the development of tendinopathy. This extreme plantarflexion is an extrinsic risk factor also seen in other athletes like gymnasts, ice skaters, and swimmers. Although it is often described in athletes, it can occur in non-athletes as well [64]. Pain in this presentation of FHL tendinopathy is typically localized to the posterior/posteromedial ankle, around the tibio-talar joint [81].

Classification of FHL tenosynovitis is done by anatomic location, rather than severity [43].

- Zone I: Posterior to the ankle joint
- Zone II: From the tarsal tunnel to the knot of Henry
- Zone III: From the knot of Henry to the FHL insertion at the plantar aspect of the distal phalanx of the hallux

The site of symptoms can vary from case to case due to the multiple areas along the tendon's anatomic course that could be involved. The most common area of tenosynovitis is at the posterior ankle, at the site of the tarsal tunnel. The second most common location is at the hallux sesamoids, followed by the knot of Henry [43]. The increased friction at these sites leads to a cycle of repetitive microtrauma which ultimately leads to tissue changes such as tenosynovitis, longitudinal tears, and irregular nodularity within the tendon [49]. The presenting symptoms will correlate to the location of the constriction or pseudo-entrapment. Table 15.8 shows differential diagnosis for FHL tendinopathy.

There have been two major theories put forward regarding the development of tenosynovitis at the tarsal tunnel. The first deals with excessive plantarflexion. When the foot is in full plantarflexion, like in ballet dancing, there are abnormal stresses on the FHL tendon within the tunnel [80]. The second deals with the anatomic variant of a low-lying muscle belly which may be transplaced distally into the tunnel when the great toe is placed into dorsiflexion [49].

Another clinical presentation for tendinopathy of the FHL may be what is known as triggering of the great toe, or hallux saltans [49]. This occurs due to stenosing tenosynovitis of the FHL [47]. Stenosing tenosynovitis of the FHL may also present as a "pseudo hallux rigidus," due to the limited excursion of the tendon due to the surrounding inflammation of the sheath [47]. This finding is typically seen when the patient's foot is placed into dorsiflexion, placing the maximal amount of pull on the tendon body.

Table 15.8 Differential diagnosis for flexor hallucis longus tendinopathy [43, 47, 49, 80]

Location	Differential
Posterior ankle	Achilles tendinopathy, posterior impingement syndrome, Sheperd's fracture, inflammatory or infectious arthritis
Midfoot	Tarsal tunnel syndrome, sinus tarsi syndrome, peroneal tendinopathy, stress fracture, Morton's neuroma
Base of great toe	Sesamoiditis, fractures, avascular necrosis, gout, osteoarthritis or inflammatory arthritis, turf toe

There also appears to be a relationship between FHL tenosynovitis and the presence of an os trigonum [52]. The presence of this accessory ossicle can lead to dysfunction in the normal ankle dorsiflexion/plantarflexion motion, making the tendon more prone to injury and inflammation. Partial tears have also been reported due to the presence of the os trigonum [82].

FHL tendinopathy with inflammation at the knot of Henry can lead to "jogger's foot," or medial plantar neuritis, which is due to irritation of the medial plantar nerve secondary to their close anatomic proximity (Fig. 15.9). The patient typically reports aching, burning, or numbness localized to the sole or the medial aspect of the foot, which is the region of skin innervated by the medial plantar nerve (Fig. 15.10) [52].

Physical Examination

Initially the exam should begin with inspection. The patient may have an impaired, or antalgic gait, as the FHL plays an important role in loading the first MTP joint [57]. Then, continue to observe the patient's feet for any other signs of possible FHL involvement as mentioned above. The patient may present with dyskinetic motions at the great toe due to hallux saltans [49].

There are four key areas of palpation along the course of the FHL that should be examined for any tenderness: the posterior ankle, sustentaculum tali, the plantar aspect of the midfoot and finally at the level of the sesamoids as the tendon traverses the inter-sesamoid ligament. These areas should be examined with the ankle and the

Fig. 15.9 Cutaneous innervation of the plantar foot

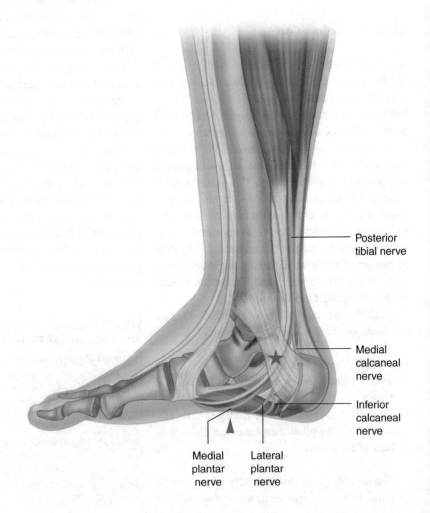

Posterior tibial nerve

Medial calcaneal nerve

Inferior calcaneal nerve

Medial plantar nerve

Lateral plantar nerve

Fig. 15.10 Anatomic
relationship between the
FHL tendon and medial
plantar nerve

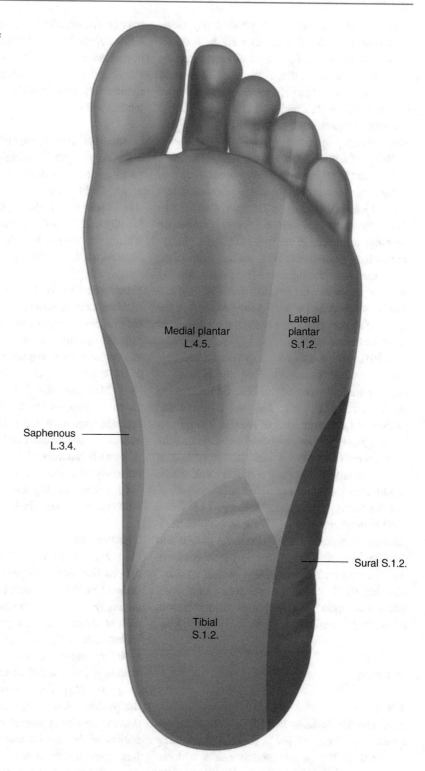

Medial plantar
L.4.5.

Lateral
plantar
S.1.2.

Saphenous
L.3.4.

Sural S.1.2.

Tibial
S.1.2.

great toe held in neutral to prevent any plantarflexion at the MTP joint, as well as in dorsiflexion to place the FHL tendon under tension [49]. We do caution that it may be difficult to accurately palpate the FHL tendon given its close proximity to the PTT and the FDL tendon. Using bedside ultrasound may be a useful tool to aid in more precise palpation [83].

Range of motion should be checked at the ankle and the first MTP joint. There may be restriction in active and passive dorsiflexion at the ankle and subtalar joints depending on the severity of the tendinopathy. There may also be a notable decrease in the range of motion at the first MTP joint, consistent with a pseudo hallux rigidus. Active dorsiflexion at the ankle and the first MTP simultaneously may also reproduce the patient's pain [8]. Pain can also be reproduced by having the patient flex the great toe against resistance while the ankle is held in plantarflexion [49].

A FHL stretch test can also be performed during the examination [49]. This test is used to evaluate the influence of the FHL on the motion of the first MTP joint. The test assesses the motion of the hallux in both maximal dorsiflexion and plantarflexion. It should be noted that the MTP should be stabilized during the maneuver as to prevent any plantarflexion at the joint, which would affect tendon excursion and tension. A positive test is pain localized to the first MTP or a notable decrease in dorsiflexion at the first MTP joint by 20 degrees when the ankle is placed into dorsiflexion [49]. A positive test also confirms that the patient has a "pseudo hallux rigidus," meaning the joint has normal range of motion when the ankle is placed into plantarflexion, relieving the tension placed on the FHL tendon.

Imaging

X-Ray

Radiographic findings in FHL tendinopathy are typically nonspecific [61]. Soft-tissue swelling localized to the posteromedial ankle with an associated effusion may be seen. Fractures of the calcaneus, medial malleolus, or os trigonum which have been implicated in FHL tendinopathy

may be visualized [23]. Overall radiographs have a low degree of confidence in diagnosis of tendinopathies as the actual tendon itself cannot be visualized. It is helpful to identify ancillary information that may clue the clinician toward FHL tendon pathology.

Computed Tomography

CT is a more precise imaging modality as it provides information about the FHL tendon as well as any fluid within the synovial sheath [61]. It should be noted that approximately 20% of healthy individuals may have CT findings of fluid within the tendon sheath since the sheath has communications with the ankle joint itself [61].

Magnetic Resonance Imaging

MRI appears to provide the most information to the clinician in regard to the tendon health. It can provide information regarding the signal intensity of the tendon, the fiber composition, the size of the tendon, as well as any surrounding edema [84]. MRI can also help differentiate between partial and complete tears of the tendon [61]. As touched upon earlier, there have been cases of an accessory muscle belly or low-lying muscle belly that can be sources of FHL irritation. These can be easily visualized via MRI [61]. As a result, MRI offers the highest degree of confidence when trying to identify FHL tendon injuries.

Ultrasound

US is becoming more and more common in clinical practice for the diagnosis of various musculoskeletal pathologies such as tendinopathies. One advantage of US is the ability to examine the patient dynamically to potentially explain the hallux saltans if present [85]. The FHL tendon is typically identified via a posterior approach, scanning just medial to the Achilles tendon in long axis [85]. This allows for visualization of the posterior joint recess as well. The FHL tendon can also be examined in short axis around the region of the medial malleolus. Here, dynamic flexion-extension at the hallux can be used to assess the tendon as it curves around the posterior aspect of the talus bone. US allows for the visualization of the tendon, its size, echogenicity, and any associated fluid collections [61]. US can depend on the skill and interpretation of the operator, but can provide a moderate to high degree of confidence, and saves the patient from radiation exposure they would otherwise receive from radiographs and CTs [61].

Treatment

Conservative

Conservative treatment of FHL tendinopathy involves rest aimed to reduce the inflammation in the tendon and its surrounding structures. Most clinicians attempt 6 months of non-surgical treatment prior to any consideration of surgical consultation [64]. Typical treatment consists of protection, relative rest, ice, compression, elevation, medications, and rehabilitative exercise modalities (PRICEMM) [43, 47, 49, 64, 80, 86].

Physical therapy typically aims to relieve the inflammation/edema within the soft tissues, stretching and mobilization of the restricted joints, progressive strengthening, balance and proprioception [87]. Physical therapy can also include other modalities such as phonophoresis and iontophoresis, though insufficient evidence exists in regard to their efficacy in FHL tendinopathy [88].

Michelson et al. created a specific treatment protocol involving FHL stretches that simultaneously dorsiflex the ankle and the first MTP joint to maximize the excursion of the tendon. The stretch was performed by having the patient stand in front of a wall with a book under the hallux, passively placing the first MTP joint into dorsiflexion. Then the patient leans forward using the wall for support, allowing for passive dorsiflexion at the ankle. This is followed by active knee flexion further stretching the tendon. This position is held for 10 seconds. The exercise was performed in the study for 10 repetitions in sets of three to four daily. The height of the book was further increased as the patients progressed [49]. They reported a success rate of 64% with non-operative management over 18 weeks which included the FDL stretches as well as oral NSAIDs and immobilization.

Depending on the severity of the symptoms, immobilization is also recommended; however, the exact length is unknown and may depend on the individual patient and their prior activity level. Immobilization was performed in the Michelson study which included 81 patients, 27 which were athletes [43, 47, 49, 64, 80, 87, 88]. If the patient did not respond to the stretching protocol after 6 weeks, they were placed in a walking boot as a night splint for 6 weeks. If there was still no improvement the patient was immobilized for 23.5 hours again for 6 weeks. Thirty-nine of the 81 patients required some form of immobilization; however, it was not specified how many needed the aggressive immobilization. Once the conservative measures failed, 23 patients underwent operative management.

Unfortunately, there have been no good quality outcome studies in regard to determining the best protocol in these patients. These treatment protocols tend to have a high failure/recurrence rate. These high failure rates may be related to poor patient compliance to treatment protocols, continued use of improper technique when dancing, inaccurate diagnosis or severe local impingement of the FHL tendon at ankle, knot of Henry or the sesamoids [89]. The success rate of conservative treatment including a combination of physical therapy, use of oral NSAIDS and bracing is approximately 46–64% [49, 77]. Failure rates have been published ranging from 40–100% [49, 64].

Interventional

Corticosteroid injections have also been performed to help in conservative management of FHL tendinopathy. These procedures are typically performed with or without fluoroscopic guidance [90]. With ultrasonography becoming more common in daily practice, newer techniques have been described [91]. These techniques allow direct visualization of the soft tissues as well as the adjacent neurovascular bundle. One study found ultrasound to have 100% accuracy in FHL peritendinous injections in 10 cadavers [92]. They also prevent the patient from the unwanted effects of ionizing radiation they would otherwise be exposed to under fluoroscopy [91].

Operative

As mentioned above, conservative management may fail. In such cases, surgery may be indicated. The surgical approach varies depending on several factors: the location of the impingement, any injuries to the surrounding osseous structures, and the preference of the surgeon. Initially, the open technique was utilized from a posterior and a medial approach [47, 49, 77, 80]. The goal of surgery is to debride the tendon, repair any tears, and tenosynovectomy of the sheath. If the location of the entrapment is at the posteromedial ankle, then release of the tunnel is indicated. If there is presence of a bony impediment such as an os trigonum, that must also be addressed by removing it.

The posteromedial open approach is the technique recommended by most authors, as this allows for direct visualization and protection of the tibial nerve [47, 49, 80]. This approach begins just posterior to the medial malleolus. The medial approach requires three to 6 months of recuperation time [49, 80]. The reported rate of tibial nerve injury is 6.7% via the medial open approach.

The alternative technique is a posterolateral approach, which involves making an incision posterior to the lateral malleolus and anterior to the lateral border of the Achilles tendon [49]. An os trigonum can be more easily visualized and removed using this approach [52]. This approach also allows the direct visualization of the musculotendinous junction and upper portions of the tarsal tunnel [52]. Although the tibial nerve is less likely to be damaged, the sural nerve may be injured in this approach. The sural nerve should be identified and protected during the surgery [49].

The typical postoperative protocol for both approaches involves immobilization with a CAM boot and weight-bearing as tolerated for 2 weeks. The patient is allowed to remove the boot to perform active range of motion at the ankle and first MTP joint as pain permits. After 2 weeks, immobilization is discontinued and the patient will then begin physical therapy [47, 49, 77, 80]. The focus of the postoperative rehabilitation program is to strengthen the FHL as well as improve the range of motion of the great toe and ankle with the goal of improving overall function and gait. Patients have 10–13 weeks of physical therapy on average. Full recovery can take up to 6 months in certain cases [49, 77, 80, 82, 93, 94]. In the athletic population rehabilitation is also focused on proprioception, coordination, and muscle strength of not only the ankle but also the trunk stabilizers in order to allow dancers to perform at their preinjury level [82, 95].

More recently, the endoscopic approach has been described [43, 77, 82, 93]. Endoscopy provides some clear advantages when compared to the open approach including decreased postoperative pain, decreased scar formation, and earlier return to activities [43, 77, 93]. The average time to recover and return to sport is 6 to 8 weeks with the endoscopic approach [49, 82]. Two portals are created on either side of the Achilles tendon, 15 mm above the calcaneal tuberosity [52]. Just as with the open approach, the goal is to debride the tendon and release the tunnel [43, 77, 93]. Tibial nerve injury is reported to be as high as 11.1% via this method, but it was noted that all patients fully recovered function at 1-year follow-up [94]. Injury to the sural nerve has been reported to be anywhere from 3.4% to 8.3% via the endoscopic approach, versus 6.3% to 19.5% in the open approach [93]. Postoperative infection rates with endoscopy were 3.3–6.7%, versus 2.4% in the open approach [94]. When considering the athlete population both open and endoscopic approaches have been shown to provide success rates as high as 90% in dancers [95].

Flexor Digitorum Longus

Introduction/Anatomy

The FDL originates from the medial side of the posterior surface of the distal tibial shaft. As it travels down into the foot and ankle, it wraps around the medial malleolus and passes through the tarsal tunnel [96]. The tendon then continues down the plantar aspect of the foot, crossing from medial to lateral, before it splits off into four smaller tendons (Fig. 15.11a). As it crosses from medial to lateral, it crosses under the FHL tendon at the "master knot of Henry." A fibrous connection between the two tendons can be found here as mentioned earlier. These connections can be very complex and multiple anatomical variations have been found in cadaveric studies. The most common relationship between the two tendons involves a proximal to distal connection from the FHL to the FDL [97]. The four terminal slips of the FDL tendon then go on to insert at the plantar aspects of the bases of the distal phalanx of the lateral four toes (Fig. 15.11b) [1]. There have been reports of anatomic variants of the FDL including one case of bilateral accessory FDLs leading to the development of bilateral posterior tarsal tunnel syndrome [98].

The vascular supply to the FDL is provided by the muscular branch of the posterior tibial artery [1]. The FDL muscle is innervated by the tibial nerve (S2-S3). The primary function of the FDL is to flex the lateral toes, 2–5. It also aids in plan-

tarflexion and inversion of the ankle joint [1]. It supports the talocalcaneal joint along with the other surrounding muscles, tendons, and ligaments [99].

Flexor Digitorum Longus Tendinopathy

A 19-year-old female gymnast presents with chief complaint of right medial and plantar foot pain while jumping during her floor routine for 1 month. On physical exam she had tenderness to palpation at the medial foot and along the plantar second to fifth MTPs. She had pain in the plantar foot with resisted second to fifth toe flexion and with single leg jump.

Clinical Presentation

Although the FDL can suffer from injury just as any other muscle/tendon, there has not been much published in the literature in regard to

Fig. 15.11 (a, b): FDL anatomy and the origin and insertion of the flexor digitorum longus

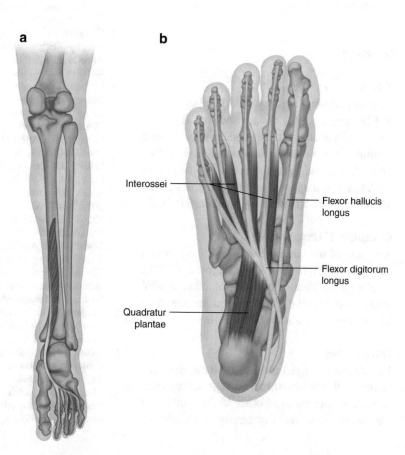

a

b

Interossei

Flexor hallucis longus

Flexor digitorum longus

Quadratur plantae

specifics. Disorders of the FDL are considerably less common than the other tendons of the medial foot [10]. There is pathology that can occur at the master knot of Henry, where the FDL and FHL cross paths (jogger's foot), which is discussed in the prior section. No other syndrome is associated with tendinopathy of the FDL.

Physical Examination

Physical examination is similar to evaluation of other medial ankle tendinopathies and can start with observation and evaluation of gait. The patient may have pain to palpation along the course of the tendon. Range of motion and strength testing of the ankle and digits should be done. The patient may have pain with resisted toe flexion of the lesser toes. There have been no special tests established for evaluation of FDL tendinopathy.

Imaging

X-Ray
As with FHL tendinopathy, radiographic findings in FDL tendinopathy are nonspecific. It can be used to visualize edema secondary to soft tissue swelling, as well as to rule out underlying fractures. Again, radiographs have a low degree of confidence in diagnosis of tendinopathies as the actual tendon itself cannot be visualized [61].

Computed Tomography
A review of the current literature did not reveal any uses of CT to aid in the diagnosis of FHL tendinopathy. Though as with the other medial ankle tendons, one could expect to see fluid within the tendon sheath of the FHL.

Ultrasound
Ultrasound has been used to evaluate the FDL tendon [10]. The ultrasound findings are typically consistent with those of other tendinopathies of the medial foot. Initially tenosynovitis can be

seen, followed by signs of degradation of the tendon body itself [10]. There will be presence of increased Doppler activity around the FDL tendon. MRI has also been used in the diagnosis of FDL tendinopathies, especially at the location of the knot of Henry [43].

Treatment

There are no specific treatment protocols that have been developed for the conservative management of FDL injuries, but relative rest, immobilization, orthotics, anti-inflammatories, and physical therapy may be used.

References

1. Standring S, editor. Gray's anatomy. 39th ed. London: Churchill Livingstone; 2011.
2. Wheeless CR, editor. Wheeless' textbook of orthopaedics [cop. 1996–2009]. Brooklandville: Data Trace Publishing Co.
3. D'Antoni AV. Clinically oriented anatomy, 7th edition, by Keith L. Moore, Arthur F. Dalley II, and Anne M. R. Agur, Baltimore: Lippincott Williams & Wilkins; Lower Limb 2014.
4. Bloome D, Marymont J, Varner K. Variations on the insertion of the posterior tibialis tendon: a cadaveric study. Foot Ankle Int. 2003;24:780.
5. Martin B. Observations on the muscles and tendons of the medial aspect of the sole of the foot. J Anat. 1964;98:437–53.
6. Deland JT, de Asla RJ, Sung IH, Ernberg LA, Potter HG. Posterior tibial tendon insufficiency: which ligaments are involved? Foot Ankle Int. 2005;26:427–35.
7. Kitaoka HB, et al. Stability of the arch of the foot. Foot Ankle Int. 1997;18(10):644–8.
8. Myerson MS. Adult acquired flat foot deformity. J Bone Joint Surg. 1996;78A:780–92.
9. Gluck GS, Heckman DS, Parekh SG. Tendon disorders of the foot and ankle, part 3: the posterior tibial tendon. Am J Sports Med. 2010;38:2133–44.
10. Chapter: 24. In: McNally E, editor. Practical musculoskeletal ultrasound. 2nd ed. Churchill Livingstone; London, United Kingdom. p. 269–301, 301–14.
11. Johnson KA, Strom DE. Tibialis posterior tendon dysfunction. Clin Orthop Relat Res. 1989;239:196–206.
12. Myerson MS. Adult acquired flatfoot deformity: treatment of dysfunction of the posterior tibial tendon. Instr Course Lect. 1997;46:393–405.

13. Mosier SM, Pomeroy G, Manoli AII. Pathoanatomy and etiology of posterior tibial tendon dysfunction. Clin Orthop Relat Res. 1999;365:12–22.

14. Choi YS, Lee KT, Kang HS, Kim EK. MR imaging findings of painful type II accessory navicular bone: correlation with surgical and pathologic studies. Korean J Radiol. 2004;5:274–9.

15. Manske MC, McKeon KE, Johnson JE, McCormick JJ, Klein SE. Arterial anatomy of the tibialis posterior tendon. Foot Ankle Int. 2015;36(4):436–43.

16. Holmes JB Jr, Mann RA. Possible epidemiological factors associated with rupture of the posterior tibial tendon. Foot Ankle Int. 1992;13:70–9.

17. Funk DA, Cass JR, Johnson KA. Acquired adult flat foot secondary to posterior tibial – tendon pathology. J Bone Joint Surg Am. 1986;68(1):95–102.

18. Bluman EM, Title CI, Myerson MS. Posterior tibial tendon rupture: a refined classification system. Foot Ankle Clin. 2007;12:233–49, v.

19. Abousayed MM, et al. Classifications in brief: Johnson and Strom classification of adult-acquired flatfoot deformity. Clin Orthop Relat Res. 2016;474(2):588–93. PMC. Web. 27 Apr. 2017.

20. Deland JT. The adult acquired flatfoot and spring ligament complex: pathology and implications for treatment. Foot Ankle Clin. 2001;6:129–35, vii.

21. McCormack AP, Niki H, Kiser P, Tencer AF, Sangeorzan BJ. Two reconstructive techniques for flatfoot deformity comparing contact characteristics of the hindfoot joints. Foot Ankle Int. 1998;19:452–61.

22. Raikin SM, Winters BS, Daniel JN. The RAM classification: a novel, systematic approach to the adult-acquired flatfoot. Foot Ankle Clin. 2012;17:169–81.

23. Komiya K, Terada N. Entrapment of the Flexor Hallucis Longus tendon by direct impalement in the osseofibrous tunnel under the sustentaculum tali: an extremely rare complication of a calcaneal fracture. JBJS Case Connector. 2014;4:e100–4. Web. 25 Apr. 2017.

24. Houck JR, et al. Ankle and foot kinematics associated with stage II PTTD during stance. Foot Ankle Int/Am Orthop Foot Ankle Soc [and] Swiss Foot Ankle Soc. 2009;30(6):530–9. PMC. Web. 28 Apr. 2017.

25. Hintermann B, Gachter A. The first metatarsal rise sign: a simple, sensitive sign of tibialis posterior tendon dysfunction. Foot Ankle Int. 1996;17:236–41.

26. Slovenkai MP. Clinical and radiographic evaluation. Foot Ankle Clin. 1997;2:241–60.

27. Banks AS, Downey MS, Martin DE, et al. McGlamry's comprehensive textbook of foot and ankle surgery. Philadelphia: Lippincott Williams & Wilkins; 2001. ISBN:0683304712.

28. Kong A, Van Der Vliet A. Imaging of tibialis posterior dysfunction. Br J Radiol. 2008;81:826–36.

29. Younger AS, Sawatzky B, Dryden P. Radiographic assessment of adult flatfoot. Foot Ankle Int. 2005;26:820–5.

30. Schreibman KL, Gilula LA. Ankle tenography. Radiol Clin N Am. 1998;36(4):739–56.

31. Rosenberg ZS, Cheung Y, Jahss MH, Noto AM, Norman A, Leeds NE. Rupture of posterior tibial tendon: CT and MR imaging with surgical correlation. Radiology. 1988;169:229–35.

32. Conti S, Michelson J, Jahss M. Clinical significance of magnetic resonance imaging in preoperative planning for reconstruction of posterior tibial tendon ruptures. Foot Ankle. 1992;13(4):208–14. https://doi.org/10.1177/107110079201300408.

33. Rosenberg ZS, Beltran J, Bencardino JT. Radiological Society of North America: MR imaging of the ankle and foot. Radiographics. 2000;20:S153–79.

34. Edwards MR, Jack C, Singh SK. Tibialis posterior dysfunction. Curr Orthop. 2008;22:185–92.

35. Xarchas KC, Oikonomou L. A missing flexor Hallucis Longus muscle and tendon in a young female patient: a case report of a rare anomaly. J Foot Ankle Surg. 2016;55(1):181–2.

36. Miller SD, Van Holsbeeck M, Boruta PM, Wu KK, Katcherian DA. Ultrasound in the diagnosis of posterior tibial tendon pathology. Foot Ankle Int. 1996;17:555–8.

37. Arnoldner MA, Gruber M, Syre S, et al. Imaging of posterior tibial tendon dysfunction–comparison of high-resolution ultrasound and 3T MRI. Eur J Radiol. 2015;84:1777–81.

38. Chen YJ, Liang SC. Diagnostic efficacy of ultrasonography in stage I posterior tibial tendon dysfunction: sonographic-surgical correlation. J Ultrasound Med. 1997;16(6):417–23.

39. Ha S, Hong SH, Paeng JC, Lee DY, Cheon GJ, Arya A, et al. Comparison of SPECT/CT and MRI in diagnosing symptomatic lesions in ankle and foot pain patients: diagnostic performance and relation to lesion type. PLoS One. 2015;10(2):e0117583.

40. Lin D, Williams C, Zaw H. A rare case of an accessory flexor hallucis longus causing tarsal tunnel syndrome. Foot Ankle Surg. 2014;20(3):e37–9.

41. Nielsen MD, Dodson EE, Shadrick DL, et al. Nonoperative care for the treatment of adult-acquired flatfoot deformity. J Foot Ankle Surg. 2011;50(3):311–4.

42. Neville CG, Houck JR, Flemister AS. Science behind the use of orthotic devices to manage posterior tibial tendon dysfunction. Tech Foot Ankle Surg. 2008;7(2):125–33.

43. Lui TH, Chow FY. "Intersection syndrome" of the foot: treated by endoscopic release of master knot of Henry. Knee Surg Sports Traumatol Arthrosc. 2011;19(5):850–2. Epub 2011 Feb 3.

44. Chao W, Wapner KL, Lee TH, et al. Nonoperative management of posterior tibial tendon dysfunction. Foot Ankle Int. 1996;17(12):736–41.

45. Havenhill TG, Toolan BC, Draganich LF. Effects of a UCBL orthosis and a calcaneal osteotomy on tibiotalar contact characteristics in a cadaver flatfoot model. Foot Ankle Int. 2005;26:607–13.

46. Arangio GA, Salathe EP. A biomechanical analysis of posterior tibial tendon dysfunction, medial displacement calcaneal osteotomy and flexor digitorum longus transfer in adult acquired flat foot. Clin Biomech. 2009;24:385–90.

47. Gould N. Stenosing tenosynovitis of the flexor hallucis longus tendon at the great toe. Foot Ankle. 1981;2:46–8.

48. Kulig K, Reischl SF, Pomrantz AB, et al. Nonsurgical management of posterior tibial tendon dysfunction with orthoses and resistive exercise: a randomized controlled trial. Phys Ther. 2009;89(1):26–37. https://doi.org/10.2522/ptj.20070242.

49. Michaelson J, Dunn L. Tenosynovitis of the flexor hallucis longus; a clinical study of the spectrum of presentation and treatment. Foot Ankle Int. 2005;26(4):291–303.

50. Wasielewski NJ, Kotsko KM. Does eccentric exercise reduce pain and improve strength in physically active individuals with symptomatic lower extremity tendinosis: a systematic review. J Athl Train. 2007;42(3):409–21.

51. Tsai WC, Tang FT, Hsu CC, Hsu YH, Pang JH, Shiue CC. Ibuprofen inhibition of tendon cell proliferation and upregulation of the cyclin kinase inhibitor p21CIP1. J Orthop Res. 2004;22(3):586–91.

52. Petchprapa CN, Rosenberg ZS, Sconfienza LM, Cavalcanti CF, Vieira RL, Zember JS. MR imaging of entrapment neuropathies of the lower extremity. Part 1. The pelvis and hip. Radiographics. 2010;30:983–100.

53. Taylor DW, Petrera M, Hendry M, Theodoropoulos JS. A systematic review of the use of platelet-rich plasma in sports medicine as a new treatment for tendon and ligament injuries. Clin J Sport Med. 2011;21(4):344–52.

54. O'Connor K, Baumhauer J, Houck JR. Patient factors in the selection of operative versus nonoperative tr posterior tibial tendon dysfunction. Foot Ankle Int. 2010;31(3):197–202. https://doi.org/10.3113/FAI.2010.0197.

55. Teasdall RD, Johnson KA. Surgical treatment of stage I posterior tibial tendon dysfunction. Foot Ankle Int. 1994;15(12):646–8. https://doi.org/10.1177/107110079401501203.

56. Chow HT, Chan KB, Lui TH. Tendoscopic debridement for stage I posterior tibial tendon dysfunction. Knee Surg Sports Traumatol Arthrosc. 2005;13(8):695–8. https://doi.org/10.1007/s00167-005-0635-8.

57. Kirane YM, Michelson JD, Sharkey NA. Contribution of the flexor hallucis longus to loading of the first metatarsal and first metatarsophalangeal joint. Foot Ankle Int. 2008;29(4):367–77. https://doi.org/10.3113/FAI.2008.0367.

58. Christensen JC, Lanier TD. Tendoscopy of the ankle. Clin Podiatr Med Surg. 2011;28:561–70. https://doi.org/10.1016/j.cpm.2011.05.003.

59. Bernasconi A, Sadile F, Welck M, Mehdi N, Laborde J, Lintz F. Role of tendoscopy in treating stage II posterior Tibial tendon dysfunction. Foot Ankle Int. 2018;39(4):433–42. https://doi.org/10.1177/1071100717746192. Epub 2018 Feb 16. PubMed PMID: 29451811.

60. Myerson MS, Corrigan J. Treatment of posterior tibial tendon dysfunction with flexor digitorum longus tendon transfer and calcaneal osteotomy. Orthopedics. 1996;19(5):383–8.

61. Flexor Hallucis Longus tendon injury imaging: overview, radiography, computed tomography. Emedicine.medscape.com. N. p. 2017.

62. Fayazi AH, Nguyen HV, Juliano PJ. Intermediate term follow-up of calcaneal osteotomy and flexor digitorum longus transfer for treatment of posterior tibial tendon dysfunction. Foot Ankle Int. 2002;23(12):1107–11.

63. Pomeroy GC, Pike RH, Beals TC, Manoli A. 2nd acquired flatfoot in adults due to dysfunction of the posterior tibial tendon. J Bone Joint Surg Am. 1999;81:1173–82.

64. Sammarco GJ, Cooper PS. Flexor hallucis longus tendoninjury in dancers and nondancers. Foot Ankle Int. 1998;19:356–62.

65. Parsons S, Naim S, Richards PJ, McBride D. Correction and prevention of deformity in type II tibialis posterior dysfunction. Clin Orthop Relat Res. 2010;468(4):1025–32. https://doi.org/10.1007/s11999-009-1122-1.

66. Mann RA. Flatfoot in adults. In: Mann RA, Coughlin MJ, editors. Surgery of the foot and ankle, vol. 1. 6th ed. St. Louis: The CV Mosby Co; 1993. p. 757–84.

67. Song SJ, Deland JT. Outcome following addition of peroneus brevis tendon transfer to treatment of acquired posterior tibial tendon insufficiency. Foot Ankle Int. 2001;22(4):301–4.

68. Kohls-Gatzoulis J, et al. Tibialis posterior dysfunction: a common and treatable cause of adult acquired flatfoot. BMJ. 2004;329(7478):1328–33. Print.

69. Kitaoka HB, Patzer GL. Subtalar arthrodesis for posterior tibial tendon dysfunction and pes planus. Clin Orthop Relat Res. 1997;(345):187–94.

70. Myerson M. Reconstructive foot and ankle surgery: management of complications. Philadelphia: Elsevier/Saunders; 2010. Print.

71. Bluman EM, Dowd T. The basics and science of tendon transfers. Foot Ankle Clin. 2011;16:385–99.

72. Silver RL, de la Garza J, Rang M. The myth of muscle balance. A study of relative strengths and excursions of normal muscles about the foot and ankle. J Bone Joint Surg Br. 1985;67:432–7.

73. Hansen ST, Clark W. Tendon transfer to augment the weakened tibialis posterior mechanism. J Am Podiatr Med Assoc. 1988;78(8):399–402.

74. Aronow MS. Tendon transfer options in managing the adult flexible flatfoot. Foot Ankle Clini N Am. 2012;17:205–26.

75. Goldner JL, Keats PK, Bassett FH 3rd, et al. Progressive talipes equinovalgus due to trauma or degeneration of the posterior tibial tendon and medial plantar ligaments. Orthop Clin North Am. 1974;5:39–51.

76. Pretterklieber B. The high variability of the chiasma plantare and the long flexor tendons: anatomical aspects of tendon transfer in foot surgery. Ann Anat. 2017;211:21–32. https://doi.org/10.1016/j.aanat.2017.01.011. Epub 2017 Feb 3. PubMed PMID: 28163203.

77. Rungprai C, et al. Disorders of the Flexor Hallucis Longus and Os Trigonum Rungprai. Clin Sports Med. 2015;34(4):741–59.

78. Mao H, Shi Z, Wapner KL, Dong W, Yin W, Xu D. Anatomical study for flexor hallucis longus tendon transfer in treatment of Achilles tendinopathy. Surg Radiol Anat. 2015;37(6):639–47.

79. O'sullivan E, Carare-Nnadi R, Greenslade J, Bowyer G. Clinical significance of variations in the interconnections between flexor digitorum longus and flexor hallucis longus in the region of the knot of Henry. Clin Anat. 2005;18(2):121–5.

80. Hamilton WG, Geppert MJ, Thompson FM. Pain in the posterior aspect of the ankle in dancers. Differential diagnosis and operative treatment. J Bone Joint Surg. 1996;78A:1491–500.

81. Kolettis GJ, Micheli LJ, Klein JD. Release of the flexor hallucis longus tendon in ballet dancers. J Bone Joint Surg. 1996;78(9):1386–90.

82. Corte-Real NM, Moreira RM, Guerra-Pinto F. Arthroscopic treatment of tenosynovitis of the flexor hallucis longus tendon. Foot Ankle Int. 2012;33:1108.

83. Mehta P, Rand EB, Visco CJ, Wyss J. Resident accuracy of musculoskeletal palpation with ultrasound verification. J Ultrasound Med. 2018;37:1719–24. https://doi.org/10.1002/jum.14523.

84. Lo LD, et al. MR imaging findings of entrapment of the flexor hallucis longus Tendon. PubMed – NCBI. Ncbi.nlm.nih.gov. N. p. 2017.

85. Maeseneer MD, Marcelis S, Jager T, et al. Sonography of the normal ankle: a target approach using skeletal reference points. AJR Am J Roentgenol. 2009;192:487–95.

86. Murrell GA. Understanding tendinopathies. Br J Sports Med. 2002;36(6):392–3.

87. Albisetti W, Ometti M, Pascale V, De Bartolomeo O. Clinical evaluation and treatment of posterior impingement in dancers. Am J Phys Med Rehabil. 2009;88(5):349–54.

88. Senécal I, Richer N. Conservative management of posterior ankle impingement: a case report. J Can Chiropr Assoc. 2016;60(2):164.

89. Russell JA. Preventing dance injuries: current perspectives. Open Access J Sports Med. 2013;4:199–210. Published 2013 Sep 30. https://doi.org/10.2147/OAJSM.S36529.

90. Sofka CM, Collins AJ, Adler RS. Use of ultrasonographic guidance in interventional musculoskeletal procedures: a review from a single institution. J Ultrasound Med. 2001;20:21–6.

91. Mehdizade A, Adler RS. Sonographically guided flexor Hallucis longus tendon sheath injection. J Ultrasound Med. 2007;26:233–7. https://doi.org/10.7863/jum.2007.26.2.233.

92. Reach JS, Easley ME, Chuckpaiwong B, Nunley JA. Accuracy of ultrasound guided injections in the foot and ankle. Foot Ankle Int. 2009;30(3):239–42. [ISSN: 1071-1007].

93. Guo QW, Hu YL, Jiao C, et al. Open versus endoscopic excision of a symptomatic os trigonum: a comparative study of 41 cases. Arthroscopy. 2010;26:384–90.

94. Marotta JJ, Micheli LJ. Os trigonum impingement in dancers. Am J Sports Med. 1992;20:533–6.

95. Rietveld ABMB, Hagemans FMT. Operative treatment of posterior ankle impingement syndrome and flexor Hallucis longus tendinopathy in dancers open versus endoscopic approach. J Dance Med Sci. 2018;22(1):11–8. https://doi.org/10.12678/1089-313X.22.1.11. PubMed PMID: 29510785.

96. Sarrafian SK. Anatomy of the foot and ankle: descriptive, topographic, functional. 2nd ed. Philadelphia: JB Lippincott; 1993.

97. Mao H, et al. Anatomical study for flexor hallucis longus tendon transfer in treatment of Achilles tendinopathy. PubMed – NCBI.

98. Schmidt-Hebbel A, Elgueta J, Villa A, Mery P, Filippi J. Síndrome del túnel del tarso posterior bilateral por músculo flexor digitorum longus accesorio; reporte de un caso y descripción de técnica quirúrgica. Rev Esp Cir Ortop Traumatol. 2017;61:117–23.

99. Sarrafian SK. Biomechanics of the subtalar joint complex. Clin Orthop Relat Res. 1993;290:17–26.

Achilles Tendon

16

Stephen Schaaf, Ma Calus V. Hogan,
and Adam S. Tenforde

Abbreviation

CT   Computed tomography
MRI   Magnetic resonance imaging
US   Ultrasound
NSAID Non-steroidal anti-inflammatory drug

Introduction

Achilles tendon injury is one of the most common musculoskeletal conditions in athletes. The annual incidence of Achilles tendon injuries has been reported as 9–11%, and an estimated lifetime risk of 52% in runners [1, 2]. The majority of Achilles tendon injuries are managed non-surgically [3]. However, up to 29% of cases can be chronic and interfere with sports [4]. Achilles tendon injuries are classically defined by the location of the pathology, separating the most distal 2 cm segment as "insertional" and more proximal segment as "mid-portion or non-insertional" [5]. However, more recently, the terminology to classify Achilles tendon injury is based on clinical symptoms and histopathology. Achilles tendinopathy by definition is a clinical syndrome of pain, with or without swelling, and impaired performance [6].Chronic Achilles tendinopathy is largely devoid of frank swelling. Achilles tendinopathy can be divided further into Achilles tendonitis and tendinosis based on histopathologic findings (Fig. 16.1) [7, 8]. Reduced tensile strength of the tendon may predispose an Achilles tendon to partial tears and spontaneous rupture [9].

S. Schaaf (✉)
Department of Physical Medicine and Rehabilitation,
University of Pittsburgh, Pittsburgh, PA, USA
e-mail: schaafs@upmc.edu

M. C. V. Hogan
Department of Orthopedic Surgery, University of
Pittsburgh, Pittsburgh, PA, USA
e-mail: hoganmv@upmc.edu

A. S. Tenforde
Department of Physical Medicine and Rehabilitation,
Harvard Medical School, Cambridge, MA, USA

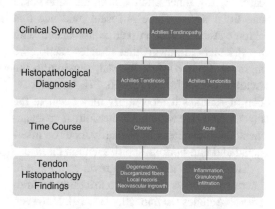

Fig. 16.1 Terminology for Achilles tendinopathy, tendinosis, and tendonitis

Anatomy

The Achilles tendon fibers arise from the rostral end of both the gastrocnemius and soleus muscles. Although the strongest and thickest tendon in the human body, the Achilles tendon is believed to be at anatomical risk for injuries due to crossing both the knee and ankle joint and sustaining up to 12.5 times the body weight during high-impact activities, such as running, jumping, or landing [8, 10, 11].

The Achilles tendon lacks a true tendon sheath and is surrounded by an areolar tissue called paratenon [12].The paratenon normally lubricates tendon tissue but can become inflamed and a source of pain. The retrocalcaneal bursa is deep and the retroachilles bursa is superficial at the insertion of the Achilles tendon. Both bursae can be a source of heel pain when inflamed [13].

The plantaris tendon can serve as a cofactor for mid-portion Achilles tendinopathy due to abnormal medial contact resulting in adhesions and tendon pain [14].

The vascular supply to the Achilles tendon arises from branches of both the posterior tibial artery and the peroneal artery. The mid-portion area receives relatively less blood supply compared to the distal portion of the tendon, which might explain why midportion tendinopathy is five times more frequent than insertional cases [3, 15]. Innervation is from the sural nerve and tibial nerve. There is recent evidence that chronic Achilles tendon pain is associated with neovascular ingrowth that creates neo-nerve ingrowth from Kager's fat pad, sensitizing the Achilles tendon further [12, 16, 17]. A third location of Achilles tendon injury may occur at the myotendinous junction. Discussion of management in this chapter will primarily focus on insertional and mid-portion Achilles tendon disease.

The plantaris tendon has grown as a topic of interest due to its reported contribution to mid-portion Achilles tendinopathy [18, 19]. However, a plantaris injury can be seen as an isolated clinical condition. Specifically, around one-third of plantaris injuries occur with no involvement of the Achilles tendon [19, 20]. The majority of plantaris injuries are reported as acute tendinopa-

thy [20]. Tears and ruptures of the plantaris can also occur, most often at the myotendinous junction along the upper part of the gastrocnemius and more rarely at the mid-substance of the tendon [21]. In the authors' collective experience, these injuries rarely require further interventional treatments or surgery.

Case

A 41-year-old male marathon runner without significant past medical history presents with 9 months of persistent right heel pain. His primary care physician had previously diagnosed him with Achilles tendinitis and instructed him to refrain from running and start physical therapy. He underwent 6 weeks of physical therapy without definitive improvement. Subsequently, he was sent to a sports medicine specialist for further evaluation. History was notable for unresolving right heel pain provoked by initial loading on his right leg. Pertinent positives from physical exam include an area of focal tenderness and thickening along the mid-portion of the right Achilles tendon, symptom reproduction with a right single heel raise, and a negative Thompson test. Diagnostic ultrasound of the right Achilles demonstrated a hypoechoic area within the midportion of the tendon with loss of fibrillar architecture, fusiform thickening, neovascularization on color Doppler, and sonopalpation tenderness (Figs. 16.2 and 16.3).

Clinical Presentation

Achilles tendinopathy is usually diagnosed using history and physical examination. Pain is the primary symptom resulting in a patient seeking medical treatment. Patients most often complain of pain in the Achilles tendon that is worse with loading. The pain and stiffness may be most notable on initiating activity, such as in the morning or starting exercise. In the early stage of Achilles tendinopathy, patients have pain following strenuous activities. Those in the later phase report pain accompanying all activities which may even

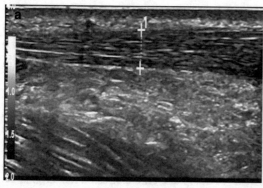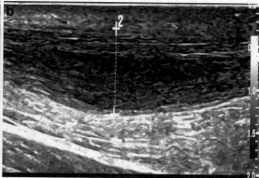

Fig. 16.2 Long axis view of the Achilles tendon on musculoskeletal ultrasound. (**a**) Demonstrates normal Achilles tendon which appears as echogenic fibrillary lines with homogeneous thickness typically 4–7 mm. (**b**) Demonstrates Achilles tendinopathy which will appear hypoechoic with loss of fibrillar architecture and fusiform thickening of the tendon

Fig. 16.3 Long axis view of the Achilles tendon on musculoskeletal ultrasound with color Doppler. Neovascularization is seen, which is the development of new blood vessels within the tendon and can indicate Achilles tendinopathy. Healthy tendon will be largely devoid of blood vessels

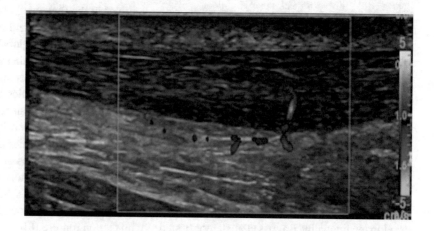

occur at rest [3, 22]. Achilles tendon rupture is typically described by patients as experiencing a sudden snap in the heel region, followed by pain and difficulty with weight bearing on the affected leg [8].

Achilles tendinopathy ultimately results from excessive load on the tendon often accompanied by other factors predisposing to tendon disease [17]. Intrinsic and extrinsic individual risk factors have been identified in Achilles tendinopathy (Table 16.1) [23]. Male gender and ages greater than 60 with age-related reduced vascularity of the tendon have been associated with increased risk of Achilles tendon disorders [4, 12, 24]. Several biomechanical malalignments have been implicated in the pathogenesis of Achilles tendon diseases [25]. Forefoot hyperpronation can cause

"whipping" mechanics of the Achilles tendon during running, resulting in micro-tears along the medial portion of the tendon that can precipitate tendinopathy [12]. In contrast, cavus foot deformity may cause lateral Achilles tendinopathy by placing excessive stress on the Achilles tendon during loading [26]. Subtalar joint immobility can increase the tension of the Achilles tendon during movement [4].

External to the Achilles, other alternations of the kinetic chain can contribute to abnormal mechanics. Altered neuromotor control of the gluteus medius and maximus is associated with Achilles tendinopathy [27]. There is increasing awareness of the clinical importance of the foot core, a concept that describes the Achilles tendon function as part of a system defined as both

Table 16.1 Intrinsic and extrinsic risk factors for Achilles tendinopathy [4, 12, 23–28, 30]

Risk factors of Achilles tendinopathy
Intrinsic 1. Male gender
2. Advanced age (Above 60 years old)
3. Biomechanical malalignments
(i) Forefoot hyperpronation
(ii) Cavus foot
(iii) Subtalar joint immobility
(iv) Gluteal muscle weakness
(v) Foot core weakness
Extrinsic 1. Training errors
(i) Sudden increase in running mileage or intensity
(ii) Change in terrain
(iii) Running on hard or sloped surfaces
2. Improper footwear
(i) Insufficient heel height
(ii) Rigid soles
(iii) Inadequate shock absorption
(iv) Wedging from uneven wear

small and large muscle complexes with neuromotor control systems that all contribute to overall function of the foot. Foot core contributes to foot and lower extremity stability and function, as well as to proper loading of the Achilles tendon [28]. Footwear contributes to tendon properties. For example, wearing minimalist shoes places an increased load and stress on the Achilles tendon leading to stiffness [29]. Lastly, certain Achilles tendon loading activities lead to a higher risk to develop tendinopathy. Bayliss et al. demonstrated that jumping exposes the Achilles tendon to more force and stress resulting in stiffness [30]. Lorimer et al. identified large peak break force, which can be seen in runners with altered gait mechanics, as negative for tendon health [25].

Physical Examination

Clinical exam should start with inspection of the Achilles tendon which may reveal focal thickening. On palpation, an area of focal tenderness is most often present. Swelling, warmth, or erythema along the tendon is more consistent with an inflammatory process seen in acute Achilles tendonitis/paratenonitis. Tendon pain may be elicited with both active and passive plantar flexion of the ankle [22]. Paratenonitis may be associated with crepi-

tus on examination. Paratendinitis (tendon sheath nodules) do not move with passive plantar/dorsi flexion, while tendinopathy does. The Thompson test has a 96% to 98% positive predictive value in detecting an Achilles tendon rupture [31]. This test is performed by placing the patient in a prone position and the examiner squeezing the middle third of the calf muscle. Passive plantar flexion of the foot should be seen as a normal response when the calf muscle is squeezed (Fig. 16.4). Single heel leg raise or a hop test on the affected tendon may be performed [32]. Repetitive calf raises can be helpful to evaluate for calf and tendon endurance to repetitive loads, and typically 30 single leg calf raises are a good benchmark for adequate plantar foot strength for most sport activities. Other muscles in the foot should be evaluated to ensure adequate foot strength, and single leg balance testing is helpful to assess global foot and ankle function. Additionally, examination for biomechanical faults in the lower extremity should be accessed including basic mechanics with single leg squat test. Differential diagnosis for Achilles tendinopathy should be comprehensive (Table 16.2), with further imaging modalities being used to rule out these differential diagnoses.

With tendon disruption, there is absence of a plantar flexion response. In addition, a palpable gap in the Achilles tendon is commonly observed with tendon rupture [8].

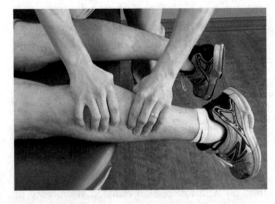

Fig. 16.4 Thompson test. Performed by placing the patient in a prone position with the examiner squeezing the middle third of the calf muscle. A normal response as depicted results in passive plantar flexion of the ankle when the calf muscle is squeezed. With tendon disruption, there is absence of a plantar flexion response

Table 16.2 Differential diagnosis for Achilles tendinopathy

Achilles tendinopathy differential diagnosis	
Pathologic process	Condition
Bone	Haglund's deformity
	Os trigonum
	Ankle joint osteoarthritis
	Osteochondritis of the talus
	Stress fracture of the distal tibia or calcaneus
	Sever's disease
Muscle/tendon	Complete or partial rupture of the Achilles tendon
	Accessory soleus muscle
	Posterior tibialis tendon rupture
	Plantar fasciitis
	Tenosynovitis of the flexor hallucis longus
	Plantaris tendon tear
Nerve	Tarsal tunnel syndrome
	Sural neuropathy
Inflammatory	Retrocalcaneal bursitis
	Infection

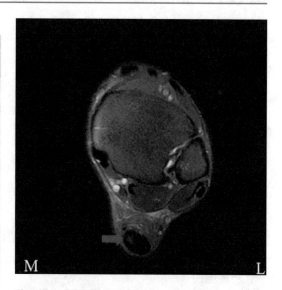

Fig. 16.5 MRI T2-weighted fat saturated image of the left lower extremity. Red arrow points to an area of increased signal within the Achilles tendon, which is indicative of Achilles tendinopathy. M medial, L lateral

Diagnostic Studies

Plain Films and CT Scan

X-rays and computed tomography [33] scans have low utility in the diagnosis of Achilles tendinopathy, given the limited detail of soft tissue and tendon structures [34, 35]. However, these imaging techniques may reveal bone conditions associated with posterior heel pain. Haglund's deformity is a posterosuperior bony outgrowth arising from the calcaneal tuberosity that can contribute to pain or predispose to posterior ankle impingement. Calcaneal apophysitis, also known as Sever's disease, is caused by painful inflammation of the calcaneal growth plate in children. Additionally, these imaging modalities may identify mineralization of the tendon [34].

Magnetic Resonance Imaging

Magnetic resonance imaging (MRI) provides excellent soft tissue and tendon detail [34]. A healthy Achilles tendon will display low signal on conventional MRI, reflecting compact tendon structure and minimal water content. Conversely, tendinosis results in increased T2 signal within the tendon, as well as tendon thickening and fusiform tendon shape (Fig. 16.5). MRI is the preferred imaging technique when tendon rupture is suspected and if high-quality ultrasound is not readily available [34]. Increased signal on MRI in cases of tendinosis may also help predict chronicity of symptoms and clinical outcomes [36].

Ultrasound

Musculoskeletal ultrasound [37] is a cost-effective, readily available diagnostic imaging modality that can evaluate Achilles tendon disease. Normal Achilles tendon appears as echogenic fibrillary lines in long axis view and appears homogeneous in thickness, typically 4–7 mm [34, 36]. Tendinosis will appear hypoechoic with loss of fibrillar architecture and fusiform thickening of the tendon (Fig. 16.2) [35]. With careful examination, both partial and full thickness tears can be visualized [34, 35]. Ultrasound can also be performed dynamically (asking the patient to actively engage plantar flexor of the foot) to evaluate for tendon retraction seen in more significant Achilles tendon tears. Additional ultrasound findings of tendinosis include neovascularization, which is the development of new blood vessels within the tendon, and are visualized on color Doppler (Fig. 16.3). Whereas healthy tendon will be largely devoid of blood vessels, neovascularization can be a sign of chronic tendon irritation and is associated with greater pain and worse functional outcomes when identified in cases of tendinosis [34, 35, 38]. Thus, ultrasound serves as a reliable imaging modality to locate Achilles tendon abnormalities and estimate severity [39]. Limitations in ultrasound include reduced accuracy compared to MRI for evaluating Achilles tendon morphology and cross-sectional area as well as the ability to detect pathology may be user dependent [40].

Treatments

Conservative

Conservative management of Achilles tendinopathy is successful in most cases, which is usually employed for 3–6 months before advancing to alternative and more invasive treatments (Fig. 16.6) [34]. Approximately one-quarter of cases fail conservative treatment [41]. Conservative management includes relative rest with avoidance of tendon loading, shoe wear modifications, heel lifts, and taping, as well as stretching [41]. Short courses of nonsteroidal anti-inflammatories (NSAIDs) with any combination of these treatments may also be beneficial in the acute stages of tendinopathy to help reduce pain and inflammation [42]. Strengthening the tendon through progressive loading is standard treatment of Achilles tendinopathy and other tendon disease. Eccentric loading of the tendon may encourage healing by improving tendon collagen fiber orientation and by restoring leg muscle strength [16]. This program includes 3 sets of 15 slow repetitions of eccentric unilateral loading usually performed standing on the step of a staircase. For eccentric Achilles tendon loading, the patient first places all body weight on the forefoot of the affected leg with the ankle

joint in plantar flexion. The calf muscle is then loaded by having the patient lower the heel past neutral into dorsiflexion. Patients are instructed to spend approximately 3 seconds completing each repetition. One exercise is performed with a straight knee and one with a bent knee, twice a day (morning and evening), 7 days a week, for 12 consecutive weeks. Load is increased gradually using a weighted backpack as pain diminishes. This type of eccentric muscle training program termed the "Alfredson Protocol" for mid-portion Achilles tendinopathy has reported success rate of up to 90% (Fig. 16.7) [43, 44], although in our clinical experience, success rate is lower. In addition, long-term benefits of this program have been shown with improved pain relief and physical function for patients with Achilles tendinopathy at 5 years of follow-up [45]. In contrast, eccentric loading programs for insertional Achilles tendinopathy have lower success rates of 32% [46]. A published modification to this program for insertional Achilles tendinopathy was suggested by Jonsson et al. to reduce the dorsiflexion component. With this modified program, patients with insertional tendinopathy performed ankle eccentric exercises by slowly lowering the foot from a plantar-flexed position to a flat surface, rather than on a raised box or platform. Elimination of dorsiflexion was proposed to reduce the compression forces between the pathologic tendon, bursa, and bone from posterior impingement [46].

Additionally, treatment of all Achilles tendon disorders should also include rehabilitation exercises that improve the kinetic chain and lower muscle activity such as in the tibialis anterior, rectus femoris, gluteus medius, and the foot core [27, 28, 47].

Topical glyceryl trinitrate (GTN) patches can be considered as an adjunct for Achilles tendinopathy. GTN is a prodrug of endogenous nitric oxide and stimulates collagen synthesis by wound fibroblasts, and thus promotes tendon healing by improving blood supply. Daily 1.25 mg per 24 hours GTN patches, combined with conservative modalities, were able to reduce pain and increase activity levels in cases of non-

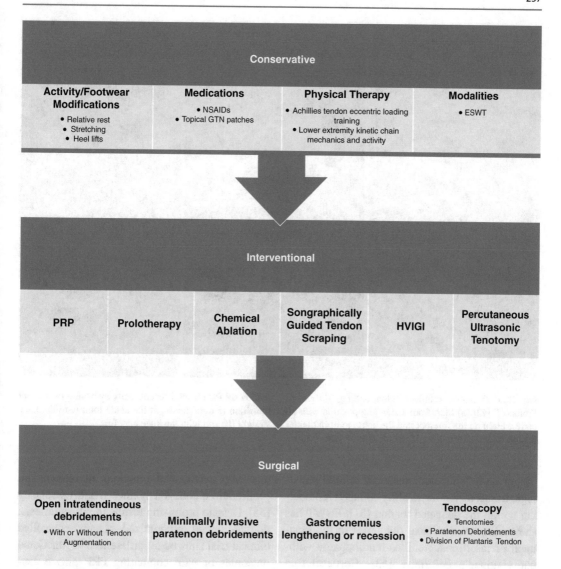

Fig. 16.6 Management of Achilles tendinopathy. Conservative measures are typically utilized for 3–6 months. Choice of treatment after conservative measures is patient specific, with interventional treatments serving as an

alternative to surgery. GTN glyceryl trinitrate, ESWT extracorpeal shock wave therapy, PRP platelet-rich plasma, HVIGI high-volume image-guided injections

insertional Achilles tendinopathy [48]. However, a repeat study failed to support this clinical benefit of GTN patches [49]. Side effects include light headedness or headaches associated with more systemic vasodilation effects, especially in those with low blood pressure. The medication should not be used in patients taking nitrate-containing compounds for vascular conditions including cardiac disease or erectile dysfunction.

Interventional

Extracorporeal shock wave therapy (ESWT) can be considered an interventional modality in the treatment of Achilles tendinopathy [50]. ESWT involves the delivery of acoustic energy waves to pathologic tendon in Achilles tendinopathy [51, 52]. The mechanism of action is still not completely understood, but ESWT is thought to

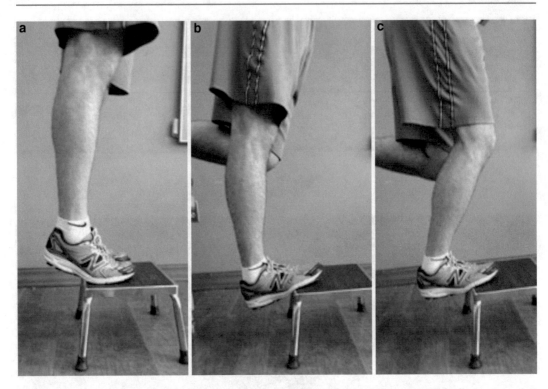

Fig. 16.7 Eccentric Achilles tendon loading, "Alfredson Protocol." [43] (**a**) Start from a standing position with all body weight on the forefoot and the ankle joint in plantar flexion of the affected leg. The calf muscle and Achilles tendon are then loaded eccentrically by having the patient transition to dorsiflexion at the ankle joint with the knee straight (**b**) and with the knee bent (**c**)

trigger an inflammatory response around patho-logic tissue, triggering healthy collagen remodel-ing within the damaged tendon [51]. ESWT has shown improved clinical outcomes in the treat-ment of insertional Achilles tendinopathy with-out Haglund's deformity [53]. Corticosteroid injections are not recommended for treatment of Achilles tendinopathy due to concern for tendon rupture [16]. Steroids may further alter appropri-ate healing by inhibiting formation of favorable, tendon-healing collagen cells [54]. However, other forms of non-steroid injection treatment are reasonable to consider for refractory cases of tendon disease and are delivered using ultra-sound image guidance (Fig. 16.6). Platelet-rich plasma (PRP) therapy has been proposed as a possible treatment for mid-portion Achilles ten-dinopathy. Preparation of PRP is from platelets derived from whole blood via cell separation techniques. The PRP is injected into the area of tendinopathy, triggering a release of growth fac-

tors with established functions in tendon cell proliferation, collagen synthesis, and vascularity [55]. Despite promising results in pilot studies, a double-blinded, randomized, placebo-controlled clinical trial showed no differences in functional outcomes or pain comparing PRP plus eccen-tric exercise to lidocaine injection plus eccen-tric exercise [56–59]. Additionally, there were no differences in sonographic tendon appear-ance nor degree of neovascularization at follow-up between the PRP and placebo groups [60]. There are limitations to the protocol design that make this study difficult to interpret the value of use in PRP for patients with refractory disease. Additional studies of PRP with repeated injec-tions, different concentrations, variable activation techniques, and long-term outcomes for Achilles tendinopathy are underway [61].

Dextrose hyperosmolar injections, known as prolotherapy injections, have been shown to result in reduction in pain, improvement in function, patient satisfaction, and sonographic appearance of the tendon. The exact mechanism of prolotherapy is unknown; the hypermolar injection is thought to cause an immune-mediated healing cascade and result in proliferation of healthy tendon tissue [62, 63]. Synergy of prolotherapy and eccentric exercise programs has been documented [64]. However, most studies did not include adequate controls to investigate relative efficacy [62, 63, 65].

Additional interventions target neovascularization. Chemical ablation is an injection of a sclerosing agent polidocanol. Polidocanol injections target the intimal layer of the vascular wall, leading to vessel micro-thrombosis [38]. The nerves around the tendon which act as pain generators are proposed to be affected through elimination of blood supply or direct action of the sclerosing agent. Polidocanol was shown to be superior to an injection of anesthetic for decreasing pain and increasing patient satisfaction in treatment for Achilles tendinosis, with maximum benefit achieved with multiple injections [38, 66]. Note this treatment has not received US Food and Drug Administration (FDA) approval.

Tendon scraping is direct separation of neovessels with a scalpel or needle and has shown early success in treating Achilles tendinopathy [67, 68]. Open tendon scraping technique with a scalpel compared to percutaneous scraping with a needle performed under sonographic guidance was shown to be equivalent in improvement of pain, complication rate, and patient satisfaction [68]. Additionally, tendon scraping allowed for quicker progression with return to full tendon loading as compared to prolotherapy and polidocanol injections [68, 69].

High-volume image-guided injections (HVIGI) target neovascularization associated with Achilles tendinosis [70]. For this intervention, large volumes, approximately 20 mL to 50 mL, in a combination of local anesthetic and normal saline are injected adjacent to the damaged tendon. This is thought to generate local mechanical effects leading to stretching and breaking of neovessels and resulting in the disruption of neurogenic inflammation [71, 72]. These injections were shown to be effective in decreasing pain and improving function at 3 weeks following intervention and had sustained benefits at 1-year follow-up [70, 71].

Sonographically guided percutaneous tenotomy and debridement, or simply, percutaneous ultrasonic tenotomy (PUT), is an emerging technology for treatment of recalcitrant mid-portion Achilles tendinosis. This technology is based on the concept of phacoemulsification, in which ultrasonic energy is utilized to emulsify and remove pathologic tissue [51]. This intervention has shown favorable results in animal models and may soon be studied in clinical trials of refractory Achilles tendinopathy [73].

In summary, many non-surgical interventions have been proposed for refractory Achilles tendinopathy. However, the relative efficacy of these interventions is limited by small sample sizes, few randomized control trials, and inconsistent study outcome variables. As a result, consensus on efficacy and applicability has not been reached for these interventions. Selection of these interventions is patient and physician dependent, with insurance coverage and cost being factored.

Operative

Minimally invasive techniques, such as paratenon debridement, focus on paratendinous tissues and elimination of neovascularization. Open techniques, such as intratendineous debridement, address the diseased area of the tendon itself and may involve augmentation of the tendon, including flexor hallucis longus tendon transfer, in severe cases [74, 75]. However, more recent evidence has shown mixed results for surgical treatment of Achilles tendinopathy with flexor hallucis longus tendon transfer, especially for insertional cases [76, 77]. Gastrocnemius lengthening or recession to offload the Achilles tendon, which can be done open or in a minimally invasive approach, is another recognized technique [74]. There is no significant difference between open versus minimally invasive surgery for Achilles tendinopathy in terms of success rates, patient satisfaction, or return to full tendon loading activities at 3–6 months following surgery [74, 78].

Tenotomies, paratenon debridements, and division of the plantaris tendon when indicated can all be performed endoscopically in experienced hands [79–81]. Tendoscopy may have lower rates of surgical complications, but return to full tendon loading activities by 3 months remains the same as other surgical techniques [80]. If an acute Achilles tendon rupture occurs, non-operative management may be considered; however, operative treatment remains to be the most common recommendation for active patients [8]. Both conservative and non-operative treatment options when compared resulted in similar patient satisfaction, return to sports, and tendon strength [82]. Operative management though resulted in decreased tendon re-rupture rate [82]. Several surgical techniques can be used for tendon rupture repair including open (with or without augmentation) and less invasive techniques such as percutaneous and mini-open repairs [8]. Minimally invasive techniques are increasing in popularity and utilization due to similar outcomes with a lower incidence of wound breakdown and healing complications [83, 84]. Further, resection of Haglund's deformity and retrocalcaneal bursectomy may also be considered with insertional Achilles tendinopathy with associated anatomical sources of pain.

References

1. Lopes AD, Hespanhol Junior LC, Yeung SS, Costa LO. What are the main running-related musculoskeletal injuries? A systematic review. Sports Med. 2012;42(10):891–905.
2. Kujala UM, Sarna S, Kaprio J. Cumulative incidence of Achilles tendon rupture and tendinopathy in male former elite athletes. Clin J Sport Med. 2005;15(3):133–5.
3. Paavola M, Kannus P, Paakkala T, Pasanen M, Jarvinen M. Long-term prognosis of patients with Achilles tendinopathy. Am J Sports Med. 2000;28(5):634–42.
4. Kvist M. Achilles tendon injuries in athletes. Ann Chir Gynaecol. 1991;80(2):188–201.
5. van Dijk CN, van Sterkenburg MN, Wiegerinck JI, Karlsson J, Maffulli N. Terminology for Achilles tendon related disorders. Knee Surg Sports Traumatol Arthrosc. 2011;19(5):835–41.
6. Maffulli N, Khan KM, Puddu G. Overuse tendon conditions: time to change a confusing terminology. Arthroscopy. 1998;14(8):840–3.
7. Puddu G, Ippolito E, Postacchini F. A classification of Achilles tendon disease. Am J Sports Med. 1976;4(4):145–50.
8. Uquillas CA, Guss MS, Ryan DJ, Jazrawi LM, Strauss EJ. Everything Achilles: knowledge update and current concepts in management: AAOS exhibit selection. J Bone Joint Surg Am. 2015;97(14):1187–95.
9. Józsa LG, Kannus P. Human tendons: anatomy, physiology, and pathology. Champaign, IL: Human Kinetics; 1997. ix, 574 p.
10. Komi PV. Relevance of in vivo force measurements to human biomechanics. J Biomech. 1990;23 Suppl 1:23–34.
11. Komi PV, Fukashiro S, Jarvinen M. Biomechanical loading of Achilles tendon during normal locomotion. Clin Sports Med. 1992;11(3):521–31.
12. Kader D, Saxena A, Movin T, Maffulli N. Achilles tendinopathy: some aspects of basic science and clinical management. Br J Sports Med. 2002;36(4):239–49.
13. McGarvey WC, Palumbo RC, Baxter DE, Leibman BD. Insertional Achilles tendinosis: surgical treatment through a central tendon splitting approach. Foot Ankle Int. 2002;23(1):19–25.
14. Masci L, Spang C, van Schie HT, Alfredson H. How to diagnose plantaris tendon involvement in midportion Achilles tendinopathy – clinical and imaging findings. BMC Musculoskelet Disord. 2016;17:97.
15. Carr AJ, Norris SH. The blood supply of the calcaneal tendon. J Bone Joint Surg Br. 1989;71(1):100–1.
16. Alfredson H, Cook J. A treatment algorithm for managing Achilles tendinopathy: new treatment options. Br J Sports Med. 2007;41(4):211–6.
17. Cook JL, Purdam CR. Is tendon pathology a continuum? A pathology model to explain the clinical presentation of load-induced tendinopathy. Br J Sports Med. 2009;43(6):409–16.
18. Alfredson H. Midportion Achilles tendinosis and the plantaris tendon. Br J Sports Med. 2011;45(13):1023–5.
19. Calder JD, Freeman R, Pollock N. Plantaris excision in the treatment of non-insertional Achilles tendinopathy in elite athletes. Br J Sports Med. 2015;49(23):1532–4.
20. Pollock N, Dijkstra P, Calder J, Chakraverty R. Plantaris injuries in elite UK track and field athletes over a 4-year period: a retrospective cohort study. Knee Surg Sports Traumatol Arthrosc. 2016;24(7):2287–92.
21. Spang C, Alfredson H, Docking SI, Masci L, Andersson G. The plantaris tendon: a narrative review focusing on anatomical features and clinical importance. Bone Joint J. 2016;98-B(10):1312–9.
22. Paavola M, Kannus P, Jarvinen TA, Khan K, Jozsa L, Jarvinen M. Achilles tendinopathy. J Bone Joint Surg Am. 2002;84-A(11):2062–76.
23. Saltzman CL, Tearse DS. Achilles tendon injuries. J Am Acad Orthop Surg. 1998;6(5):316–25.
24. Kannus P, Niittymaki S, Jarvinen M, Lehto M. Sports injuries in elderly athletes: a three-year prospective, controlled study. Age Ageing. 1989;18(4):263–70.

25. Lorimer AV, Hume PA. Achilles tendon injury risk factors associated with running. Sports Med. 2014;44(10):1459–72.

26. Den Hartog BD. Insertional Achilles tendinosis: pathogenesis and treatment. Foot Ankle Clin. 2009;14(4):639–50.

27. Franettovich Smith MM, Honeywill C, Wyndow N, Crossley KM, Creaby MW. Neuromotor control of gluteal muscles in runners with Achilles tendinopathy. Med Sci Sports Exerc. 2014;46(3):594–9.

28. McKeon PO, Hertel J, Bramble D, Davis I. The foot core system: a new paradigm for understanding intrinsic foot muscle function. Br J Sports Med. 2015;49(5):290.

29. Histen K, Arntsen J, L'Hereux L, Heeren J, Wicki B, Saint S, et al. Achilles tendon properties in minimalist and traditionally shod runners. J Sport Rehabil. 2016:1–16.

30. Bayliss AJ, Weatherholt AM, Crandall TT, Farmer DL, McConnell JC, Crossley KM, et al. Achilles tendon material properties are greater in the jump leg of jumping athletes. J Musculoskelet Neuronal Interact. 2016;16(2):105–12.

31. Maffulli N. The clinical diagnosis of subcutaneous tear of the Achilles tendon. A prospective study in 174 patients. Am J Sports Med. 1998;26(2):266–70.

32. Hutchison AM, Evans R, Bodger O, Pallister I, Topliss C, Williams P, et al. What is the best clinical test for Achilles tendinopathy? Foot Ankle Surg. 2013;19(2):112–7.

33. Kelsey JL, Bachrach LK, Procter-Gray E, Nieves J, Greendale GA, Sowers M, et al. Risk factors for stress fracture among young female cross-country runners. Med Sci Sports Exerc. 2007;39(9):1457–63.

34. Wijesekera NT, Calder JD, Lee JC. Imaging in the assessment and management of Achilles tendinopathy and paratendinitis. Semin Musculoskelet Radiol. 2011;15(1):89–100.

35. Jacobson JA. Fundamentals of musculoskeletal ultrasound. Philadelphia, PA: Elsevier/Saunders; 2013.

36. Khan KM, Forster BB, Robinson J, Cheong Y, Louis L, Maclean L, et al. Are ultrasound and magnetic resonance imaging of value in assessment of Achilles tendon disorders? A two year prospective study. Br J Sports Med. 2003;37(2):149–53.

37. Tenforde AS, Nattiv A, Barrack MT, Kraus E, Kim B, Kussman A, et al. Distribution of bone stress injuries in elite male and female collegiate endurance runners. Med Sci Sports Exerc. 2015;47(5S):905.

38. Alfredson H, Ohberg L. Sclerosing injections to areas of neo-vascularisation reduce pain in chronic Achilles tendinopathy: a double-blind randomised controlled trial. Knee Surg Sports Traumatol Arthrosc. 2005;13(4):338–44.

39. Paavola M, Paakkala T, Kannus P, Jarvinen M. Ultrasonography in the differential diagnosis of Achilles tendon injuries and related disorders. A comparison between pre-operative ultrasonography and surgical findings. Acta Radiol. 1998;39(6):612–9.

40. Bohm S, Mersmann F, Schroll A, Makitalo N, Arampatzis A. Insufficient accuracy of the ultrasound-based determination of Achilles tendon cross-sectional area. J Biomech. 2016;49(13):2932–7.

41. Alfredson H, Lorentzon R. Chronic Achilles tendinosis: recommendations for treatment and prevention. Sports Med. 2000;29(2):135–46.

42. Maquirriain J, Kokalj A. Acute Achilles tendinopathy: effect of pain control on leg stiffness. J Musculoskelet Neuronal Interact. 2014;14(1):131–6.

43. Alfredson H, Pietila T, Jonsson P, Lorentzon R. Heavy-load eccentric calf muscle training for the treatment of chronic Achilles tendinosis. Am J Sports Med. 1998;26(3):360–6.

44. Beyer R, Kongsgaard M, Hougs Kjaer B, Ohlenschlaeger T, Kjaer M, Magnusson SP. Heavy slow resistance versus eccentric training as treatment for Achilles tendinopathy: a randomized controlled trial. Am J Sports Med. 2015;43(7):1704–11.

45. van der Plas A, de Jonge S, de Vos RJ, van der Heide HJ, Verhaar JA, Weir A, et al. A 5-year follow-up study of Alfredson's heel-drop exercise programme in chronic midportion Achilles tendinopathy. Br J Sports Med. 2012;46(3):214–8.

46. Jonsson P, Alfredson H, Sunding K, Fahlstrom M, Cook J. New regimen for eccentric calf-muscle training in patients with chronic insertional Achilles tendinopathy: results of a pilot study. Br J Sports Med. 2008;42(9):746–9.

47. Azevedo LB, Lambert MI, Vaughan CL, O'Connor CM, Schwellnus MP. Biomechanical variables associated with Achilles tendinopathy in runners. Br J Sports Med. 2009;43(4):288–92.

48. Paoloni JA, Appleyard RC, Nelson J, Murrell GA. Topical glyceryl trinitrate treatment of chronic noninsertional Achilles tendinopathy. A randomized, double-blind, placebo-controlled trial. J Bone Joint Surg Am. 2004;86-A(5):916–22.

49. Kane TP, Ismail M, Calder JD. Topical glyceryl trinitrate and noninsertional Achilles tendinopathy: a clinical and cellular investigation. Am J Sports Med. 2008;36(6):1160–3.

50. Rasmussen S, Christensen M, Mathiesen I, Simonson O. Shockwave therapy for chronic Achilles tendinopathy: a double-blind, randomized clinical trial of efficacy. Acta Orthop. 2008;79(2):249–56.

51. Langer PR. Two emerging technologies for Achilles tendinopathy and plantar fasciopathy. Clin Podiatr Med Surg. 2015;32(2):183–93.

52. Gerdesmeyer L, Mittermayr R, Fuerst M, Al Muderis M, Thiele R, Saxena A, et al. Current evidence of extracorporeal shock wave therapy in chronic Achilles tendinopathy. Int J Surg. 2015;24(Pt B):154–9.

53. Wu Z, Yao W, Chen S, Li Y. Outcome of extracorporeal shock wave therapy for insertional Achilles tendinopathy with and without Haglund's deformity. Biomed Res Int. 2016;2016:6315846.

54. Zhang J, Keenan C, Wang JH. The effects of dexamethasone on human patellar tendon stem cells:

implications for dexamethasone treatment of tendon injury. J Orthop Res. 2013;31(1):105–10.

55. de Mos M, van der Windt AE, Jahr H, van Schie HT, Weinans H, Verhaar JA, et al. Can platelet-rich plasma enhance tendon repair? A cell culture study. Am J Sports Med. 2008;36(6):1171–8.

56. Sampson S, Gerhardt M, Mandelbaum B. Platelet rich plasma injection grafts for musculoskeletal injuries: a review. Curr Rev Musculoskelet Med. 2008;1(3–4):165–74.

57. Mishra A, Woodall J Jr, Vieira A. Treatment of tendon and muscle using platelet-rich plasma. Clin Sports Med. 2009;28(1):113–25.

58. Sanchez M, Anitua E, Orive G, Mujika I, Andia I. Platelet-rich therapies in the treatment of orthopaedic sport injuries. Sports Med. 2009;39(5):345–54.

59. de Vos RJ, Weir A, van Schie HT, Bierma-Zeinstra SM, Verhaar JA, Weinans H, et al. Platelet-rich plasma injection for chronic Achilles tendinopathy: a randomized controlled trial. JAMA. 2010;303(2):144–9.

60. de Vos RJ, Weir A, Tol JL, Verhaar JA, Weinans H, van Schie HT. No effects of PRP on ultrasonographic tendon structure and neovascularisation in chronic midportion Achilles tendinopathy. Br J Sports Med. 2011;45(5):387–92.

61. Filardo G, Kon E, Di Matteo B, Di Martino A, Tesei G, Pelotti P, et al. Platelet-rich plasma injections for the treatment of refractory Achilles tendinopathy: results at 4 years. Blood Transfus. 2014;12(4):533–40.

62. Maxwell NJ, Ryan MB, Taunton JE, Gillies JH, Wong AD. Sonographically guided intratendinous injection of hyperosmolar dextrose to treat chronic tendinosis of the Achilles tendon: a pilot study. AJR Am J Roentgenol. 2007;189(4):W215–20.

63. Ryan M, Wong A, Taunton J. Favorable outcomes after sonographically guided intratendinous injection of hyperosmolar dextrose for chronic insertional and midportion achilles tendinosis. AJR Am J Roentgenol. 2010;194(4):1047–53.

64. Yelland MJ, Sweeting KR, Lyftogt JA, Ng SK, Scuffham PA, Evans KA. Prolotherapy injections and eccentric loading exercises for painful Achilles tendinosis: a randomised trial. Br J Sports Med. 2011;45(5):421–8.

65. Sanderson LM, Bryant A. Effectiveness and safety of prolotherapy injections for management of lower limb tendinopathy and fasciopathy: a systematic review. J Foot Ankle Res. 2015;8:57.

66. Willberg L, Sunding K, Ohberg L, Forssblad M, Fahlstrom M, Alfredson H. Sclerosing injections to treat midportion Achilles tendinosis: a randomised controlled study evaluating two different concentrations of Polidocanol. Knee Surg Sports Traumatol Arthrosc. 2008;16(9):859–64.

67. Alfredson H. Low recurrence rate after mini surgery outside the tendon combined with short rehabilitation in patients with midportion Achilles tendinopathy. Open Access J Sports Med. 2016;7:51–4.

68. Alfredson H. Ultrasound and Doppler-guided mini-surgery to treat midportion Achilles tendinosis: results of a large material and a randomised study comparing two scraping techniques. Br J Sports Med. 2011;45(5):407–10.

69. Alfredson H, Ohberg L, Zeisig E, Lorentzon R. Treatment of midportion Achilles tendinosis: similar clinical results with US and CD-guided surgery outside the tendon and sclerosing polidocanol injections. Knee Surg Sports Traumatol Arthrosc. 2007;15(12):1504–9.

70. Humphrey J, Chan O, Crisp T, Padhiar N, Morrissey D, Twycross-Lewis R, et al. The short-term effects of high volume image guided injections in resistant non-insertional Achilles tendinopathy. J Sci Med Sport. 2010;13(3):295–8.

71. Maffulli N, Spiezia F, Longo UG, Denaro V, Maffulli GD. High volume image guided injections for the management of chronic tendinopathy of the main body of the Achilles tendon. Phys Ther Sport. 2013;14(3):163–7.

72. Wheeler PC, Mahadevan D, Bhatt R, Bhatia M. A comparison of two different high-volume image-guided injection procedures for patients with chronic noninsertional Achilles tendinopathy: a pragmatic retrospective cohort study. J Foot Ankle Surg. 2016;55(5):976–9.

73. Kamineni S, Butterfield T, Sinai A. Percutaneous ultrasonic debridement of tendinopathy-a pilot Achilles rabbit model. J Orthop Surg Res. 2015;10:70.

74. Lohrer H, David S, Nauck T. Surgical treatment for Achilles tendinopathy – a systematic review. BMC Musculoskelet Disord. 2016;17:207.

75. Maffulli N, Binfield PM, Moore D, King JB. Surgical decompression of chronic central core lesions of the Achilles tendon. Am J Sports Med. 1999;27(6):747–52.

76. Schon LC, Shores JL, Faro FD, Vora AM, Camire LM, Guyton GP. Flexor hallucis longus tendon transfer in treatment of Achilles tendinosis. J Bone Joint Surg Am. 2013;95(1):54–60.

77. Hunt KJ, Cohen BE, Davis WH, Anderson RB, Jones CP. Surgical treatment of insertional Achilles tendinopathy with or without flexor hallucis longus tendon transfer: a prospective, randomized study. Foot Ankle Int. 2015;36(9):998–1005.

78. Tallon C, Coleman BD, Khan KM, Maffulli N. Outcome of surgery for chronic Achilles tendinopathy. A critical review. Am J Sports Med. 2001;29(3):315–20.

79. Cychosz CC, Phisitkul P, Barg A, Nickisch F, van Dijk CN, Glazebrook MA. Foot and ankle tendoscopy: evidence-based recommendations. Arthroscopy. 2014;30(6):755–65.

80. Maquirriain J. Surgical treatment of chronic Achilles tendinopathy: long-term results of the endoscopic technique. J Foot Ankle Surg. 2013;52(4):451–5.

81. Pearce CJ, Carmichael J, Calder JD. Achilles tendinoscopy and plantaris tendon release and division in the treatment of non-insertional Achilles tendinopathy. Foot Ankle Surg. 2012;18(2):124–7.

82. Weber M, Niemann M, Lanz R, Muller T. Nonoperative treatment of acute rupture of the Achilles tendon: results of a new protocol and comparison with operative treatment. Am J Sports Med. 2003;31(5):685–91.

83. Lim J, Dalal R, Waseem M. Percutaneous vs. open repair of the ruptured Achilles tendon – a prospective randomized controlled study. Foot Ankle Int. 2001;22(7):559–68.

84. Bhattacharyya M, Gerber B. Mini-invasive surgical repair of the Achilles tendon – does it reduce postoperative morbidity? Int Orthop. 2009;33(1):151–6.

Plantar Fascia

Vince Si and Melody Hrubes

Abbreviations

BMI	Body mass index
ESWT	Extracorporeal shockwave therapy
FDL	Flexor digitorum longus
FGF	Fibroblast growth factor
FHL	Flexor hallucis longus
MRI	Magnetic resonance imaging
MTP	Metatarsophalangeal
NSAID	Nonsteroidal anti-inflammatory drug
PDGF	Platelet-derived growth factor
PRP	Platelet rich plasma
TGF-®	Transforming growth factor beta
US	Ultrasound
VEGF	Vascular endothelial growth factor

Introduction

Plantar fasciopathy is one of the most common disorders of the foot and results in more than one million patient visits per year to physicians' offices [1]. Approximately 10% of people are predicted to develop plantar heel pain in their lifetime affecting a wide range of populations from the geriatric to the pediatric athletic population, but peak inci-dence occurs between 40 years and 60 years of age [2, 3]. This condition is also seen relatively frequently in military personnel [4, 5]. Family practitioners, internists, and orthopedists commonly evaluate and treat plantar fasciitis with an esti-mated annual cost of 284 million dollars [1, 6].

Historically, plantar faciopathy was called plan-tar fasciitis, and was described as an inflammatory process of the plantar fascia at its origin induced by repetitive excess loads during running or secondary to periosteal inflammation [7, 8]. More recently, the underlying pathology is felt to be degenerative, therefore the name "plantar fasciopathy" or "plan-tar fasciosis" was created. Gross observation of surgical specimens demonstrated marked thicken-ing and fibrosis, while histologic analysis revealed collagen necrosis, angiofibroblastic hyperplasia, matrix calcification, and myxoid degeneration without evidence of an inflammatory response [9]. This shift from an inflammatory etiology to a degenerative etiology has implications regarding management of this condition. For example, corti-costeroid injections may be helpful in short-term symptomatic treatment but could also accelerate the degenerative process while increasing the risk of rupture [10].

Anatomy

The plantar fascia is a broad, fibrous aponeurosis spanning the plantar structures of the foot deep to the subcutaneous tissue and calcaneal fat pad.

V. Si
Department of Sports Medicine, Redwood City Medical Center, Redwood City, CA, USA

M. Hrubes (✉)
Rothman Orthopedics, New York, NY, USA

© Springer Nature Switzerland AG 2021
K. Onishi et al. (eds.), *Tendinopathy*, https://doi.org/10.1007/978-3-030-65335-4_17

There are three distinct bands: medial, central, and lateral. The medial and central bands originate at the medial calcaneal tuberosity; the lateral band attaches to the lateral process of the calcaneal tuberosity. The proximal fibers blend with the periosteum of the calcaneus and Achilles tendon. Pain typically associated with plantar fasciopathy is located in the region of the medial calcaneal tuberosity. Distally, the plantar fascia divides into five slips that insert on each of the proximal phalanges merging with the transverse metatarsal ligaments and flexor tendon sheaths (Fig. 17.1a).

Biomechanically, the foot and the plantar fascia act as a structural truss, with the calcaneus, midtarsal joint, and metatarsals forming the arch of the truss (medial longitudinal arch). The plantar fascia acts as the tie-rod connecting the calcaneus to the phalanges. During quiet standing, ground reaction forces travel down the tibia and flatten the medial longitudinal arch; the plantar fascia resists this collapse of the foot maintaining the medial longitudinal arch by its tensile strength [7].

During normal gait, the plantar fascia helps maintain the arch by contributing to the appropriate amount and sequencing of pronation and supination during the gait cycle. The foot pronates when progressing from heel strike to midstance. This increases the distance between the calcaneus and metatarsals applying tension to the plantar fascia which acts as a shock absorber to prevent foot collapse [11]. Dorsiflexion of the metatarsophalangeal joints, particularly at the first metatarsophalangeal (MTP) joint, causes an increase in plantar fascia tension and medial longitudinal arch height due to the windlass mechanism [7, 12]. The progression from midstance to toe-off results in supination of the foot and dorsiflexion of the MTP joints, activating the windlass mechanism and results in a rigid lever arm (Fig. 17.1b). This allows forward body propulsion [11]. Pronation and supination are vital to a normal gait, and the plantar fascia plays an important role in both motions. Any imbalance results in inefficient foot function, increased forces across the plantar fascia, and potential pathology.

Plantar Fasciopathy

A 23-year-old recreational runner presents with 6-month history of worsening medial plantar heel pain after she started increasing her training mileage for her first full marathon. Her job also involves standing for extended periods of time, and the pain worsens towards the end of her work day. She also complains of pain with the first few steps in the morning which abates shortly after. She does not remember any injuries or trauma to the foot. She takes no medications and has no other medical problems. Upon visual examination, there is no swelling, bruising or redness around the heel. She exhibits pes planus bilaterally and increased pronation during examination of her gait. On physical examination, she has tenderness to palpation along the medial heel.

Clinical Presentation

Patients with plantar fasciopathy classically present with insidious isolated medial plantar heel pain with initial weight bearing, either with the first steps in the morning or after prolonged sitting. After several minutes of activity, the pain usually subsides but will return later in the day as the duration of weight bearing activity increases [13]. The typical pain is characterized as a sharp sensation localized to the plantar heel. Patients may limp to avoid weight bearing through the heel. Often, the history will include a recent increase in their exercise program, a change in footwear, or a change in exercise surface [3]. Phases are classified by the chronicity of symptoms. The acute phase is the first 4 weeks after symptom onset. The subacute phase spans 4 weeks to 3 months with heel pain increasing during activity, and a dull pain present at rest. After 3 months, the condition is considered chronic and pain may begin to interfere with most weight-bearing activities [14]. Up to one-third of patients experience bilateral symptoms [6].

The etiology of plantar faciopathy is not completely understood but is considered multifactorial with several risk factors implicated. Therefore, a thorough evaluation of the patient

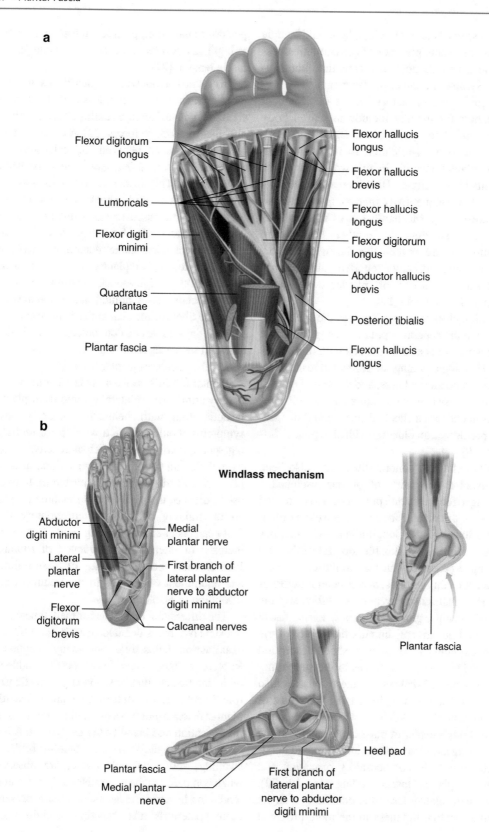

Fig. 17.1 (**a**) Normal anatomy. (**b**) Windlass mechanism

with suspected plantar fasciopathy should include inquiry regarding presence of comorbidities, recreational and occupational activities, constitutional symptoms, and prior treatments.

Significant risk factors for the development of plantar fasciopathy include increased body weight and body mass index (BMI) [15, 16]. Studies show a 1.4-fold increase in the probability of plantar fasciitis in overweight or obese patients [17]. A higher BMI increases mechanical load, consequentially increasing plantar fascia stress [18]. Mechanical load increases as prolonged standing is another risk factor. Patients who are on their feet during the majority of the workday reported significantly increased symptoms of plantar fasciopathy compared to controls [19].

Peak incidence occurs between the ages of 40 and 60 in the general population, suggesting that increasing age is also associated with this condition. Histologic findings of degenerative changes, increased fascia thickness, and decreased elasticity are consistent with aging. These changes result in decreased shock absorbing abilities and may predispose an older individual to plantar fasciitis [20].

Biomechanical abnormalities have also been suggested as the cause of plantar fasciopathy. Prolonged foot pronation predisposes to increased forces on the plantar fascia; these patients often have a lower medial longitudinal arch (i.e., pes planus), with a more flexible foot. Excessive and prolonged pronation can lead to muscle fatigue, posterior chain tightness, and structural deformities. Proximal muscle weakness, particularly the gluteus medius, gluteus minimus, tensor fascia latae, and quadriceps, impairs the ability of the lower extremity to assist with shock absorption and produces increased forces to the supporting foot structures. Weakness in these muscles also decreases distal control, increasing the degree of foot pronation [11]. Ankle dorsiflexion is required for the body's center of mass to advance over the foot during a normal gait cycle. Decreased dorsiflexion results in compensatory pronation and increased plantar fascia loading [11, 19, 20]. Because the plantar fascia has continuity with the Achilles tendon, tightness in the more proximal posterior chain (i.e., gastrocnemius/soleus, hamstrings) also results in increased load and plantar fascia tension [21].

In contrast, a foot with a higher medial longitudinal arch (pes cavus) is a less compliant, more rigid foot with a decreased ability to act as a shock absorber to dissipate forces [22]. A cavus foot has a shorter distance between the calcaneus and metatarsals, resulting in a shorter, less distensible plantar fascia. This decrease in elasticity is associated with decreased shock absorption and increased plantar fascia tension similar to a stretch on a bowstring during heel strike and midstance [11]. Biomechanical studies demonstrated a cavus foot predicted higher plantar fascia loads while running [22]. A high medial longitudinal arch is also associated with limited ankle dorsiflexion. Since the fibers of the plantar fascia have continuity with the Achilles tendon, decreased ankle dorsiflexion increases tension in the Achilles tendon which also increases plantar fascia [11].

Plantar fasciitis is also associated with inflammatory arthritides. Bilateral symptoms of plantar fasciitis along with rheumatologic or systemic symptoms should initiate a workup for underlying spondyloarthropathy, such as reactive arthritis, ankylosing spondylitis, or psoriatic arthritis [2, 3, 23]. Extrinsic factors contributing to overuse injuries of the plantar fascia include training errors, training surfaces, inappropriately firm footwear, heel-strike running gait, and/or an increase in intensity or frequency of running. Identification and modification of these training and equipment errors aids in the treatment and resolution of plantar fasciitis.

The differential diagnosis for medial heel pain is extensive, but a detailed history and physical examination helps rule out many diagnoses. Rupture of the plantar fascia occurs suddenly with athletic activities or secondary to corticosteroid injections. In contrast to plantar fasciitis, plantar fascia rupture occurs rapidly with a tearing sensation and inability to bear weight. A loss of medial longitudinal arch height, bruising, swelling, and a palpable defect are observed when compared to the contralateral foot. Achilles tendinopathy and infracalcaneal bursitis presents more posteriorly after repetitive activities and worsens throughout the day. The posterior heel is tender to palpation; swelling and erythema can also be present. The plantar fat pad is in a similar anatomic location to the plantar fascia and atrophy causes pain. Plantar fat pad atrophy predominantly affects the elderly with pain and tenderness primarily in the central heel with noticeable atrophy of the heel pad. The posterior tibial tendon courses along the medial heel and dysfunction here causes medial heel pain. Patients with posterior tibialis dysfunction have a loss of arch height and difficulty with single limb heel rise. The tendon is tender to palpation posterior to the medial malleolus and distally to its insertion on the navicular and medial cuneiform. Similarly, the flexor digitorum longus (FDL) and flexor hallucis longus (FHL) are also in close anatomic proximity to the plantar fascia; palpation of these tendons is painful with limitations in range of motion of the metatarsophalangeal joints.

Stress reaction of the calcaneus also presents similarly to plantar fasciitis; however, pain is typically exacerbated with repetitive weight-bearing exercises. Stress reaction/fracture of the calcaneus can be distinguished by reproducing pain with the squeeze test (mediolateral compression of the calcaneus). Sever's disease is an apophysitis of the calcaneus is seen mainly in the pediatric population with running and jumping activities. Pain is also reproduced with a squeeze test but plain radiographs may help to differentiate it from stress fractures of plantar fasciopathy.

Neurogenic etiologies of medial heel pain include tarsal tunnel syndrome which presents with burning pain or paresthesia along the distribution of the posterior tibial and plantar nerves. Symptoms are reproduced with Tinel's test along the nerve. Entrapment of Baxter's nerve, which is the first branch of the lateral plantar nerve, can be seen with plantar fasciopathy, but in addition to plantar fascia pain, Baxter's neuropathy presents with paresthesia and weakness of the abductor digiti quinti. Compression of the medial plantar nerve where the flexor hallucis longus and flexor digitorum longus tendons cross each other at the knot of Henry along the medial plantar foot is known as Jogger's foot, which presents as neuropathic pain along the medial longitudinal arch and toes 1–3. Jogger's foot is often aggravated by improper shoes and rigid orthotics. Lumbosacral radiculopathy presents with pain that radiates down the leg to heel with weakness in the ankle. Neural tension signs are positive, such as the straight leg raise or slump test. Peripheral neuropathy is typically symmetric and bilateral with sensory abnormalities in a stocking distribution.

Systemic causes should also be considered, such as underlying infection and malignancy. These etiologies will present with concomitant constitutional symptoms, like fevers, chills, nocturnal pain, weight loss, and history of prior malignancy. Bilateral symptoms suggest systemic inflammatory arthritis, particularly if coexisting signs and symptoms exist, such as back pain, morning stiffness, inflammatory joint complaints, and/or psoriasis (Table 17.1).

Physical Examination

A thorough physical examination will help to distinguish plantar fasciopathy from other conditions in the differential diagnosis of heel pain. The exam should begin with a visual inspection of the patient's body habitus, stance, and gait with special attention paid to the medial longitudinal arch (neutral, planus, and cavus) and whether any compensatory behaviors, such as a limp, is present. Neurologic and vascular examination of the proximal lower extremities and lower back should also be performed to screen for biomechanical abnormalities, radiculopathy, peripheral neuropathy, or vascular etiologies. A lumbosacral nerve root impingement can cause radiating leg pain, dermatomal numbness and tingling, and weakness in the ankle. Diminished sensation of bilateral feet in a stocking distribution is consistent with peripheral neuropathy. Diminished pulses in the dorsalis pedis and posterior tibial arteries and delayed capillary refill suggest peripheral vascular disease which causes leg and foot pain during ambulation. The range of motion of the lumbar spine should also be assessed if there is a concern for underlying ankylosing spondylitis.

Table 17.1 Differential diagnosis of medial heel pain

Diagnosis	Distinguishing characteristics	Physical exam findings
Plantar fascia rupture	Sudden, tearing pain, inability to bear weight	Loss of arch height, bruising, swelling, palpable defect
Stress reaction/fracture of calcaneus	Excessive or repetitive weight-bearing exercises	Positive squeeze test, tender calcaneus
Infracalcaneal bursitis	Worsens with repetitive activities and throughout the day	Swelling and erythema of posterior heel
FDL, FHL tenosynovitis	Worsens with repetitive exercises	Tender along tendons, painful MTP ROM
Posterior tibialis dysfunction	Unable to do single limb heel rise	Tender along tendon, navicular, and medial cuneiform
Fat pad atrophy	Affects elderly, pain in central heel	Central heel tenderness, heel pad atrophy
Achilles tendinopathy	Worsens after repetitive or excessive activities	Heel cord tightness, insertional tenderness
Sever's disease	Affects pediatric population, running, jumping activities	Positive squeeze test, XR to differentiate from stress fracture
Tarsal tunnel syndrome	Neuropathic pain of posterior tibial and plantar nerves	Positive Tinel's test along the nerve
Baxter's neuropathy	Paresthesias and numbness	Weakness of abductor digiti quinti
Jogger's foot	Paresthesias and burning	Positive Tinel's along abductor hallucis near navicular
Lumbosacral radiculopathy	Pain radiates down the leg to heel	Dermatomal sensory disturbance, ankle weakness, positive neural tension signs
Peripheral neuropathy	Diffuse neuropathic foot pain, numbness, paresthesias	Sensory loss in a stocking distribution
Inflammatory arthritis	Bilateral presentation, associated symptoms of back stiffness, joint pain	Limited lumbar ROM, joint effusion, or skin changes
Infection	Fevers, chills, nocturnal pain	Localized swelling, erythema, discharge
Malignancy	Deep bone pain, nocturnal pain, constitutional symptoms, prior malignancy	Weight loss/cachexia, bony tenderness, XR to assess for metastasis

A more focused visual assessment of the heel and foot should be made to identify any deformity, bruising, swelling, erythema, or skin breakdown. Both active and passive range of motion should be assessed in the affected and contralateral foot, and the examiner should note any deficits, particularly in the ankle, midfoot, and first MTP range of motion. Passive dorsiflexion of the toes often exacerbates plantar fascia pain as this stretches the entire plantar fascia.

Palpation should be directed toward the foot's bony prominences, tendinous insertions, and ligamentous insertions. Proximal plantar fasciitis will have tenderness over the medial aspect of the calcaneal tuberosity, and distal planar fasciopathy will have tenderness more distally (Fig. 17.2). A palpable defect at the calcaneal tuberosity with

swelling and ecchymosis suggests plantar fascia rupture [2]. A squeeze test of the calcaneus is performed by medial and lateral heel compression, and if positive, suggests calcaneal stress fracture. The fat pad of the heel is palpated more proximally and centrally than the origin of the plantar fascia, and tenderness with softening in this area suggests fat pad atrophy. The flexor digitorum longus and flexor hallucis longus tendons should also be palpated as these structures lie close to the plantar aponeurosis. Point tenderness along these tendons, especially if associated with painful resisted toe flexion, indicates tenosynovitis and differentiates it from plantar fasciopathy.

Tarsal tunnel syndrome, a posterior tibial compression neuropathy, can often be mistaken for plantar fasciopathy and vice versa. Whereas plantar

Fig. 17.2 Locations of tenderness for diagnoses of heel pain

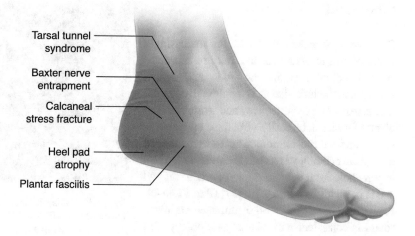

Tarsal tunnel syndrome

Baxter nerve entrapment

Calcaneal stress fracture

Heel pad atrophy

Plantar fasciitis

fasciopathy will have pain with passive toe dorsiflexion, tarsal tunnel syndrome is exacerbated by percussion of the nerve within the tarsal tunnel, reproducing numbness and tingling with radiation to the plantar heel. The lateral plantar nerve (Baxter's nerve), due to its close proximity to the medial calcaneal tubercle, is prone to entrapment and can coexist with plantar fasciitis, thus making it difficult to distinguish between the two diagnoses.

Diagnostic Workup

X-Ray

A diagnosis of plantar fasciopathy is often made clinically with history and physical examination. Imaging, therefore, plays a limited role in routine clinical practice, but it may be useful to rule out other cause of heel pain when the diagnosis is unclear or improvement is limited. Plain radiographs are usually normal in plantar fasciopathy, although there may be a heel spur or plantar calcaneal calcification, but these are nonspecific as they also occur in asymptomatic patients (Fig. 17.3) [24, 25]. X-rays can help rule out bony abnormalities, such as stress fractures or other rare bony lesions [3]; a "fluffy periostitis" can be suggestive of spondyloarthropathy.

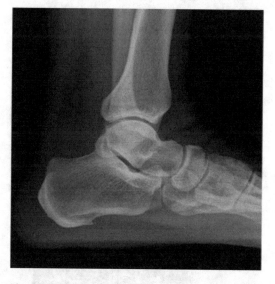

Fig. 17.3 Calcaneal spur seen on lateral weight bearing view of the left foot

Magnetic Resonance Imaging

If plain radiographs are normal, and the suspicion for a stress reaction is high, magnetic resonance imaging (MRI) can be helpful in differentiating between plantar fasciitis and a stress reaction. Bone scan is an alternative diagnostic test; however, MRI is preferred as it can assess other etiologies within the differential and lacks radiation exposure [26].

Ultrasound

Diagnostic ultrasound (US) is an increasingly effective tool to assess for a variety of musculo-skeletal pathologies in the foot and ankle. Advantages include that it is noninvasive, radiation free, safe, cost-effective, and portable. The plantar fascia can be easily visualized under ultrasound, and the most common measurement used to indicate pathology is its thickness. It is seen as a hyperechoic band deep to the hypoechoic fat pad and is normally 2–4 mm thick [27] (Fig. 17.4a–c). Plantar fascia thickness >4.0 mm seen on ultrasound is consistent with plantar fasciopathy [28] (Fig. 17.5). Other features assessed by US include the fascia echogenicity, neovascularization, peri-fascial fluid, bony spurs, partial or full-thickness tears, or other etiologies under the differential diagnosis, such as nerve impingement [28, 29]. The sensitivity of diagnostic US ranges from 65% to 80.9% and specificity 75–85.7% for detecting

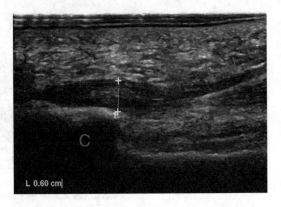

Fig. 17.5 Plantar fasciitis. Long axis ultrasound shows a thickened low reflective plantar fascia at its calcaneal origin (between callipers). More distally, the plantar fascia shows normal thickness (arrows). C calcaneus

plantar fasciopathy accurately [3, 30–32]. When examining the plantar fascia with US, comparison to the contralateral side is recommended, particularly if the symptoms are unilateral. The limitations of ultrasound include clinician experience, comfort, and technique.

Magnetic resonance imaging (MRI) offers superior soft-tissue contrast resolution and is useful in plantar fascia diagnosis and presurgical planning but is expensive when compared to plain radiography and US. Normal plantar fascia demonstrates a hypointense signal on both T1- and T2-weighted sequences [33]. Abnormal findings on MRI that suggests plantar fasciitis include plantar fascia thickening >3 mm, edema within and surrounding the fascia on T2-weighted images, and increased intrafacial T1-signal, and marrow edema of the calcaneal tuberosity [34] (Fig. 17.6a–d). Fascial thickening is typically fusiform in nature rather than nodular, indicative of plantar fibromatosis [33]. Findings on MRI must be clinically correlated as the above findings, particularly fascial thickening, perifascial edema, and calcaneal spurs, are also found in asymptomatic, healthy individuals [35]. High signal intensity on T2-weighted images involving the muscles innervated by the medial or lateral plantar nerves can also be suggestive of tarsal tunnel syndrome or an isolated medial or lateral neuropathy.

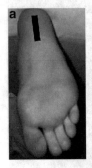
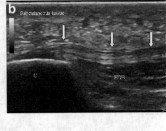
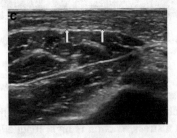

Fig. 17.4 Plantar fascia: (**a**) transducer position and corresponding (**b**) longitudinal ultrasound image of the plantar fascia calcaneal origin. The hypoechoic muscle belly of the flexor digitorum brevis (FDB) is identified directly deep to the plantar fascia in the midline. (**c**) Transverse ultrasound image of the plantar fascia midfoot. C calcaneus

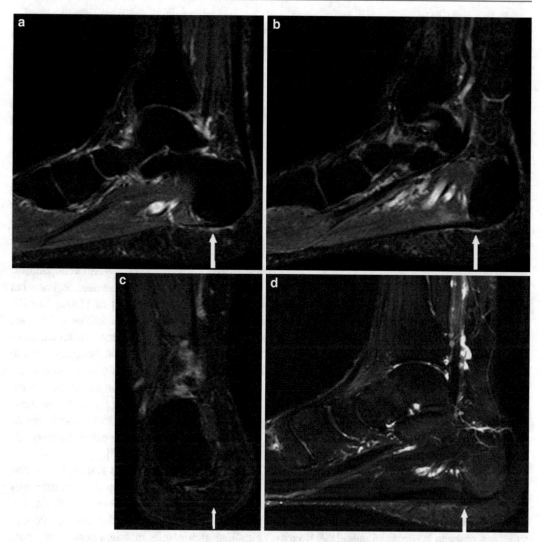

Fig. 17.6 Sagittal STIR MRI (**a**) shows a subtle thickening of the lateral cord of proximal plantar fascia (*arrow*) with a high signal area of edema in the adjacent subcutaneous fat. Sagittal STIR MRI (**b**) depicts greater thickening of the medial cord of the proximal plantar fascia (*arrow*). Coronal T2*-weighted MRI (**c**) shows heterogeneous signal and thickening of the plantar fascia (*arrow*). Sagittal STIR MRI (**d**) in another patient with plantar fasciitis shows a thickened proximal area of plantar fascia (*arrow*) without marked edema in adjacent subcutaneous fat. In the chronic stage of plantar fasciitis, plantar thickness may increase and soft-tissue edema may decrease

Electrodiagnostics

When an underlying or concomitant neuropathy is of concern, electrodiagnostic studies can be utilized. Lumbosacral nerve root compression (L5, S1) can refer to the plantar heel with an absent or delayed H-reflex on nerve conduction studies and active denervation and/or chronic reinnervation in L5/S1 innervated muscles including lumbosacral paraspinal muscles on needle electromyography [36]. Distal tarsal tunnel syndrome is also fairly common and often seen with chronic plantar fasciitis. The terminal branches of the tibial nerve, the medial plantar, lateral plantar, and medial calcaneal nerve can be irritated deep to the proximal plantar fascia and abductor hallucis muscle. Nerve conduction studies may show conduction block of the plantar nerves but can frequently be negative and are not as sensitive as with carpal tunnel syndrome.

However, axonal injury is more common in tarsal tunnel syndrome than the demyelination more predominant in carpal tunnel syndrome and needle electromyography should always be tested to assess for denervation in the abductor hallucis or abductor digiti quinti [37].

Heel pain is also seen in systemic conditions, such as seronegative arthritis, gout, diffuse idiopathic skeletal hyperostosis, rheumatoid arthritis, and fibromyalgia. More rarely, benign and malignant tumors, infection, and vascular insufficiency may also be etiologies for heel pain [13]. As previously mentioned, if concern for an underlying systemic condition exists, appropriate laboratory testing and additional radiographic imaging should be ordered.

Treatment

Conservative

A variety of therapeutic options exist for the treatment of plantar fasciitis; however, managing plantar fasciopathy can be challenging as the cause is multifactorial, and treatment should be focused on identifying and correcting these numerous factors.

In the acute phase (<4 weeks) of plantar fasciitis when inflammation is most predominant, a regimen of rest, ice, compression, elevation (RICE) and a stretching program is beneficial initially. A stretching exercise program targeting the gastrocnemius–soleus complex and the medial longitudinal arch has been shown to be beneficial in reducing symptoms [38]. A randomized, placebo-controlled study performed by Donley et al. in 2007 demonstrated that when compared to a placebo, nonsteroidal anti-inflammatory drugs (NSAIDs) provided significant reduction in pain and disability up to 6 months [39]. However, the use of NSAIDs may be limited by its potentially gastrointestinal, renal, and cardiovascular side effects. Furthermore, NSAID use is also controversial in acute tendon pathology as it interrupts the inflammatory cascade, interfering with the natural healing process [40, 41].

Formal physical therapy augments a plantar fasciitis home exercise program with a targeted exercise program, myofascial release, biomechanical correction. Myofascial trigger points and tightness of the posterior chain contribute to increased plantar fascia tension. Soft tissue manual therapy, usually performed by physical therapists with the Graston or Astym techniques, aims to release and relieve these trigger points, which are painful, palpable, taut bands of muscle. Several studies demonstrate that the addition of trigger point manual therapy to a self-stretching program results in significantly better outcomes in pain and function [42, 43]. Trigger points unresponsive to soft tissue release techniques can respond to techniques that target deeper into the muscle, such as dry needling, trigger point injections, or cupping. Modalities, such as cryotherapy and iontophoresis, can also complement the treatment regimen but are insufficient for treatment of plantar fasciitis alone. Studies show that modalities offer good short-term relief but do not have sustained long-term benefits [44, 45]. Physical therapists can also correct any gait abnormalities or functional weakness that has been identified on physical examination, such as hip abductor and core weakness, posterior chain tightness, and foot intrinsic muscle weakness that predisposed the patient to the development of plantar fasciitis [46].

Foot orthotics can be used to treat plantar fasciitis to help correct any anatomic abnormalities identified, such as pes cavus or pes planus. For pes cavus type deformities, the high medial longitudinal arch results in a less compliant, more rigid foot. Therefore, orthotic inserts should be softer and more accommodative inserts to help dissipate ground reaction forces and reduce tension along the plantar fascia. Conversely, a pes planus foot has a lower medial longitudinal arch resulting in a more compliant, softer foot. Consequently, this foot type will benefit from firmer inserts that provide adequate medial longitudinal arch support [14]. Regardless of the foot type, arch supports with a heel cup can be helpful in all patients with plantar fasciitis by decreasing the degree of dorsiflexion necessary for appropriate gait mechanics [47, 48]. When comparing prefabricated foot orthotics to custom molded foot orthotics, no significant difference in reduction of pain or improved function has been found.

The key in finding the correct insert is that the patient feels immediate comfort and does not require a "breaking in" period [49, 50]. Night splints are another orthotic device that are designed to prevent and correct passive contracture of the plantar fascia and the gastrocnemius-soleus complex by keeping the foot in neutral or slight dorsiflexion. The application of night splints with foot inserts has been shown to be more effective than with foot inserts alone [51].

Certain shoe types can predispose patients to developing plantar fasciitis, particularly if it is a negative drop shoe which can increase the strain on the Achilles complex, or if the shoe has a stiff sole which increases forces through the foot at heel strike. Moreover, shoes with high mileage also increases the risk for plantar fasciitis as the cushioning and support decreases; the need for shoe replacement is typically recommended after approximately 300–500 miles of use. Shoe modifications, such as the addition of a rocker bottom sole, can decrease the tension in the plantar fascia by minimizing the windlass mechanism [52].

Interventional

Patients who have not responded satisfactorily to nonsurgical treatment options and are in the subacute phase may benefit from more aggressive options, including injections. Multiple injectates are utilized for the treatment of plantar fasciitis, which can be injected with or without ultrasound guidance. Several studies demonstrated that ultrasound guidance provides superior accuracy, decreased plantar fascia thickness, maintenance of calcaneal fat pad thickness, and improved pain symptoms when compared to unguided procedures [30, 53–55] (Fig. 17.7a, b).

Corticosteroid injections, such as triamcinolone, to the thickened, painful region of the plantar fascia are common choice as a first injectate and often provide significant short-term pain relief. Ultrasound studies of corticosteroid injections demonstrated improvement of the hypoechogenicity seen prior to the injection, but the calcaneal fat pad thickness decreased significantly, and the mechanical properties of the heel did not change [54]. The use of corticosteroid injections, especially multiple injections, is not recommended. Frequent use increases the risk of heel fat pad atrophy and plantar fascia rupture due to the catabolic effects of corticosteroids [56]. Fat pad atrophy compromises subcalcaneal cushioning, increasing pain and risk of calcaneal fractures. Corticosteroids suppress proteoglycan production and collagen synthesis within tendons and ligaments, increasing the risk of plantar fascia ruptures in up to 10% of study subjects who received a corticosteroid injection [57, 58]. Multiple corticosteroid injections should be avoided, and the patients should be counseled to restrict running and jumping activities for at least 1–2 weeks.

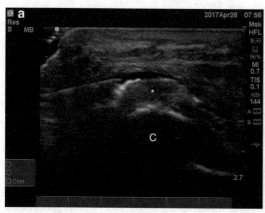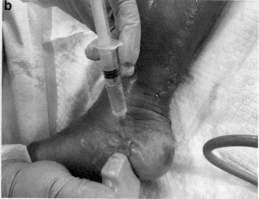

Fig. 17.7 Ultrasound-guided (**a**) injection of the right plantar fascia performed in a short axis view of the plantar fascia (*) overlying the calcaneus (**c**). The needle is guided in an in-plane approach (**b**)

Orthobiologic injection therapy, such as platelet rich plasma (PRP) and prolotherapy, are promising treatment options for chronic tendinopathies and fasciopathies. PRP is a solution-containing plasma rich in platelets obtained from centrifuged autologous whole blood. Platelet-rich plasma is thought to induce tissue inflammation and regeneration by introducing growth factors stored in the alpha granules of platelets, such as transforming growth factor beta (TGF-®), vascular endothelial growth factor (VEGF), and platelet-derived growth factor (PDGF) [59]. Prolotherapy induces a wound healing cascade via hyperosmolar dextrose, an osmotic shock agent, typically diluted with normal saline or lidocaine to produce a localized inflammatory response. The goal of inducing a wound healing cascade is to deposit new collagen [60]. A recent systematic review of PRP injections for the treatment of chronic plantar fasciitis concluded that PRP may be of benefit compared to conservative treatment and steroid injections. However, further high-quality research is required as the current studies are limited, and there are still variations in the protocol and preparation of PRP solutions [59]. Prolotherapy also demonstrated beneficial effects in chronic plantar fasciitis that were not statistically different when compared to PRP [61]. Orthobiologic injection therapy, when compared to corticosteroid injections, does not increase the risk of plantar fascia rupture. However, the cost of preparing and performing these injections, particularly PRP, is a limiting factor.

Extracorporeal shockwave therapy (ESWT) has been approved by the US Food and Drug Administration for the treatment of plantar fasciitis since 2000. The mechanism of action involves sound waves directed toward the injured area, causing microtrauma and inducing regeneration of damaged fascia by inducing neovascularization, hyperemia, and collagen synthesis [62]. ESWT also reduces pain symptoms by destroying unmyelinated sensory pain fibers [14, 62]. A meta-analysis reviewing randomized-controlled trials of ESWT demonstrated that it was effective and safe in the treatment of chronic plantar fasciitis when compared to controls [62]. Complications

and side effects were minimal and most commonly include pain along the calcaneal area, erythema, swelling, and bruising; no serious side effects were observed. Similar to regenerative injections, the use of ESWT may be limited by costs and insurance coverage; however, it should be considered in refractory cases prior to considering surgical management.

More recently, minimally invasive percutaneous ultrasonic fasciotomy procedures have been developed with promising outcomes, including reduced pain, improved clinical outcomes, and low complication rates. Percutaneous ultrasonic fasciotomy is a technique that uses a small probe and ultrasonic energy to ablate soft tissues which, similar to orthobiologic injection techniques, induces a healing response, angiogenesis, and increases VEGF and fibroblast growth factor (FGF) [63, 64]. Moreover, the procedure likely produces an anesthetic effect by modulation of local sensory fibers. The fasciotomy is performed in a grid-like pattern over the most painful aspect of the plantar surface and can be performed through an open incision with direct visualization or percutaneously with ultrasound guidance. Radiofrequency microfasciotomy/tenotomy is another procedure. When compared with open and endoscopic plantar fasciotomy, radiofrequency microtenotomy is effective in pain reduction, functional improvement, and patient satisfaction. The primary complication observed was persistent heel pain after 1 year in 7.3% of study subjects [64].

Operative

A vast majority, approximately 90–96%, of plantar fasciitis cases resolve with nonoperative treatment. Most surgeons recommend waiting a minimum of 6–18 months before considering surgery [65]. If the symptoms of plantar fasciitis are refractory to conservative treatment or chronic in nature, surgical options include open fasciotomies, endoscopic fasciotomies, and microtenotomy. Historically, open procedures consisted of either partial or complete release of the plantar fascia and decompression of the first branch of the lateral plantar nerve. If present, resection of an associated heel spur or release of the abductor hallucis fascia is also performed. Endoscopic procedures also have the goal of performing a partial transection of the plantar fascia but provide quicker healing time and faster return to activity when compared to open procedures [66]. Both surgeries require 2–6 weeks of protected weight bearing in a walker boot postoperatively. Complications remain a major limitation of both open and endoscopic procedures, with rates as high as 58% in open procedures and 41% in endoscopic [63]. The most common complications are superficial and deep infections, complex regional pain syndrome, persistent scar pain, and numbness [63].

Conclusion

Plantar fasciopathy is a common foot disorder resulting in medial plantar heel pain that can become debilitating. Accurate diagnosis through physical examination and imaging can lead to appropriate and timely management. Successful treatment of plantar fasciopathy is often multifactorial, including footwear modification, biomechanical optimization through physical therapy, and at times requires procedures such as injections, ESWT, tenotomies, or surgical release. Current research in the management of plantar fasciopathy shows promise to improve management in the future for even better patient outcomes.

References

1. Riddle DL, Schappert SM. Volume of ambulatory care visits and patterns of care for patients diagnosed with plantar fasciitis: a national study of medical doctors. Foot Ankle Int. 2004;25(5):303–10.
2. Rosenbaum AJ, DiPreta JA, Misener D. Plantar heel pain. Med Clin North Am. 2014;98(2):339–52.
3. Buchbinder R. Clinical practice. Plantar fasciitis. N Engl J Med. 2004;350(21):2159–66.
4. Kibler WB, Goldberg C, Chandler TJ. Functional biomechanical deficits in running athletes with plantar fasciitis. Am J Sports Med. 1991;19(1):66–71.
5. Sadat-Ali M. Plantar fasciitis/calcaneal spur among security forces personnel. Mil Med. 1998;163(1):56–7.
6. Tong KB, Furia J. Economic burden of plantar fasciitis treatment in the United States. Am J Orthop (Belle Mead NJ). 2010;39(5):227–31.
7. Hicks JH. The mechanics of the foot. II. The plantar aponeurosis and the arch. J Anat. 1954;88(1):25–30.
8. Sewell JR, Black CM, Chapman AH, Statham J, Hughes GR, Lavender JP. Quantitative scintigraphy in diagnosis and management of plantar fasciitis (calcaneal periostitis): concise communication. J Nucl Med. 1980;21(7):633–6.
9. Lemont H, Ammirati KM, Usen N. Plantar fasciitis: a degenerative process (fasciosis) without inflammation. J Am Podiatr Med Assoc. 2003;93(3):234–7.
10. Suzue N, Iwame T, Kato K, Takao S, Tateishi T, Takeda Y, et al. Plantar fascia rupture in a professional soccer player. J Med Investig. 2014;61(3–4):413–6.
11. Bolgla LA, Malone TR. Plantar fasciitis and the windlass mechanism: a biomechanical link to clinical practice. J Athl Train. 2004;39(1):77–82.
12. Fuller EA. The windlass mechanism of the foot. A mechanical model to explain pathology. J Am Podiatr Med Assoc. 2000;90(1):35–46.
13. Thomas JL, Christensen JC, Kravitz SR, Mendicino RW, Schuberth JM, Vanore JV, et al. The diagnosis and treatment of heel pain: a clinical practice guideline-revision 2010. J Foot Ankle Surg. 2010;49(3 Suppl):S1–19.
14. Berbrayer D, Fredericson M. Update on evidence-based treatments for plantar fasciopathy. PM R. 2014;6(2):159–69.
15. Rano JA, Fallat LM, Savoy-Moore RT. Correlation of heel pain with body mass index and other characteristics of heel pain. J Foot Ankle Surg. 2001;40(6):351–6.
16. Irving DB, Cook JL, Young MA, Menz HB. Obesity and pronated foot type may increase the risk of chronic plantar heel pain: a matched case-control study. BMC Musculoskelet Disord. 2007;8:41.
17. Frey C, Zamora J. The effects of obesity on orthopaedic foot and ankle pathology. Foot Ankle Int. 2007;28(9):996–9.
18. van Leeuwen KD, Rogers J, Winzenberg T, van Middelkoop M. Higher body mass index is associated with plantar fasciopathy/'plantar fasciitis': systematic review and meta-analysis of various clinical and imaging risk factors. Br J Sports Med. 2016;50(16):972–81.
19. Riddle DL, Pulisic M, Pidcoe P, Johnson RE. Risk factors for plantar fasciitis: a matched case-control study. J Bone Joint Surg Am. 2003;85-A(5):872–7.
20. Beeson P. Plantar fasciopathy: revisiting the risk factors. Foot Ankle Surg. 2014;20(3):160–5.
21. Stecco C, Corradin M, Macchi V, Morra A, Porzionato A, Biz C, De Caro R. Plantar fascia anatomy and its relationship with Achilles tendon and paratenon. J Anat. 2013;223(6):665–76.

22. Ribeiro AP, Sacco IC, Dinato RC, João SM. Relationships between static foot alignment and dynamic plantar loads in runners with acute and chronic stages of plantar fasciitis: a cross-sectional study. Braz J Phys Ther. 2016;20(1):87–95.

23. Geppert MJ, Mizel MS. Management of heel pain in the inflammatory arthritides. Clin Orthop Relat Res. 1998;349:93–9.

24. Prichasuk S, Subhadrabandhu T. The relationship of pes planus and calcaneal spur to plantar heel pain. Clin Orthop Relat Res. 1994;306:192–6.

25. Lareau CR, Sawyer GA, Wang JH, DiGiovanni CW. Plantar and medial heel pain: diagnosis and management. J Am Acad Orthop Surg. 2014;22(6):372–80.

26. Dobrindt O, Hoffmeyer B, Ruf J, Seidensticker M, Steffen IG, Zarva A, et al. MRI versus bone scintigraphy. Evaluation for diagnosis and grading of stress injuries. Nuklearmedizin. 2012;51(3):88–94.

27. Gibbon WW, Long G. Ultrasound of the plantar aponeurosis (fascia). Skelet Radiol. 1999;28(1):21–6.

28. Draghi F, Gitto S, Bortolotto C, Draghi AG, Ori Belometti G. Imaging of plantar fascia disorders: findings on plain radiography, ultrasound and magnetic resonance imaging. Insights Imaging. 2017;8(1):69–78.

29. Radwan A, Wyland M, Applequist L, Bolowsky E, Klingensmith H, Virag I. Ultrasonography, an effective tool in diagnosing plantar fasciitis: a systematic review of diagnostic trials. Int J Sports Phys Ther. 2016;11(5):663–71.

30. Mohseni-Bandpei MA, Nakhaee M, Mousavi ME, Shakourirad A, Safari MR, Vahab Kashani R. Application of ultrasound in the assessment of plantar fascia in patients with plantar fasciitis: a systematic review. Ultrasound Med Biol. 2014;40(8):1737–54.

31. Argerakis NG, Positano RG, Positano RC, Boccio AK, Adler RS, Saboeiro GR, et al. Ultrasound diagnosis and evaluation of plantar heel pain. J Am Podiatr Med Assoc. 2015;105(2):135–40.

32. Sabir N, Demirlenk S, Yagci B, Karabulut N, Cubukcu S. Clinical utility of sonography in diagnosing plantar fasciitis. J Ultrasound Med. 2005;24(8):1041–8.

33. Lawrence DA, Rolen MF, Morshed KA, Moukaddam H. MRI of heel pain. AJR Am J Roentgenol. 2013;200(4):845–55.

34. Grasel RP, Schweitzer ME, Kovalovich AM, Karasick D, Wapner K, Hecht P, et al. MR imaging of plantar fasciitis: edema, tears, and occult marrow abnormalities correlated with outcome. AJR Am J Roentgenol. 1999;173(3):699–701.

35. Ehrmann C, Maier M, Mengiardi B, Pfirrmann CW, Sutter R. Calcaneal attachment of the plantar fascia: MR findings in asymptomatic volunteers. Radiology. 2014;272(3):807–14.

36. Callaghan BC, Burke JF, Feldman EL. Electrodiagnostic tests in polyneuropathy and radiculopathy. JAMA. 2016;315(3):297–8.

37. Gould JS. Tarsal tunnel syndrome. Foot Ankle Clin. 2011;16(2):275–86.

38. DiGiovanni BF, Nawoczenski DA, Lintal ME, Moore EA, Murray JC, Wilding GE, et al. Tissue-specific plantar fascia-stretching exercise enhances outcomes in patients with chronic heel pain. A prospective, randomized study. J Bone Joint Surg Am. 2003;85-A(7):1270–7.

39. Donley BG, Moore T, Sferra J, Gozdanovic J, Smith R. The efficacy of oral nonsteroidal anti-inflammatory medication (NSAID) in the treatment of plantar fasciitis: a randomized, prospective, placebo-controlled study. Foot Ankle Int. 2007;28(1):20–3.

40. Lu Y, Li Y, Li FL, Li X, Zhuo HW, Jiang CY. Do different cyclooxygenase inhibitors impair rotator cuff healing in a rabbit model? Chin Med J. 2015;128(17):2354–9.

41. Hammerman M, Blomgran P, Ramstedt S, Aspenberg P. COX-2 inhibition impairs mechanical stimulation of early tendon healing in rats by reducing the response to microdamage. J Appl Physiol (1985). 2015;119(5):534–40.

42. Renan-Ordine R, Alburquerque-Sendín F, de Souza DP, Cleland JA, Fernández-de-Las-Peñas C. Effectiveness of myofascial trigger point manual therapy combined with a self-stretching protocol for the management of plantar heel pain: a randomized controlled trial. J Orthop Sports Phys Ther. 2011;41(2):43–50.

43. Wynne MM, Burns JM, Eland DC, Conatser RR, Howell JN. Effect of counterstrain on stretch reflexes, hoffmann reflexes, and clinical outcomes in subjects with plantar fasciitis. J Am Osteopath Assoc. 2006;106(9):547–56.

44. Gudeman SD, Eisele SA, Heidt RS, Colosimo AJ, Stroupe AL. Treatment of plantar fasciitis by iontophoresis of 0.4% dexamethasone. A randomized, double-blind, placebo-controlled study. Am J Sports Med. 1997;25(3):312–6.

45. Osborne HR, Allison GT. Treatment of plantar fasciitis by LowDye taping and iontophoresis: short term results of a double blinded, randomised, placebo controlled clinical trial of dexamethasone and acetic acid. Br J Sports Med. 2006;40(6):545–9; discussion 9.

46. Cleland JA, Abbott JH, Kidd MO, Stockwell S, Cheney S, Gerrard DF, et al. Manual physical therapy and exercise versus electrophysical agents and exercise in the management of plantar heel pain: a multi-center randomized clinical trial. J Orthop Sports Phys Ther. 2009;39(8):573–85.

47. Pfeffer G, Bacchetti P, Deland J, Lewis A, Anderson R, Davis W, et al. Comparison of custom and prefabricated orthoses in the initial treatment of proximal plantar fasciitis. Foot Ankle Int. 1999;20(4):214–21.

48. Uden H, Boesch E, Kumar S. Plantar fasciitis – to jab or to support? A systematic review of the current best evidence. J Multidiscip Healthc. 2011;4:155–64.

49. Landorf KB, Keenan AM, Herbert RD. Effectiveness of foot orthoses to treat plantar fasciitis: a randomized trial. Arch Intern Med. 2006;166(12):1305–10.

50. Baldassin V, Gomes CR, Beraldo PS. Effectiveness of prefabricated and customized foot orthoses made from low-cost foam for noncomplicated plantar fasciitis: a randomized controlled trial. Arch Phys Med Rehabil. 2009;90(4):701–6.
51. Lee WC, Wong WY, Kung E, Leung AK. Effectiveness of adjustable dorsiflexion night splint in combination with accommodative foot orthosis on plantar fasciitis. J Rehabil Res Dev. 2012;49(10):1557–64.
52. Lin SC, Chen CP, Tang SF, Wong AM, Hsieh JH, Chen WP. Changes in windlass effect in response to different shoe and insole designs during walking. Gait Posture. 2013;37(2):235–41.
53. Kane D, Greaney T, Shanahan M, Duffy G, Bresnihan B, Gibney R, et al. The role of ultrasonography in the diagnosis and management of idiopathic plantar fasciitis. Rheumatology (Oxford). 2001;40(9):1002–8.
54. Tsai WC, Wang CL, Tang FT, Hsu TC, Hsu KH, Wong MK. Treatment of proximal plantar fasciitis with ultrasound-guided steroid injection. Arch Phys Med Rehabil. 2000;81(10):1416–21.
55. Yucel I, Yazici B, Degirmenci E, Erdogmus B, Dogan S. Comparison of ultrasound-, palpation-, and scintigraphy-guided steroid injections in the treatment of plantar fasciitis. Arch Orthop Trauma Surg. 2009;129(5):695–701.
56. Brinks A, Koes BW, Volkers AC, Verhaar JA, Bierma-Zeinstra SM. Adverse effects of extra-articular corticosteroid injections: a systematic review. BMC Musculoskelet Disord. 2010;11:206.
57. Wong MW, Tang YY, Lee SK, Fu BS. Glucocorticoids suppress proteoglycan production by human tenocytes. Acta Orthop. 2005;76(6):927–31.
58. Acevedo JI, Beskin JL. Complications of plantar fascia rupture associated with corticosteroid injection. Foot Ankle Int. 1998;19(2):91–7.
59. Franceschi F, Papalia R, Franceschetti E, Paciotti M, Maffulli N, Denaro V. Platelet-rich plasma injections for chronic plantar fasciopathy: a systematic review. Br Med Bull. 2014;112(1):83–95.
60. Di Paolo S, Gesualdo L, Ranieri E, Grandaliano G, Schena FP. High glucose concentration induces the overexpression of transforming growth factor-beta through the activation of a platelet-derived growth factor loop in human mesangial cells. Am J Pathol. 1996;149(6):2095–106.
61. Kim E, Lee JH. Autologous platelet-rich plasma versus dextrose prolotherapy for the treatment of chronic recalcitrant plantar fasciitis. PM R. 2014;6(2):152–8.
62. Sun J, Gao F, Wang Y, Sun W, Jiang B, Li Z. Extracorporeal shock wave therapy is effective in treating chronic plantar fasciitis: a meta-analysis of RCTs. Medicine (Baltimore). 2017;96(15):e6621.
63. Lucas DE, Ekroth SR, Hyer CF. Intermediate-term results of partial plantar fascia release with microtenotomy using bipolar radiofrequency microtenotomy. J Foot Ankle Surg. 2015;54(2):179–82.
64. Chou AC, Ng SY, Su DH, Singh IR, Koo K. Radiofrequency microtenotomy is as effective as plantar fasciotomy in the treatment of recalcitrant plantar fasciitis. Foot Ankle Surg. 2016;22(4):270–3.
65. Conflitti JM, Tarquinio TA. Operative outcome of partial plantar fasciectomy and neurolysis to the nerve of the abductor digiti minimi muscle for recalcitrant plantar fasciitis. Foot Ankle Int. 2004;25(7):482–7.
66. Saxena A. Uniportal endoscopic plantar fasciotomy: a prospective study on athletic patients. Foot Ankle Int. 2004;25(12):882–9.

Office-Based Mechanical Procedures for Tendons

18

Jesse Charnoff and Joshua B. Rothenberg

Abbreviations

CET	Common extensor tendon
HVIGI	High-volume image guided injection
LHBT	Long head of the bicep tendon
MTS	Mechanical tendon scraping
NSAID	Non-steroidal anti-inflammatory drug
PNT	Percutaneous needle tenotomy
PUT	Percutaneous ultrasonic tenotomy
US	Ultrasound
VAS	Visual analog scale

Introduction

With accumulating experiences in use of musculoskeletal ultrasound (US) and evolving technologies in equipment, office-based procedures have diversified in recent years [1]. In this chapter, we discuss micro-invasive mechanical tendon procedures. The evolving nature of these procedures has led to new emerging advancements in technology and technique, with some early successes.

J. Charnoff (✉)
Department of Physiatry, Hospital for Special Surgery, New York, NY, USA

J. B. Rothenberg
Orthopedic Group, Baptist Health North Medical Group, Boca Raton Regional Hospital, Boca Raton, FL, USA

Ultrasound Imaging Findings in Tendinopathy

Ultrasound (US) represents a cost-effective, readily available imaging modality that is used to image and characterize tendons and fascia. When scanning the body area in question, one should examine for signs of pathology. Sonographic findings of tendinopathy may include thickened and hypoechoic ("darker than usual") tissues. Occasionally, hyperechoic tissue is seen, typically suggestive of intra-tendinous calcifications and ossifications. Finally, an anechoic area indicates an area of tissue void or a tear, although this is sometimes difficult to tell apart from an area of advanced chronic tendinopathy. Color Doppler allows for an observation of neovascularization, a sign of either ongoing tenosynovitis, or chronic tendinopathy (Fig. 18.1a–g). It is important for the sonographer to remember the dynamic nature of US. Specifically, in the case of a tear, one can examine the extent of the injury under stress, as well as in both the short and long axis to determine the extent of the injury. When unilateral evaluation is inconclusive, side to side comparison of the same tendon can also be considered [2–4]. It is important to remember to use US as an extension of traditional clinical encounters as US may not detect a 100% of tendinopathy due to its technological limitation.

High-Volume Image-Guided Injection

Background

First described by Crisp et al. and by Chan et al. in 2008, high-volume image-guided injection (HVIGI) is a tendon procedure that is performed in an office/outpatient setting under sonographic guidance, which remains important for procedure safety and accuracy. HVIGI has historically been used to treat recalcitrant Achilles and patellar tendinopathies but newer research has addressed shoulder impingement and trochanteric bursitis [4–11]. The injectate often varies among physicians and corticosteroids have traditionally been employed. Due to well-known risks, such as tendon rupture and tendon degeneration, corticosteroid may not be ideal [12]. As discussed later, mechanical tendon scraping (MTS) is sometimes used in conjunction with HVIGI for maximum results [13].

Mechanism of Action

Since the 1970's, it has been well documented that "tendinitis" is associated with a degenerative process [14, 15], which has now been "renamed" appropriately as tendinosis to emphasize the pathologic finding of degeneration [13, 14, 16, 17]. Nirschl first used the term "angiofibroblastic

Fig. 18.1 (a) Normal common extensor tendon. Long axis view of the common extensor tendon origin at the lateral epicondyle, shows normal tendon fibrillar texture. The hyperechoic appearance of bone on the image represents the radius (left, R) and lateral epicondyle (right, LE). (*Images obtained from Dr. Joshua Rothenberg, DO (Konika Minolta Ultrasound Machine)*). (b) Hypoechoic tensor fasciae lata tendon: Long axis view of the tensor fasciae lata (TFL) insertion at the anterior superior iliac spine (ASIS), shows hypoechogenicity consistent with tendinopathic changes. (*Images obtained from Dr. Joshua Rothenberg, DO (Konika Minolta Ultrasound Machine)*). (ci) Thickened Achilles tendon: Long axis view of tendon thickening (Achilles tendon). (*Images obtained from Dr. Joshua Rothenberg, DO (Konika Minolta Ultrasound Machine)*). (cii) Short axis view of tendon thickening (Achilles tendon). (*Images obtained from Dr. Joshua Rothenberg, DO (Konika Minolta Ultrasound Machine)*). (ciii) Short axis view of tendon thickening (Achilles tendon). On the left image, this is a sonographic image of the right Achilles tendon showing diffuse thickening when compared with the right image, which is a view of the left Achilles tendon. (*Images obtained from Dr. Joshua Rothenberg, DO (Konika Minolta Ultrasound Machine)*). (d) Intratendinous supraspinatus calcification: Long axis view of intratendinous calcification (supraspinatus tendon). The hyperechoic region represents the bony insertional point on the greater tuberosity (GT). (*Images obtained from Dr. Joshua Rothenberg, DO (Konika Minolta Ultrasound Machine)*). (ei) Partial thickness supraspinatus tear: Short axis view of a partial thickness tear (supraspinatus tendon). The hyperechoic region represents the bony insertional point on the greater tuberosity (GT). (*Images obtained from Dr. Joshua Rothenberg, DO (Konika Minolta Ultrasound Machine)*). (eii) Long axis view of a partial thickness tear (supraspinatus tendon). The hyperechoic region represents the bony insertional point on the greater tuberosity (GT). (*Images obtained from Dr. Joshua Rothenberg, DO (Konika Minolta Ultrasound Machine)*). (fi) Full thickness supraspinatus/Achilles tears: Short axis view of full thickness supraspinatus tear. The hyperechoic region represents the bony insertional point on the greater tuberosity (GT). (*Images obtained from Dr. Joshua Rothenberg, DO (Konika Minolta Ultrasound Machine)*). (fii) Long axis view of full thickness supraspinatus tear. The hyperechoic region represents the bony insertional point on the greater tuberosity (GT). (*Images obtained from Dr. Joshua Rothenberg, DO (Konika Minolta Ultrasound Machine)*). (fiii) Short axis view of full thickness Achilles tendon tear. (*Images obtained from Dr. Joshua Rothenberg, DO (Konika Minolta Ultrasound Machine)*). (fiiii) Long axis view of full thickness Achilles tendon tear. (*Images obtained from Dr. Joshua Rothenberg, DO (Konika Minolta Ultrasound Machine)*). (fiiiii) Short axis view of full thickness tendon tear (Achilles tendon). On the left image, this is a sonographic image of the right Achilles tendon showing an anechoic region void of tendon, compared with the right image, which is a view of the patient's intact left Achilles tendon. (*Images obtained from Dr. Joshua Rothenberg, DO (Konika Minolta Ultrasound Machine)*). (fiiiiii) Long axis view of full thickness tendon tear (Achilles tendon). On the left image, this is a sonographic image of the right Achilles tendon showing an anechoic region void of tendon, compared with the right image, which is a view of the patient's intact left Achilles tendon. (*Images obtained from Dr. Joshua Rothenberg, DO (Konika Minolta Ultrasound Machine)*). (g) Modified Ohberg grade XXX of Achilles tendon: Short axis view of tendon hyperemia, associated with neovascularization (Achilles tendon). (*Images obtained from Dr. Joshua Rothenberg, DO (Konika Minolta Ultrasound Machine)*) tendinosis" to describe tissue and the histologic changes it incurs [18, 19]. The literature explains that neurogenic inflammation may also play a role in addition to the degenerative process seen in tendinosis [13, 20, 21]. Inflammatory mediators are found surrounding the tendons, which may play a role in promoting neovascularization. The new vessels are thought to be associated with new nerves, or neonerves, which are theorized to be the genesis of pain [20–23].

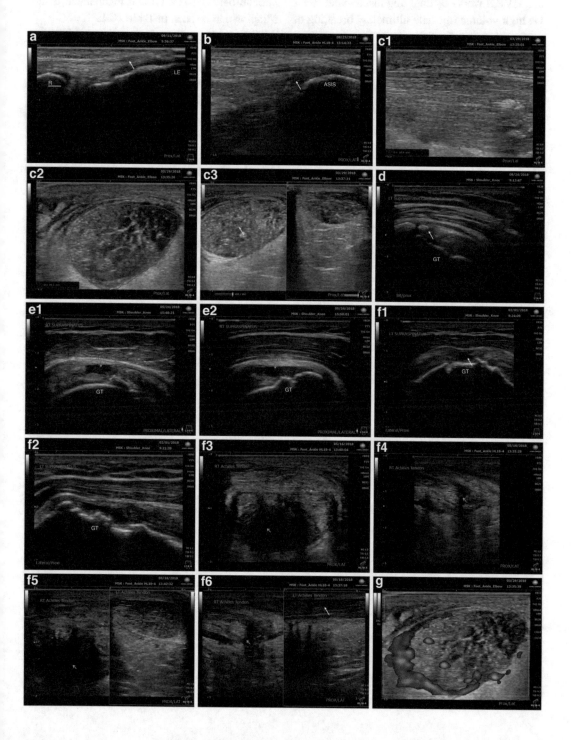

Ohberg and Alfredson hypothesized that targeting of neovessels under image guidance may be a therapeutic target of mechanical procedures resulting in neovessel ablation and a reduction in neurogenic inflammation [2, 24]. It is postulated that HVIGI works by applying mechanical stress via high volume injectate ultimately breaking or occluding abnormal neovessels, attenuating neurogenic inflammation, and disrupting the accompanying nerve mediated tendinopathic pain [4, 6, 20, 21, 25].

A summary of the literature review and a comparison between HVIGI and mechanical tendon scraping can be seen in Table 18.1.

Table 18.1 A summary of literature review

A: High-volume image-guided injection					
Author year	1. Diagnosis treated 2. Location of injection 3. Injection used for treatment	Average duration of symptoms (months) prior to intervention	Sample size (No. of tendons)	Outcome measurements	Results
Crisp et al. (2008) [5]	1. Patellar tendinopathy 2. Patellar/Hoffa fat pad interface 3. 10 ml of 0.5% bupivacaine, 25 mg of hydrocortisone, between 12 and 40 ml of normal saline determined by the clinician based on the amount of resistance encountered	Unknown	9	Pain VAS, function VAS, VISA-P	Pain VAS scores improved significantly by 56 mm at 2 weeks post-procedure Function VAS scores improved significantly by 58 mm at 2 weeks post-procedure VISA-P scores improved significantly from a baseline score of 46 to 68 at 9 months
Morton et al. (2014) [4]	1. Patellar tendinopathy 2. Patellar/Hoffa fat pad interface 3. 10 ml of 0.5% bupivacaine, 25 mg of hydrocortisone, and 30 ml of normal saline, with variability of volume based on clinician judgment	Retrospective – 18.9 Prospective – 20.8	20	VISA-P, return to sport	At 12 weeks post-procedure, VISA-P score showed statistically significant improvement-with a mean improvement of 18.5 There was no statistical significant difference in VISA-P mean change between 12 weeks and 9 month follow-up 37.5% of subjects returned to full sport at 12 weeks Post-procedure protocol included eccentric strengthening rehabilitation program at 4 days post-procedure, non-impact aerobic exercise at 7 days post-procedure, and returned to sport at 12 days post-procedure at the earliest, depending on individual patient factors and clinical response

Table 18.1 (continued)

A: High-volume image-guided injection

Author year	1. Diagnosis treated 2. Location of injection 3. Injection used for treatment	Average duration of symptoms (months) prior to intervention	Sample size (No. of tendons)	Outcome measurements	Results
Maffulli et al. (2016) [7]	1. Patellar tendinopathy 2. Patellar/Hoffa fat pad interface 3. 10 ml of 0.5% bupivacaine, 62,500 IU of aprotinin, and 40 ml of normal saline was used for the injections	18.4	32	Pain VAS, VISA-P, function VAS, return to play at same level as before symptom onset	15 months post-procedure, pain VAS, function VAS and VISA-P scores were significantly improved from baseline. Of the 32 subjects described by the investigators as being physically active, 72% of these patients returned to sport by 15 months post-procedure at the same level as before symptom onset. The average number of injections was 1.8. Patients were allowed to walk on the injected leg immediately but advised to rest from strenuous activity for 3–4 days. Patients returned to their referring clinicians 2 weeks after the injection for advice about further physiotherapy and return to sport. They were then instructed to begin an eccentric loading program under the guidance of a chartered physiotherapist
Chan et al. (2008) [6]	1. Midportion Achilles tendinopathy 2. Achilles tendon/Kager fat pad interface 3. A 10 ml of bupivacaine, 25 mg of hydrocortisone, and up to 40 ml of normal saline	35.8	30	VISA-A, VAS	VISA-A significantly improved from baseline at 30 weeks post-procedure, with a mean change of 31.4. VAS scores significantly improved at 4 weeks by 51 mm, and 48 mm at 30 weeks post-procedure

(continued)

Table 18.1 (continued)

	1. Diagnosis treated 2. Location of injection 3. Injection used for treatment	Average duration of symptoms (months) prior to intervention	Sample size (No. of tendons)	Outcome measurements	Results
A: High-volume image-guided injection					
Author year					
Humphrey et al. (2010) [8]	1. Midportion Achilles tendinopathy 2. Achilles tendon/ Kager fat pad interface 3. Mixture of 10 ml of 0.5% bupivacaine and 25 mg of hydrocortisone, followed by 4 × 10 ml of normal saline	11.8	11	VISA-A, tendon neovascularization grade, maximal tendon thickness on sonography	There was statistically significant difference between baseline and 3-week follow-up in all outcome measures post-procedure VISA-A scores significantly improved at 3 weeks post-procedure; no long term follow-up Investigator determined sonographic changes noted for decreases in neovascularization and tendon thickness Patients were allowed to walk on the injected leg immediately, but were strictly advised to refrain from high impact activity for 72 hours. After this period, they were instructed to re-start heavy eccentric loading physiotherapy regime twice daily until they stopped their sporting career. Six Patients attended a 3-week follow-up for repeated data collection of all the outcome measures and advice on return to sport

Table 18.1 (continued)

A: High-volume image-guided injection

Author year	1. Diagnosis treated 2. Location of injection 3. Injection used for treatment	Average duration of symptoms (months) prior to intervention	Sample size (No. of tendons)	Outcome measurements	Results
Restighini and Yeoh (2012) [64]	1. Midportion Achilles tendinopathy 2. Area of maximal tendon thickness. Anterior to the Achilles tendon 3. 25 mg of hydrocortisone, 5 ml of 1% lidocaine and up to 40 ml of normal saline	17	32	VAS, VISA- A, mean maximal tendon diameter, mean Ohberg neovascularity scores	Mean VAS scores decreased significantly from baseline to 1-month review and was maintained at 3-month review ($6.6 \rightarrow 3.2 \rightarrow 2.9$) VISA-A scores significantly improved at 1-month and 3-month review Significant decrease in mean maximal tendon diameter from baseline to 3-month review Significant decrease in mean Ohberg neovascularity scores between baseline and 3-month review Post-injection patients were advised to refrain from exercise for 3 days but allowed to partake in normal activities of daily living. For a further 3 days they were advised to return to their eccentric program of exercise only. Then 3 days of eccentric exercise and low-impact exercise were followed by a slow return to normal exercise as pain allowed. The eccentric exercise program was to be continued for 3 months

(continued)

Table 18.1 (continued)

A: High-volume image-guided injection					
Author year	1. Diagnosis treated 2. Location of injection 3. Injection used for treatment	Average duration of symptoms (months) prior to intervention	Sample size (No. of tendons)	Outcome measurements	Results
Maffulli et al. (2013) [9]	1. Midportion Achilles tendinopathy 2. Achilles tendon/ Kager fat pad interface 3. 10 ml of 0.5% bupivacaine, 62,500 U of aprotinin, and up to 40 ml of normal saline If symptoms persisted at 2 weeks repeat injection with 10 ml of 0.5% bupivacaine, 25 mg of hydrocortisone acetate, and up to 40 ml of normal saline	13.4	94	VISA-A	At 12 months post-procedure, VISA-A scores significantly improved from 41.7 to 74.6 ($p = 0.003$) At 12 months there was no evidence of an association between maximal tendon thickness and VISA-A score and number of injections at final follow-up At 12 months there was no evidence of an association between neovascularization grade at final follow-up and VISA-A score and number of injections At 12 months 68% of athletes returned to sport at their desired level After 72 hours, they were instructed by a research fellow to restart heavy eccentric loading under the guidance of a chartered physiotherapist. Patients returned to their referring clinicians 2 weeks post-injection for advice about further physiotherapy and returning to sport
Wheeler (2014) [65]	1. Midportion Achilles tendinopathy 2. Achilles tendon/ Kager fat pad interface 3. 10 ml of 1% lidocaine and 40 ml of sterile saline	Unknown	14	VAS, VISA-A	Statistically significant average reduction of 6.1 points on 10 point visual analog scale at 347 day follow-up Statistically significant average improvement of 41 on the VISA-A at 347 day follow-up *First published date on HVIGI without the use of corticosteroid of aprotinin

Table 18.1 (continued)

A: High-volume image-guided injection					
Author year	1. Diagnosis treated 2. Location of injection 3. Injection used for treatment	Average duration of symptoms (months) prior to intervention	Sample size (No. of tendons)	Outcome measurements	Results
Wheeler et al. (2016) [26]	1. Midportion Achilles tendinopathy 2. Achilles tendon/ Kager fat pad interface 3a. 10 ml of 1.0% lignocaine, followed by 40 ml of sterile saline delivered via a series of 10 ml syringes 3b. 3–5 ml of 1% lignocaine was used to anesthetize the area. Needle tenotomy was performed over the area of tendinosis (unknown number of fenestrations). The needle was than directed to the tendon fat pad interface where a mixture of 10 ml of lidocaine and 20 ml of normal saline where injected	Unknown	34	VISA-A, 0–10 pain rating score	Group 3a had a statistically significant improvement in VISA-A from 30% to 64% at a mean follow-up duration of 281 days Group 3b VISA-A scores improved from 31% to 37%, but was not found to be statistically significant Post-procedure VISA A scores when compared between 3a and 3b groups was found to be statistically significant Pain rating scores (0–10) were only collected for 3a pre- 7.6 and post-procedure- 3.0. The difference of 4.6 was found to be statistically significant Investigation design and data collection flaws inhibited the author from declaring an association between the different injection techniques and better VISA-A score

(continued)

Table 18.1 (continued)

A: High-volume image-guided injection					
Author year	1. Diagnosis treated 2. Location of injection 3. Injection used for treatment	Average duration of symptoms (months) prior to intervention	Sample size (No. of tendons)	Outcome measurements	Results
Wheeler et al. (2018) [66]	1. Midportion Achilles tendinopathy 2. Achilles tendon/ Kager fat pad interface 3. Single ultrasound-guided HVIGI (10 ml of 1% lidocaine and 40 ml of sterile saline)	32.7	41	VAS, VISA-A, MOXFQ	At 6 weeks, 3 months and 6 months the VAS (pain) score significantly decreased from baseline 6.74 to 3.58 → 3.57 → 3.50, respectively At 6 weeks, 3 months and 6 months the VISA-A significantly improved when compared to baseline, from 35% to 52% → 51% → 52% ,respectively. Following the procedure, the patient was advised about a structured rehabilitation program, which normally involves relative rest/light activities only for 24 hours, before restarting the static stretches for 48 hours, and progression back into the eccentric strengthening-based rehabilitation exercises after approximately 72 hours depending on symptoms

Abbreviations: *VISA-P* Victorian Institutes of Sport Assessment-Patellar Tendon, *VISA-A* Victorian Institutes of Sport Assessment-Achilles Tendon, *VAS* visual analog scale, *MOXFQ* Manchester-Oxford Foot Questionnaire

Table 18.1 (continued)

B: Mechanical Tendon Scraping (MTS)					
Author year	1. Diagnosis treated 2. Location of procedure 3. Description of procedure	Average duration of symptoms (months) prior to intervention	Sample size (# of tendons)	Outcome measurements	Results
Alfredson et al. (2007) [29]	1. Midportion Achilles tendinopathy 2. Achilles tendon/ Kager fat pad interface 3a. Polidocanol (10 mg/ml) injection for a total of 1–2 ml over area of neovascularization 3b. A longitudinal skin incision (1–2 cm) was placed on the lateral side of the Achilles midportion, the sural nerve was kept aside and the tendon was carefully identified. In the region with tendon changes and high blood flow (marked by skin markers) the tendon was completely released from the ventral soft tissue, by sharp dissection with a knife	3a – 33 3b – 23	Group 3a – 9 Group 3b – 10	Pain during tendon-loading activity, pain VAS during sport activity, patient satisfaction	At 12 weeks 80% of group 3b reported satisfaction with the treatment and back to their previous level of recreational or sport activity. Of note, 4 of the 8 patients returned to previous recreational or sport activity at 6 weeks post-procedure At 12 weeks VAS during recreational or sport activity in group 3b had significantly decreased from 75 to 21 One patient suffered an operative wound At 6 month follow-up 100% of group 3b were satisfied with their treatment and had returned to previous level of activity After treatment: Day 1, there was rest with the foot in elevated position. Day 2, range of motion exercises and short walks were instituted. Day 3–7, the patients were allowed to gradually increase walking activity. Day 8–14, light bicycling was added. After 2 weeks, the sutures were taken, and free activity was allowed

(continued)

Table 18.1 (continued)

B: Mechanical Tendon Scraping (MTS)					
Author year	1. Diagnosis treated 2. Location of procedure 3. Description of procedure	Average duration of symptoms (months) prior to intervention	Sample size (# of tendons)	Outcome measurements	Results
Alfredson (2011) [30]	1. Midportion Achilles tendinopathy 2. Achilles tendon/Kager fat pad interface 3a. A longitudinal skin incision (1–2 cm) was placed on the lateral side of the Achilles midportion, the sural nerve was kept aside and the tendon was carefully identified. In the region with tendon changes and high blood flow (marked by skin markers) the tendon was completely released from the ventral soft tissue, by sharp dissection with a knife 3b. A 14-gauge needle inserted medial or lateral depending on the area of changes. Tendon was released from ventral soft tissue by scraping with the sharp side of the needle, staying close to the ventral tendon 3c. Large group of patients who had undergone the mini open procedure not part of randomization	Large group of mini open procedures-not reported *Randomized study* Mini open procedure-74 PMTS- 82	37 total randomized Mini open- 18 PMTS- 19 Mini open not randomized-88	VAS, patient satisfaction, difference in outcomes of the two different approaches, adverse events	At mean follow-up of 18 months post-procedure, VAS during the Achilles tendon loading significantly decreased from baseline of 77 to 2, with patient satisfaction in 89% of 111 tendons treated The PMTS group had a good clinical result in 74% of tendons, with patients back in full Achilles tendon loading activity Means VAS in the PMTS group statistically significantly improved from 75 at baseline to 2 post-procedure There were no significant differences in outcomes between the open surgical scalpel and PMTS groups in the randomized arm of the study One partial Achilles tendon rupture related to a major trauma was reported, although it is not clear whether this patient was in the open surgical or PMTS group Patients all followed the same post-procedure protocol that included-Day 1: rest, elevated foot. Day 2, ROM exercises, light stretching and short walks. Day 3–7: gradually increased walking activity. Day 8–14, light bicycling. After 2 weeks: sutures out, gradually increased load up to free activity on pain and depending on discomfort

Table 18.1   (continued)

B: Mechanical Tendon Scraping (MTS)

Author year	1. Diagnosis treated 2. Location of procedure 3. Description of procedure	Average duration of symptoms (months) prior to intervention	Sample size (# of tendons)	Outcome measurements	Results
Hall and Rajasekaran (2016) [31]	1. Patellar tendinopathy 2. Patellar/Hoffa fat pad interface 3. An 18-gauge, 2-inch needle with a medial approach. A 5 ml of 1% lidocaine was used for local anesthesia. 20 ml of sterile saline was used to assist the separation via hydrodissection	6	1	VAS, VISA-P, return to sport, Blazina scale score	At 4 weeks post-procedure, the patient had fully returned to sport At 6 month follow-up his VISA-P score improved from 34 to 95, VAS (0–10) score improved from 10 to 1, Blazina score improved from 5 to 1 Patient remained asymptomatic at 11 month follow-up
Bedi et al. (2016) [32]	1. Focal noninsertional Achilles tendinopathy 2. Achilles tendon/ Kager fat pad interface 3. Medial approach to the area of tendinopathy. Plantaris tendon and any soft tissue adhesions to the Achilles tendon were released with sharp dissection	All had greater than 6 months of symptoms	17	VISA-A, return to full training/ competition at 12 weeks, ultrasound tissue characterization	At 12 week follow-up 15/17 tendons returned to full training/ competition VISA-A scores significantly improved after >6 months post-procedure from 51 to 95 All of the subjects in this study were either professional or semiprofessional running athletes Patients were non-weight-bearing for 48 hours and were then able to weightbear as tolerated with crutches. After 2 weeks, patients commenced cycling and eccentric exercises. Running was commenced at 4–6 weeks and return to full training was allowed after 8 weeks

Abbreviations: *PMTS* percutaneous mechanical tendon scraping

Table 18.1 (continued)

| C: Percutaneous needle tenotomy | | | | | |
Author year	1. Diagnosis treated 2. Injection(s) used for treatment	Average duration of symptoms (months) prior to intervention	Sample size (# of tendons)	Outcome measurements	Results
McShane et al. (2006) [33]	1. Elbow common extensor tendon 2. 1 ml of corticosteroid + either 6 mg of betamethasone or 40 mg of triamcinolone acetonide, mixed with 2 ml of 0.5% bupivacaine	9	61	Patient perceived outcomes- pain over the past week, pain that woke the patient at night, worst level of pain over the past week (none, mild, moderate, severe), adverse events, personal recommendation to others	Average time of follow-up was 28 months at which time 80% of patients reported an "excellent" or "good" outcome 81.4% of patients reported having no pain at rest over the past week 93.2% never had pain that woke them up at night post-procedure No adverse events were reported 85.5% of patients reported they would refer a friend or close relative
McShane et al. (2008) [35]	1. Elbow common extensor tendon 2. Bupivacaine & sodium bicarbonate was used as local anesthetic in the skin, subQ, CET and periosteum of the lateral epicondyle	43/55 (78.1) symptomatic for greater than 9 months	55	Patient perceived outcomes including pain experienced in week prior to interview, pain woke patient at night, over previous week the worst level of pain, functional difficulty with tasks, personal recommendation to others, adverse events	Average time to follow-up was 22 months at which time 92.3% of patients reported excellent or good outcomes 80.8% reported no pain experienced at rest in week prior to interview 96.2% never had pain wake them at night 92.7% stated that they had none or mild functional difficulty with tasks 90% would refer a close friend or family member Zero adverse events reported *PNT without steroids was found to be effective
Zhu et al. (2008) [67]	1. Elbow common extensor tendon 2. A 16-gauge needle was used for fenestration. A 1 ml mixture of 25 mg prednisone acetate and 1% lidocaine was injected to the fenestrated tendon. If symptoms were not relieved, the procedure was repeated 2–3 times at 1–2 week intervals	3.2	76	Patient perceived outcomes, VAS, sonographically demonstrated neovascularization, adverse events	At completion of the study 87% of patients reported excellent or good outcomes VAS scores significantly decreased at 3, 6, 12, and 24 week examinations No reported adverse events Patients were treated with NSAIDs s/p procedure to alleviate pain

Table 18.1 (continued)

C: Percutaneous needle tenotomy

Author year	1. Diagnosis treated 2. Injection(s) used for treatment	Average duration of symptoms (months) prior to intervention	Sample size (# of tendons)	Outcome measurements	Results
Housner et al. (2009) [36]	1. Patellar, Achilles, proximal gluteus medius, proximal iliotibial band, proximal hamstring tendon, common elbow extensor tendon, and proximal rectus femoris 2. A 22-gauge needle was used to pierce the diseased tissue under sonographic guidance, 3–6 ml of lidocaine: bupivacaine mixture was injected during procedure	53	14	VAS, adverse events	VAS scores noted at the 4 and 12 week follow-up appointments were significantly lower than at baseline $(5.8 \rightarrow 2.4 \rightarrow 2.2)$ No statistical significant difference was observed between 4 and 12 weeks post-procedure There were no reported complications *PNT without steroids was found to be effective
Housner et al. (2010) [40]	1. Patellar tendinopathy 2. A 22-gauge needle was used to pierce the diseased tissue under sonographic guidance, 6 ml of lidocaine: bupivacaine mixture was injected during procedure	20	47	Patient perceived outcomes, return to sport with no or mild pain, adverse events	Average time to follow-up was 45 months and 81% of patients reported excellent or good outcomes 72% of patients were able to return to desired activity level One patient suffered a ruptured patellar tendon at 6 weeks post-procedure *PNT without steroids was found to be effective
Jacobson et al. (2015) [39]	1. Gluteus medius tendons, gluteus minimus tendons, hamstring tendons, and tensor fascia lata tendon 2. A 1% lidocaine local anesthetic was used prior to the fenestration process and during the procedure as needed, a 20- or 22-gauge spinal needle was used for fenestration. The inner trocar was removed prior to fenestration	29	22 tendons (21 patients)	Patient perceived improvement	At an average follow-up of 70 days 45% reported marked improvement, 37% reported some improvement, 9% reported no change, and 9% reported worsening symptoms Patients avoided NSAIDs for 2 weeks prior to procedure

(continued)

Table 18.1 (continued)

Author year	Diagnosis treated	Average duration of symptoms (months) prior to intervention	Sample size (No. of tendons)	Outcome measurements	Results
D: Percutaneous ultrasonic tenotomy					
Elattrache & Morrey (2013) [45]	Patellar tendinopathy	Not reported	16	Return to previous level of play, patient reported improvement	A total of 63% of the subjects returned to the prior level of activity or competition A total of 93% of subjects expressed some level of improvement
Koh et al. (2013) [49] & Seng et al. (2015) [47]	Elbow common extensor tendinopathy	Median duration of symptoms- 12.5, mean- unknown	20	VAS, DASH, DASH- Work, sonographic appearance of tendon, patient satisfaction, personal recommendation to others, adverse events	VAS score showed statistically significant improvement when comparing baseline to week 1, and continued to show significant improvement at 1,3,6, and 12 months, respectively VAS score improved from 1 year to 3 years but was not statistically significant Post-procedure, DASH compulsory findings were noted to improve throughout the year, but only the following differences were found to be statistically significant: (1) From baseline to 1 month, (2) 3–6 months, (3) 1–3 years DASH-Work had significant decreases as compared with baseline at 1 month. At 3,6,12, and 36 months there was a linear decrease At least 85% of tendons showed improved morphologic characteristics at 6 months post-procedure 95% of patients endorsed satisfaction at 1 year, 80% would recommend this procedure to a friend At 3 year follow-up 100% of patients reported satisfaction, 100% would recommend this procedure to a friend No complications were noted

Table 18.1 (continued)

D: Percutaneous ultrasonic tenotomy

Author year	Diagnosis treated	Average duration of symptoms (months) prior to intervention	Sample size (No. of tendons)	Outcome measurements	Results
Barnes, Beckley, and Smith (2015) [44]	Common extensor and common flexor/pronator tendinopathy	6 months or more	12 (CET) 7 (CFPT) Case series	VAS, QuickDASH, MEPS, complications	VAS statistically significantly improved from baseline by week 6. Statistically significant changes were noted at 3, 6, and 12 months compared with baseline (pretreatment VAS, 6.4; 6 weeks, 2.6; 3 months, 0.9; 6 months, 1.7; 12 months, 0.7) QuickDASH statistically significantly improved from baseline by week 6. statistically improved further by 3 months, and remained stable thereafter (pretreatment Q-DASH, 44.1; 6 weeks, 30.1; 3 months, 13.8; 6 months, 16.4; 12 months, 8.6) MEPS improved significantly by 6 weeks, and this improvement was maintained throughout the 12-month follow-up period No complications were noted
Patel (2015) [46]	Plantar fasciitis	19	12 Case series	AOFAS, Symptom resolution	Average AOFAS improved from 30->88 at 3 month follow-up 11/12 patients reported resolution of symptoms at 3 month follow-up All subjects reported they were pain free at 24 months follow-up
Razdan et al. (2015) [68]	Plantar fasciitis	4 months or more	100	FADI, would recommend to a friend	FADI scores significantly improved from 59 preprocedure to 71 at 2 weeks, 83 at 6 weeks, and 90 at 24 weeks post-procedure At 6 month follow-up 98% of those who could be reached (53 patients) indicated they would recommend the procedure to a friend

(continued)

Table 18.1 (continued)

D: Percutaneous ultrasonic tenotomy

Author year	Diagnosis treated	Average duration of symptoms (months) prior to intervention	Sample size (No. of tendons)	Outcome measurements	Results
Battista et al. (2018) [69]	Elbow common extensor tendinopathy	21.4	7	ASES, VAS	Statistically significant improvement in ASES scores that were first noted at 6 weeks were maintained at the 3, 6, 12, and 24-month follow-up times Baseline ASES score 55.6 improved to 94.1 at 2 year follow-up The preoperative mean VAS score significantly improved from baseline 7.9, to mean postoperative VAS score of 1.1 at 2 year follow-up

Abbreviations: *AOFAS* American Orthopaedic Foot and Ankle Society Scores, *CET* elbow common extensor tendinopathy, *CFPT* elbow common flexor/pronator tendinopathy, *DASH* Disabilities of the Arm, Shoulder, Hand Score, *MEPS* Mayo Elbow Performance Scale, *QuickDASH* shortened version of DASH score, *VAS* visual analog scale, *ASES* American shoulder elbow surgeons, *FADI* Foot and Ankle Disability Index

Procedural Technique: Mid-Portion Achilles Tendinopathy with Neovascularization

I. Equipment
   (a) Needles
       (i) Smallest bore needle for local anesthetics (generally 30-gauge or 27-gauge)
       (ii) 18-gauge or 20-gauge needle for HVIGI
   (b) Injectate
       (i) 2–4 ml of 1.0% lidocaine for local anesthesia
       (ii) 10 ml of 0.5% ropivacaine and up to 40 ml of normal saline for HVIGI
   (c) High-frequency linear array transducer

Injectate volumes have ranged in the literature from four injections of 10 ml to one injection with 20–40 ml. Only one study has examined the difference in efficacy of different injectate volumes and they were unable to definitively state that one injectate volume was superior to another due to confounding variables [26]. Our clinical experience is that with the more fluid used, the greater is chance of post-procedure discomfort. (Ropivacaine when used alone as compared with lidocaine and bupivacaine has the least toxic effect on tenocytes. Ropivacaine when used with dexamethasone potentiated ropivacaine tenocyte toxicity; [27, 28]).

II. Authors' preferred technique
   (a) Patient positioning and approach
       (i) Prone positioning with the foot in neutral position off the edge of the table, using lateral to medial approach.
   (b) Pre-procedure scan
       (i) Examine the tendon under US in order to delineate the target area.

(ii) If hyperemia is not seen, we recommend using the area of most severe sonopalpation tenderness.

(iii) Identify the sural nerve, tibial nerve, and posterior tibial artery and avoid.

(c) Sterile preparation

(i) Apply sterile gloves, and then sterilely prepare a large area beyond the target site.

(ii) Sterilely drape the area.

(iii) Apply a sterile transducer cover kit followed by sterile gel to the probe.

(d) Anesthetic

(i) Insert the anesthetic needle under continuous sonographic visualization in plane to the transducer while viewing the Achilles tendon in short axis. Anesthetize the skin, subcutaneous tissue, and the interface between the Kager's fat pad and Achilles tendon (Figs. 18.2 and 18.3).

(ii) Consider using a gel stand-off/oblique stand-off technique to ensure accurate needle entry point with good needle visualization. This technique can help to adjust the entry point prior to the needle contact with the patient's skin.

(e) HVIGI

(i) Insert an 18- or 20-gauge needle at the same entry point with the same needle trajectory as the anesthetic needle using continuous sonographic visualization (Fig. 18.4).

(ii) Guide the injection needle to the target area deep to Achilles tendon, superficial to the fat pad.

(iii) After a confirmation of an accurate needle tip placement at the interface, injectate is introduced under constant pressure on the syringe.

(iv) Color Doppler might show disappearance of neovessels. Though in cases of HVIGI, this might happen at a later time and not during the procedure.

(v) Current literature does not specify the speed at which the injectate should be administered. Based on the theorized mechanism of action, no conclusive recommendation can be given, as no study has compared speed, efficacy, and complication rates.

(f) Post-procedure protocol

There is currently no data regarding outcomes based on different post-procedure protocols. Several studies have described their protocols [4, 7–10]. We recommend the following protocol based on our clinical experiences:

(i) Weight bear as tolerated after the procedure, using crutches as needed. The patient should be advised to refrain from high impact activity for 72 hours.

(ii) After 72 hours post-procedure, non-impact aerobic exercise may be done with a progressive isometric to isotonic strengthening program while avoiding eccentric loading and stretching until the second week post-procedure.

(iii) At the start of the second week post-procedure, an eccentric exercise program may be considered.

(iv) If the patient is progressing well after 2 weeks post-injection they can consider return to sport [13].

(v) Eccentric exercise has been shown to have similar disruptive effect on neovascularization disruption and should be used by patients after 1-week post-procedure [7, 8, 24].

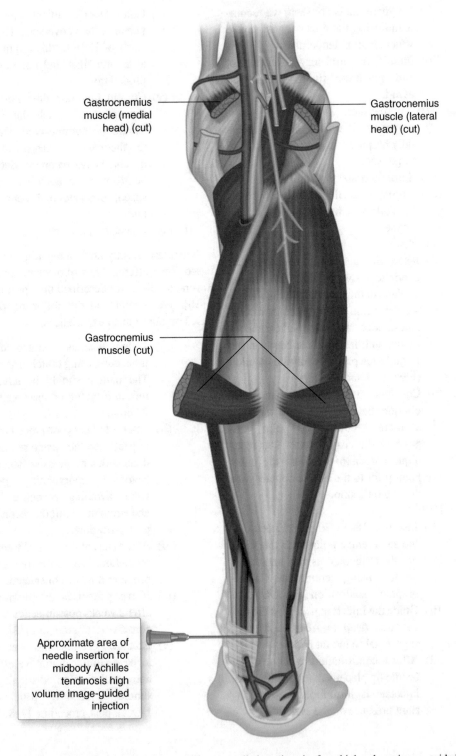

Gastrocnemius muscle (medial head) (cut)

Gastrocnemius muscle (lateral head) (cut)

Gastrocnemius muscle (cut)

Approximate area of needle insertion for midbody Achilles tendinosis high volume image-guided injection

Fig. 18.2 The given figure demonstrates the approximate needle insertion site for a high volume image-guided injection in the midbody Achilles tendon

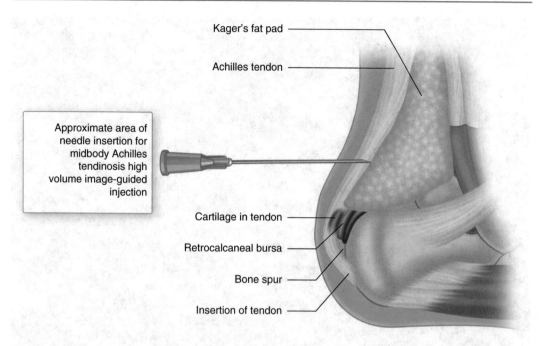

Fig. 18.3 The given figure demonstrates that the needle should be positioned between the Achilles tendon and Kager's fat pad when administering a high volume image-guided injection of the midbody Achilles tendon

Mechanical Tendon Scraping

Background

Mechanical tendon scraping (MTS) was first described for midportion Achilles tendinopathy by Alfredson and colleagues in 2007 [29]. The procedure was initially surgical. In the original procedure, ultrasound was used to identify the area of maximal neovascularization followed by surgically releasing the tendon from any ventral soft tissue adhesions with a scalpel via direct visualization. Alfredson later did a study comparing the mini-open surgical technique to a percutaneous version of the procedure performed using a 14-gauge needle under sonographic guidance without creating an opening for visualization [30]. The study found that the ultrasound-guided procedure resulted in 89% of patients reporting satisfaction with the proce-

dure, along with an average reduction of about 7 in a 10-point visual analog scale (VAS). The study also documented that there was no significant difference between the mini-open and the ultrasound-guided technique [30], concluding that the ultrasound-guided technique may be superior both from the complication and ease-of-access standpoints. The theorized mechanism of MTS is similar to HVIGI as it is believed to target neovascularization; however, some clinicians note that MTS is better tolerated as compared with HVIGI. They theorize that less volume of injectate is required, leading to less patient discomfort throughout the procedure [31]. MTS has produced good results in regard to both satisfaction and return to play, ranging from 80% to 100% [29].

(Refer to Table 18.1.)

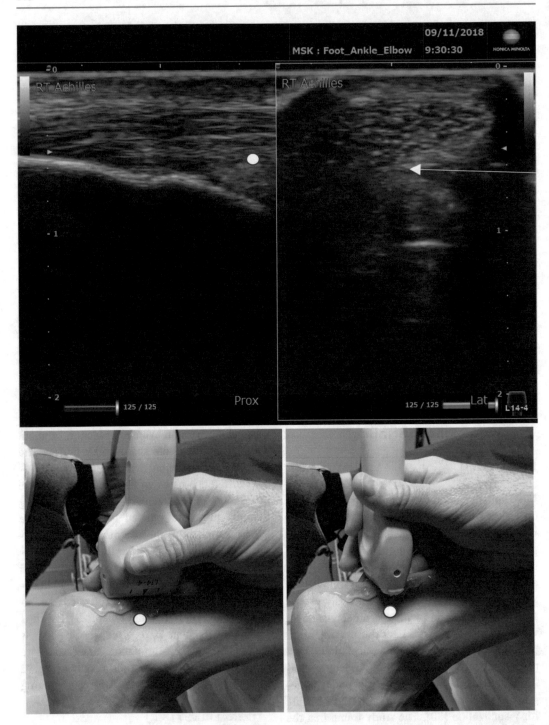

Fig. 18.4 Long axis view (on the left) and short axis view (on the right) of the Achilles tendon close to its insertional point on the calcaneus, with Kager's fat pad deep to the Achilles tendon (seen better on the top right). Circle on the Achilles tendon in long axis (top left) represents a long axis out-of-plane approach of needle for HVIGI. This is done proximal to the calcaneal bone, seen as a hyperechoic signal, and deep to the fibrillar pattern of the Achilles tendon. On the top left image, the needle enters from lateral to medial out-of-plane. Arrow (top right) indicates a short axis in-plane approach of needle for HVIGI (author's preferred technique), deep to the Achilles tendon. On the top right image, the needle enters from lateral to medial in-plane. On the bottom left and right images, the circle represents the entry point of the needle. (*Images obtained from Dr. Joshua Rothenberg, DO (Konika Minolta Ultrasound Machine)*)

Mechanism of Action

As discussed here for HVIGI, the procedure targets neurogenic inflammation secondary to neurovascular ingrowth and neovascularization [6, 13, 24, 30]. In MTS, the scraping technique is used to mechanically disrupt neovessels and accompanying neonerves, most classically using a needle tip. Color Doppler is used to localize the procedure in order to minimize the procedure-associated traumas. MTS has been studied for mid-portion Achilles and, to a lesser extent, for patellar tendinopathy [29–32].

Procedural Technique – Mid-Portion Achilles Tendinopathy with Neovascularization

I. Equipment
   (a) Needles
      (i) Smallest bore needle for local anesthetics (generally 30-gauge or 27-gauge)
      (ii) 18-gauge needle for MTS
      (iii) #11 blade for a stab incision
   (b) Injectate
      (i) 3–5 ml of 1% lidocaine for local anesthesia
      (ii) Up to 20 ml of sterile normal saline for separation of fat pad from tendon
   (c) High-frequency linear array transducer
II. Authors' preferred technique
   (a) Patient positioning and approach
      (i) Prone positioning with the foot in neutral position off the edge of the table, using lateral to medial approach.
   (b) Pre-procedure scan
      (i) Examine the tendon under US in order to delineate the target area.
      (ii) If hyperemia is not seen, we recommend using the area of most severe sonopalpation tenderness.
      (iii) Ensure that vital structures including the sural nerve is identified and mapped out prior to the procedure to limit potential complications.
   (c) Sterile preparation
      (i) Apply sterile gloves, and then sterilely prepare (may use chlorhexidine applicator or betadine swabs) a large area beyond the target site.
      (ii) Sterilely drape the area.
      (iii) Apply a sterile transducer cover kit followed by sterile gel to the probe.
   (d) Anesthetic
      (i) Insert the anesthetic needle under continuous sonographic visualization in plane to the transducer while viewing the Achilles tendon in short axis. Anesthetize the skin, subcutaneous tissue, and the interface between the Kager's fat pad and Achilles tendon (Figs. 18.2 and 18.3).
      (ii) Consider using a gel stand-off/oblique stand-off technique to ensure accurate needle entry point with good needle visualization. This technique can help to adjust the entry point prior to the needle contact with the patient's skin.
   (e) Percutaneous MTS
      (i) Insert an 18- or 20-gauge needle at the same entry point with the same needle trajectory as the anesthetic needle using continuous sonographic visualization.
      (ii) Guide the injection needle to the target area deep to Achilles tendon, superficial to the fat pad (Fig. 18.4).
      (iii) After confirmation of accurate needle tip placement at the interface, a swiping motion of the needle in a cephalo-caudad direction is performed with the bevel of the needle pointing toward the fat pad.
      (iv) Up to 20 ml of sterile normal saline can help assist the tendon-fat pad separation via HVIGI.
      (v) Unlike HVIGI, neovascularization disappears immediately with MTS. Frequently check color Doppler as disappearance of the

flow indicates the end of the procedure.

(f) Post-procedure protocol

    (i) There is currently no data regarding outcomes based on different post-procedure protocols. Several studies have described their protocols [29–31].

    (ii) We recommend that patients' weight-bear as tolerated after the procedure, using crutches as needed for any post-procedure discomfort.

    (iii) Starting post-procedure day 1, a conservative program of light active range of motion, stretching, and isometric exercises may be employed.

    (iv) At the start of week two, non-impact aerobic exercise may be done with isotonic strengthening. This can be progressed with the supervision of an experienced trainer or physical therapist to an eccentric exercise program.

    (v) If the patient is progressing well after 2 weeks post-injection, they can consider full tendon loading [31].

    (vi) If patient is able to tolerate full loading of tendon, with minimal or no discomfort, they can return to sport [13, 30, 31].

    (vii) MTS tends to be a more direct procedure and a potentially quicker recovery time. Rehab protocol may need slight adjustments if the two procedures are done together and largely depends on the progress of the patient at each phase. Patients should use pain as a navigator and communicate with their physician when concerns arise regarding advancing stages of rehab.

Percutaneous Needle Tenotomy

Background

Percutaneous needle tenotomy (PNT) is an office-based tendon procedure now most commonly performed under sonographic guidance. Sonographically guided PNT was first described by McShane and colleagues in 2006 to treat chronic common extensor tendinopathy of the elbow [33]. Prior to this indication, needle tenotomy was performed using landmark guidance, termed "dry needling," to emphasize it did not involve the injection of other products. Although not implied by its definition, PNT has since been combined with injectates such as lidocaine, corticosteroids, or orthobiologics (see Chap. 19 on details regarding orthobiologics) [1, 13, 34]. McShane's study found, however, PNT without corticosteroid was both safe and efficacious [35]. Additionally, further studies agree on PNT's effectiveness in treating tendinopathy [1, 36, 37]. Today, large-scale randomized controlled trials are still lacking and further studies are warranted.

Mechanism of Action

PNT involves the fenestration of pathologic tissue to induce acute changes to the pathologic environment by causing injury. This is believed to lead to the mobilization of scar tissue and the chronic degenerative tendon, while causing local bleeding and fibroblast proliferation, which may translate to the release of growth factors, new collagen formation, and ultimately healing [13]. It is hypothesized that PNT helps facilitate the change of the local tendon environment from a chronic degenerative state to an acute injury state that is capable of healing [13, 33, 35, 36], however the exact cellular benefit has yet to be elucidated.

Procedural Technique: Elbow Common Extensor Tendon (CET) Tendinosis

I. Equipment
  (a) Needles
     (i) Smallest bore needle for anesthetics (generally 30-gauge or 27-gauge)
     (ii) Large bore (usually 18- or 20-gauge) needle used for PNT [1, 33]
  (b) Injectate
     (i) 2–4 ml of 1.0% lidocaine for local anesthesia
  (c) High-frequency linear array transducer
II. Authors preferred technique
  (a) Patient positioning and approach
     (i) Supine positioning with elbow flexed to 60° and the pronated forearm resting on the patient's abdomen (a pillow under the arm might help the patient with comfort), using distal to proximal approach.
  (b) Pre-procedure scan
     (i) Examine the tendon under US in order to delineate the target area.
     (ii) If tendon thickening, loss of hyper-echoic fibrillar echotexture, hypoechoic or anechoic appearance is not seen, we recommend using the area of the most severe sonopalpation tenderness.
     (iii) Ensure that vital structures including the posterior interosseous nerve (PIN) and radial collateral ligament are identified and mapped out prior to the procedure to limit potential complications. Note that only approximately 50% of the CET makes up the total footprint of the lateral epicondyle. The radial collateral ligament lies deep to the common extensor tendon and can be damaged [13, 38].
     (iv) Consider marking your needle trajectory path and any vital structures to avoid with a sterile marker on the skin.

  (c) Sterile procedure
     (i) Apply sterile gloves, and then sterilely prepare (may use chlorhexidine applicator or betadine swabs) a large area beyond the target site.
     (ii) Sterilely drape the area.
     (iii) Apply a sterile transducer cover kit followed by sterile gel to the probe.
  (d) Anesthetic
     (i) Insert the anesthetic needle under continuous sonographic visualization in plane to the transducer while viewing the CET tendon in long axis. Anesthetize the skin, subcutaneous tissue, and the peritendinous region (Figs. 18.5 and 18.6).
  (e) PNT
     (i) Insert the tenotomy needle at the same entry point as the anesthetic.
     (ii) Under continuous sonographic monitoring, the needle is advanced into the area of tendinopathy.
     (iii) It is recommended that both orthogonal and transverse views of the CET are used to ensure coverage of the entire tendinopathic regions (Fig. 18.7).
     (iv) In the PNT literature, the number of passes into the tendon, termed fenestrations, listed ranges from 20 to 40 per tendon [13, 39]. There is not a clear distinction between different tendons and different number of fenestrations required. However, some authors have stated that softening of the abnormal tendon is an indication that proper fenestration has occurred [13, 33, 35, 39, 40].
     (v) It is recommended that a syringe with anesthetic is attached to the needle throughout the procedure. The anesthetic is to be used as needed if the patient experiences pain. The amount of anesthetic should be as limited as possible secondary to the known tenocyte toxicity of anesthetics [27, 28].

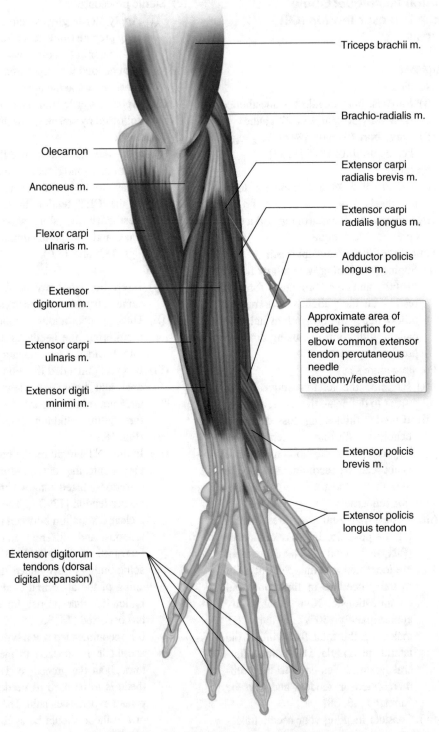

Triceps brachii m.

Brachio-radialis m.

Olecarnon

Anconeus m.

Extensor carpi
radialis brevis m.

Extensor carpi
radialis longus m.

Flexor carpi
ulnaris m.

Adductor policis
longus m.

Extensor
digitorum m.

Approximate area of
needle insertion for
elbow common extensor
tendon percutaneous
needle
tenotomy/fenestration

Extensor carpi
ulnaris m.

Extensor digiti
minimi m.

Extensor policis
brevis m.

Extensor policis
longus tendon

Extensor digitorum
tendons (dorsal
digital expansion)

Fig. 18.5 The given figure demonstrates the approximate needle insertion site for percutaneous need tenotomy/fenestration of the elbow common extensor tendons

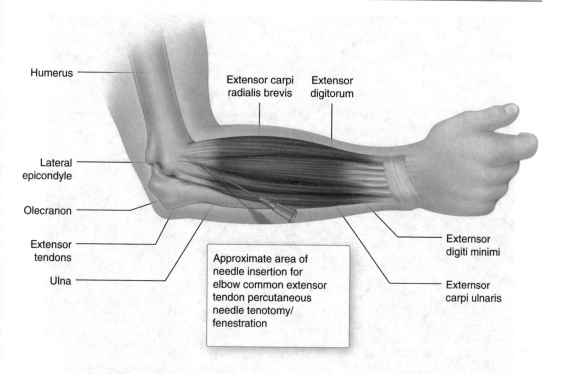

Humerus

Extensor carpi
radialis brevis

Extensor
digitorum

Lateral
epicondyle

Olecranon

Extensor
tendons

Ulna

Approximate area of
needle insertion for
elbow common extensor
tendon percutaneous
needle tenotomy/
fenestration

Externsor
digiti minimi

Externsor
carpi ulnaris

Fig. 18.6 The given figure demonstrates the approximate needle insertion site for percutaneous need tenotomy/fenestration of the elbow common extensor tendons

(vi) When the procedure has been completed, the needle is removed, pressure is maintained, and a sterile adhesive dressing is applied.

(f) Post-procedure protocol

  (i) There is currently no data regarding outcomes based on different post-procedure protocols. Several studies have described their protocol in varying detail [1, 21, 33, 35, 36].

  (ii) We recommend following the post-PNT protocol described by Finnoff and colleagues in 2011, however, no current standard protocol exists [1].

  (iii) Days 0–2: Non-weight-bearing for lower extremity procedures, sling for upper extremity procedures. Patients are encouraged to perform active range of motion multiple times per day and ice, compression, and elevation.

  (iv) Days 3–14: Weight-bearing activity as tolerated in walking boot (ankle/foot procedures), knee immobilizer (knee procedures), or 50% weight-bearing with crutches (hip procedures) for lower extremity procedures. Continue ice, compression, elevation, active range of motion.

  (v) Weeks 2–4: Multiplanar isometric exercises with passive stretching. Wean out of boot, knee immobilizer, or off crutches for lower extremity procedure. Stationary bike with light resistance.

  (vi) Weeks 4–6: Isotonic exercises, elliptical machine or stationary bike with moderate resistance.

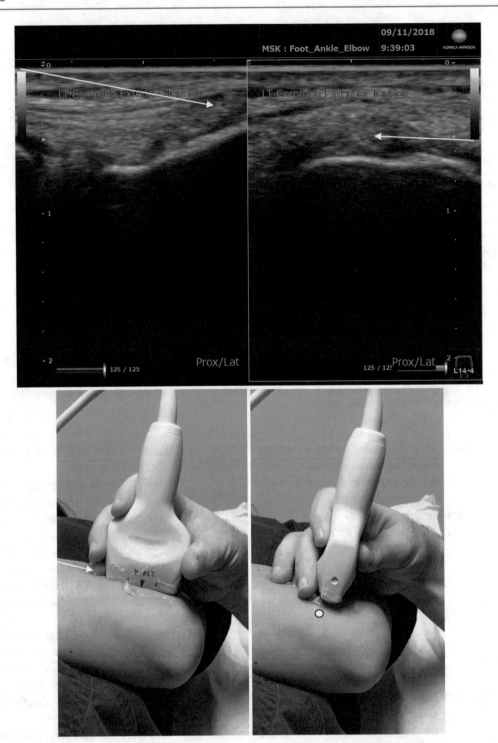

Fig. 18.7 Long axis view (on the left) and short axis view (on the right) of the common extensor tendon close to its origin on the lateral epicondyle. Arrows (top left, bottom left) correspond to the direction of the needle from a distal to proximal in-plane approach of percutaneous needle tenotomy (PNT) directed at the common extensor tendon origin (author's preferred technique). Arrow (top right), and circle (bottom right) indicates a lateral to medial in-plane approach of needle for needle tenotomy. (*Images obtained from Dr. Joshua Rothenberg, DO (Konika Minolta Ultrasound Machine)*)

(vii) Weeks 6–10: Eccentric exercises. Walking program progressing to jogging and may stand and use heavy resistance while bicycling.

(viii) Weeks 10–12: Plyometrics and sports-specific training.

(ix) Week 12: Unrestricted activity [1].

(x) NSAID use pre- and post-procedure is something that is debated in the academic community. There are currently no trials that clearly show with or without NSAIDs as superior or inferior. However, because of the mechanism of action previously described, we recommend our patients to avoid NSAIDs for 1 week prior to the procedure and at least 2 weeks post-procedure to avoid inhibiting the inflammatory stage of tendon healing [1, 13].

Percutaneous Ultrasonic Tenotomy

Background

Percutaneous ultrasonic tenotomy (PUT) is a microinvasive procedure that can be performed in an office or ambulatory surgical center. The technology used in PUT was inspired from the principles of phacoemulsification used in cataracts surgery [41, 42]. PUT using Tenex, one of the currently available devices, is FDA-approved for the treatment of tendinopathy since 2011. This gave physicians the opportunity to perform targeted tendon debridement without having to perform open or arthroscopic/tendoscopic tenotomy [43, 44]. The Tenex hand-held piece has a two main parts. The inner metal part vibrates back and forth rapidly with ultrasonic energy emitted into a <1 mm semi-circumferential focal zone at the tip of the device to debride tendinopathy tissues. The outer part is shaped like a tube and is connected to a saline irrigation system and this part is used to aspirate debrided tissues [44–46] (Fig. 18.8). With advances in US technology we can now identify the area most affected by tendinopathy, and consequently, diagnostic US experience is an essential part of successful completion of PUT [47, 48].

Mechanism of Action

The TX1 and TX2 systems (Tenex Health, Lake Forest, California) are the devices being used to perform PUT, with the only difference being the length of the MicroTip. The TX2 has a longer MicroTip to reach deeper structures, particularly in the shoulder and hip, while the TX1 has the advantage of a shorter MicroTip. The device consists of a console that controls the fluid and ultrasonic energy being delivered to the probe. The effective device size is approximately that of a conventional 32-mm 18-gauge needle [13]. During PUT, the ultrasonic vibrating tip is directed at the angiofibroblastic tissue of tendinopathy under continuous sonographic guidance. Tendinopathic tissue becomes emulsified and subsequently debrided/suctioned away [13, 49]. The majority of the published research has been on epicondylosis, patellar tendinosis, plantar fasciitis, and, more recently, insertional Achilles tendinosis [50]. To date all of the studies are case series. The former three demonstrate immediate and prolonged patient satisfaction and sonographic improvement for up to 3 years [44–47, 49]. It is theorized that the pain evoked by the necrotic tendon is mediated by cytokines, which are removed by this process providing immediate pain relief. In addition, it is hypothesized that the space created by the ultrasonic tenotomy allows for a more normal environment leading to a healing response as compared with the impaired tendon healing due to degenerative tissues [44]. Zhang et al. demonstrated that platelet-rich plasma was unlikely to reverse tendinopathic conditions in an in vitro model, however, was not likely to worsen the condition [51]. The removal of the chronic degenerated tissue also likely eliminates the neovascularization and coinciding neonerves that are implicated in neurogenic inflammation

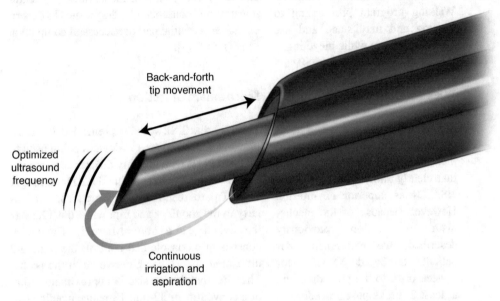

Back-and-forth
tip movement

Optimized
ultrasound
frequency

Continuous
irrigation and
aspiration

Fig. 18.8 The given figure illustrates the hand-held piece used in percutaneous ultrasonic tenotomy with Tenex. The inner part vibrates and introduces destructive energy into a <1 mm semi-circumferential focal zone at the tip of the device. The outer part aspirates the emulsified tissue [46]

[20, 21]. Animal models have shown that the PUT procedure promotes the growth of normal tendon architecture when applied to areas of degenerated tendon [52].

Procedural Details: Patellar Tendinopathy

I. Equipment
  (a) Needles
    (i) Smallest bore needle for local anesthetics (generally 30-gauge or 27-gauge)
    (ii) 18-gauge needle for fenestration
    (iii) #11 blade for a stab incision
    (iv) TX-1 disposable handpiece for PUT
  (b) Injectate
    (i) 2–4 ml of 1.0% lidocaine for local anesthesia
  (c) High frequency linear array transducer
II. Authors preferred technique
  (a) Patient positioning and approach
    (i) Supine positioning with a pillow under the knee (30–45° of flexion),

using distal lateral to proximal medial approach
  (b) Pre-procedure scan
    (i) Examine the tendon under US in order to delineate the target area.
    (ii) If hypoechoic or anechoic area is not seen, we recommend using the area of most severe sonopalpation tenderness (Figs. 18.9 and 18.10).
    (iii) Consider marking your needle trajectory path and any vital structures, such as the fibular nerve, with a sterile marker on the skin.
  (c) Sterile procedure
    (i) Apply sterile gloves and then sterilely prepare (may use chlorhexidine applicator or betadine swabs) a large area beyond the target site.
    (ii) Steriley drape the area.
    (iii) Apply a sterile transducer cover kit followed by sterile gel to the probe.
  (d) Anesthetic
    (i) Insert the anesthetic needle under continuous sonographic visualization in plane to the transducer while view-

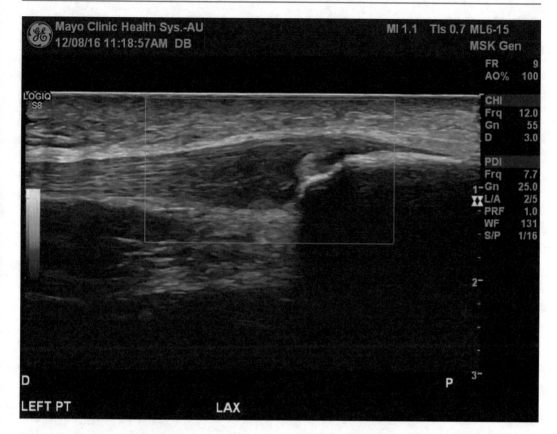

Fig. 18.9 The given ultrasound image demonstrates patellar tendinosis in the longitudinal axis. Note the loss of fibular tendon and the edema near the site of insertion.

P = patellar tendon, Pa = patella, * = tendinopathic portion of patellar tendon

ing the patellar tendon in short axis. Anesthetize the skin, subcutaneous tissue, the tendon, and the interface between Hoffa's fat pad and the patellar tendon (Fig. 18.11).

(e) Needle fenestration

(i) A #11 blade knife is used to pierce the skin wheal and incise the fascia, which is followed by a passage of an 18-gauge needle.

(f) PUT

(i) The PUT device is the size of an 18-gauge needle with a blunted tip and cannot enter the pathological area without this incision (Fig. 18.12).

(ii) Once the PUT device is visualized at the tip of the pathological area, the device is activated via a foot pedal.

(iii) The device should be guided throughout the pathological area while minimizing the irritation to the healthy tendon tissue [45]. The literature has described the device being used for 30–50 s of ultrasonic energy in most instances to adequately treat the lesion. However, some authors have used up to 100–120 s for more diffuse tendinopathy [43–45]. Improper placement of the tip may result in poorer outcomes.

(iv) Note that ossified tissues are not removable by this technique, however, the TX-Bone, is an ultrasound device, which may be considered to emulsify, fragment, or aspirate hard tissues [53].

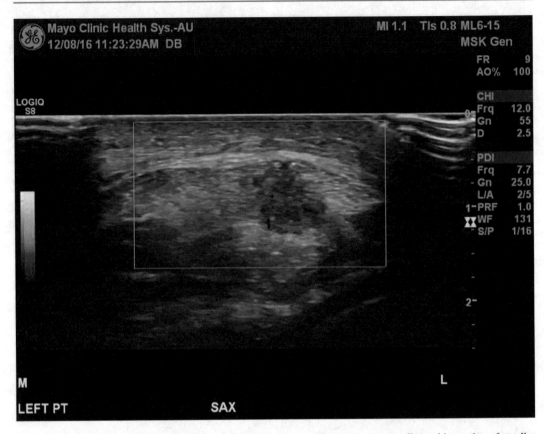

Fig. 18.10 The given ultrasound image demonstrates patellar tendinosis in the short axis. Note the loss of fibular tendon and the edema near the site of insertion. P = patellar tendon, * = tendinopathic portion of patellar tendon, H = Hoffa fat pad

    (v) Wound closure is done using a sterile adhesive dressing.
(g) Post-procedure protocol
    (i) Ice is recommended for the night of the procedure along with acetaminophen or acetaminophen/codeine.
    (ii) There is currently no data regarding outcomes based on different post-procedure protocols.
    (iii) The authors of this chapter advise following recommendations regarding post-procedure activity from Peck and colleagues [13].
    (iv) Toe-touch weight bearing on the treated limb using a knee immobilizer and crutches for 1 week. After 1–2 weeks of the procedure, the patient can progress to 50% partial weight bearing.

    (v) Patients should be instructed to perform active knee range-of-motion exercises starting at 2 days post-procedure and continue for the first 2 weeks post-procedure.
    (vi) After week 2, we recommend following the same post-procedure protocol used for PNT. Please refer to PNT post-procedure stages v–ix [1, 13].
    (vii) NSAID use pre- and post-procedure is something that is debated in the academic community. There are currently no trials that clearly show with or without NSAIDs as superior or inferior. However, because of the

Fig. 18.11 The given figure demonstrates the approximate needle/probe insertion site for percutaneous ultrasonic tenotomy of the patellar tendon

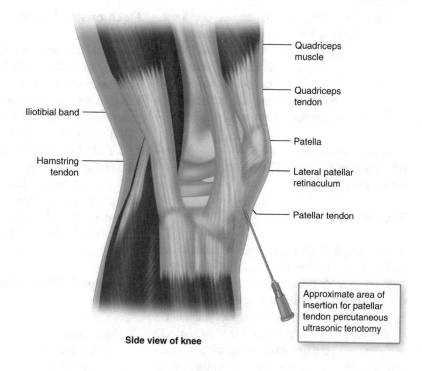

Quadriceps muscle

Quadriceps tendon

Iliotibial band

Patella

Hamstring tendon

Lateral patellar retinaculum

Patellar tendon

Approximate area of insertion for patellar tendon percutaneous ultrasonic tenotomy

Side view of knee

Fig. 18.12 The given illustration shows the proper technique of the probe entering the small incision over the patellar tendon for percutaneous needle tenotomy

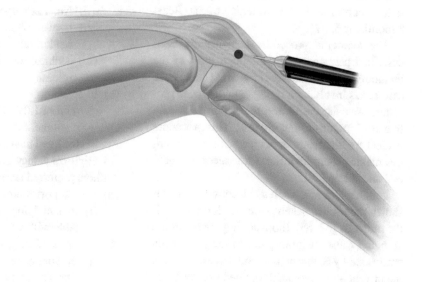

mechanism of action previously described we recommend our patients to avoid NSAIDs for 1 week prior to the procedure and at least 2 weeks post-procedure to avoid inhibiting the inflammatory stage of tendon healing [1, 13].

Biceps and Iliopsoas Tendon Releases

Background

The biceps and iliopsoas tendon releases are advanced procedures and confirmation prior to proceeding with these procedures is necessary. Oftentimes a lidocaine challenge may be helpful in determining the source of the pain generator.

The long head of the bicep tendon (LHBT) is a common pain generator in shoulder pathology [54–56]. Bicep tenotomy is indicated for patients with shoulder pain who have rotator cuff tears or biceps-labral pathology that have failed conservative treatments of at least 3 months [56, 57].

The tenotomy procedure has recently been described percutaneously, although most of the literature involves cadavers [58–61]. There is one case series involving a living patient whose procedure was successful and the patient was pain free at 15 months follow-up [59]. This procedure is ideal for a patient population with comorbidities making them high risk for surgery and general anesthesia [59].

Another musculoskeletal location that has shown pain relief benefit from tendon release is the iliopsoas [62, 63]. Iliopsoas impingement is a common cause of groin pain. In the pilot study performed by Sampson and colleagues, a patient underwent sonographically guided percutaneous iliopsoas tenotomy and had complete pain resolution at 9 weeks [63]. Percutaneous bicipital and iliopsoas release done with ultrasound are evolving procedures that have limited data regarding its safety and efficacy [59, 60, 63] .

Mechanism of Action

The LHBT is associated with shoulder pain, particularly in patients who have rotator cuff tears. The mechanism for pain associated with the LHBT is unclear. However, Walch noted that his patients who had pathology associated with LHBT experienced pain relief with rupture of the LHBT. He decided that in these patients who have failed other options, he would perform the rupture of the tendon himself (tenotomy) in an attempt to provide relief [56]. Since that time, tenotomy has proven to provide patients with relief via an unclear mechanism [55–57].

Procedural Details: Bicep Tendon Release

I. Equipment
   (a) Needles
      (i) Smallest bore needle for local anesthetics (generally 30-gauge or 27-gauge)
      (ii) No. 11 Scalpel for stab incision
      (iii) Beaver 6900 mini-blade for Bicep tendon release
      (iv) Arthrex hook knife for Bicep tendon release
   (b) Injectate
      (i) 4 ml of 1.0% lidocaine, 1 ml of triamcinolone, 0.5 ml of 0.2% ropivacaine for local anesthesia
   (c) High-frequency linear array transducer
II. Authors preferred technique
   (a) Patient positioning
      (i) Patient lying supine on examination table with arm supinated
   (b) Pre- procedure scan
      (i) Sonographic evaluation with the transducer placed over the anterior aspect of the arm, locating the LHBT (Figs. 18.13 and 18.14). The performing physician should identify the transverse humeral ligament (THL) and the superior aspect of the pectora-

lis major tendon insertion on the humerus. A mark should be made of the skin with sterile marker inferior to the THL and 1 cm superior to the pectoralis major as this is considered the safe zone (Fig. 18.15). Although not expressed in literature, the authors suggest marking the region of the musculocutaneous nerve for proper safety.

(ii) Cadaver studies have shown complications including iatrogenic (blade) injuries on the cartilage of the humeral head, lacerations of the supraspinatus tendon, and subscapularis tendon. Therefore, it is vital to visualize these structures prior to the procedure [58, 60, 61].

(c) Sterile procedure

(i) Apply sterile gloves and then sterilely prepare (may use chlorhexidine appli-

cator or betadine swabs) a large area beyond the target site (Fig. 18.16).

(ii) Sterilely drape the area.

(iii) Apply a sterile transducer cover kit followed by sterile gel to the probe.

(d) Anesthetic

(i) Insert the anesthetic needle under continuous sonographic visualization in plane to the transducer while viewing the biceps tendon in short axis. Anesthetize the skin, subcutaneous tissue, the tendon, and the long head of biceps sheath.

(e) Tendon release

(i) A #11 blade knife is used to make a 0.5 cm superficial incision where the anesthetic was injected. A Beaver 6900 mini-blade creates a track to the LHBT and frees the biceps tendon undersurface from periosteum (Fig. 18.17).

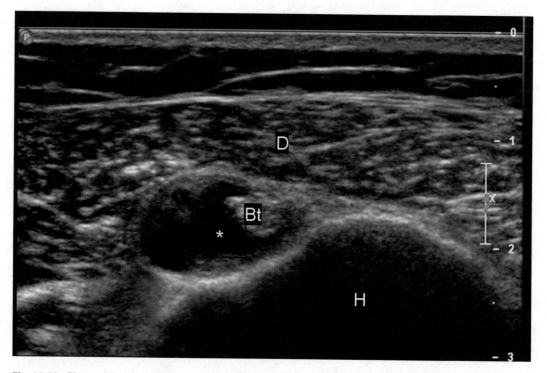

Fig. 18.13 Short axis image demonstrating severe long head biceps tenosynovitis with effusion (asterisks) and tenosynovial thickening (arrow) Bt = long head biceps tendon; H = humerus; D = deltoid

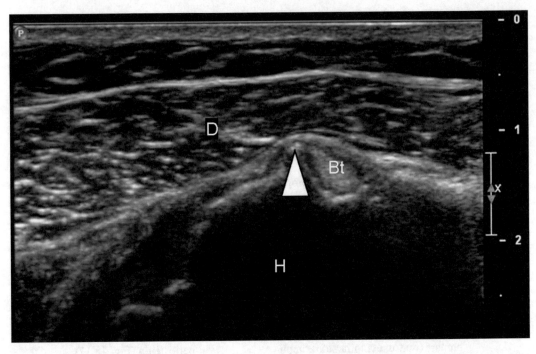

Fig. 18.14 Note hypertrophic bony osteophytes at proximal groove (arrowhead) resulting in impingement of the biceps tendon. Right side of image is lateral. Bt = long head biceps tendon; H = humerus; D = deltoid

Fig. 18.15 The given illustration demonstrates the anatomy involved in a percutaneous bicipital tendon release. Note the area that is considered the safe entry zone as to avoid injury

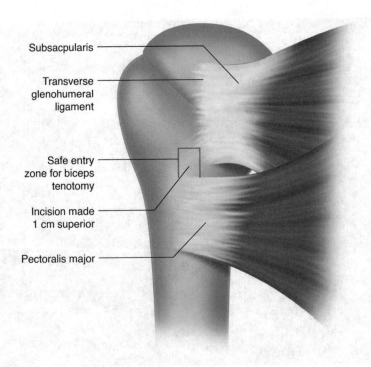

(ii) The ultrasound probe is visualizing the tendon in the short axis, when the Arthrex hook knife is advanced toward the long head of the tendon. The hook knife is advanced under the tendon and is placed between the bone and bicep tendon (Figs. 18.18 and 18.19). Once this is confirmed sonographically, the knife is rotated and pulled through the tendon until resistance is lost (Fig. 18.20). A fluid gap now created between tendon ends should be sonographically confirmed (Figs. 18.21 and 18.22). Upon completion of tenotomy, inject 1 ml of triamcinolone and 0.5 ml of 0.2% ropivacaine into the tendon sheath for pain and inflammation control [59].

(iii) Sonographic examination of surrounding soft tissue should be performed to ensure no iatrogenic injury occurred.

(iv) Monitor for hematoma formation secondary to an injury to the circumflex artery or any vasculature.

(v) Wound closure is done using a sterile adhesive dressing.

(f) Post-procedure protocol

(i) Percutaneous bicep tendon release does not have a clear timeline in the literature for recovery. However, one case report shows complete resolution of patient's symptoms at 15 month post-procedure follow-up [59].

(Technique described by Dr. Hall)

Fig. 18.16 Note patient positioning and that the procedure is performed using sterile technique. (Images provided by Dr. Mederick Hall)

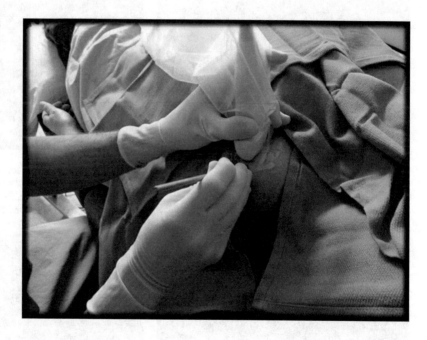

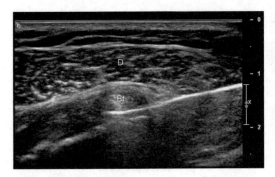

Fig. 18.17 The ultrasound image depicts a Beaver 6900 mini-blade (arrows) used to create a tract down to the long head biceps tendon and free the undersurface for introduction of the hook knife. (Images provided by Dr. Mederick Hall)

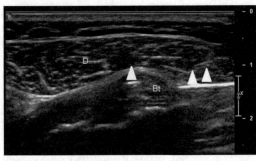

Fig. 18.20 An Arthrex hook knife is introduced through the incision and guided under the tendon Fig. 18.19 and rotated to engage the tendon in this figure, after which the knife is pulled and the tendon is released. (Images provided by Dr. Mederick Hall)

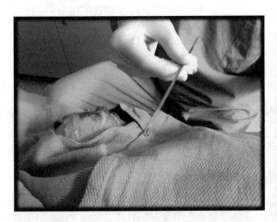

Fig. 18.18 An Arthrex hook knife is then introduced through the incision and guided under the tendon. (Images provided by Dr. Mederick Hall)

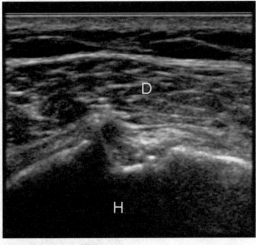

Fig. 18.21 The ultrasound image is a short axis image at the same location as Fig. 18.17 demonstrating the absence of tendon within the groove. Right side of imaging is lateral. (Images provided by Dr. Mederick Hall)

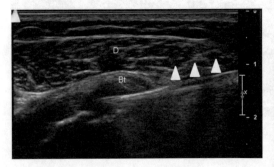

Fig. 18.19 An Arthrex hook knife is then introduced through the incision and guided under the tendon. (Images provided by Dr. Mederick Hall)

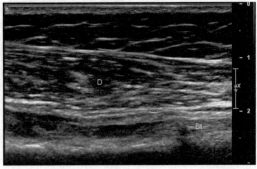

Fig. 18.22 The given ultrasound image is the long axis image demonstrating the retracting bicep tendon stump. Right side of image is distal. Bt = long head biceps tendon; H = humerus; D = deltoid. (Images provided by Dr. Mederick Hall)

References

1. Finnoff JT, Fowler SP, Lai JK, Santrach PJ, Willis EA, Sayeed YA, et al. Treatment of chronic tendinopathy with ultrasound-guided needle tenotomy and platelet-rich plasma injection. PM R. 2011;3(10):900–11.
2. Ohberg L, Alfredson H. Ultrasound guided sclerosis of neovessels in painful chronic Achilles tendinosis: pilot study of a new treatment. Br J Sports Med. 2002;36(3):173–5; discussion 6–7.
3. Del Buono A, Chan O, Maffulli N. Achilles tendon: functional anatomy and novel emerging models of imaging classification. Int Orthop. 2013;37(4):715–21.
4. Morton S, Chan O, King J, Perry D, Crisp T, Maffulli N, et al. High volume image-guided injections for patellar tendinopathy: a combined retrospective and prospective case series. Muscles Ligaments Tendons J. 2014;4(2):214–9.
5. Crisp T, Khan F, Padhiar N, Morrissey D, King J, Jalan R, et al. High volume ultrasound guided injections at the interface between the patellar tendon and Hoffa's body are effective in chronic patellar tendinopathy: a pilot study. D bil Rehabil. 2008;30(20–22):1625–34.
6. Chan O, O'Dowd D, Padhiar N, Morrissey D, King J, Jalan R, et al. High volume image guided injections in chronic Achilles tendinopathy. Disabil Rehabil. 2008;30(20–22):1697–708.
7. Maffulli N, Del Buono A, Oliva F, Testa V, Capasso G, Maffulli G. High-volume image-guided injection for recalcitrant patellar tendinopathy in athletes. Clin J Sport Med. 2016;26(1):12–6.
8. Humphrey J, Chan O, Crisp T, Padhiar N, Morrissey D, Twycross-Lewis R, et al. The short-term effects of high volume image guided injections in resistant non-insertional Achilles tendinopathy. J Sci Med Sport. 2010;13(3):295–8.
9. Maffulli N, Spiezia F, Longo UG, Denaro V, Maffulli GD. High volume image guided injections for the management of chronic tendinopathy of the main body of the Achilles tendon. Phys Ther Sport. 2013;14(3):163–7.
10. Morton S, Chan O, Ghozlan A, Price J, Perry J, Morrissey D. High volume image guided injections and structured rehabilitation in shoulder impingement syndrome: a retrospective study. Muscles Ligaments Tendons J. 2015;5(3):195–9.
11. Morton S, Chan O, Price J, Pritchard M, Crisp T, Perry JD, et al. High volume image-guided injections and structured rehabilitation improve greater trochanter pain syndrome in the short and medium term: a combined retrospective and prospective case series. Muscles Ligaments Tendons J. 2015;5(2):73–87.
12. Coombes BK, Bisset L, Brooks P, Khan A, Vicenzino B. Effect of corticosteroid injection, physiotherapy, or both on clinical outcomes in patients with unilateral lateral epicondylalgia: a randomized controlled trial. JAMA. 2013;309(5):461–9.
13. Peck E, Jelsing E, Onishi K. Advanced ultrasound-guided interventions for tendinopathy. Phys Med Rehabil Clin N Am. 2016;27(3):733–48.
14. Puddu G, Ippolito E, Postacchini F. A classification of Achilles tendon disease. Am J Sports Med. 1976;4(4):145–50.
15. Khan KM, Cook JL, Bonar F, Harcourt P, Astrom M. Histopathology of common tendinopathies. Update and implications for clinical management. Sports Med (Auckland, NZ). 1999;27(6):393–408.
16. Khan KM, Cook JL, Taunton JE, Bonar F. Overuse tendinosis, not tendinitis part 1: a new paradigm for a difficult clinical problem. Phys Sportsmed. 2000;28(5):38–48.
17. Charnoff J, Naqvi U. Tendinosis (tendinitis). StatPearls. Treasure Island: StatPearls Publishing StatPearls Publishing LLC; 2018.
18. Nirschl RP. Elbow tendinosis/tennis elbow. Clin Sports Med. 1992;11(4):851–70.
19. Nirschl RP, Pettrone FA. Tennis elbow. The surgical treatment of lateral epicondylitis. J Bone Joint Surg Am. 1979;61(6a):832–9.
20. Dakin SG, Dudhia J, Smith RK. Resolving an inflammatory concept: the importance of inflammation and resolution in tendinopathy. Vet Immunol Immunopathol. 2014;158(3–4):121–7.
21. Abate M, Silbernagel KG, Siljeholm C, Di Iorio A, De Amicis D, Salini V, et al. Pathogenesis of tendinopathies: inflammation or degeneration? Arthritis Res Ther. 2009;11(3):235.
22. Alfredson H, Ohberg L, Forsgren S. Is vasculo-neural ingrowth the cause of pain in chronic Achilles tendinosis? An investigation using ultrasonography and colour Doppler, immunohistochemistry, and diagnostic injections. Knee Surg Sports Traumatol Arthrosc. 2003;11(5):334–8.
23. Andersson G, Danielson P, Alfredson H, Forsgren S. Nerve-related characteristics of ventral paratendinous tissue in chronic Achilles tendinosis. Knee Surg Sports Traumatol Arthrosc. 2007;15(10):1272–9.
24. Alfredson H, Pietila T, Jonsson P, Lorentzon R. Heavy-load eccentric calf muscle training for the treatment of chronic Achilles tendinosis. Am J Sports Med. 1998;26(3):360–6.
25. Forsgren S, Danielson P, Alfredson H. Vascular NK-1 receptor occurrence in normal and chronic painful Achilles and patellar tendons: studies on chemically unfixed as well as fixed specimens. Regul Pept. 2005;126(3):173–81.
26. Wheeler PC, Mahadevan D, Bhatt R, Bhatia M. A comparison of two different high-volume image-guided injection procedures for patients with chronic noninsertional Achilles tendinopathy: a pragmatic retrospective cohort study. J Foot Ankle Surg. 2016;55(5):976–9.
27. Piper SL, Laron D, Manzano G, Pattnaik T, Liu X, Kim HT, et al. A comparison of lidocaine, ropivacaine and dexamethasone toxicity on bovine tenocytes in culture. J Bone Joint Surg. 2012;94(6):856–62.
28. Zhang AZ, Ficklscherer A, Gulecyuz MF, Paulus AC, Niethammer TR, Jansson V, et al. Cell toxicity in fibroblasts, tenocytes, and human mesenchymal stem cells-a comparison of necrosis and apoptosis-

inducing ability in Ropivacaine, bupivacaine, and tri-amcinolone. Arthroscopy. 2017;33(4):840–8.

29. Alfredson H, Ohberg L, Zeisig E, Lorentzon R. Treatment of midportion Achilles tendinosis: similar clinical results with US and CD-guided surgery outside the tendon and sclerosing polidocanol injections. Knee Surg Sports Traumatol Arthrosc. 2007;15(12):1504–9.

30. Alfredson H. Ultrasound and Doppler-guided mini-surgery to treat midportion Achilles tendinosis: results of a large material and a randomised study comparing two scraping techniques. Br J Sports Med. 2011;45(5):407–10.

31. Hall MM, Rajasekaran S. Ultrasound-guided scraping for chronic patellar tendinopathy: a case presentation. PM R. 2016;8(6):593–6.

32. Bedi HS, Jowett C, Ristanis S, Docking S, Cook J. Plantaris excision and ventral paratendinous scraping for Achilles tendinopathy in an athletic population. Foot Ankle Int. 2016;37(4):386–93.

33. McShane JM, Nazarian LN, Harwood MI. Sonographically guided percutaneous needle tenotomy for treatment of common extensor tendinosis in the elbow. J Ultrasound Med. 2006;25(10):1281–9.

34. Chiavaras MM, Jacobson JA. Ultrasound-guided tendon fenestration. Semin Musculoskelet Radiol. 2013;17(1):85–90.

35. McShane JM, Shah VN, Nazarian LN. Sonographically guided percutaneous needle tenotomy for treatment of common extensor tendinosis in the elbow: is a corticosteroid necessary? J Ultrasound Med. 2008;27(8):1137–44.

36. Housner JA, Jacobson JA, Misko R. Sonographically guided percutaneous needle tenotomy for the treatment of chronic tendinosis. J Ultrasound Med. 2009;28(9):1187–92.

37. Mattie R, Wong J, McCormick Z, Yu S, Saltychev M, Laimi K. Percutaneous needle tenotomy for the treatment of lateral epicondylitis: a systematic review of the literature. PM R. 2017;9(6):603–11.

38. Jacobson JA, Chiavaras MM, Lawton JM, Downie B, Yablon CM, Lawton J. Radial collateral ligament of the elbow: sonographic characterization with cadaveric dissection correlation and magnetic resonance arthrography. J Ultrasound Med. 2014;33(6):1041–8.

39. Jacobson JA, Rubin J, Yablon CM, Kim SM, Kalume-Brigido M, Parameswaran A. Ultrasound-guided fenestration of tendons about the hip and pelvis: clinical outcomes. J Ultrasound Med. 2015;34(11):2029–35.

40. Housner JA, Jacobson JA, Morag Y, Pujalte GG, Northway RM, Boon TA. Should ultrasound-guided needle fenestration be considered as a treatment option for recalcitrant patellar tendinopathy? A retrospective study of 47 cases. Clin J Sport Med. 2010;20(6):488–90.

41. Kelman CD. The history and development of phaco-emulsification. Int Ophthalmol Clin. 1994;34(2):1–12.

42. Paul T, Braga-Mele R. Bimanual microincisional phacoemulsification: the future of cataract surgery? Curr Opin Ophthalmol. 2005;16(1):2–7.

43. Barnes D. Ultrasonic energy in tendon treatment. Oper Tech Orthop. 2013;23:78–83.

44. Barnes DE, Beckley JM, Smith J. Percutaneous ultrasonic tenotomy for chronic elbow tendinosis: a prospective study. J Shoulder Elb Surg. 2015;24(1):67–73.

45. Elattrache NS, Morrey BF. Percutaneous ultrasonic tenotomy as a treatment for chronic patellar tendinopathy—Jumper's knee. Oper Tech Orthop. 2013;23(2):98–103.

46. Patel MM. A novel treatment for refractory plantar fasciitis. Am J Orthop (Belle Mead, NJ). 2015;44(3):107–10.

47. Seng C, Mohan PC, Koh SB, Howe TS, Lim YG, Lee BP, et al. Ultrasonic percutaneous tenotomy for recalcitrant lateral elbow tendinopathy: sustainability and sonographic progression at 3 years. Am J Sports Med. 2016;44(2):504–10.

48. Levin D, Nazarian LN, Miller TT, O'Kane PL, Feld RI, Parker L, et al. Lateral epicondylitis of the elbow: US findings. Radiology. 2005;237(1):230–4.

49. Koh JS, Mohan PC, Howe TS, Lee BP, Chia SL, Yang Z, et al. Fasciotomy and surgical tenotomy for recalcitrant lateral elbow tendinopathy: early clinical experience with a novel device for minimally invasive percutaneous microresection. Am J Sports Med. 2013;41(3):636–44.

50. Chimenti RL, Stover DW, Fick BS, Hall MM. Percutaneous ultrasonic tenotomy reduces insertional Achilles tendinopathy pain with high patient satisfaction and a low complication rate. J Ultrasound Med. 2019;38(6):1629–35.

51. Zhang J, Wang JH. PRP treatment effects on degenerative tendinopathy - an in vitro model study. Muscles Ligaments Tendons J. 2014;4(1):10–7.

52. Kamineni S, Butterfield T, Sinai A. Percutaneous ultrasonic debridement of tendinopathy-a pilot Achilles rabbit model. J Orthop Surg Res. 2015;10:70.

53. Eisner W. FDA clears ultrasonic device from Tenex Health 2019. Available from: https://ryortho.com/breaking/fda-clears-ultrasonic-device-from-tenex-health.

54. Elser F, Braun S, Dewing CB, Giphart JE, Millett PJ. Anatomy, function, injuries, and treatment of the long head of the biceps brachii tendon. Arthroscopy. 2011;27(4):581–92.

55. Hsu AR, Ghodadra NS, Provencher MT, Lewis PB, Bach BR. Biceps tenotomy versus tenodesis: a review of clinical outcomes and biomechanical results. J Shoulder Elb Surg. 2011;20(2):326–32.

56. Szabo I, Boileau P, Walch G. The proximal biceps as a pain generator and results of tenotomy. Sports Med Arthrosc Rev. 2008;16(3):180–6.

57. Gausden EB, Taylor SA, Ramkumar P, Nwachukwu BU, Corpus K, Rebolledo BJ, et al. Tenotomy, tenodesis, transfer: a review of treatment options for

biceps-labrum complex disease. Am J Orthop (Belle Mead, NJ). 2016;45(7):E503–e11.

58. Levy B, Ducat A, Gaudin P, Maqdes A, Brasseur JL, Klouche S, et al. Ultrasound-guided percutaneous tenotomy of the long head of the biceps tendon: a non-reliable technique. Knee Surg Sports Traumatol Arthrosc. 2012;20(6):1027–30.

59. Greditzer H, Kaplan L, Lesniak B, Jose J. Ultrasound-guided percutaneous long head of the biceps tenotomy: a novel technique with case report. HSS J. 2014;10:240–4.

60. Sconfienza LM, Mauri G, Messina C, Aliprandi A, Secchi F, Sardanelli F, et al. Ultrasound-guided percutaneous tenotomy of biceps tendon: technical feasibility on cadavers. Ultrasound Med Biol. 2016;42(10):2513–7.

61. Aly AR, Rajasekaran S, Mohamed A, Beavis C, Obaid H. Feasibility of ultrasound-guided percutaneous tenotomy of the long head of the biceps tendon – a pilot cadaveric study. J Clin Ultrasound. 2015;43(6):361–6.

62. Heaton K, Dorr LD. Surgical release of iliopsoas tendon for groin pain after total hip arthroplasty. J Arthroplast. 2002;17(6):779–81.

63. Sampson MJ, Rezaian N, Hopkins JM. Ultrasound-guided percutaneous tenotomy for the treatment of iliopsoas impingement: a description of tech-

nique and case study. J Med Imaging Radiat Oncol. 2015;59(2):195–9.

64. Resteghini P, Yeoh J. High-volume injection in the management of recalcitrant mid-body Achilles tendinopathy: a prospective case series assessing the influence of neovascularity and outcome. Int Musculoskelet Med. 2012;34(3):92–100.

65. Wheeler PC. The use of high-volume image-guided injections (HVIGI) for Achilles tendinopathy – a case series and pilot study. Int Musculoskelet Med. 2014;36(3):96–103.

66. Wheeler PC, Tattersall C. Novel interventions for recalcitrant Achilles tendinopathy: benefits seen following high-volume image-guided injection or extracorporeal shockwave therapy-a prospective cohort study. Clin J Sport Med. 2020;30(1):14–9.

67. Zhu J, Hu B, Xing C, Li J. Ultrasound-guided, minimally invasive, percutaneous needle puncture treatment for tennis elbow. Adv Ther. 2008;25(10):1031–6.

68. Razdan R, Vanderwoude E. Percutaneous ultrasonic fasciotomy: a novel approach to treat chronic plantar fasciitis. J Vasc Interv Radiol. 2015;26(2):S40.

69. Battista CT, Dorweiler MA, Fisher ML, Morrey BF, Noyes MP. Ultrasonic percutaneous tenotomy of common extensor tendons for recalcitrant lateral epicondylitis. Tech Hand Up Extrem Surg. 2018;22(1):15–8.

Office-Based Orthobiologic Procedures for Tendons

19

David J. Cormier, Todd R. Hayano, Lauren Elson, and Joanne Borg-Stein

Abbreviations

ABI	Autologous blood injection
AECs	Amniotic epithelial cells
ASCs	Adipose stem cells
ATD	Adipose tissue derivatives
BMAC	Bone marrow aspirate concentrate
CTPs	Connective tissue progenators
ECM	Extracellular matrix
FDA	Food and Drug Administration
LR-PRP	PRP with elevated leukocytes
MFAT	Microfragmented adipose tissue
MSC	Mesenchymal stem cell
MSK	Musculoskeletal
PRP	Platelet-rich plasma
PSIS	Posterior superior iliac spine
RBCs	Red blood cells
SVF	Stromal vascular fraction
TSCs	Tendon-specific stem cells
WBCs	White blood cells

D. J. Cormier (✉) · T. R. Hayano
L. Elson · J. Borg-Stein
Department of Physical Medicine and Rehabilitation,
Harvard Medical School, Spaulding Rehabilitation
Hospital, Charlestown, MA, USA
e-mail: lelson@partners.org; jborgstein@partners.org

Introduction

The field of regenerative medicine and orthobiologics, defined as the use of biological tissue to optimize treatment of musculoskeletal injuries, is not new. Platelet-rich plasma (PRP) therapy has been in use on joints, ligaments, and some tendons since the 1970s. However, there has been a growing interest in the use of office-based orthobiologic treatments of tendons for four reasons. First, the emergence of the musculoskeletal (MSK) ultrasound for diagnosis and evaluation of tendons allows improved procedural outcomes by offering higher accuracy and less pain than palpation-guided injections [1]. Second, the field has seen an improved understanding of tendinopathy. As discussed in Chaps. 1 and 2, tendinopathy is a painful tendon condition caused by a combination of degeneration and inflammation [2–4]. It may take 1–2 years for a tendon to heal after an injury, the process by which is influenced by several growth factors. bFGF, BMP-12,-13,-14, CTGF, IGF-1, PDGF, and TGFB are important for tendon healing, whereas others such as IL10, IL-1, matrix metalloproteinases 1, 2, 3, and 4, and HAFCs have anti-inflammatory effects [6]. Third, our veterinary and oral surgical colleagues utilizing orthobiologics in animals have had promising outcomes [5, 7–13]. Through their research, we know that orthobiologics have the ability to augment disordered healing process and reduce scar formation contributing to the disease process of tendinopathy [6]. Orthobiologics are apparently successful, in part, because they contain growth factors associated with tendon healing [6]. Finally, there is a growing evidence demonstrating that corticosteroid injection provides short-term relief but does not alter long-term outcomes, and actually it might promote tendon degeneration, increasing the risk of tendon ruptures [14–17]. Thus, other injection alternatives are being sought [18–22]. The emerging office-based procedures for tendinopathy discussed below are currently considered an alternative to surgical intervention for patients with chronic refractory symptoms following the failure of other conservative treatment options.

PRP

Platelet-rich plasma (PRP) has become an increasingly popular regenerative therapy in musculoskeletal and sports medicine for its potential to treat and repair acute and chronic tendinopathies. PRP is an autologous plasma derivative in which the concentration of platelets is above the baseline level. Treatment with PRP involves its injection/infiltration into the affected area, which theoretically stimulates regenerative healing. Advantages of PRP relative to other office orthobiologics include ease of obtaining substrates from autologous blood, ease of performing the procedure, its low cost compared to other orthobiologics, and its demonstrated safety. Nevertheless, PRP remains controversial in the literature due to the lack of standardization in the consistency of the substrate and perhaps due to the need for a better understanding of tendinopathy as a disease entity. The inconsistencies across studies have made it difficult to fully evaluate the efficacy of this treatment option. See Table 19.1 [23–89].

Classification System

PRP remains a controversial treatment option for tendinopathy in large part because the literature on its efficacy appears inconsistent. This apparent inconsistency results from the fact that effi-

cacy can be difficult to measure since it is dependent on both the type of tendinopathy treated and the type of PRP used. Moreover, many studies fail to report the basic characteristics of the PRP preparation, such as platelet concentration/counts, the number of white blood cells (WBCs) including differential counts, the presence or absence of red blood cells (RBCs) and RBC remnants, whether there is platelet activation to provoke degranulation, and the release of the alpha granules. Studies often also fail to report the volume of PRP delivered, the specific injection location (peritendinous or intratendinous), the needle size, whether there was mechanical trauma, and whether ultrasound guidance was used.

As a result of this inconsistent reporting, previous publications had attempted to create standardized criteria that would allow studies to be accurately analyzed and compared. For example, some authors classify PRP into leukocyte-rich vs leukocyte-poor preparations. Leukocyte-rich preparations have a neutrophil concentration higher than baseline, while leukocyte-poor preparations have a neutrophil concentration lower than baseline. Delong et al. developed a system called PAW classification, which categorizes platelet levels (with the most efficacious being around two to three times above baseline), the presence of activation, the white blood cell count, and the presence of neutrophils [90]. Mishra et al. also described a classification system that focused on platelet concentration, WBC count, and activation [91]. These classification systems have been criticized for their failures to evaluate the role of red blood cell counts and the detrimental effect of RBC remnants, to review newer technology/methods available, to account for volumes of PRP, and to appreciate the importance of neutrophils' presence [92]. Thus, Mautner et al. developed a classification system that calls for documentation of the concentration of platelets, leukocytes, and red blood cells [93]. The Mautner classification PRLA is the most widely used classification system at the time of this publication [93] (see Table 19.2), but still others exist. For example, Lana et al. describe a system MARSPILL that includes the methods

Table 19.1 PRP studies

Lateral epicondyle tendinopathy	
Peerbooms ([23] and 2011)	Randomized control trials have demonstrated the efficacy of PRP for treating chronic LET with 1-year and 2-year improvements superior in function and pain compared to steroid injection
Thanasas et al. [24]	PRP was superior to autologous blood injection (ABI) at reducing pain at 6 weeks, but inferior to ABI at improving function by 6 months
Krough (2013)	PRP was no different when compared to steroid or saline at reducing pain and improving function at 3 months, inferior to steroid at improving pain and function at 1 month and associated with greater post-injection pain
Nasser et al. [26]	PRP compared against glucocorticoid and saline injections showed that PRP was significant in pain reduction and led to more homogenous tendon healing than corticosteroid and saline after 3 months of follow-up
IMPROVE Trial (expected in June 2018, trial closed)	Multicenter RCT comparing autologous PRP, autologous whole blood, dry needle fenestration, and physical therapy alone on pain and quality of life in patients with LET
Achilles tendinopathy	
De Vos [28] and De Jonge [29]	RCTs did not demonstrate significant differences in outcomes of clinical function, tendon healing, or return to sport times at either 6 months or 1 year between PRP and saline injection
Schepull et al. [30]	Reported PRP injections did not improve mechanical properties or functional performance of the Achilles tendon up to 1 year after surgical repair of an acute rupture compared to no PRP injection
Gaweda [31], Volpi [32], Finnoff et al. [33], Owens et al. [34], Monto [55], Ferrero et al. [36], Deans et al. [37], Gosens et al. [38], Kearney et al. [39], Mautner et al. [40], Filardo et al. [41], Murawski et al. [42], Filardo et al. [43], Charousset et al. [44], and Oloff et al. [45]	Multiple studies for chronic Achilles tendinopathy, including case series, pilot studies, and retrospective studies, have reported promising results for the efficacy of PRP injections with lasting improvements in functional outcomes at 4 years
DeVos [46]	PRP did not provide significantly different neovascularization response or ultrasonographically assessed change in tendon structure over 6 months compared to saline injection in chronic Achilles tendinopathy
Zou et al. [47]	PRP is safe and effective for surgical repair of acute tendon mid-tear rupture and may improve early-midterm postoperative functional recovery
Krough et al. [48]	A single PRP injection vs. saline (placebo) after 3 months did not show any difference in pain, but it did demonstrate significant difference in tendon thickness. However, noted to have a large dropout rate
Patellar tendinopathy	
Kon et al. [49], Volpi et al. [32], Ferrero et al. [36], Gosens et al. [38], Mautner et al. [40], Filardo et al. [41], Charousset et al. [44]	Multiple studies demonstrate results from case series and retrospective studies to have shown promise for PRP injection to improve function in patients with chronic patellar tendinopathy, with lasting effects in functional outcomes at 4 years
De Almeida et al. [50] and Cervellin et al. [51]	RCTs for the application of PRP to patellar tendinopathy harvest sites for ACL reconstruction were found to provide significant reduction in postoperative pain, greater donor patellar tendon healing at 6 months, and greater function at 12 months
Vetrano [52]	10 cc of single spin, non-activated PRP provided by a 22-gauge needle without anesthetic showed that athletes with chronic patellar tendinopathy responded positively to both PRP and ESWT, but PRP had significantly greater improvements in pain and functional outcomes.
Dragoo [52]	Ultrasound-guided PRP injection administered with dry needling accelerated recovery from patellar tendinopathy relative to dry needling alone, but benefits to pain and function dissipated after 3 months without improvement to quality of life

(continued)

Table 19.1 (continued)

Kaux et al. [54] and Zayni et al. [55]	Studies have demonstrated efficacy of PRP for treating patellar tendinopathy, with superior outcomes at 1 year compared to ECSW therapy
Kaux et al. [56]	Comparison between single infiltration vs. double infiltrations of PRP demonstrated improvement of symptoms by both procedures on chronic patellar tendinopahty previously unresponsive to other treatments out to at least 1 year, but there was no difference between single vs. double infiltration
Scott et al. [89]	RCT with 1-year follow-up evaluated that exercise, LR PRP, LP-PRP is no more effective than saline
Rotator cuff tendinopathy	
Gumina et al. [57]	PRP improved repair integrity for large tears without an associated improvement in function and had lower rates of re-tears for small to large tears at 1 year
Randelli et al. [58] and Malavolta et al. [59]	Intra-operative local application of autologous PRP to arthroscopic repair sites of complete rotator cuff tears has been associated with significantly less pain within the first postoperative month and greater strength within the first 3 months compared with standard repair alone. It showed benefits more pronounced for less extensive tears; however, benefits to pain, function, and healing were not seen beyond a year
Jo [60] and Hak [61]	Reported early, underpowered studies demonstrating no significant benefit to pain or function of PRP augmentation during arthroscopic rotator cuff repair
Rodeo et al. [62] and Carr et al. [63]	Not only reported no significant benefit from PRP but also suggested potential negative effects on rotator cuff healing
Hamstring	
Reurink et al. [65]	A single-blinded RCT demonstrated that PRP significantly reduced pain intensity over 10 weeks and accelerated return to sport by 16 days for acute hamstring partial tears
Reurink et al. [64, 65]	US-guided intramuscular injections of PRP vs. saline, both combined with rehab for acute hamstring injuries, showed no significant difference between groups in reinjury rates at 2 months or 1 year nor return to sport at 6 months or 1 year
Fader et al. [66]	18 patients with chronic proximal hamstring tendinopathy treated with ultrasound-guided PRP demonstrated that 10 patients had 80% or greater improvement to pain at 6 months and an overall average improvement of 63% for all patients
Hamilton et al. [67]	Large, double-blinded RCTs showed that PRP injections provided no significant benefit when compared with intensive rehab alone for return to sport, muscle strength, or reinjury rates after 2 and 6 months in acute hamstring injuries
Plantar fasciopathy	
Ragab and Othman [68], Martinelli et al. [69], and Kumar et al. [70]	Early cohort studies have reported the benefit of PRP on improving pain, function, and tissue structure for chronic plantar fasciopathy
Lee and Ahmad and [71], Omar et al. [72], Aksahin et al. [73], Mautner et al. [40], Say et al. [74], Monto et al. [75], Shetty et al. [76], and Jain et al. [77]	Comparisons in efficacy between PRP an d corticosteroid injection without a placebo control which showed variable results. Results ranged from PRP providing greater early pain reduction and functional improvement with lasting effects at 1 and 2 years; others reported equally effective results between PRP and corticosteroids at 3 and 6 months and finally others demonstrated less effective results for PRP in reducing pain at 3 months
Kim and Lee [78]	PRP was as effective as prolotherapy in reducing pain and improving function at 6 months for plantar fasciopathy
Mahindra et al. [79]	Reported a double-blinded RCT comparing PRP vs. corticosteroid which showed that PRP was as effective as or more effective than corticosteroid when compared with normal saline in reducing pain and improving functional scores at 3 months of follow-up for chronic plantar fasciopathy
Gill et al. [80]	Compared PRP vs. conservative treatment of NSAIDs and footpads with follow-up at 2, 4, 8, 12, and 52 weeks, which concluded that PRP injections for plantar fasciitis were statistically significant compared to conservative treatment in improvements to pain through the VAS scale.
Gluteus Medius	
Lee et al. [81]	Case series with 21 total patients which reported improvements to all mean outcome measures and were both clinically and statistically significant at a mean post-injection follow-up of 19.7 months

Table 19.2 Recommendations from Mautner et al. [93]

Platelets	2.5× – 3× baseline was identified as most ideal concentration
	Need to document actual platelet concentration and quantity of PRP delivered
Leukocytes	Pro-inflammatory effects of WBCs, particularly neutrophils, which may lead to excessive inflammation and counterproductive
	Some phagocytic properties of WBCs may be beneficial in chronic tendinopathy, but could also result in excessive inflammation and additional tissue damage in the setting of chronic, uncontrolled inflammatory states
	Monocytes: Role in balancing the pro-inflammatory and anti-inflammatory balance of the healing process
	Lymphocytes: Initiate cell-to-cell interactions and modulate tissue healing via the release of bioactive molecules
	Higher concentrations of leukocytes may be beneficial in specific MSK conditions (chronic tendinosis)
Red blood cells	Alters pH environment
	Highly supportive evidence for promoting inflammation and chondrocyte death
	Low spin centrifugation systems = minimal to no RBCs
	High spin centrifugation systems = 5–15% Hct
	New double spin suspension method = high platelet concentration but little to no RBCs
	PLRA classification is the only system that includes RBCs
Activators: Thrombin, calcium, and collagen	Recombinant human thrombin and synthetic peptides may offer more sustained release growth factors upon activation
	Overactivation can develop into a bivalent network, which is unstable
	A tetramolecular network enhances the adherence of cells, and growth factors have a sustained slower release
	Most studies on tendinopathy have not used activators

and cycles of procuring the PRP injectate and a much more detailed report of content delivered to the site of injection [94]. While this may be the most complete system available to date, the extensive profile of the classification may not be practical.

Mechanism of Action

PRP contains a higher-than baseline concentration of platelets. Its mechanism of action is yet to be elucidated but believed to be multifactorial. One such proposed mechanism of action is the activation of platelets resulting in the release of growth factors that are regenerative to tendon tissues. Several of these growth factors attract mesenchymal stem cells, macrophages, and fibroblasts, which, in combination, orchestrate the removal of degenerative and necrotic tissue and tissue regeneration and healing [93, 95]. PRP with elevated

leukocytes (LR-PRP) is associated with pro-inflammatory effects, as well as elevated catabolic cytokines including interleukin-1β, tumor necrosis factor-α, and metalloproteinases [96, 97].

Procedure

Peripheral blood comprises 93% RBCs, 6% platelets, and 1% leukocytes. PRP is typically prepared by centrifugation to separate its components and concentrate platelets above baseline levels [98].

First, the physician draws ~15–120 cc of the patient's own peripheral blood. Care must be taken during the blood draw as small needle may cause premature activation. The blood should be aspirated slowly to avoid overagitation. Once the blood draw is complete, the process of centrifugation begins. The first spin should be at 900 g for 5 minutes to concentrate the platelets and separate the RBCs and leukocytes. The final concentration of platelets is typically 2–3 times more than the baseline. If a second spin is used, it would be at 1500 g for approximately 15 minutes for the purpose of creating a buffy coat and further concentrating the platelets. The final concentration after a second spin is typically about 3–8× baseline.

Once the product is obtained, it must be properly placed in appropriate syringes. Different types of materials can affect the final platelet products. Polypropylene is considered the best material to use for platelet preparation because glass and polystyrene may lead to premature platelet activation or alter morphology.

Prior to injection, an anesthetic may be administered; however, it should be selected carefully because anesthetics may create a more acidic environment that interferes with the efficacy of the treatment. Commonly used local anesthetics such as lidocaine and ropivacaine decrease platelet aggregation to varying degrees [98]. In a meta-analysis of 18 randomized clinical trials pertaining to PRP for various tendinopathies, Fitzpatrick et al. concluded that an injection of 1–2 cc of local anesthetic prior to administration of a leukocyte-rich PRP (>1% of volume injected), superficial to the injection target, in a single injection, with a peppering technique, and under ultrasound guidance was most beneficial for tendinopathy [99].

Kits

There are many commercially available systems for in-office PRP treatment. These systems create varying PRP characteristics because of their platelet capture efficiency, isolation method, speed of centrifugation, and type of collection tube system [100]. In one study looking at seven different centrifugation systems, six of the seven systems produced platelet concentration levels higher than 3× baseline (range 3×–9×). Only one system produced a platelet concentration lower than 3× (0.52× baseline) [101]. In terms of cost, these kits range from $50 to $500 [99]. Newer technology has emerged that uses not only cen-

trifugation but also light spectrometry as part of the process of separating out the cells.

Additional Considerations

There are many patient-specific factors that can impact a PRP treatment. A high-fat meal has been shown to increase peripheral platelet concentration in healthy volunteers compared with fasting periods [99]. Circadian rhythms also affect platelet concentrations and function with increased platelet concentration in the afternoon and decreased platelet activation from noon to midnight [99]. The most important factor might be age. Aging patients have fewer stem cells and their tendon-specific stem cells (TSCs) may of be poor quality. Age may also diminish PRP treatment efficacy. Moderate exercise may also increase the number of stem cells [102].

With regard to pathology, the stage of tendinopathy must be considered. Healthy tendon tissue displays predominantly type 1 parallel collagen fibers, among cellular components, including mature tendon cells or tenocytes and tendon-specific stem/progenitor cells (TSCs) within a well-organized extracellular matrix (ECM) composed of proteoglycans, glycoproteins, and elastin [103]. The first stage is the inflammatory phase which is characterized by acute inflammation as pro-inflammatory cytokines attract blood cells to initiate the repair of injured tissues and generally last 5–7 days [103]. In the early stage of inflammation and differentiation (formation of non-tendinous tissues), PRP may be used to suppress inflammation and reduce pain leading to enhanced function. In animal studies, it has shortened the inflammatory phase with additional benefits of increasing the ratio of type I to type III collagen and increasing ECM synthesis, resulting in faster healing [104–106]. Additionally, PRP has been shown to increase angiogenesis and vessel density as early as 2 weeks [107]. Since reduced vascularity of tendons is a major factor in their limited healing capacity, PRP-associated angiogenesis also contributes to accelerated tendon healing [107]. Zhang et al. demonstrated that after acute tendon injury PRP induced tenogenic differentiation of TSCs and suppressed non-tenocyte differentiation, but when PRP was applied to TSCs from tendons that had already undergone non-tenogenic differentiation, PRP was unable to reverse the undesirable differentiation that had already occurred [108, 109]. Thus in the later stages, tendons become severely degenerated with lipid deposits, proteoglycan production increases, and calcifications are present. PRP may be less effective at that point because it is unable to improve degeneration in tendons and debridement may be needed to allow the TSCs to renew [102].

Summary

PRP continues to evolve as a less invasive therapy which promotes regeneration of tendinous tissue. As research concerning PRP has evolved, the potential to reduce pain and provide long-term connective tissue healing, with minimal complications and adverse effects, has been demonstrated with treatment of common extensor tendinopathy and patellar tendinopathy [110]. See Table 19.1 [23–89]. There is still, however, little evidence to show benefit for Achilles, rotator cuff, gluteal, and proximal hamstring tendinopathies. As measurement of outcomes becomes more standardized and follow-up longer in duration, a more accurate evaluation of its therapeutic efficacy will be possible. In addition to this standardization, further investigation is warranted to optimize overall cellular composition and to provide parameters specific to each tendon, the optimal composition of PRP based on the stage of tendinopathy, and standardized documentation for equivalent comparisons. Patient physiologic and genetic factors should continue to be considered and investigated as well.

Autologous Blood Injection

Autologous blood injection (ABI) is a relatively new treatment for tendinopathy that delivers an injection of whole blood to the site of tendon injury to speed the healing process. The first study was done by Edwards et al. in 2003 for lateral epicondylopahty [82]. ABI is hypothesized to deliver humoral mediators in a streamlined process to stimulate healing. The advantages of ABI include ease of obtaining whole blood, ability to perform the technique without a kit, speed at which it can be done since there is no centrifugation, and demonstrated safety. ABI studies have shown mixed results as to efficacy, though several studies have confirmed a reduction in tendon pain following treatment. Unfortunately, there have been few studies to date within sports medicine because the World Anti-Doping Agency currently bans the use of ABIs as a treatment modality. Further study is needed with respect to the use of ABI in connection with non-organized sports to assess the potentially negative impact of all of the substrates within whole blood.

Classification System

To the authors knowledge, there are no current classification or quantification systems in use for ABI.

Mechanism of Action

It is hypothesized that whole blood contains a variety of components that aid in healing, including growth factors that act as humoral mediators, and biological catalysts, including transforming growth factor-β and basic fibroblast growth factor, which promote the healing cascade of tissue repair and regeneration [82, 111–113]. In addition, cells such as macrophages, fibroblasts, and mesenchymal stem cells are able to migrate to the location of injury and aid in the removal of degenerative and necrotic tissues, thereby enhancing tissue regeneration and healing [83]. To date, no ABI studies have discussed or evaluated the specific blood product components as either beneficial or harmful when injected together. Platelets, while not at supra-physiologic concentration like PRP, may be beneficial, while RBCs may be harmful in the same way they detract from the efficacy of PRP. Physiologic concentrations of WBCs may also be helpful for their ability to produce inflammatory reactions that are beneficial for tendon healing.

Procedure

Prior to the procedure, ultrasound is performed to assess and visualize the tendon injury. A small amount of blood (~2–3 cc) is drawn in standard aseptic draws utilizing a 21-gauge butterfly needle. The affected area and ultrasound setup are then sterilized and readied for injection, and a local anesthetic is given via ultrasound guidance in a plane longitudinal to the tendon. Optional dry needling may also be performed prior to injection. Dry needling creates fenestrations which cause internal bleeding, in turn, more strongly stimulating the healing process. Ultrasound is used once again to visualize the location of injury and the needle is then inserted via ultrasound guidance using an in-plane approach longitudinal to the tendon and the autologous blood is delivered. In a cadaveric study, Evens et al. found that at both volumes of 1 ml and 3 ml, the injectate distributed equally across 97% of the intratendinous area of the common extensor tendon with no difference demonstrated between single-shot or fenestrated injection techniques [114].

Kits

To the authors' knowledge, there are no standardized kits. The procedure is completed by standard blood draw, butterfly needle extension, tubing, and syringe.

Additional Considerations and Evidence of Efficacy

While there have been several randomized controlled trials that have compared ABI with PRP, studies on lateral epicondylopathy are the most predominant [24, 83, 115, 116]. These studies have their limitations including heterogenicity

and methodologic approaches which demonstrate the need for further study. There are three studies comparing AB with corticosteroid for lateral epicondylopathy [117–119] [24, 83–88, 115–119], which have demonstrated promising long-term results in favor of ABI but with study limitations including low power and heterogenicity of the studies. No cost-benefit or efficacy studies are there to evaluate ABI injection compared to PRP injections. Some clinicians consider ABI as an alternative because it is cheaper; a clinician does not need to utilize a trademarked or patented kit. A meta-analysis by Arirachakaran found that ABI had the highest risk of adverse effect which included injection site pain and skin reactions [120] (see Table 19.3).

Summary

The use of ABIs as a treatment modality is still controversial. The majority of the studies that exist on it currently have looked at the common extensor tendon for lateral epicondylopathy, with some early encouraging results in low powered studies. There is a dearth of literature for other tendons. See Table 19.3 [24, 83–88, 115–119]. As the body of ABI research develops, including whether ABI is indicated for specific tendons, we will be able to better determine its utility in pain reduction and tissue repair. The tentative research available to date reveals that while ABI is effective for reducing tendon pain, it comes with the potential risks of pain or bruising at the injection site.

Mesenchymal Stem Cell

Mesenchymal stem cell (MSC) therapy has emerged as a treatment option for musculoskeletal disorders. These cells influence tendon healing due to the paracrine effect from secretomal molecules, [121] which provide signaling cells and growth factors such as those present in the bone marrow aspirate [122]. Mesenchymal stem cells have the ability to differentiate and proliferate into osteocytes, chondrocytes, myocytes, fibroblast, adipocytes, astrocytes, and stromal

Table 19.3 Autologous blood injection studies

Evidence comparing autologous blood injection vs. platelet-rich plasma

Edwards and Calandruccio [82]	Prospective study showed 79% (22 of 28 patients) patients, in whom non-surgical modalities had failed in treating lateral epicondylopathy and patients were relieved completely of pain even during strenuous activity after an average follow-up period of 9.5 months.
Creaney et al. [83]	Reported comparable success between ABI and PRP in a double-blinded, randomized trial of 150 patients with lateral epicondylopathy after 6 months of follow-up, in which physical therapy such as eccentric loading had previous failed
Thanasas et al. [24]	Showed a significant difference in pain reduction at 6 weeks with PRP superior to ABI, but no difference at later time points (3 and 6 months) in chronic lateral epicondylopathy
Pearson [88]	Proposed evidence for small short-term symptomatic improvement in use of ABI compared to standard rehabilitation treatment for Achilles tendinopathy. However, the author suggests for further double-blinded studies with longer follow-ups and larger sample for more accuracy
Krough et al. (2013)	Performed a systematic review of 17 studies that demonstrated ABI, PRP, and corticosteroids were more effective than placebo
Ahmad et al. [85]	Showed in an RCT that PRP was more effective than ABI in terms of non-response rate, conversion to surgery rates, and VAS pain scores at a 6 week time point for lateral epicondylopathy
Chou et al. [86]	Reported no difference between efficacy in ABI and PRP in treating lateral epicondylopathy but ABI to be more effective than corticosteroid injection
Vahdatpour et al. [87]	Reported PRP and ABI had similar effectiveness for the treatment of chronic plantar fasciitis in the short term (3 months of follow-up)

Summary: ABI and PRP seem to provide short-term pain relief which is more effective than standard rehabilitation treatment and corticosteroids, but they have not shown long-term benefits at 3 and 6 months of follow-up. Both treatments show no significant difference between each other regarding pain reduction, but further studies are needed.

Evidence comparing autologous blood injection vs. corticosteroid

Kazemi et al. [117]	Showed in an RCT that ABI vs steroid showed significantly better effects compared to steroid in outcome measures including Quick Dash and pain in maximum grip at 4 Weeks and all outcome measures, including quick Dash, VAS, pain and strength in maximum grip PPT. D15:T15
Singh et al. [118]	RCT demonstrated no difference between ABI and steroid at 6 weeks, but there was significant improvement in PRETEE at 12 weeks
Dojode et al. [119]	Reported that corticosteroid showed statistically significant decrease in pain at 1 week and 4 weeks, but at 12 weeks the VAS and Nirschl scores were Significantly lower in the AB group. AB had 90% retention of improvement

cells [123, 124]. These cells have been harvested from bone marrow [7], adipose tissue [125], synovium [126], and muscle [127] for the treatment of tendon diseases. This chapter will focus specifically on two emerging in-office procedures by which mesenchymal stem cells can be obtained: bone marrow aspiration and adipose tissue aspiration.

BMAC

Bone marrow aspirate concentrate (BMAC) has emerged as a treatment option for osteoarthritis and tendinopathy in part because it was the first tissue type from which MSC was isolated and it has an extensive track record of safety in harvesting from our hematology and oncology colleagues. Moreover, the growth factors and mesenchymal stem cells have shown significant efficacy in treating tendon injury [7–13]

Food and Drug Administration (FDA) regulations stipulate that a biological material is not a drug if it is only minimally manipulated such that the processing (aliquoting, rinsing, freezing, and removal of microscopic debris) does not alter the original characteristics of the tissue. Examples of more than minimal manipulation include cell isolation, cell expansion, and enzymatic digestion. With BMAC, the homologous substance used for the repair, reconstruction, replacement, or supplementation of the recipient's tissues performs the same basic function as the original biological material, and the processing of the product does not involve the combination of another substance with the cells or tissues. Further, there is minimal systemic effect, meaning that BMAC is not considered a drug [128]

Classification System

To date there is no current classification system used specifically for BMAC MSC injection options. Current classification systems have focused on the harvest site of the MSCs.

Mechanism of Action

BMAC has a yield of 0.01–0.001% concentration of mesenchymal stem cells among all nucleated cells in the aspiration [129]. Mesenchymal stem cells have the ability to differentiate and proliferate into progenitors of different mesenchymal tissue. The process of transdifferentiation describes the differentiation of the stem cells by signaling from distant and local tissues [130, 131]. These stem cells have unique cell surface markers, adhesion molecules, cytokines, growth factors, and receptions which have anti-inflammatory and immunomodulatory properties [19]. Due to the lack of major histocompatibility complex II, molecular expression allows them to have hypo-immunogenicity [132]. Patient selection is an important consideration as it has been demonstrated that the yield of stem cells within the bone marrow aspirate decreases with age [133–135].

Procedure

A formal office consultation should include an evaluation of whether BMAC is the appropriate procedure for the patient and confirmation that the patient has no contraindications such as active infections, cancer, rheumatologic conditions requiring immunomodulation, anticoagulation that cannot be held, or immune compromise [136]. Medications such as prednisone, statins, and NSAIDs must be stopped prior to BMAC [136]. Patient education and counseling should include a review of the current literature, expense, benefits, risks, and need for active rehabilitation. During the initial consultation, it is critical to set expectations with regard to pain, function, range of motion, and durability. The patient should also be advised that following the procedure, he or she will need to work with a physical therapist to address proper biomechanics, strength, and mechanical loading considerations.

Harvest sites have been reported from the anterior and posterior iliac crest, proximal tibia, and calcaneus; however, the highest yield of mesenchymal stem cells comes from the posterior superior iliac spine (PSIS), making it the most common and recommended site [136, 137, 143].

When choosing the approach and thus proper patient positioning, the practitioner should consider any patient-specific complications involving respiratory, cardiovascular, and musculoskeletal systems [136]. For PSIS extraction, the patient should be placed in the prone position and the practitioner should seek the PSIS landmark through palpation. Ultrasound guidance is used to confirm the location. When using ultrasound, the authors recommend scanning the PSIS in the short axis until the PSIS is visualized at the most parallel (flat) hyperechoic linear structure. See Fig. 19.1. Patient size and BMI may impact needle and trocar sizing.

Following identification of the proper location for harvest, the area is marked and cleaned in a sterile fashion. Local anesthetic is provided with a

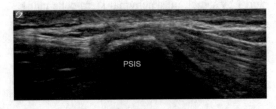

Fig. 19.1 Ultrasound PSIS

25-gauge, 2-inch needle, by forming a skin wheel and advancing the needle down to just touch the bone cortex. Then a long-acting anesthetic, such as ropivacaine due to the cytotoxic effects of other anesthetics [138], is injected into the tract, superior to the periosteum, using a 14-gauge, 1.5-inch needle so as to achieve longer duration post-procedure pain control. When withdrawing, in lieu of using a scalpel, the 14-gauge needle can be used to continue to create a skin wheel and open the skin access point. A scalpel blade may also be used to create an entry site.

Clinics typically choose between commercially available manual needles or commercially available power driver needles to core into the PSIS. See Fig. 19.2. These trocar options allow for physician preference, taking into consideration the size, age, and bone density of the patient. Once the outer cortex is breached, there is a soft inner cortex. Whether the practitioner should use a needle or trocar depends not only on clinician preference but also on considerations for bone age and health. Bone hardness will typically diminish with age. Thus, in individuals 55 years or older or in those having a diagnosis of osteoporosis, the cortex will be easier to breach and using a manual needle may help prevent over-penetration [136].

An initial aspiration is obtained to confirm placement. A heparin flush is then provided and the BMAC can be extracted in a 10 cc syringe prefilled with 2-3 cc of heparin. This is repeated at two other sites to obtain 30 cc of BMAC mixture from one PSIS side. The procedure is then repeated on the contralateral PSIS.

The anecdotal safe volumes of BMAC to yield per procedure range from 50 ml in a small woman or child to 60–70 ml for an average size adult to 120 ml for large individuals [136]. The authors recommend 60 ml of divided BMAC because drawing smaller volumes (~10 cc) from many sites has been reported to increase the mesenchymal stem cell yield as compared to larger volumes from a single site [138–141]. The most common complication during the procedure is clotting. This renders the stem cells trapped and unable to be used. Generous use of heparin will help reduce this complication. The trocars also need to be thoroughly heparinized.

Kits

There are many commercially available kits that focus on centrifugation at this time. A study by Hedge et al. compared three of the commercially available systems evaluating the number and concentration of progenitor cells achieved both before and after centrifugation and the percentage of progenitor cells salvaged after centrifugation. They found no difference in the percent yield of connective tissue progenitors (CTPs), or the number and concentration of the CTPs, but one system did have high percent yield of CTPs [142]. To date there have been no further system comparison studies. Progenitor cells account for a small population within the bone marrow (0.001–0.01%) after centrifugation [142]. A recent study by Nazal et al. examined the CTP from the ilium which revealed a cell concentration of 879.3 stem cells/cc of BMAC, a mean CTP prevalence of 34.1 stem cells/million nucleated cells, and a mean number of 2.97 days to form colonies [144]. They found that the harvest site was found to have a CTP concentration similar to or exceeding other published harvest sites [144].

Additional Considerations and Evidence of Efficacy

The safety and efficacy of BMAC therapy has been documented for the past 20–30 years through its use in hematology and oncology

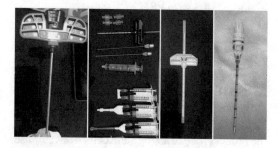

Fig. 19.2 Trocar options

[145]. More recent studies have demonstrated its safety profile within musculoskeletal uses specific to arthritis [146, 147]. BMAC treatment has a similar safety profile to other injectable procedures [146]. Concerns for neoplasm risk have been voiced, but a multicenter analysis by Centeno et al. consisting of 2372 patients undergoing autologous stem cell therapy demonstrated no higher neoplasm risk as compared to the general public over a 9 year span [146]. It is important to consider that this study had a very low follow-up rate.

BMAC research has been focused on osteochondral pathology. There have been small prospective studies for lateral epicondylitis, patellar tendinopathy, and rotator cuff tendinopathy that have demonstrated promising results [149–152]. See Table 19.4. Singh et al. studied 30 adult patients with untreated tennis elbow, assessing their condition at 6 and 12 weeks. They demonstrated statistically significant pain and functional improvement in a small prospective study, though they acknowledge limitations of the lack of a control group and short follow-up. There was also lack of injection image guidance and cell count description [149]. Pascual-Garrido et al. studied eight patients who failed prior patellar tendinopathy treatment. They were able to include hematologic analysis and use image guidance for their injections. They demonstrated statistically significant improvements in the KOOS score for patellar tendinopathy, with continued improvements during the first year.

Table 19.4 BMAC evidence

Lateral epicondylopathy	
Singh et al. [149]	Prospective study demonstrated significant pain and functional improvement at 12 weeks
Patellar tendinopathy	
Pascual-Garrido et al. [150]	Case series demonstrated statistically significant improvements in KOOS out to 1 year
RTC and shoulder OA	
Centeno et al. [151]	Improvements in DASH but heterogeneous study treated with PRP and prolotherapy
Hernigou et al. [152]	Augmented rotator cuff repair has a risk of absence of healing when MSCs concentration was lower than 1500 per milliliter

Although the improvements plateaued at 1 year, the authors followed up 5 years later, and the patients had no recurrence. This study was limited due to the lack of a control group and low power [150]. Centeno et al. looked at 115 shoulders with glenohumeral osteoarthritis and rotator cuff tears. They had three different outcome scales which demonstrated promising results with improvement in DASH outcome scores for rotator cuff arthropathy. This study had several limitations including the dichotomy of glenohumeral osteoarthritis with the rotator cuff tear and the use of combination therapy with PRP and prolotherapy injections being used in addition to BMAC [151]. A French study by Hernigou et al. evaluated BM-MSCs with arthroscopic repair of rotator cuff tears with regard to re-tear rates with correlation to the number of MSCs received. The authors determined that there was a risk of absence of healing when the MSCs concentration was lower than 1500 per milliliter [152]. Further research has also demonstrated that PRP plays a role in augmenting BMAC. Kim et al. suggested that PRP enhances proliferation and migration of tendon-derived stem cells to aid in the rotator cuff tendon tear healing, suggesting that PRP plays a role in providing a scaffold for the BMAC [153].

Summary

In summary, current evidence for BMAC MSC injections for the treatment of tendinopathy is still emerging but has shown some early promising results. More high-quality heterogeneous studies are needed. In addition, further analysis is needed to determine the beneficial effect of combining BMAC with PRP.

Adipose Tissue Derivatives

Adipose tissue derivatives are increasing in popularity due to the ease of the procedure to obtain them and their wider availability [19]. In the past, the process for extracting stem cells from adipose tissue required enzymatic manipulation, which under current FDA rulings is regulated as a drug. Adipose tissue derivatives follow the same regulatory rules as previously discussed with regard to BMAC. However, only one recent commercial product has been FDA cleared, while the other commercial options have not.

Classification System

Adipose tissue derivatives (ATD) include microfragmented adipose tissue (MFAT) and/or stromal vascular fraction (SVF). Nomenclature regarding ATDs has been ambiguous in the literature. MFAT is generated using a combination of washing and passing harvested ATD through a size-reduction filter to mechanically break up the adipose tissue. SVF is typically obtained in three ways. The first involves centrifugation with enzymatic digestion, usually with collagenase. The second is centrifugation and enzymatic digestion with the addition of mechanical separation using a size-reduction filter, and the last is centrifugation and mechanical separation [154]. Recent FDA guidance documents suggest that devices that utilize mechanical processing to resize particles of fat without enzymes are thought to comply with these regulations by staying within the bounds of minimal manipulation; however, whether or not minimally manipulated adipose tissue injected into joints or tendons constitutes homologous use is still debated [154].

Mechanism of Action

Adipose tissue derivatives contain mesenchymal stem cells that have the ability to differentiate into musculoskeletal tissues including chondrocytes or tenocytes and may also contain supportive cells that can modulate the microenvironment and attract cells involved in regeneration and repair [154]. Lipoaspirate has been shown to yield a final product containing MSCs at a 100- to 1000-fold higher concentration per cubic meter when compared to products from bone marrow [155]. Initial research on ATDs focused on human adipose stem cells (ASCs) which were

first isolated, cultured, expanded, and characterized by Zuk et al. in 2001 [156]. ASCs are MSCs that can differentiate toward osteogenic, chondrogenic, adipogenic, and myofanic lineages and express cell markers such as CD90, CD73, CD105, and CD44 and are negative for CD45(hematopoetic cell marker) and CD31 (marker of angiogenesis). Culture-expanded ASCs are thought to be beneficial in treating musculoskeletal conditions due to their direct differentiation into cartilage and tendon. However, culture and expansion of ASC cannot be performed in most clinics. Additionally, expanded ASCs do not contain supportive cells, which are now thought to be beneficial in the treatment of musculoskeletal tissues as they modulate the micro-environment though paracrine effects. Supportive cells include perivascular smooth muscle cells, endothelial cells, pericytes, fibroblasts, and immune cells, and they release growth factors that modulate proinflammatory cytokines, increase tissue angiogenesis and blood flow, and decrease cell death and fibrosis [154]. Docheva et al. have suggested that BMAC MSCs are more prone to differentiate into osteogenic and chondrogenic cells compared to adipose-derived mesenchymal stem cells [6]. Thus, for the treatment of tendinopathy, adipose-derived mesenchymal stems cells have shown upregulated expression of tendon-related markers and have been found comparable to BMAC in terms of scaffold adherence and proliferation potential [6].

Procedure

Adipose tissue is known to display varying characteristics depending on the sites of harvesting. For example, adipose tissue can be harvested from the joint fat pads, the abdomen, which is reported to be resistant to apoptosis, the arm, which is suggested to have the highest yield of cells, or the inguinal region, which is reported to have the greatest plasticity [157]. The most common locations for adipose tissue harvesting in MSK practice have been the abdomen, flanks, and thighs. Once the harvest site is identified, a field block using tumescent fluid should be initiated. Once the field block is obtained, the practitioner utilizes a commercially available kit that contains a processing canister, a lipo-aspiration cannula, a vacuum syringe, and other necessary syringes. Using the kit, the lipo-aspiration cannula is inserted into the selected site, and in a series of advancements and retractions in a circular field, the adipose tissue is collected. Depending on which kit is being used, the steps of the procedure differ and are dependent on the final product, MFAT or SVF.

Kits

Currently the kit options are divided into three categories: MFAT, SVF enzymatic, and SVF mechanical. See Table 19.5. No direct comparison of each kit has been performed. Bora et al. have demonstrated that centrifugation with enzymatic separation has higher efficiency compared to centrifugation with mechanical separation alone in obtaining SVF [158]. Lastly, due to FDA regulations, only one commercially available kit

Table 19.5 Adipose kits [154]

MFAT:
  Lipogems® (Lipogems International S.p.A., Italy)
  Tulip NanoSpinTM (Tulip Medical, USA)
SVF, enzymatic:
  AdipoCellTM (US Stem Cell Inc., USA)
  Celution® (Cytori Inc., USA)
  Icellator® X (Tissue Genesis LLC, USA)
  Lipo-Kit GT (Medikan International Inc., South Korea)
  Multi Station or Cha-StationTM (PNC International Co., Ltd., Korea) myStem® (MyStem LLC, USA Q-Graft® (HumanMed AG, Germany)
  RevolveTM/GID 700TM (LifeCell Corporation, USA/GID Group, Inc., USA) StempeutronTM (Stempeutics Research Pvt. Ltd., India).
SVF, mechanical:
  Fastkit (Fastem) (CORIOS Soc. Coop., Italy)
  Harvest AdiPrep® Adipose Concentration System (Termo BCT Inc., USA Q-Graft® (HumanMed AG, Germany)
  StromaCellTM (MicroAire Surgical Instruments, LLC, USA)
  Stromed (Cell Innovations Inc., Australia)

is compliant, at this time, with the FDA requirements in the United States to obtain adipose tissue for orthopedic use [159].

Additional Considerations and Evidence of Efficacy

Safety profiles for liposuction cases have reported no deaths and a complication rate of 0.068 per 1000 cases [160]. When assessing the current literature, challenges remain with regard to homogenicity as some of the studies are of enzymatically digested adipose-derived MSCs which are different from MFAT or SVF. In a study by Lee et al., adipose-derived MSCs were used for the treatment of lateral epicondylosis with defects seen on the ultrasound. They obtained their adipose derivatives by SVF enzymatic digestion. They demonstrated that adipose-derived stem cells were safe and effective for improving elbow pain according to visual analog scores and performance under the Mayo Elbow Performance Index. The tendon structural defect was found to have improved at ultrasound examination follow-up at 52 weeks [161]. In a case series of 18 subjects by Striano et al., the authors evaluated chronic shoulder pain due to rotator cuff tear and glenohumeral osteoarthritis and found significant improvements in all time points to 1 year when using MFAT treatment option [162]. Usuelli et al. evaluated Achilles tendinopathy in an RCT of PRP versus mechanical SVF. They found that the SVF had faster improvement with a significantly better outcome with regard to VAS, VISA-A and AOFAS hindfoot scale, no significant difference between PRP and Adipose groups at 30 day follow up [163]. Wang et al. demonstrated a case series of 20 consecutive patients using patellar tendon cells that were expanded by in vitro culture and found improvement in structural integrity (via MRI comparisons) and functional outcomes [164]. Lastly in a study by Jang et al., BMAC vs SVF cell concentrations were compared, revealing that SVF had 10 times more

MSCs and BMAC had six times more leukocytes [165]. MSC in bone marrow is about 1/10,000 mononucleated cells and adipose is higher per cubic meter in adipose aspirate than bone marrow aspirate.

Summary

In summary, ATDs are becoming more commonly used by physicians to treat musculoskeletal conditions non-surgically. Literature reviews have demonstrated heterogeneity in promising, but low-quality clinical studies in support of the use of ATDs. See Table 19.6. MFAT and SVF are easy to use in the clinic and contain ASCs plus supportive cells that modulate the microenvironment and are thought to lead to tissue regeneration and healing, but additional evidence is needed. Future studies, including randomized clinical trials and reports on data from large registries, should focus on standardizing procedures, including injectate content (i.e., cell count, exosome count, use of mechanical or enzymatic fragmentation, use of additional injectates), frequency of injections, use of guidance during the procedures, outcome measures, and rehabilitation protocols for determining optimum protocols for the use of ATDs and for pooling of data.

Table 19.6 Adipose derivatives evidence

RTC tear and OA	
Striano et al. [162]	MFAT – Case series evaluated numeric pain scores and the ASES demonstrated significant improvement at all time points to 1 year
Achilles	
Usuelli et al. [163]	Mechanical SVF – RCT prp versus SVF. The SVF had faster improvement with a significantly better outcome with regard to VAS, VISA-A, and AOFAS hindfoot scale, and no significant difference between PRP and adipose groups at 30 day follow-up
Lateral Epicondylopathy	
Lee et al. [161]	Enzymatic SVF case series: 79% improved pain scores, improved functional performance, and reduced structural tendon defects on US exam up to 1 yr

Placental Products

Placental products are another emerging option in the field of orthobiologics. Placental tissues have been used to treat burns and wounds for over a century and their regenerative potential has been studied in treating hepatic, cardiac, and neurologic disorders [166]. Amniotic membranes have been shown to have antibacterial, pain reducing, anti-inflammatory, and soft-tissue healing properties [166, 167]. The placental tissue utilized in initial evaluations was harvested from full-term pregnancies to reduce controversy over its source [163]. The neonatal stem cells from such amniotic fluid, amnion, chorion, umbilical cord tissue, and blood provide a source from which MSCs can be isolated [163]. Neonatal placental MSCs have higher proliferative and differential potential than adult stem cells isolated from other types of tissues [169]. As many of the emerging techniques involve a time commitment to perform the procedure and obtain the desired product, other alternative and efficient means are being developed. However, the use of placental products remains controversial at this time because the isolation and expansion of cells from these tissues are considered by the FDA to involve more than "minimal" manipulation [166].

Commercially available products are made with proprietary processes for cleaning, sterilizing, and drying human amniotic/chorionic membranes into a powder form that can be mixed with saline to create an injectate that can be stored at room temperature for up to 5 years. Off-the-shelf products (like the many options of viscosupplementation) are a convenient and efficient option for treatment. Although some have hypothesized that placental products have the potential to contain growth factors that are similar to the other regenerative options, that hypothesis is not without controversy. Indeed, studies have shown that there are no live cells contained in these commercial products due to the process of preserving and sterilizing the tissues [170, 171]. Moreover, while MSCs are easy to isolate from amniotic fluid, they are present at very low numbers and must be expanded in culture and preserved for storage and long-term shelf-life. This process is not FDA approved. As a result, there are no placental based MSC drugs in the United States. Furthermore, it is possible that the beneficial effects observed following the use of such products are not the result of the MSCs but rather the result of the placental extracellular matrix and/or the growth factors and cytokines present in the tissue [170, 171].

Classification System

To date there is no consensus on a proposed classification system. One approach would be breaking the placental tissues down into their derivatives anatomically for improved nomenclature. First, there is the amniotic membrane, which consists of two cellular layers: a single layer of amniotic epithelial cells (AECs) called the epithelial layer (which is attached to the basement membrane) and an outer mesenchymal layer that contains fibroblasts and amniotic membrane MSCs [172]. Stem cells have been isolated from both of these layers. The AEC layer is known to be clonogenic, meaning that it can differentiate into cells of all three germline lineages [166]. The amniotic membrane MSCs are known to have a higher proliferative rate than other MSCs from adult sources [173].

The second placental product is amniotic fluid, which provides nutrients that are essential for fetal growth and health. Kaviani et al. identified MSCs in amniotic fluid and attempted to use them for tissue engineering in 2001 [174]. Roubelakis et al. demonstrated that cells in the amniotic fluid have the ability to differentiate into cells of adipogenic, osteogenic, myogenic, and endothelial lineages and that the MSCs derived from that amniotic fluid expressed markers characteristic of MSCs [166, 173].

The third placental product is the chorionic membrane, which is the outermost layer of placental tissue, consisting of the chorionic mesenchyme and the trophoblast layer that encapsulates the amniotic tissue and embeds into the mother's endometrium [166]. Stem cells can be isolated from both the chorionic villi and the chorionic membrane [166]. Chorionic MSCs have higher proliferative potential than bone marrow-derived MSCs [175].

The fourth placental product is the umbilical cord tissue, which connects the mother and child. MSCs have been isolated from all subsections of the umbilical cord, which is composed of umbilical epithelium and a connective substance known as Wharton's jelly [166]. Umbilical cord MSCs have an immunosuppressive capacity and multilineage differentiation potential. They also have the same biomarkers that are consistent with the other MSC derivations (CD73, CD90, CD105) [166].

The final placental product source is the umbilical cord blood. The cells in this blood operate to exchange oxygen and nutrients between the mother and the child. The majority of stem cells in the umbilical cord blood are CD34 positive hematopoietic stem cells. Although the MSCs are present in much lower numbers than in bone marrow, adipose tissue, and other sources, they are thought to have a higher potential for expansion than MSCs derived from those other sources [166].

Mechanism of Action

Amniotic suspension allografts are derived from human amniotic membrane as well as human amniotic fluid-derived cells. Some of these products have been found to have anti-inflammatory factors such as IL-10 and IL-1, matrix metalloproteinases, hyaluronic acid, proteoglycans, and growth factors which stimulate epithelial cell migration, proliferation, and other metabolic processes including protein and collagen synthesis [167, 168, 176]. Amniotic surface epithelial cells are thought to have immunocompatability due to the lack of tissue HLA antibodies [177].

Procedure

As with any orthobiologic procedure, ultrasound guidance for accuracy of placement is recommended. The products are available in an off-the-shelf syringe and the injection is performed as any other conventional injection.

Kits

There are multiple placental injectable options commercially available, designed for off the shelf usage. There have been no comparison studies evaluating the different commercially available options. Each has a reconstitution method.

Additional Considerations and Evidence of Efficacy

Most of the emerging literature with regard to the use of amniotic products involves applications in the foot and ankle. See Table 19.7. Zelen et al. published a small prospective randomized comparative study that established feasibility with promising results [170]. Hanselman et al. conducted a randomized double-blinded pilot study for the treatment of plantar fasciitis and found that the results from amniotic products were promising and comparable to steroids [171]. Werber also found promising results in treating

Achilles tendinosis and plantar fasciosis [178]. Gelhorn et al. published a case series of 40 patients with chronic tendinosis or arthropathy who underwent an injection of micronized dehydrated human amniotic/chorionic membrane which demonstrated clinical effectiveness in reducing pain and improving function. The study did have limitations though, including heterogeneous patient selection, lack of a control group, and lack of physical therapy standardization [179].

Summary

In summary, current research on placental-derived products is limited. Use of these products has shown promising results, but current clinical considerations are limited in the United States due to FDA regulations. At least two companies have been notified by the FDA that their placental allograft formulation does not meet HCT/P requirements. Moreover, there is continued controversy concerning the manipulation of live cells, and to date, the research has demonstrated that no live cells persist in the sterilized and formulated final products.

Table 19.7 Placental products evidence

Lower extremity tendinopathy	
Lullove (2015)	Single-site, retrospective case series using placental tissue matrix: VAS pain score improvement at weeks 4 and 5
Warner and Lasyone (2014)	Single-site retrospective case series, open foot and ankle surgical repair with supplementation of amniotic membrane and umbilical cord. Post-op AOFAS rating scale improved at 32 weeks
Werber [178]	Prospective open label case series with amniotic membrane and amniotic fluid. Significant VAS reduction by 4 weeks and mild pain at week 12
Zelen et al. [170]	RCT single-blinded compared low dose with high dose of mdHACM to saline placebo. AOFAS and Wong Baker FACES and SF-36 showed improvement at all time points up to 8 weeks
Hanselman et al. [171]	RCT double-blinded amniotic membrane to corticosteroid. Using FHSQ as the primary outcome and VAS as secondary outcome, showed no significant differences after 1 injection, but there was significant improvement with 2 injections of amniotic membrane compared to 2 injections of corticosteroid. VAS percentage improvement at 12 weeks statistically greater in the steroid group
Multiple sites	
Gellhorn and Han [179]	Retrospective case series using dehydrated amnion/chorion membrane allograft for tendinopathy and arthritis clinically effective in reducing pain and improving function

Summary

In conclusion, there is promise and potential for orthobiologics in the treatment of tendinopathy, a prevalent condition leading to impaired quality of life in the general population and performance in athletes and disability in the working population. Traditional measures such as PT, corticosteroid injections, or even surgical debridement are sometimes unsuccessful in relieving pain and improving function. Office-based procedures, especially PRP, are becoming widely available. However, before we can confidently recommend such procedures prior to implementation of surgical options, we need additional research and understanding on the mechanism of both tendinopathy and the various orthobiological procedures. Further research including multicenter-sized randomized controlled studies, allowing for larger sample sizes, needs to be completed.

References

1. Rand E, Welbel R, Visco CJ. Fundamental considerations for ultrasound-guided musculoskeletal interventions. Phys Med Rehabil Clin N Am. 2016;27:539–53.
2. Chen J, Wang A, Xu J, Zheng M. In chronic lateral epicondylitis, apoptosis and autophagic cell death occur in the extensor carpi radialis brevis tendon. JSES. 2010;19(3):355–62.
3. Khan KM, Cook JL, Bonar F, Harcourt P, Astrom M. Histopathology of common tendinopathies: update and implications for clinical management. Sports Med. 1999;27:393–408.
4. Soslowsky LJ, Thomopoulos S, Tun S, et al. Overuse activity injuries the supraspinatus tendon in an animal model: a histologic and biomechanical study. JSES. 2000;9:79–84.
5. Goodship AE, Birch HL, Wilson AM. The pathobiology and repair of tendon and ligament injury. Vet Clin North Am Equine Pract. 1994;10:323–49.
6. Docheva D, et al. Biologics for tendon repair. Adv Drug Deliv Rev. 2015;84:222–39.
7. Ouyang HW, Goh JC, Lee EH. Viability of allogenic bone marrow stromal cells following local delivery into patella tendon in rabbit model. Cell Transplant. 2004;13:649–57.
8. Chong AK, Ang AD, Goh JC, et al. Bone Marrow-derived mesenchymal stem cells influence early tendon-healing in a rabbit Achilles tendon model. JBJS. 2007;89(1):74–81.
9. Smith RK. Autogenous stem cell implantation. Vet Surg. 2004;33:199–201.
10. Smith RK, Korda M, Blunn GW, Goodship AE. Isolation and implantation of autologous equine mesenchymal stem cells from bone marrow into the superficial digital flexor tendon as a potential novel treatment. Equine Vet J. 2003;35:99–102.
11. Smith RK, Webbon PM. Harnessing the stem cell for the treatment of tendon injuries: heralding a new dawn. Br J Sports Med. 2005;39:582–4.
12. Gulotta LV, Kovacervic D, Packer JD, Deng XH, Rodeo SA. Bone marrow-derived mesenchymal stem cells transduced with scleraxis improve rotator cuff healing in a rat model. Am J Sports Med. 2011;39(6):1282–9.
13. Yokoya S, Mochizuki Y, Natsu K, Omae H, Nagata Y, Ochi M. Rotator cuff regeneration using a bioabsorbable material with bone marrow derived mesenchymal stem cells in a rabbit model. Am J Sports Med. 2012;40(6):1259–68.
14. Gottlieb NL, Riskin WG. Complications of local corticosteroid injections. JAMA. 1980;243:1547–8.
15. Neustadt DH. Complications of local corticosteroid injections. JAMA. 1981;246:835–6.
16. Yamada K, Masuko T, Iwasaki N. Rupture of the flexor digitorum profundus tendon after injections of insoluble steroid for a trigger finger. J Hand Surg Eur Vol. 2011;36:77–8.
17. Mills SP, Charalambous CP, Hayton MJ. Bilateral rupture of the extensor pollicis longus tendon in a professional goalkeeper following steroid injections for extensor tenosynovitis. Hand Surg. 2009;14:135–7. [PubMed] [Google Scholar].
18. Pattanittum P, Turner T, Green S, Buchbinder R. Non-steroidal anti-inflammatory drugs (NSAIDs) for treating lateral elbow pain in adults. Cochrane Database Syst Rev. 2013;5:CD003686.
19. Obaid H, Connell D. Cell therapy in tendon disorders. AJSM. 2010;38(10):2123–32.
20. Smidt N, Van der Windt DAWM, Assendel WJJ, Devillé WL, JMK O-dB, Bouter LM. Corticosteroid injections, physiotherapy, or a wait-and-see policy for lateral epicondylitis: a randomised controlled trial. Lancet. 2002;359(9307):657–62.
21. Bisset L, Smidt N, van der Windt DA, et al. Conservative treatments for tennis elbow—do subgroups of patients respond differently? Rheumatology. 2007;46(10):1601–5.
22. Kahlenberg CA, Knesek M, Terry MA. New developments in the use of biologics and other modalities in the management of lateral epicondylitis. BioMed Res Int. 2015;2015(5):439309.
23. Peerbooms JC, Sluimer J, Bruijn DJ, et al. Positive effect of an autologous platelet concentrate in lateral epicondylitis in a double-blind randomized controlled trial: platelet-rich plasma versus corticosteroid injection with a 1-year follow-up. Am J Sports Med. 2010;38(2):255–62.
24. Thanasas C, Papadimitriou G, Charalambidis C, et al. Platelet-rich plasma versus autologous whole blood for the treatment of chronic lateral elbow epi-

condylitis: a randomized controlled clinical trial. Am J Sports Med. 2011;39(10):2130–4.

25. Krogh TP, Fredberg U, Stengaard-Pedersen K, et al. Treatment of lateral epicondylitis with platelet-rich plasma, glucocorticoid, or saline: a randomized, double-blind, placebo-controlled trial. Am J Sports Med. 2013;41(3):625–35.

26. Nasser MT, El Yasaki A, Ezz El Mallah R, Abdelazeem AM. Treatment of lateral epicondylitis with platelet-rich plasma, glucocorticoid, or saline. A comparative study. Egypt Rheumatol Rehabil. 2017;44(1)

27. Chiavaras MM, Jacobson JA, Carlos R, et al. IMpact of Platelet Rich plasma OVer alternative therapies in patients with lateral Epicondylitis (IMPROVE): protocol for a multicenter randomized controlled study: a multicenter, randomized trial comparing autologous platelet-rich plasma, autologous whole blood, dry needle tendon fenestration, and physical therapy exercises alone on pain and quality of life in patients with lateral epicondylitis. Acad Radiol 2014;21(9):1144–55.

28. de Vos RJ, Weir A, van Schie HT, et al. Platelet-rich plasma injection for chronic Achilles tendinopathy: a randomized controlled trial. JAMA. 2010;303(2):144–9.

29. de Jonge S, de Vos RJ, Weir A, et al. One-year follow-up of platelet-rich plasma treatment in chronic Achilles tendinopathy: a double-blind randomized placebo- controlled trial. Am J Sports Med. 2011;39(8):1623–9.

30. Schepull T, Kvist J, Norrman H, et al. Autologous platelets have no effect on the healing of human Achilles tendon ruptures: a randomized single-blind study. Am J Sports Med. 2011;39(1):38–47.

31. Gaweda K, Tarczynska M, Krzyzanowski W. Treatment of Achilles tendinopathy with platelet-rich plasma. Int J Sports Med. 2010;31(8):577–83.

32. Volpi P, Quaglia A, Schoenhuber H, et al. Growth factors in the management of sport-induced tendinopathies: results after 24 months from treatment. A pilot study. J Sports Med Phys Fitness. 2010;50(4):494–500.

33. Finnoff JT, Fowler SP, Lai JK, et al. Treatment of chronic tendinopathy with ultrasound-guided needle tenotomy and platelet-rich plasma injection. PM R. 2011;3(10):900–11.

34. Owens RF Jr, Ginnetti J, Conti SF, et al. Clinical and magnetic resonance imaging outcomes following platelet rich plasma injection for chronic midsubstance Achilles tendinopathy. Foot Ankle Int. 2011;32(11):1032–9.

35. Monto RR. Platelet rich plasma treatment for chronic Achilles tendinosis. Foot Ankle Int. 2012;33(5):379–85.

36. Ferrero G, Fabbro E, Orlandi D, et al. Ultrasound-guided injection of platelet-rich plasma in chronic Achilles and patellar tendinopathy. J Ultrasound. 2012;15(4):260–6.

37. Deans VM, Miller A, Ramos J. A prospective series of patients with chronic Achilles tendinopathy treated with autologous-conditioned plasma injections combined with exercise and therapeutic ultrasonography. J Foot Ankle Surg. 2012;51(6):706–10.

38. Gosens T, Den Oudsten BL, Fievez E, et al. Pain and activity levels before and after platelet-rich plasma injection treatment of patellar tendinopathy: a prospective cohort study and the influence of previous treatments. Int Orthop. 2012;36(9):1941–6.

39. Kearney RS, Parsons N, Costa ML. Achilles tendinopathy management: a pilot randomised controlled trial comparing platelet-rich plasma injection with an eccentric loading programme. Bone Joint Res. 2013;2(10):227–32.

40. Mautner K, Colberg RE, Malanga G, et al. Outcomes after ultrasound-guided platelet-rich plasma injections for chronic tendinopathy: a multicenter, retrospective review. PM R. 2013;5(3):169–75.

41. Filardo G, Kon E, Di Matteo B, et al. Platelet-rich plasma for the treatment of patellar tendinopathy: clinical and imaging findings at medium-term follow-up. Int Orthop. 2013;37(8):1583–9.

42. Murawski CD, Smyth NA, Newman H, et al. A single platelet-rich plasma injection for chronic midsubstance Achilles tendinopathy: a retrospective preliminary analysis. Foot Ankle Spec. 2014;7(5):372–6.

43. Filardo G, Kon E, Di Matteo B, et al. Platelet-rich plasma injections for the treatment of refractory Achilles tendinopathy: results at 4 years. Blood Transfus. 2014;12(4):533–40.

44. Charousset C, Zaoui A, Bellaiche L, et al. Are multiple platelet-rich plasma injections useful for treatment of chronic patellar tendinopathy in athletes? A prospective study. Am J Sports Med. 2014;42(4):906–11.

45. Oloff L, Elmi E, Nelson J, et al. Retrospective analysis of the effectiveness of platelet-rich plasma in the treatment of Achilles tendinopathy: pretreatment and posttreatment correlation of magnetic resonance imaging and clinical assessment. Foot Ankle Spec. 2015;8(6):490–7.

46. de Vos RJ, Weir A, Tol JL, et al. No effects of PRP on ultrasonographic tendon structure and neovascularisation in chronic midportion Achilles tendinopathy. Br J Sports Med. 2011;45(5):387–92.

47. Zou J, Mo X, Shi Z, Li T, Xue J, Mei G, Li X. A prospective study of platelet-rich plasma as biological augmentation for acute Achilles tendon rupture repair. Biomed Res Int. 2016;2016(January 2014):1–8.

48. Krogh TP, Ellingsen T, Christensen R, Jensen P, Fredberg U. Ultrasound-guided injection therapy of Achilles tendinopathy with platelet-rich plasma or saline: a randomized, blinded, placebo-controlled trial. Am J Sports Med. 2016;44(8):1990–7.

49. Kon E, Filardo G, Delcogliano M, et al. Platelet-rich plasma: new clinical appli- cation: a pilot study for treatment of jumper's knee. Injury. 2009;40(6):598–603.

50. de Almeida AM, Demange MK, Sobrado MF, et al. Patellar tendon healing with platelet-rich plasma: a prospective randomized controlled trial. Am J Sports Med. 2012;40

51. Cervellin M, de Girolamo L, Bait C, et al. Autologous platelet-rich plasma gel to reduce donor-site morbidity after patellar tendon graft harvesting for anterior cruciate ligament reconstruction: a randomized, controlled clinical study. Knee Surg Sports Traumatol Arthrosc. 2012;20(1):114–20. (6):1282–8.

52. Vetrano M, Castorina A, Vulpiani MC, et al. Platelet-rich plasma versus focused shock waves in the treatment of jumper's knee in athletes. Am J Sports Med. 2013;41(4):795–803.

53. Dragoo JL, Wasterlain AS, Braun HJ, et al. Platelet-rich plasma as a treatment for patellar tendinopathy: a double-blind, randomized controlled trial. Am J Sports Med. 2014;42(3):610–8.

54. Kaux JF, Bruyere O, Croisier JL, et al. One-year follow-up of platelet-rich plasma infiltration to treat chronic proximal patellar tendinopathies. Acta Orthop Belg. 2015;81(2):251–6.

55. Zayni R, Thaunat M, Fayard JM, et al. Platelet-rich plasma as a treatment for chronic patellar tendinopathy: comparison of a single versus two consecutive injections. Muscles Ligaments Tendons J. 2015;5(2):92–8.

56. Kaux JF, Croisier JL, Forthomme B, Le Goff C, Buhler F, Savanier B, et al. Using platelet-rich plasma to treat jumper's knees: exploring the effect of a second closely-timed infiltration. J Sci Med Sport. 2016;19(3):200–4.

57. Gumina S, Campagna V, Ferrazza G, et al. Use of platelet-leukocyte membrane in arthroscopic repair of large rotator cuff tears: a prospective randomized study. J Bone Joint Surg Am. 2012;94(15):1345–52.

58. Randelli P, Arrigoni P, Ragone V, et al. Platelet rich plasma in arthroscopic rotator cuff repair: a prospective RCT study, 2-year follow-up. J Shoulder Elb Surg. 2011;20(4):518–28.

59. Malavolta EA, Gracitelli ME, Ferreira Neto AA, et al. Platelet-rich plasma in rotator cuff repair: a prospective randomized study. Am J Sports Med. 2014;42(10):2446–54.

60. Jo CH, Kim JE, Yoon KS, et al. Does platelet-rich plasma accelerate recovery after rotator cuff repair? A prospective cohort study. Am J Sports Med. 2011;39(10):2082–90.

61. Hak A, Rajaratnam K, Ayeni OR, et al. A double-blinded placebo randomized controlled trial evaluating short-term efficacy of platelet-rich plasma in reducing postoperative pain after arthroscopic rotator cuff repair: a pilot study. Sports Health. 2015;7(1):58–66.

62. Rodeo SA, Delos D, Williams RJ, et al. The effect of platelet-rich fibrin matrix on rotator cuff tendon healing: a prospective, randomized clinical study. Am J Sports Med. 2012;40(6):1234–41.

63. Carr AJ, Murphy R, Dakin SG, et al. Platelet-rich plasma injection with arthroscopic acromioplasty for chronic rotator cuff tendinopathy: a randomized controlled trial. Am J Sports Med. 2015;43(12):2891–7.

64. Reurink G, Goudswaard GJ, Moen MH, et al. Platelet-rich plasma injections in acute muscle injury. N Engl J Med. 2014;370(26):2546–7.

65. Reurink G, Goudswaard GJ, Moen MH, et al. Rationale, secondary outcome scores and 1-year follow-up of a randomised trial of platelet-rich plasma injections in acute hamstring muscle injury: the Dutch Hamstring Injection Therapy Study. Br J Sports Med. 2015;49(18):1206–12.

66. Fader RR, Mitchell JJ, Traub S, et al. Platelet-rich plasma treatment improves outcomes for chronic proximal hamstring injuries in an athletic population. Muscles Ligaments Tendons J. 2015;4:461Y6.

67. Hamilton B, Tol JL, Almusa E, et al. Platelet-rich plasma does not enhance return to play in hamstring injuries: a randomised controlled trial. Br J Sports Med. 2015;49(14):943–50.

68. Ragab EM, Othman AM. Platelets rich plasma for treatment of chronic plantar fasciitis. Arch Orthop Trauma Surg. 2012;132(8):1065–70.

69. Martinelli N, Marinozzi A, Carni S, et al. Platelet-rich plasma injections for chronic plantar fasciitis. Int Orthop. 2013;37(5):839–42.

70. Kumar V, Millar T, Murphy PN, et al. The treatment of intractable plantar fasciitis with platelet-rich plasma injection. Foot (Edinb). 2013;23(2–3):74–7.

71. Lee TG, Ahmad TS. Intralesional autologous blood injection compared to corticosteroid injection for treatment of chronic plantar fasciitis. A prospective, randomized, controlled trial. Foot Ankle Int. 2007;28(9):984–90.

72. Omar AS, Ibrahim ME, Ahmed AS, et al. Local injection of autologous platelet rich plasma and corticosteroid in treatment of lateral epicondylitis and plantar fasciitis: randomized clinical trial. Egypt Rheumatol. 2012;34:43–9.

73. Aksahin E, Dogruyol D, Yuksel HY, et al. The comparison of the effect of corticosteroids and platelet-rich plasma (PRP) for the treatment of plantar fasciitis. Arch Orthop Trauma Surg. 2012;132(6):781–5.

74. Say F, Gurler D, Inkaya E, et al. Comparison of platelet-rich plasma and steroid injection in the treatment of plantar fasciitis. Acta Orthop Traumatol Turc. 2014;48(6):667–72.

75. Monto RR. Platelet-rich plasma efficacy versus corticosteroid injection treatment for chronic severe plantar fasciitis. Foot Ankle Int. 2014;35(4):313–8.

76. Shetty VD, Dhillon M, Hegde C, et al. A study to compare the efficacy of corticosteroid therapy with platelet-rich plasma therapy in recalcitrant plantar fasciitis: a preliminary report. Foot Ankle Surg. 2014;20(1):10–3.

77. Jain K, Murphy PN, Clough TM. Platelet rich plasma versus corticosteroid injection for plantar fasciitis: a comparative study. Foot (Edinb). 2015;25(4):235–7.

78. Kim E, Lee JH. Autologous platelet-rich plasma versus dextrose prolotherapy for the treatment

of chronic recalcitrant plantar fasciitis. PM R. 2013;6(2):152–8.

79. Mahindra P, Yamin M, Selhi HS, et al. Chronic plantar fasciitis: effect of platelet-rich plasma, corticosteroid, and placebo. Orthopedics. 2016;39(2):e285–9.

80. Gill SPS. A randomized controlled study to evaluate the effectiveness of local platelet rich plasma (PRP) injection for the management of the cases of planter fasciitis – final outcome of 179 cases at 12 months. Indian J Appl Res. 2016;6(November):59–64.

81. Lee JJ, Harrison JR, Boachie-Adjei K, Vargas E, Moley PJ. Platelet-rich plasma injections with needle tenotomy for gluteus medius tendinopathy: a registry study with prospective follow-up. Orthop J Sports Med. 2016;4(11):2325967116671692.

82. Edwards SG, Calandruccio JH. Autologous blood injections for refractory lateral epicondylitis. J Hand Surg. 2003;28(2):272–8.

83. Creaney L, Wallace A, Curtis M, et al. Growth factor-based therapies provide additional benefit beyond physical therapy in resistant elbow tendinopathy: a prospective, single-blind, randomised trial of autologous blood injections versus platelet-rich plasma injections. Br J Sports Med. 2011;45(12):966–71.

84. Krogh TP, Bartels EM, Ellingsen T, et al. Comparative effectiveness of injection therapies in lateral epicondylitis: a systematic review and network meta- analysis of randomized controlled trials. Am J Sports Med. 2013;41(6):1435–46.

85. Ahmad Z, Brooks R, Kang SN, Weaver H, Nunney I, Tytherleigh-Strong G, Rushton N. The effect of platelet-rich plasma on clinical outcomes in lateral epicondylitis. J Arthrosc Relat Surg. 2013;29(11):1851–62.

86. Chou L-C, Liou T-H, Kuan Y-C, Huang Y-H, Chen H-C. Autologous blood injection for treatment of lateral epicondylosis: a meta-analysis of randomized controlled trials. Phys Therapy Sport. 2016;18(2016):68–73.

87. Babak Vahdatpour B, Kianimehr L, Ahrar MH. Autologous platelet-rich plasma compared with whole blood for the treatment of chronic plantar fasciitis; a comparative clinical trial. Adv Biomed Res. 2016;5:84.

88. Pearson J. Autologous blood injection to treat Achilles tendinopathy? A randomized controlled trial. J Sport Rehab. 2012;21:218.

89. Scott A, LaPrade RF, Harmon KG, et al. Platelet-rich plasma for patellar tendinopathy: a randomized controlled trial of leukocyte-rich PRP or leukocyte-poor PRP versus saline. AJSM. 2019;47(7):1654–61.

90. Delong JM, Russell RP, Mazzocca AD. Platelet-rich plasma: the PAW classification system. J Arthrosc Relat Surgry. 2012;28(7):998–1009.

91. Mishra A, Harmon K, Woodall J, Vieira A. Sports medicine applications of platelet rich plasma. Curr Pharm Biotechnol. 2012;13(March 2016):1185–95.

92. Everts PA, Malanga GA, Paul RV, Rothenberg JB, Stephens N, Mautner KR. Assessing clinical implications and perspectives of the pathophysiological effects of erythrocytes and plasma free hemoglobin in autologous biologics for use in musculoskeletal regenerative medicine therapies. A review. Regen Ther. 2019;11:56–64. Published 2019 May 10. https://doi.org/10.1016/j.reth.2019.03.009.

93. Mautner K, Malanga GA, Smith J, Shiple B, Ibrahim V, Sampson S, Bowen JE. A call for a standard classification system for future biologic research: the rationale for new PRP nomenclature. PMR. 2015;7(4):S53–9.

94. Lana, et al. Contributions for classification of platelet rich plasma – proposal of a new classification: MARSPILL. Regen Med. 2017;12(5):565–74.

95. Zhou Y, Wang J, et al. PRP treatment efficacy for tendinopathy: a review of basic science studies. Bio Med Res Int. 2016:1–8.

96. Dragoo JL, Braun HJ, Durham JL, Ridley BA, Odegaard JI, Luong R, et al. Comparison of the acute inflammatory response of two commercial platelet-rich plasma systems in healthy rabbit tendons. Am J Sports Med. 2012;40:1274–81.

97. Sundman EA, Cole BJ, Fortier LA. Growth factor and catabolic cytokine concentrations are influenced by the cellular composition of platelet-rich plasma. Am J Sports Med. 2011;39:2135–40.

98. Lansdown DA, Fortier LA. Platelet rich plasma: formulations, preparations, constituents, and their effects. Oper Tech Sports Med. 2017;25(1):7–12.

99. Fitzpatrick J, Bulsara M, Zheng MH. The effectiveness of platelet-rich plasma in the treatment of tendinopathy: a meta-analysis of randomized controlled clinical trials. Am J Sports Med. 2016:363546516643716.

100. Le ADK, Enweze L, DeBaun MR, Dragoo JL. Current clinical recommendations for use of platelet-rich. Plasma Curr Rev Musculoskeletal Med. 2018;11(4):624–34.

101. Kushida S, Kakudo N, Morimoto N, et al. Platelet and growth factor concentrations in activated platelet-rich plasma: a comparison of seven commercial separation systems. J Artif Organs. 2014;17:186–92.

102. Wang JHC, Nirmala X. Application of tendon stem/progenitor cells and platelet-rich plasma to treat tendon injuries. Oper Tech Orthop. 2016;26(2):68–72.

103. Neph A, Schroeder A, Enseki KR, et al. Role of mechanical loading for platelet-rich plasma treated Achilles tendinopathy. Curr Sports Med Reports. 2020;

104. Yuan T, Zhang CQ, Wang JH. Augmenting tendon and ligament repair with platelet-rich plasma (PRP). Muscles Ligaments Tendons J. 2013;3(3):139–49. Epub 2013/12/25. PubMed PMID: 24367773; PubMed Central PMCID: PMCPMC3838322.

105. Zhang J, Yuan T, Wang JH. Moderate treadmill running exercise prior to tendon injury enhances wound healing in aging rats. Oncotarget. 2016;7(8):8498–512. Epub 2016/02/18. https://doi.org/10.18632/oncotarget.7381. PubMed PMID: 26885754; PubMed Central PMCID: PMCPMC4890982.

106. Takamura M, Yasuda T, Nakano A, Shima H, Neo M. The effect of platelet-rich plasma on Achilles tendon healing in a rabbit model. Acta Orthop Traumatol Turc. 2017;51(1):65–72. Epub 2016/12/29. https://doi.org/10.1016/j.aott.2016.12.001. PubMed PMID: 28027872; PubMed Central PMCID: PMCPMC6197299.

107. Lyras DN, Kazakos K, Verettas D, Polychronidis A, Tryfonidis M, Botaitis S, et al. The influence of platelet-rich plasma on angiogenesis during the early phase of tendon healing. Foot Ankle Int. 2009;30(11):1101–6. Epub 2009/11/17. https://doi.org/10.3113/FAI.2009.1101.

108. Zhang J, Middleton KK, Fu FH, Im HJ, Wang JH. HGF mediates the anti-inflammatory effects of PRP on injured tendons. PLoS One. 2013;8(6):e67303. Epub 2013/07/11. https://doi.org/10.1371/journal.pone.0067303. PubMed PMID: 23840657; PubMed Central PMCID: PMCPMC3696073.

109. Zhang J, Wang JH. PRP treatment effects on degenerative tendinopathy – an in vitro model study. Muscles Ligaments Tendons J. 2014;4(1):10–7. Epub 2014/06/17. PubMed PMID: 24932441; PubMed Central PMCID: PMCPMC4049643.

110. Neph A, Onishi K, Wang JH. Myths and facts of in-office regenerative procedures for tendinopathy: literature review. Am J Phys Med Rehabil. 2018. Epub 2018/11/16; https://doi.org/10.1097/PHM.0000000000001097.

111. Maffulli N, Longo UG, Denaro V. Novel approaches for the management of tendinopathy. J Bone Joint Surg Am. 2010;92:2604–13.

112. Iwasaki M, Nakahara H, Nakata K, Nakase T, Kimura T, Ono K. Regulation of proliferation and osteochondrogenic differentiation of periosteum-derived cells by transforming growth factor-beta and basic fibroblast growth factor. J Bone Joint Surg Am. 1995;77:543–54.

113. Rabago D, Best TM, Zgierska AE, Zeisig E, Ryan M, Crane D. A systematic review of four injection therapies for lateral epicondylosis: prolotherapy, polidocanol, whole blood and platelet-rich plasma. Br J Sports Med. 2009;43:471–81.

114. Evans JP, Metz J, Anaspure R, et al. The spread of Injectate after ultrasound guided lateral elbow injection – a cadaveric study. J Exper Orthopaed. 2018;5:27.

115. Raeissadat SA, Rayegani SM, Hassanabadi H, Rahimi R, Sedighipour L, Rostami K. Is platelet-rich plasma superior to whole blood in the management of chronic tennis elbow: 1 year randomized clinical trial. BMC Sports Sci Med Rehabil. 2014;6(1):12. https://doi.org/10.1186/2052-1847-6-12.

116. Raeissadat SA, Sedighipour L, Rayegani SM, Bahrami MH, Bayat M, Rahimi R. Effect of platelet-rich plasma (PRP) versus autologous whole blood on pain and function improvement in tennis elbow: a randomized clinical trial. Pain Res Treat. 2014; https://doi.org/10.1155/2014/191525.

117. Kazemi M, Azma K, Tavana B, Rezaiee Moghaddam F, Panahi A. Autologous blood versus corticosteroid local injection in the short-term treatment of lateral elbow tendinopathy: a randomized clinical trial of efficacy. Am J Phys Med Rehabil. 2010;89(8):660–7.

118. Singh A, Gangwar DS, Shekhar. Autologous blood versus corticosteroid local injection for treatment of lateral epicondylosis: a randomized clinical trial. Online J Health Allied Sci. 2013;12(2):11.

119. Dojode CM. A randomised control trial to evaluate the efficacy of autologous blood injection versus local corticosteroid injection for treatment of lateral epicondylitis. Bone Joint Res. 2012;1(8):192–7.

120. Arirachakaran A, Sukthuayat A, Sisayanarane T, et al. Platelet-rich plasma versus autologous blood versus steroid injection in lateral epicondylitis:systematic review and network meta-analysis. J Orthopaed Traumatol. 2016;17:101–12.

121. Baraniak PR, McDevitt TC. Stem cell paracrine actions and tissue regeneration. Regen Med. 2010;5:121–43.

122. Rubio-Azpeitia E, Sanchez P, Delgado D, Andia I. Adult cells combined with platelet-rich plasma for tendon healing. Orthop J Sports Med. 2017;5(2):1–11.

123. Caplan AI. Mesenchymal stem cells. J Orthop Res. 1991;9:641–50.

124. Pittenger MF, Mackay AM, Beck SC, et al. Multilineage potential of adult human mesenchymal stem cells. Science. 1999;284(5411):143–7.

125. da Silva ML, Chagastelles PC, Nardi NB. Mesenchymal stem cells reside in virtually all post-natal organs and tissues. J Cell Sci. 2006;119:2204–13.

126. De Bari C, Dell'Accio F, Tylzanowski P, Luyten FP. Multipotent mesenchymal stem cells from adult human synovial membrane. Arthritis Rheum. 2001;44:1928–42.

127. Williams JT, Southerland SS, Souza J, Souza J, Calcutt AF, Cartledge RG. Cells isolated from adult human skeletal muscle capable of differentiating into multiple mesodermal phenotypes. Am Surg. 1999;65:22–6.

128. www.fda.gov 21st Century Cures Act (Public Law 114–255).

129. Bocker W, Yin Z, Drosse I, Haasters F, Rossmann O, Wierer M, Popov C, Locher M, Mutschler W, Docheva D, Schieker M. Introducing a single-cell-derived human mesenchymal stem cell line expressing hTERT after lentiviral gene transfer. J Cell Mol Med. 2008;12:1347–59.

130. Wakitani S, Saito T, Caplan AI. Myogenic cells derived from rat bone marrow mesenchymal stem cells exposed to 5-azacytidine. Muscle Nerve. 1995;18:1417–26.

131. Young RG, Butler DL, Weber W, et al. Use of mesenchymal stem cells in a collagen matrix for Achilles tendon repair. J Orthop Res. 1998;16:406–13.

132. Uccelli A, Moretta L, Pistoia V. Immunoregulatory function of mesenchymal stem cells. Eur J Immunol. 2006;36:2566–73.

133. Stanulis-Prager B. In-vitro studies of aging. Clin Geriatric Med. 1983;5:23–40.

134. Dressler MR, Butler DL, Boivin GP. Effects of age on the repair ability of mesenchymal stem cells in rabbit tendon. J Orthop Res. 2005;23:287–93.

135. Cristofalo VJ. Cellular biomarkers of aging. Exp Gerontol. 1988;23:297–307.

136. Friedlis MF, Centeno CJ. Performing a Better Bone Marrow Aspiration. Phys Med Rehabil Clin N Am. 2016;27:919–39.

137. Marx RE, Tursun R. A qualitative and quantitative analysis of autologous human multipotent adult stem cells derived from three anatomic areas by marrow aspi ration: tibia, anterior ilium, and posterior ilium. Int J Oral Maxillofac Implants. 2013;28(5):e290–4.

138. Rahnama R, Wang M, Dang AC, et al. Cytotoxicity of local anesthetics on human mesenchymal stem cells. J Bone Joint Surg. 2013;95(2):132–7.

139. Batinic D, Marusic M, Pavletic Z, et al. Relationship between differing volumes of bone marrow aspirates and their cellular composition. Bone Marrow Transplant. 1990;6(2):103–7.

140. Muschler GF, Boehm C, Easley K. Aspiration to obtain osteoblast progenitor cells from human bone marrow: the influence of aspiration volume. J Bone Joint Surg Am. 1997;79(11):1699–709.

141. Fennema EM, Renard AJS, Leusink A, et al. The effect of bone marrow aspiration strategy on the yield and quality of human mesenchymal stem cells. Acta Orthop. 2009;80(5):618–21.

142. Hedge V, Shonuga O, Ellis S, et al. A prospective comparison of 3 approved systems for autologous bone marrow concentration demonstrated nonequivalency in progenitor cell number and concentration. J Orthop Trauma. 2014;28(10):591–8.

143. Chahla J, Mannava S, Cinque ME, et al. Bone marrow aspirate concentration harvesting and processing technique. Arthrosc Tech. 2017;6(2):e441–5.

144. Nazal MR, McCarthy MBR, Mazzocca AD. Connective tissue progenitor analysis of bone marrow aspirate concentrate harvested from the body of the ilium during arthroscopic acetabular labral repair. Arthroscopy. 2020. piiS0749–8063(19)31166–1.

145. Bosi A, Bartolozzi B. Safety of bone marrow stem cell donation: a review. Transplant Proc. 2010;42(6):2192–4.

146. Centeno CJ, Al-Sayegh H, Freeman MD, et al. A multi-center analysis of adverse events among two thousand, three hundred and seventy two adult patients undergoing adult autologous stem cell therapy for orthopaedic conditions. Int Ortho (SICOT). 2016;40:1755–65.

147. Lalu MM, McIntyre L, Pugliese C, et al. Safety of cell therapy with mesenchymal stromal cells (SafeCell): a systematic review and meta-analysis of clinical trials. PLoS One. 2012;7:e47559.

148. Centeno C, Pitts J, Al-Sayegh H, et al. Efficacy of autologous bone marrow concentrate for knee osteoarthritis with and without adipose graft. Biomed Res Int. 2014;2014:370621.

149. Singh A, Gangwar DS, Singh S. Bone marrow injection: a novel treatment for tennis elbow. J Nat Sc Biol Med. 2014;5(2):389–91.

150. Pascual-Garrido C, Rolon A, Makino A. Treatment of chronic patellar tendinopathy with autologous bone marrow stem cells: a 5-year-followup. Stem Cells Int. 2012;

151. Centeno CJ, Al-Sayegh H, Bashir J, et al. A prospective multi-site registry study of a specific protocol of autologous bone marrow concentrate for the treatment of shoulder rotator cuff tears and osteoarthritis. J Pain Res. 2015;8:269–76.

152. Hernigou P, Flouzat Lachaniette CH, Delambre J, et al. Biologic augmentation of rotator cuff repair with mesenchymal stem cells during arthroscopy improves healing and prevents further tears: a case-controlled study. Int Orthop. 2014;38:1811–8.

153. Kim SJ, Song DH, Park JW, et al. Effect of bone marrow aspirate concentrate-platelet-rich plasma on tendon-derived stem cells and rotator cuff tendon tear. Cell Transplant. 2017;26:867–78.

154. Schroeder A, Rubin P, Kokai L, et al. Use of adipose-derived orthobiologics for musculoskeletal injuries: a narrative review. PM&R xx. 2020:1–12.

155. Aust L, Devlin B, Foster SJ, et al. Yield of human adipose-derived adult stem cells from liposuction aspirates. Cytotherapy. 2004;6(1):7–14.

156. Zuk PA, Zhu M, Mizuno H, et al. Multilineage cells from human adipose tissue: implications for cell-based therapies. Tissue Eng. 2001;7(2):211–28.

157. Jurgens, JFM W, et al. Effect of tissue-harvesting site on yield of stem cells derived from adipose tissue: implications for cell-based therapies. Cell Tissue Res. 2008;332(3):415–26.

158. Bora P, Majumdar AS. Adipose tissue-derived stromal vascular fraction in regenerative medicine: a brief review on biology and translation. Stem Cell Res Ther. 2017;8(1):145.

159. Bianchi F, Maioli M, Leonardi E, et al. A new non-enzymatic method and device to obtain a fat tissue derivative highly enriched in pericyte-like elements by mild mechanical forces from human lipoaspirates. Cell Transplant. 2013;22(11):2063–77.

160. Housman TS, et al. The safety of liposuction: results of a national survey. Dermatol Surg. 2002;

161. Lee SY, Kim W, Lim C, Chung SG. Treatment of lateral epicondylosis by using allogeneic adipose-dervied mesenchymal stem cells: a pilot study. Stem Cells. 2015;33:2995–3005.

162. Striano RD, Malanga G, Bilbool N, Azatullah K. Refractory shoulder pain with osteoarthritis, and rotator cuff tear, treated with micro-fragmented adipose tissue. J Orthop Spine Sports Med. 2018;2(1):014.

163. Usuelli FG, Grassi M, Maccario C, et al. Intratendinous adipose-derived stromal vascular fraction (SVF) injection provides a safe, effica-

cious treatment for Achilles tendinopathy: results of a randomized controlled clinical trial at a 6-month follow-up. Knee Surg Sports Traumatol Arthrosc. 2018;26(7):2000–10.

164. Wang A, Breidahl W, Mackie KE, et al. Autologous tenocyte injection for the treatment of severe, chronic resistant lateral epicondylitis: a pilot study. Am J Sports Med. 2013;41(12):2925–32.

165. Jang Y, Koh YG, Choi YJ, et al. Characterization of adipose tissue-derived stromal vascular fracture for clinical application to cartilage regeneration. In Vitro Cell Dev Biol Anim. 2015;51(2):142–50.

166. McIntyre JA, Jones IA, Danilkovich A, et al. The placednta applications in orthopaedic sports medicine. AJSM. 2018;46(1):234–47.

167. Niknejad H, Peirovi H, Jorjani M, et al. Properties of the amniotic membrane for potential use in tissue engineering. Eur Cell Mater. 2008;15:88–99.

168. Parolini O, Solomon A, Evangelista M, Soncini M. Human term placenta as a therapeutic agent: from the first clinical applications to future perspectives. In: Berven E, editor. Human placenta: structure and development. Hauppauge, NY: Nova Science; 2010. p. 1–48.

169. Park S, Koh S-E, Hur CY, Lee W-D, Lim J, Lee Y-J. Comparison of human first and third trimester placental mesenchymal stem cell. Cell Biol Int. 2013;37(3):242–9.

170. Zelen C, Poka A, Andrews J. Prospective, randomized, blinded, comparative study of injectable micronized dehydrated amniotic/chornionic membrane allograft for plantar fasciitis – A feasibility study. Foot Ankle Int. 2013;34(10):1332–9.

171. Hanselman AE, Tidwell JE, Santrock RD. Cryopreserved human amniotic membrane injection for plantar fasciitis: a randomized, controlled, double-blind pilot study. Foot Ankle Int. 2015;36:151–8.

172. Pappa KI, Anagnou NP. Novel sources of fetal stem cells: where do they fit on the developmental continuum? Regen Med. 2009;4(3):423–33.

173. Roubelakis MG, Trohatou O, Anagnou NP. Amniotic fluid and amniotic membrane stem cells: marker discovery. Stem Cells Int. 2012;2012(11):107836–9.

174. Kaviani A, Perry TE, Dzakovic A, Jennings RW, Ziegler MM, Fauza DO. The amniotic fluid as a source of cells for fetal tissue engineering. J Pediatr Surg. 2001;36(11):1662–5.

175. Poloni A, Maurizi G, Serrani F, et al. Human AB serum for generation of mesenchymal stem cells from human chorionic villi: comparison with other source and other media including platelet lysate. Cell Prolif. 2012;45(1):66–75.

176. Lynch SE, Nixon JC, Colvin RB, et al. Role of platelet-derived growth factor in wound healing: synergistic effects with other growth factors. Proc Natl Acad Sci U S A. 1987;84:7696–700.

177. Adinolfi M, Akle CA, Mccoll I, et al. Expression of HLA antigens, beta 2-microglobulin and enzymes by human amniotic epithelial cells. Nature. 1982;295(5847):325–7.

178. Werber B. Amniotic tissues for the treatment of chronic plantar fasciosis and Achilles tendinosis. J Sports Med. 2015;2015:219896.

179. Gellhorn AC, Han A. The use of dehydrated human amnion/chorion membrane allograft injection for the treatment of tendinopathy or arthritis: a case series involving 40 patients. PM R. 2017;9(12):1236–43.

Office-Based Chemical Procedures for Tendons

Caroline Schepker, Xiaoning Yuan,
Zachary Bailowitz, and Christopher Visco

Introduction

The term "prolotherapy" stems from a neologism coined in the 1930s to describe what was believed to be a "proliferative" therapy. Throughout the early twentieth century, prolotherapy began with the use of irritating injectates introduced into various subcutaneous and soft tissue structures to stimulate healing [1]. Early clinical applications were aimed at addressing ligamentous laxity, joint instability, and hernia repair [2]. The theoretical basis underlying prolotherapy originated from an even earlier observation that healing could be stimulated through an inflammatory response. Reportedly, Roman gladiators utilized aggressive needling to induce sclerosis within the connective tissues supporting injured joints, such as shoulders [1].

Modern practice of prolotherapy is conventionally aimed at addressing various musculoskeletal complaints including pain, instability, and laxity attributable to either overt or microtrauma within connective tissue structures. Various hyperosmolar injectates are used, including dextrose, morrhuate sodium, polidocanol, and phenol-glycerine-glucose [3]. Dextrose is most commonly used at varying concentrations. Evidence-based protocols for injectate solutions, concentrations, and musculoskeletal indications are lacking; however, mild-to-moderate evidence exists for the use of dextrose injections to address ligamentous injuries, osteoarthritis, and tendinopathy. Polidocanol and morrhuate sodium have been used as vascular sclerosing agents. Morrhuate sodium is derived from the salts of cod liver oil [1, 4].

Prolotherapy is considered by some to fall under the umbrella of "regenerative therapies" in large part due to the genesis of additional fibrotic tissue that has been demonstrated from repeated application. However, the composition of injectate is distinct from other regenerative techniques such as platelet-rich plasma (PRP) and cellular therapies in that it lacks a biologic agent [5]. Hyperosmolar dextrose (typically 10–30%) is usually employed in highly variable injection protocols that involve different musculoskeletal structures (often ligament and/or tendon, at multiple sites) and are performed multiple times over several weeks or months. Patients who undergo

C. Schepker (✉)
Department of Physical Medicine and Rehabilitation, Weill Cornell Medical College, New York, NY, USA
e-mail: cas9219@nyp.org

X. Yuan
Department of Physical Medicine and Rehabilitation, Uniformed Services University of the Health Sciences, Bethesda, MD, USA
e-mail: xiaoning.yuan@usuhs.edu

Z. Bailowitz
Department of Orthopedics, Podiatry, & Sports Medicine, Kaiser Permanente Medical Center, Oakland, CA, USA

C. Visco
Department of Rehabilitation and Regenerative Medicine, Columbia University, New York, NY, USA
e-mail: cv2245@cumc.columbia.edu

© Springer Nature Switzerland AG 2021
K. Onishi et al. (eds.), *Tendinopathy*, https://doi.org/10.1007/978-3-030-65335-4_20

prolotherapy injections are frequently advised to avoid anti-inflammatory medications following the injections to avoid blunting of the inflammatory response, which is believed to serve as the impetus for tissue healing and repair. Vigorous activity may also be limited until resolution of expected resultant inflammation [2].

Mechanism of Action

The mechanisms underlying the therapeutic effect of prolotherapy may be multifactorial. Current theoretical models include inciting an inflammatory response that serves as a stimulus for tissue healing and repair, growth factor activation, and vascular sclerosis [5, 6]. The degree of dextrose hypertonicity in the injectate likely alters the magnitude of effect. Following administration of the hypertonic dextrose, cells shear, and lyse, causing

local tissue injury and stimulating the sequence of overlapping events that comprise wound healing [7]. Cellular debris attracts neutrophils to the site of injury in the initial inflammatory phase within 24–48 hours of injection, which debride the local "wound" environment. Macrophages follow within 72 hours of injury, which release proteolytic enzymes to break down the local extracellular matrix and secrete growth factors that recruit fibroblasts to synthesize new matrix. Fibroblast migration begins during the proliferative phase of wound healing, during which matrix components are synthesized including collagen and proteoglycans. The final phase of remodeling is a continuation of collagen synthesis and remodeling of the extracellular matrix, which occurs over a period of months. See Fig. 20.1.

In vitro studies have demonstrated effects of dextrose on various cytokines: GLUT 1–4 cell surface proteins transport dextrose into human

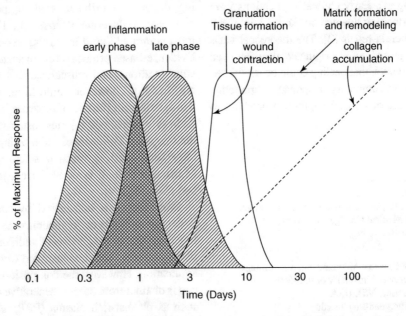

Fig. 20.1 The overlapping phases of wound healing: inflammation, granulation tissue formation, and extracellular matrix formation and remodeling. A proposed mechanism of prolotherapy is injections create a localized tissue injury, along with initiation of the inflammatory cascade, occurring over the first few days of healing. This is followed by the cell proliferation and tissue synthesis phase, consisting of angiogenesis, collagen deposition, granulation tissue formation, epithelization, and wound contraction. Finally, the tissue remodeling phase occurs

weeks to months after injury, involving collagen and extracellular matrix maturation. Time in days presented on a logarithmic scale [42]. *Summary of Wound Repair:* Inflammation: early and late inflammation lead to granulation tissue formation. Granulation tissue is rich in fibroblasts and mononuclear cells which result in healing, through a process of matrix deposition and remodeling. The new matrix is composed of collagen and other substances which are accumulated during a period of months, giving added strength to the injury (Clark 1985) cells and also interact with cytokines to signal cell growth and repair [8]. The presence of extracellular glucose and other sugar molecules has been observed to result in an upregulation of genetic expression of regulators such as connective tissue growth factor (CTGF) [9]. CTGF in turn induces cytokine pathways that promote activation of fibroblasts, chondrocytes, and nerve cells in both human and animal cells [9–12]. Studies of the effects of prolotherapy on the rat knee medial collateral ligament (MCL) have shown infiltration of leukocytes and macrophages into the ligament tissue following injection—a phenomenon that was absent when compared with saline injections and dry needling [3]. Postmortem analysis of MCL cross-sectional area following prolotherapy also revealed a significantly greater amount of ligamentous tissue as compared with the other injections. Similar studies examining the injection of morrhuate sodium into rabbit patellar and Achilles tendons demonstrated increased tendon diameter and perhaps even increased tendon tensile strength [13, 14]. However, some of these findings should be interpreted with caution, as other animal studies have failed to find a difference in tendon strength after dextrose injections as compared with no intervention [15]. Tissue tensile strength is in-part conferred by the surrounding fascia. Hyperosmolar dextrose in increasing concentration has been demonstrated to thicken this fascia and subsequently increase the tensile strength of the subsynovial connective tissue in the rabbit forepaw [16, 17].

An alternative proposed mechanism of action emphasizes possible effects on nociception. The presence of extracellular hyperosmolar dextrose causes potassium channels to open, and may result in hyperpolarization of nearby nerve cells. Hyperpolarization is associated with decreased pain perception, as it inhibits nociception [18]. Additionally, irritant solutions may result in sclerosis of local infiltrative vessels, thereby putting a halt to the maladaptive angiogenesis and hyperemia that may be observed in chronic painful tendinopathies [18].

While the mechanism of action underlying the effects of prolotherapy on both pain control and laxity is highly theoretical, multiple mechanisms may be at play at both the cellular and tissue levels.

Available Evidence for Tendinopathy

A 2015 review has identified limited evidence for the safety and efficacy of prolotherapy for various conditions, including Achilles tendinopathy, plantar fasciosis, and Osgood-Schlatter disease; however, study quality was considered to be poor [19]. A separate 2015 review assigned a level A strength of recommendation for Achilles tendinopathy and knee OA, and level B for lateral epicondylosis, Osgood-Schlatter disease, and plantar fasciosis [20]. A level A designation has a basis in "good quality patient-oriented evidence", while level B recommendations have "limited quality patient-orientated evidence" [20]. Two subsequent review articles in 2016 included level B evidence for rotator cuff tendinopathy [5].

Of the various conditions studied with regard to prolotherapy interventions, tendinopathy has been the most studied and affords the greatest available evidence. Most of these studies focus on chronic overuse tendinopathies [21–23]. The most commonly studied tendons include the Achilles tendon, the patellar tendon, and the common extensor tendon. Many researchers have proposed a common underlying pathology among all three of these tendons, as they share similar histologic and sonographic features in tendinopathy [21]. Although not technically a tendon pathology, plantar fasciopathy is often treated with similar techniques to overuse tendinopathy, and one recent randomized control trial showed efficacy of two prolotherapy treatments as compared to two saline injections [24].

Lateral epicondylosis is a common overuse injury that stems from repetitive microtrauma to the common extensor tendon, resulting in angiogenesis and neovascularization of the tendon. Given an early hypothesis that excessive angiogenesis was a primary pain generator, researchers examined the use of vessel sclerosing agents to address pain and functional limitations. Zeisig et al. performed ultrasound-guided injections of lauromacrogol, a vessel sclerosing agent, into the common extensor tendons of 36 subjects diagnosed with lateral epicondylosis. This intervention did not result in a significant improvement in pain [21]. A subsequent double-blind randomized controlled trial of 24 subjects with lateral epicondylosis (average duration of epicondylalgia: 1.9 years) compared saline injections with three injections of hypertonic glucose, morrhuate sodium, and local anesthetic over an 8-week period. While no significant differences in pain symptoms were noted in the short term (prior to the last injection), there was a significant difference favoring the prolotherapy group at 4 months, which was sustained at 1 year of follow-up [22].

Prolotherapy versus corticosteroid injection to the common extensor tendon has also been studied, in a 2011 randomized controlled trial of 17 subjects. Subjects were randomized to receive either dextrose plus phenol-glycerine-glucose plus morrhuate sodium injections or methyl-prednisolone injections. The group that received the prolotherapy injectate demonstrated greater improvements in the Visual Analog Scale (VAS) and the Disabilities of the Arm, Shoulder, and Hand (DASH) at both 3- and 6-month follow-up time points, while the methylprednisolone group showed improvement at 3 months but subsequently regressed after 6 months [25].

A trial of 44 subjects with lateral epicondylosis randomized participants to receive a 50% dextrose injection, a 50% dextrose plus 5% morrhuate sodium injection, or no injection. While both the dextrose and dextrose-plus-morrhuate sodium groups showed improvements in the Patient-Reported Tennis Elbow Evaluation score at 32-weeks as compared with the group that received no intervention, the study is limited by a lack of control injection [26]. The most recent systematic review comparing multiple injection therapies (botulinum toxin, PRP, autologous blood, corticosteroid, hyaluronate, prolotherapy, and placebo saline) for lateral epicondylosis, suggested that prolotherapy and hyaluronate injections were the most effective treatments, but both therapies required more research to validate their superiority [27].

Investigators have also attempted the use of vessel sclerosing agents in both Achilles ten-

dinopathy and patellar tendinopathy. Results were more promising with the patellar tendon than with the Achilles, however investigations of both tendons suggest that neovessels may be a potential therapeutic target. In contrast to the common extensor tendon at the elbow, the Achilles and patellar tendons have a paratenon and fat pad which readily supply neovessels that then carry neo-nociceptors. Figure 20.2 (below) demonstrates neovessels in an Achilles tendinopathy. A 2005 study by Alfredson et al. did not find a definitive improvement in symptoms of Achilles tendinopathy with ultrasound-guided lauromacrogol injections, but results suggested a trend ($p = 0.07$) [28]. However, a 2006 randomized controlled trial by Hoksrud et al. using lauromacrogol injections for chronic patellar tendinopathy did show a statistically significant improvement in pain at 16 weeks as compared with controls [29].

Further studies in Achilles tendinopathy are promising and suggest benefit, but are wrought with imperfect study designs and lack of control subjects. A study of 43 subjects with Achilles tendinopathy compared treatment with prolotherapy alone, with strictly eccentric exercise training, or a combination of the two. All three groups achieved comparable results in the short, immediate, and long term; however, the prolotherapy groups achieved favorable outcomes the fastest [30]. An uncontrolled trial used ultrasound-guided injections of dextrose and anesthetic on 36 patients with Achilles tendinopathy refractory to standard conservative care measures. A

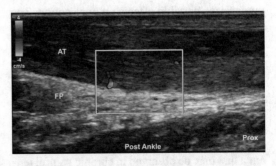

Fig. 20.2 Long axis view of the Achilles tendon seen on ultrasound using a 15–6 MHz transducer reveals neovessels supplying the undersurface and mid-substance tendinopathy from the precalcaneal fat pad. *AT* Achilles tendon, *FP* fat pad

decrease in both pain scores and neovascularity (measured as hyperemia on ultrasound) was observed in over half of the participants, however the lack of control group makes interpreting these findings difficult [31]. Indeed, three systematic reviews of interventions for Achilles tendinopathy, including prolotherapy, advised that long-term and prospective, randomized studies are still needed to strengthen recommendations for treatment [32–34].

Few studies have been published comparing prolotherapy to other regenerative therapies for tendinopathy. A single-center study of 100 cases of proximal biceps tendinopathy treated with PRP therapy or prolotherapy under sonographic guidance demonstrated no significant differences in pain and function at 1 month postprocedure [35]. However, at all subsequent time points out to 12 months, PRP was statistically superior compared to prolotherapy in terms of pain and function. A prospective randomized study of lateral epicondylosis comparing PRP, prolotherapy, extracorporeal shockwave therapy (ESWT), and physical therapy (PT) yielded better clinical outcomes in terms of function for the PRP and prolotherapy groups compared to the ESWT and PT groups, out to 18 months [36]. The authors also performed ultrasound imaging, but did not show significant differences among the four treatment groups in terms of changes in hypoechogenic area or vascularity, despite improvement in function in two of the four groups. Overall, rigorous, prospective, long-term studies comparing prolotherapy to other regenerative therapies against a control intervention remain necessary to establish higher level of evidence and support for prolotherapy treatment of tendinopathy.

Adverse Events and Side Effects

The most noteworthy side effect associated with prolotherapy injections is localized pain and stiffness at the injection site, which lasts from 12 to 96 hours after the injection [31, 37–39]. This phenomenon is often attributed to the desired inflammatory response. Yelland et al. characterized common side effects in a study of prolotherapy for low back pain: 88% reported acute-onset back pain and soreness at the injection site, few reported headaches which resolved within 1 week, and several reported leg pain with neurological features [40]. Rare adverse events reported in pooled studies included sleep disturbance, irregular menses, lumbar puncture headache, meningitis, and adhesive arachnoiditis. However, it is important to note that these were all associated with injections performed in close proximity to the axial skeleton, and that similar adverse events have not been thus far reported with appendicular tendon injections.

Sample Procedures

1. Hackett-Hemwall technique of prolotherapy [41]
   (a) Example: Shoulder
   (b) Indication: Chronic shoulder instability, pain
   (c) Solution: 15% dextrose, 0.2% lidocaine, normal saline
     • Injections: 20–40 injections per shoulder for a total of 20–30 mL of solution per shoulder
     • Tendon (0.5–1 mL each): subscapularis, rotator cuff, biceps
     • Joint: glenohumeral (5–10 mL), acromioclavicular (0.5–1 mL)
     • Bone (0.5–1 mL each): coracoid process, greater tuberosity
     • Ligament (0.5–1 mL each): acromioclavicular, coracoacromial, glenohumeral
2. Modified approach to prolotherapy treatment of focal tendinopathy
   (a) Example: Medial epicondylosis
   (b) Indication: Clinical epicondylosis with imaging confirmed tendinopathy
   (c) Solution: 10% dextrose, 0.4% lidocaine, normal saline. Total of 10 mL.
     • Injections: 1–3 injection(s) to infiltrate the proximal enthesis, pathologic area of the tendon and adjacent tissues – ulnar collateral ligament, fascia, subcutaneous tissue.
     • May be performed with ultrasound guidance, see Fig. 20.3.

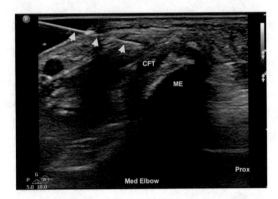

Fig. 20.3 An in-plane ultrasound-guided prolotherapy injection of medial epicondylosis. The injectate will spread to the overlying and surrounding tissue. Arrowheads: needle; *CFT* common flexor tendon, *ME* medial epicondyle

References

1. Rabago D, Best TM, Zgierska AE, et al. A systematic review of four injection therapies for lateral epicondylosis: prolotherapy, polidocanol, whole blood and platelet-rich plasma. Br J Sports Med. 2009;43(7):471–81. https://doi.org/10.1136/bjsm.2008.052761.

2. Rabago D, Slattengren A, Zgierska A. Prolotherapy in primary care practice. Prim Care. 2010;37(1):65–80. https://doi.org/10.1016/j.pop.2009.09.013.

3. Jensen KT, Rabago DP, Best TM, Patterson JJ, Vanderby R. Response of knee ligaments to prolotherapy in a rat injury model. Am J Sports Med. 2008;36(7):1347–57. https://doi.org/10.1177/0363546508314431.

4. Schepker C, Habibi B, Yao K. Prolotherapy. In: Cooper G, Herrera J, editors. Essential sports medicine. 2nd ed. Totowa: Humana Press; 2019.

5. Reeves KD, Sit RWS, Rabago DP. Dextrose prolotherapy. Phys Med Rehabil Clin N Am. 2016;27(4):783–823. https://doi.org/10.1016/j.pmr.2016.06.001.

6. Hackett GS. Ligament and tendon relaxation (skeletal disability) treated by Prolotherapy (fibro-osseous proliferation): with special reference to occipito-cervical and low back disability, trigger point pain, referred pain, headache and sciatica. Thomas; 1958.

7. Banks AR. A rationale for prolotherapy. J Orthop Med. 1991;13(3):54–9.

8. Thorens B, Mueckler M. Glucose transporters in the 21st century. Am J Physiol-Endocrinol Metab. 2010;298(2):E141–5. https://doi.org/10.1152/ajpendo.00712.2009.

9. Murphy M, Godson C, Cannon S, et al. Suppression subtractive hybridization identifies high glucose levels as a stimulus for expression of connective tissue growth factor and other genes in human mesangial cells. J Biol Chem. 1999;274(9):5830–4. https://doi.org/10.1074/jbc.274.9.5830.

10. Pugliese A, Comito G, Cantamessa C, Pollono AM, Savarino A. Comparison of different In Vitro tests for evaluating immune reactivity. Cell Biochem Funct. 1996;14(1):63–8. https://doi.org/10.1002/(SICI)1099-0844(199603)14:1<63::AID-CBF642>3.0.CO;2-D.

11. Mobasheri A, Lewis R, Maxwell JEJ, Hill C, Womack M, Barrett-Jolley R. Characterization of a stretch-activated potassium channel in chondrocytes. J Cell Physiol. 2010;223(2):511–8. https://doi.org/10.1002/jcp.22075.

12. Cigan AD, Nims RJ, Albro MB, et al. Insulin, ascorbate, and glucose have a much greater influence than transferrin and selenous acid on the in vitro growth of engineered cartilage in chondrogenic media. Tissue Eng Part A. 2013;19(17–18):1941–8. https://doi.org/10.1089/ten.tea.2012.0596.

13. Maynard JA, Pedrini VA, Pedrini-Mille A, Romanus B, Ohlerking F. Morphological and biochemical effects of sodium morrhuate on tendons. J Orthop Res. 1985;3(2):236–48. https://doi.org/10.1002/jor.1100030214.

14. Hackett GS, Henderson DG. Joint stabilization. Am J Surg. 1955;89(5):968–73. https://doi.org/10.1016/0002-9610(55)90568-7.

15. Harrison MEG. The biomechanical effects of prolotherapy on traumatized Achilles tendons of male rats. 1995.

16. Zeisig E, Öhberg L, Alfredson H. Sclerosing polidocanol injections in chronic painful tennis elbow-promising results in a pilot study. Knee Surg Sports Traumatol Arthrosc. 2006;14:1218–24. https://doi.org/10.1007/s00167-006-0156-0.

17. Yoshii Y, Zhao CD, Schmelzer JD, Low PA, An KN, Amadio PC. Effects of multiple injections of hypertonic dextrose in the rabbit carpal tunnel: a potential model of carpal tunnel syndrome development. Hand. 2014;9(1):52–7. https://doi.org/10.1007/s11552-013-9599-1.

18. Alfredson H, Ohberg L. Neovascularisation in chronic painful patellar tendinosis? Promising results after sclerosing neovessels outside the tendon challenge the need for surgery. Knee Surg Sports Traumatol Arthrosc. 2005;13(2):74–80. https://doi.org/10.1007/s00167-004-0549-x.

19. Sanderson LM, Bryant A. Effectiveness and safety of prolotherapy injections for management of lower limb tendinopathy and fasciopathy: a systematic review. J Foot Ankle Res. 2015;8(1):57. https://doi.org/10.1186/s13047-015-0114-5.

20. Covey CJ, Sineath MH, Penta JF, Leggit JC. Prolotherapy: can it help your patient? J Fam Pract. 2015;64(12):763–8.

21. Zeisig E, Fahlstrom M, Ohberg L, Alfredson H. Pain relief after intratendinous injections in patients with tennis elbow: results of a randomised study. Br J Sports Med. 2008;42(4):267–71. https://doi.org/10.1136/bjsm.2007.042762.

22. Scarpone M, Rabago DP, Zgierska A, Arbogast G, Snell E. The efficacy of prolotherapy for lateral epicondylosis: a pilot study. Clin J Sport Med. 2008;18(3):248–54. https://doi.org/10.1097/JSM.0b013e318170fc87.

23. Catapano M, Zhang K, Mittal N, Sangha H, Onishi K, de SA D. Effectiveness of dextrose prolotherapy for rotator cuff tendinopathy: a systematic review. PM & R. 2020;12:288–300.

24. Mansiz-Kaplan B, Nacir B, Pervane-Vural S, Duyur-Cakit B, Genc H. Effect of Dextrose Prolotherapy on Pain Intensity, Disability, and Plantar Fascia Thickness in Unilateral Plantar Fasciitis: A Randomized, Controlled, Double-Blind Study. Am J Phys Med Rehabil. 2020;99(4):318–24.

25. Carayannopoulos A, Borg-Stein J, Sokolof J, Meleger A, Rosenberg D. Prolotherapy versus corticosteroid injections for the treatment of lateral epicondylosis: a randomized controlled trial. PM R. 2011;3(8):706–15. https://doi.org/10.1016/j.pmrj.2011.05.011.

26. Rabago D, Lee KS, Ryan M, et al. Hypertonic dextrose and morrhuate sodium injections (Prolotherapy) for lateral epicondylosis (tennis elbow). Am J Phys Med Rehabil. 2013;92(7):587–96. https://doi.org/10.1097/PHM.0b013e31827d695f.

27. Dong W, Goost H, Lin XB, et al. Injection therapies for lateral epicondylalgia: a systematic review and Bayesian network meta-analysis. Br J Sports Med. 2016;50(15):900–8. https://doi.org/10.1136/bjsports-2014-094387.

28. Alfredson H, Öhberg L. Sclerosing injections to areas of neo-vascularisation reduce pain in chronic Achilles tendinopathy: a double-blind randomised controlled trial. Knee Surg Sports Traumatol Arthrosc. 2005;13(4):338–44. https://doi.org/10.1007/s00167-004-0585-6.

29. Hoksrud A, Öhberg L, Alfredson H, Bahr R. Ultrasound-guided sclerosis of neovessels in painful chronic patellar tendinopathy. Am J Sports Med. 2006;34(11):1738–46. https://doi.org/10.1177/0363546506289168.

30. Yelland MJ, Sweeting KR, Lyftogt JA, Ng SK, Scuffham PA, Evans KA. Prolotherapy injections and eccentric loading exercises for painful Achilles tendinosis: a randomised trial. Br J Sports Med. 2011;45(5):421–8. https://doi.org/10.1136/bjsm.2009.057968.

31. Maxwell NJ, Ryan MB, Taunton JE, Gillies JH, Wong AD. Sonographically guided intratendinous injection of hyperosmolar dextrose to treat chronic tendinosis of the Achilles tendon: a pilot study. Am J Roentgenol. 2007;189(4):W215–20. https://doi.org/10.2214/AJR.06.1158.

32. Morath O, Kubosch EJ, Taeymans J, et al. The effect of sclerotherapy and prolotherapy on chronic painful Achilles tendinopathy—a systematic review including meta-analysis. Scand J Med Sci Sports. 2018;28(1):4–15. https://doi.org/10.1111/sms.12898.

33. Maffulli N, Papalia R, D'Adamio S, Balzani LD, Denaro V. Pharmacological interventions for the treatment of Achilles tendinopathy: a systematic review of randomized controlled trials. Br Med Bull. 2015;113(1):101–15. https://doi.org/10.1093/bmb/ldu040.

34. Gross CE, Hsu AR, Chahal J, Holmes GB. Injectable treatments for noninsertional Achilles tendinosis: a systematic review. Foot Ankle Int. 2013;34(5):619–28. https://doi.org/10.1177/1071100713475353.

35. Moon YL, Ha SH, Lee YK, Park YK. Comparative studies of platelet-rich plasma (PRP) and prolotherapy for proximal biceps tendinitis. Clin Shoulder Elbow. 2011;14(2):153–8.

36. Lhee S-H, Park J-Y. Prospective randomized clinical study for the treatment of lateral epicondylitis: comparison among PRP (platelet-rich plasm), prolotherapy, physiotherapy and ESWT. J Shoulder Elb Surg. 2013;22(10):e30–1. https://doi.org/10.1016/j.jse.2013.07.018.

37. Klein RG, Eek BC, DeLong WB, Mooney V. A randomized double-blind trial of dextrose-glycerine-phenol injections for chronic, low back pain. J Spinal Disord. 1993;6(1):23-33.

38. Dechow E, Davies RK, Carr AJ, Thompson PW. A randomized, double-blind, placebo-controlled trial of sclerosing injections in patients with chronic low back pain. Rheumatology. 1999;38(12):1255–9. https://doi.org/10.1093/rheumatology/38.12.1255.

39. Iseminger T, Palaikis R. A retrospective study of prolotherapy. 1995. Cal State Polytechnic, Biological Sciences Department. Honors paper (undergraduate).

40. Yelland MJ, Glasziou PP, Bogduk N, Schluter PJ, McKernon M. Prolotherapy injections, saline injections, and exercises for chronic low-back pain: a randomized trial. Spine. 2004;29(1):9–16. https://doi.org/10.1097/01.BRS.0000105529.07222.5B.

41. Hauser RA, Hauser MA. A retrospective study on Hackett-Hemwall dextrose prolotherapy for chronic shoulder pain at an outpatient charity clinic in rural Illinois. J Prolotherapy. 2009;1(4):205–16.

42. Clark RA. Cutaneous tissue repair: basic biologic considerations. I. J Am Acad Dermatol. 1985;13(5 Pt 1):701–25. https://doi.org/10.1016/s0190-9622(85)70213-7.

Emerging Operative Procedures for Tendons

Nicola Maffulli, Alessio Giai Via, and Francesco Oliva

Introduction

Tendons are important components of the musculoskeletal system that connect muscles to bones. As tendons are of primary importance to transfer forces from muscles to bones, tendon injuries can impair not only sporting but also daily activities. Tendons pathologies can be acute (tendon rupture) or chronic. Chronic tendon injury, or tendinopathy, is characterized by pain, focal tendon tenderness, and impaired performance. The pathogenesis of tendinopathy is poorly understood, and it has been variously defined as a degenerative condition or as a failure of the healing process [1]. Tendon injury can affect people of all ages, but the exact incidence in the general population is difficult to assess, but it is estimated that approximately 30% of general practice consultations for musculoskeletal pain are related to tendon problems [2]. As tendinopathy is multifactorial in its origin and the pathogenesis is poorly understood [3], many different conservative and surgical treatments have been proposed with variable results. New emerging minimally invasive procedure for Achilles tendinopathy (AT) and acute rupture will be presented in this chapter, as the pathology is extremely common in general orthopedic practice, in sports medicine, and foot and ankle surgery. In fact, Achilles tendon injuries affect not only young and active people but also older patients. It has been estimated that more than 30% of patients have a sedentary lifestyle [4]. Even if open procedures on the AT showed satisfactory results, they have been also associated with an increased risk of local complications, as wound breakdown and infection [5]. Therefore, minimally invasive surgical techniques have been developed to reduce post-surgical complications and morbidity. Furthermore, resent research reported that minimally invasive AT surgery produced faster recovery times and shorter hospital stays compared to traditional open techniques with good functional results [6]. The recent advances in minimally invasive surgery for the most common pathologies of the AT are reported in this chapter, including high-volume injections, multiple percutaneous longitudi-

N. Maffulli (✉)
Department of Musculoskeletal Disorders,
School of Medicine and Surgery,
University of Salerno, Salerno, Italy

Mary University of London, Barts and the London School of Medicine and Dentistry, Centre for Sports and Exercise Medicine, Mile End Hospital, London, UK
e-mail: n.maffulli@qmul.ac.uk

A. G. Via
Department of Musculoskeletal Surgery,
San Camillo-Forlanini Hospital, Rome, Italy

F. Oliva
Department of Musculoskeletal Disorders, School of Medicine and Surgery, University of Salerno, Salerno, Italy

nal tenotomies, and minimally invasive Achilles tendon stripping for the management of AT, and minimally invasive AT repair.

High-Volume Injections for the Management of Achilles Tendinopathy

The source of pain associated with mid-portion AT has not been clarified yet. Traditionally, it was ascribed to inflammation, but painful Achilles and patellar tendons showed no histological evidence of inflammation. Resent researches showed an increased neuronal ingrowth accompanying the peritendinous neovascularization from the paratenon into the tendinopathic area [3, 7]. Therefore, some authors speculate that the new nerve ingrowth, changes in the peripheral neuronal phenotype, and the upregulation of local synthesis of glutamate and substance P may be responsible for the pain. Recent minimally invasive techniques, as high-volume image-guided injections (HVIGI), target the new neurovascular bundles growing from the paratenon into the Achilles tendon, and break the neovessels and nerves by producing local mechanical effects.

Technique The patient is positioned prone on the operating table with the feet protruding beyond the edge and the ankles resting on a sandbag. The tendon is examined and the area of maximum swelling and/or tenderness marked and checked again by ultrasound (US) scanning. The leg is prepared in the usual sterile fashion. All the procedure is performed under ultrasound guidance. A 21G needle is inserted from the lateral aspect of the tendon between the anterior aspect of the Achilles tendon and Kager's fat pad. A mixture of 10 mL 0.5% bupivacaine hydrochloride and 25 mg of hydrocortisone acetate is injected, immediately followed by 4 × 10 mL of normal saline. Hydrocortisone acetate is used to prevent the acute mechanical inflammatory reaction produced by the large amount of saline. The position of the needle and flow of fluid is monitored continuously by US, and the needle moved

gently across the anterior aspect of the tendon from medial to lateral. After HVIGI, the Achilles tendon can be scanned again with Colour Doppler to assess whether any neovessels remain. Patients are allowed to walk on the injected leg immediately, but they are strictly advised to refrain from high impact activity for 72 h. Then, they are instructed to restart eccentric exercises twice a day.

Outcome Good results have been reported with this technique at short term follow-up [8]. A recent randomized double-blinded prospective study showed better results of HVIGI and eccentric exercises compared to eccentric training alone in reducing pain, improving activity level, in reducing tendon thickness and intratendinous vascularity [9]. Furthermore, compared to a series of 4 PRP injections, HVIGI showed better results at short-term follow-up (6 weeks) [9]. Even if few studies are published in literature, HVIGI showed promising results at short and mid-term follow-up [10]. It seems to be safe, and to relieve pain and symptoms in most of patients. However, it warrants further investigation.

Multiple Percutaneous Longitudinal Tenotomies

The main indication for multiple percutaneous longitudinal tenotomies is intratendinous lesion smaller than 25 mm long, assessed by MRI or ultrasound, without the involvement of the paratenon.

Technique The patients are positioned prone on the operating table. The procedure is performed under ultrasound guidance. The skin and the subcutaneous tissues over the Achilles tendon are infiltrated with 10–15 mL of plain 1% lidocaine. A number 11 surgical scalpel blade is inserted into the marked area, parallel to the long axis of the tendon fibers. The cutting edge of the blade points cranially and penetrates the whole thickness of the tendon (Fig. 21.1). Keeping the blade still, a full passive ankle dorsi-flexion movement is produced. The scalpel blade is then retracted to

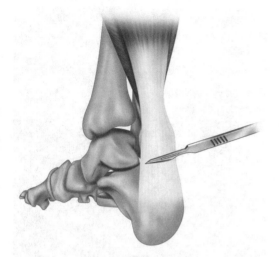

Fig. 21.1 A number 11 surgical blade is inserted into the tendinopathic area, with the cutting edge pointed cranially and parallel to the long axis of the tendon

the surface of the tendon, inclined 45° on the sagittal axis, and the blade is inserted medially through the original tenotomy. Keeping the blade still, a full passive ankle flexion is produced. Once the position of the blade is reversed of 180°, full passive plantar flexion is applied. A variable, approximately 28 mm long area of tenolysis is thus obtained through a stab wound. The whole procedure is repeated inclining the blade 45° laterally and medially to the central tenotomy (Fig. 21.2). A Steri-Strip is then applied on the stab wound. The wound is dressed with cotton swabs and a few layers of cotton wool and a dressing are applied. The procedure can be performed as an outpatient.

After surgery, early active dorsi- and plantar-flexion of the foot is encouraged. Patients are allowed to walk using elbow crutches and to weight-bear as tolerated. Full weight-bearing is allowed after 2 or 3 days. Stationary bicycling and isometric concentric and eccentric strengthening of the calf muscles are started after 4 weeks under the guidance of a trained physiotherapist. Swimming and water running are encouraged from the second week. Gentle running is started 4–6 weeks after the procedure and mileage gradually increased.

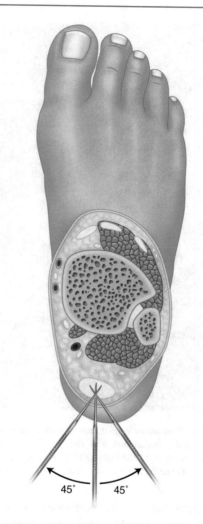

Fig. 21.2 The procedure is repeated inclining the blade 45° laterally and medially to the central tenotomy, with the cutting edge pointed cranially and caudally

Outcomes Good-to-excellent results have been reported in more than 70% of athletes with unilateral Achilles tendinopathy at 3 years follow-up [11].

Minimally Invasive Achilles Tendon Stripping

The main indication for minimally invasive Achilles tendon stripping is mid-portion Achilles tendinopathy after failed conservative treatment (3–6 months).

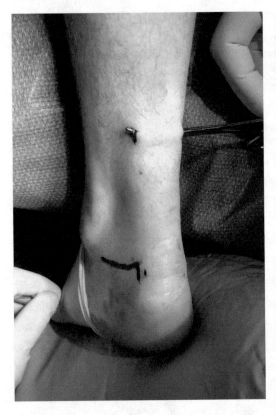

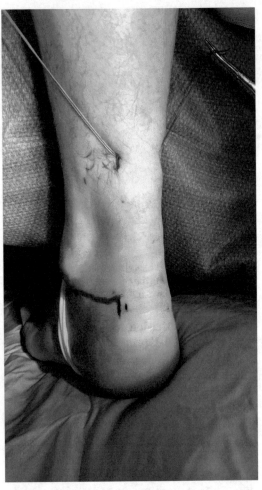

Fig. 21.3 Four small longitudinal incisions are made at the medial and lateral border of the Achilles tendon. A mosquito clamp is inserted through the proximal incisions to remove the peritendinous adhesions

Technique Surgery is performed with the patient prone, under local anesthesia. Four small (0.5-cm) longitudinal skin incisions are made, two proximal just medially and laterally the Achilles tendon, and two distal at the level of the calcaneal insertion. A mosquito clamp is inserted through the proximal incisions (Fig. 21.3) and the peritendinous adhesions anterior to the tendon are removed. A no. 1 unmounted Ethibond suture thread is doubled up and passed through the two proximal incisions, over the anterior surface of the Achilles tendon (Fig. 21.4). A suture retriever is inserted from the distal–lateral skin incision to the proximal–medial incision and the first stub of the suture is passed. Then, the suture retriever is inserted from the distal–medial skin incision to the proximal–lateral incision and the second stub of the suture is passed (Fig. 21.5). In

Fig. 21.4 A no. 1 Ethibond suture is doubled up and passed through the 2 proximal incisions, over the anterior surface of the Achilles tendon

this way, the suture is passed in an X-fashion. Finally, the Ethibond suture is retrieved distally with a gentle seesaw motion (Fig. 21.6). The tendon is thus stripped and freed from the Kager's triangle fatty tissue. The incisions can be closed with Steri-Strips, and the wounds dressed with standard dressing.

The surgery is performed as an outpatient procedure. Patients are allowed to walk with weight-bearing as tolerated after surgery. After 2 weeks, the dressing is removed, and physiotherapy is begun, focusing on proprioception, plantarflexion of the ankle, inversion, and eversion.

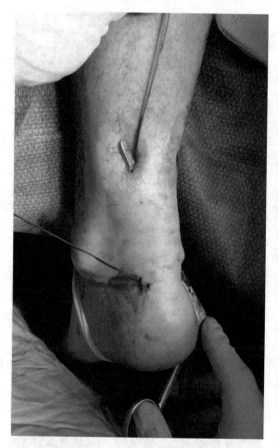

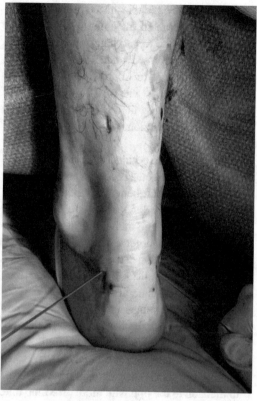

Fig. 21.6 The suture is retrieved with a gentle seesaw motion

Fig. 21.5 A suture retriever is inserted from the distal-lateral skin incision to the proximal-medial incision first, and the first stub of the suture is passed. The procedure is repeated from the distal-medial skin incision to the proximal-lateral incision and the second stub of the suture is passed in a X-fashion

Outcomes The results of this technique have been recently reported in 47 active patients [12]. A statistically significant improvement has been reported according the VISA-A questionnaire scores (Victorian Institute of Sports Assessment-Achilles scores) at final follow-up (from 53.8 to 85.3). The calf strength also statistically improved compared the preoperative score, from 313.9N to 326.9N ($p < 0.031$), with no statistically significant differences found between the operated and controlateral leg at final follow-up. Forty-one patients (85%) resume sporting activities after an average of 3.5 months (range: 2–5), and 75% of all patients returned to sport at the same pre-injury level.

Minimally Invasive Achilles Tendon Repair

Achilles tendon rupture is a common injury that orthopedic surgeons have to deal with during their clinical practice. The incidence rate ranges from 6 to 18 per 100,000 people per year, and it has been steadily increasing during the past few decades [13]. Most acute ruptures (75%) occur during recreational activities in men between 30 and 40 years old, but 25% of ruptures may occur in sedentary patients. Even if open surgery provides good strength to the repair, low re-rupture rates, and reliably good endurance and power to the gastrocnemius-Achilles tendon complex, the limit is their high rate of local complications and morbidity. Therefore, minimally invasive procedures have been successfully used to avoid local complications, such infection and wound problems.

Technique The patient is placed prone and a pillow is placed beneath the anterior aspect of the ankles to allow the feet to hang free. The procedure can be performed under local anesthesia, with 50:50 mixture of 10 mL of 2% lidocaine hydrochloride and 10 mL of 0.25% bupivacaine hydrochloride into an area 8–10 cm around the ruptured Achilles tendon.

First, a transverse incision of about 3 cm is made over the defect. Forceps is used to mobilize the tendon from beneath the subcutaneous tissues, and the tendon's stubs are cleaned up. Four longitudinal stab incisions are made proximal to the palpable defect; 2 lateral and 2 medial to the Achilles tendon. Two further longitudinal incisions are made distal to the palpable defect, one medial and one lateral the tendon (Fig. 21.7). A #2 resorbable suture is passed transversely between the two proximal stab incisions through the Achilles tendon (Fig. 21.8). The bulk of the tendon is surprisingly superficial. Each end of the suture is passed diagonally, in turn, from the stub incision to the opposite more proximal one,

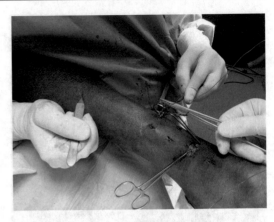

Fig. 21.8 First, a n.2 resorbable suture is passed between the two proximal incisions through the Achilles tendon

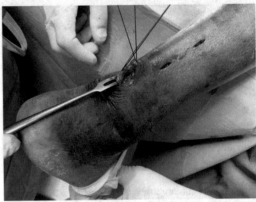

Fig. 21.9 A second n.2 resorbable suture is passed between the distal stab incisions through the tendon, and exits from the transverse incision

in an X fashion. A subsequent diagonal pass is then made to the transverse incision over the ruptured tendon. To prevent entanglement, both ends of the suture are held in separate clips. This suture is then tested for security by pulling with both ends distally. Another #2 resorbable suture is passed between the distal stab incisions through the tendon and in turn through the tendon and out of the transverse incision starting distal to the transverse passage (Fig. 21.9). The ankle is held in full plantar flexion, and, in turn, opposing ends of the sutures are tied together with a double throw knot, and then three further throws before being buried using the forceps (Fig. 21.10). A clip is used to hold the first throw of the lateral side to maintain the tension of the suture.

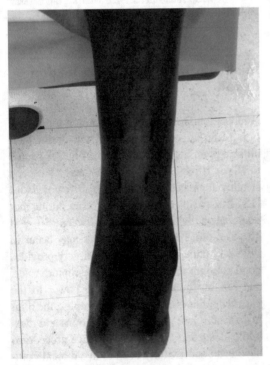

Fig. 21.7 Surgical approaches for minimally invasive Achilles tendon repair

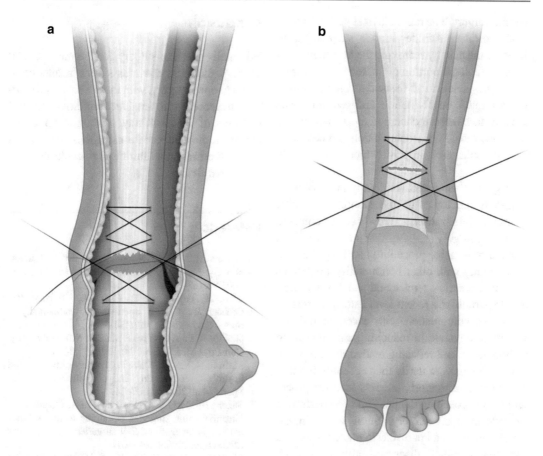

Fig. 21.10 Final configuration of the minimally invasive Achilles tendon suture. (**a**) the suture wires are passed throught the bulk of the proximal and distal tendon stubs in a X fashion, and they get out at the level of the tendon defect. (**b**) the foot is held in maximum plantarflexion, bringing near the tendon stumps, and the knots are tight

A 3-0 resorbable suture is used to close the transverse incision, and Steri-Strips to close the stabs incisions. A nonadherent dressing is applied. An anterior half cast is applied in the operating room with the ankle in physiologic equinus.

The patient is discharged the day of surgery, and weight bearing is allowed as tolerated in the cast in plantar flexion. At 2 weeks, the wounds are inspected, the cast is removed, and a boot with the ankle at 90° is used. The boot allows the patient to begin proprioception, plantar flexion, inversion, and eversion exercises. However, the patient needs the supervision of a physiotherapist to remove the boot because dorsiflexion is not allowed until 6 weeks post-surgery.

Outcomes Excellent results have been reported in 17 elite athletes after percutaneous surgical repair of Achilles tendon ruptures [14]. All patients returned to high-level competition, with an average time to return to full sport participation of 4.8 months (range 3.2–6.5).

Discussion

Achilles tendon injuries produce substantial morbidity and the current understanding of the mechanisms involved in tendon injury and repair is limited. Nonoperative treatments are the first management for AT disorders, but patients who do not respond well to conservative treatments require surgery. The rationale of HVIGI and minimally invasive Achilles tendon stripping is to improve the pain by removing the neoinnervation to the pathologic portion of the tendon, minimizing surgery-related soft tissue damage and allowing for quick rehabilitation and recovery. The limit is that these techniques are based on the hypothesis that neovascularization and neoinnervation would result in pain, which has not been proven.

A great advantage of minimally invasive techniques is the lower wound complication rate, shorter hospitalization, and lower costs compared with open surgery [15]. Another advantage is that minimally invasive procedure can be performed concurrently with other nonoperative treatments such as eccentric exercise and shock wave therapy. In particular, a recent level I study found that HVIGI in combination with eccentric training was more effective in reducing pain, improving activity level, and reducing tendon thickness and intratendinous vascularity than eccentric training alone [9]. Furthermore, the less invasive procedures do not exclude the possibility to perform a subsequent open surgery. Sural nerve injury, which manifests as paresthesia and/or pain, is a risk that should be discussed with the patient. However, the sural nerve is at risk during open or percutaneous surgery around the Achilles tendon.

Percutaneous repair of the AT is an increasingly common procedure that provides many advantages. Major advantages are less iatrogenic damage to normal tissues, lower postoperative, pain, accurate opposition of the tendon ends minimizing surgical incisions, shorter hospitalization time, lower rate of postsurgical infections, and improved cosmesis. Furthermore, a recent review showed similar clinical and functional outcomes after minimally invasive surgery for Achilles tendon ruptures compared to open repair, and the number of complications was lower compared to open surgery [16]. For these reasons, minimally invasive Achilles tendon repair is the preferred technique by the authors not only young and active people but also for patients older than 65 that are subject to higher local complication rate.

Conclusion

Minimally invasive surgery for the management of AT pathologies provides similar results compared to open surgery, with the advantages to provide decreased perioperative morbidity, decreased duration of hospital stay, and reduced costs. However, the evidence for using these techniques is low at present, and further high evidence studies are required.

References

1. Sharma P, Maffulli N. Tendon injury and tendinopathy: healing and repair. J Bone Joint Surg Am. 2005;87:187–202.
2. Kaux JF, Forthomme B, Goff CL, Crielaard JM, Croisier JL. Current opinions on tendinopathy. J Sports Sci Med. 2011;10:238–53.
3. Giai Via A, Papa G, Oliva F, Maffulli N. Tendinopathy. Curr Phys Med Rehabil Rep. 2017;11:3–00.
4. Maffulli N, Via AG, Oliva F. Chronic Achilles tendon disorders: tendinopathy and chronic rupture. Clin Sports Med. 2015;34:607–24.
5. Saxena A, Maffulli N, Nguyen A, Li A. Wound complications from surgeries pertaining to the Achilles tendon: an analysis of 219 surgeries. J Am Podiatr Med Assoc. 2008;98:95–101.
6. Maffulli N, Oliva F, Giai Via F. Minimally invasive surgery for Achilles tendon pathologies. In: Sports injuries. Springer-Verlag Berlin Heidelberg; 2014.
7. Alfredson H, Ohberg L, Forsgren S. Is vasculo-neural ingrowth the cause of pain in chronic Achilles tendinosis? An investigation using ultrasonography and colour Doppler, immunohistochemistry, and diagnostic injections. Knee Surg Sports Traumatol Arthrosc. 2003;11:334–8.
8. Maffulli N, Spiezia F, Lungo UG, Denaro V, Maffulli GD. High volume image guided injections for the management of chronic tendinopathy of the main body of the Achilles tendon. Phys Ther Sport. 2013;14:163–7.
9. Boesen AP, Hansen R, Boesen MI, Malliaras P, Langberg H. Effect of high-volume injection, platelet-rich plasma, and sham treatment in chronic Midportion Achilles tendinopathy: a randomized double-blinded prospective study. Am J Sports Med. 2017;45:2034–43.
10. Chaudhry FA. Effectiveness of dry needling and high-volume image-guided injection in the management of chronic mid-portion Achilles tendinopathy in adult population: a literature review. Eur J Orthop Surg Traumatol. 2017;27:441–8.
11. Testa V, Capasso G, Benazzo F, Maffulli N. Management of Achilles tendinopathy by

ultrasound-guided percutaneous tenotomy. Med Sci Sports Exerc. 2002;34:573–80.

12. Maffulli N, Oliva F, Maffulli GD, Giai Via A, Gougoulias N. Minimally invasive Achilles tendon stripping for the management of tendinopathy of the main body of the Achilles tendon. J Foot Ankle Surg. 2017;56(5):938–42.

13. Longo UG, Petrillo S, Maffulli N, et al. Acute Achilles tendon rupture in athletes. Foot Ankle Clin. 2013;18:319–38.

14. Maffulli N, Longo UG, Maffulli GD, et al. Achilles tendon ruptures in elite athletes. Foot Ankle Int. 2011;32:9–15.

15. Maffulli N, Giai Via, Oliva F. Achilles injuries in the athlete – noninsertional. In: Oper Tech Sports Med. Ed Cole B. https://doi.org/10.1053/j.otsm.2014.09.001

16. Del Buono A, Volpin A, Maffulli N. Minimally invasive versus open surgery for acute Achilles tendon rupture: a systematic review. Br Med Bull. 2014;109:45–54.

Correction to: Rectus Abdominis and Hip Adductor Tendons ("Athletic Pubalgia/Sports Hernia")

Gerardo Miranda-Comas, Eliana Cardozo, Svetlana Abrams, and Joseph E. Herrera

---

Correction to: Chapter 7 in: K. Onishi et al. (eds.), Tendinopathy, https://doi.org/10.1007/978-3-030-65335-4_7

Figure 7.1 belonging to Chapter 7, page 93–101, has been updated.
The labels have been updated for Figure 7.1. in the print, eBook, and MyCopy.

The updated version of this chapter can be found at https://doi.org/10.1007/978-3-030-65335-4_7

Index

Printed in the United States
by Baker & Taylor Publisher Services